Robotic Cell Manipulation

Robotic Cell Manipulation

Dong Sun
Department of Biomedical Engineering,
Centre of Robotics and Automation,
City University of Hong Kong, Hong Kong, China

ELSEVIER

ACADEMIC PRESS
An imprint of Elsevier

Academic Press is an imprint of Elsevier
125 London Wall, London EC2Y 5AS, United Kingdom
525 B Street, Suite 1650, San Diego, CA 92101, United States
50 Hampshire Street, 5th Floor, Cambridge, MA 02139, United States
The Boulevard, Langford Lane, Kidlington, Oxford OX5 1GB, United Kingdom

ISBN: 978-0-323-85259-3

For information on all Academic Press publications visit our website at https://www.elsevier.com/books-and-journals

Publisher: Mara Conner
Acquisitions Editor: Sonnini R. Yura
Editorial Project Manager: Aera F. Gariguez
Production Project Manager: Prasanna Kalyanaraman
Cover Designer: Miles Hitchen

Typeset by TNQ Technologies

To my wife—Sheryl Jiang.

Contents

Preface

Cell manipulation is a technique that uses special technical methods to shape and manipulate cells, including changing cell functions, which can help treat and fight diseases and also aid cells to regain their vitality. Traditional cell manipulation methods have limitations in accuracy, success rate, proficiency, efficiency, and consistency. Robotic cell manipulation is an emerging technology that combines robotics and micromanipulation tools to automatically and accurately complete various manipulation tasks on individual cells. The use of robotics to promote cell manipulation will provide solutions to surmount the challenges faced by traditional cell manipulation methods and promote the practical application of cell therapy.

This book introduces the combination of robotics and various micromanipulation tools, such as microneedles, optical tweezers, dielectrophoresis, electromagnetic devices, and microfluidic chips, to achieve efficient and accurate automatic cell manipulation. Using these robot-assisted operating tools, many cell manipulation tasks can be successfully completed, such as cell microinjection, cell stretching, cell transportation, cell orientation and 3D imaging, cell sorting and separation, cell stimulation and migration, cell patterning, cell adhesion, cell fusion, in vivo cell navigation and delivery, single-cell biopsy, and gene editing. These emerging technologies will allow many new and unforeseen clinical applications that were previously considered impossible.

This book is organized over three levels: operation tools from microneedles to optical tweezers, manipulation types such as microinjection and transportation, and potential medical applications across microsurgery, gene editing, and cancer treatment. The following chapters are included in the book:

Chapter 1 Introduction
Chapter 2 Cell Manipulation Tools
Chapter 3 Robotic Cell Injection
Chapter 4 Cell Stretching and Compression
Chapter 5 Cell Transport with Optical Tweezers
Chapter 6 Cell Rotation
Chapter 7 3D Image Reconstruction for Intracellular Surgery
Chapter 8 Cell Sorting and Separation
Chapter 9 Cell Stimulation and Migration Control
Chapter 10 Cell Patterning
Chapter 11 Cell Adhesion
Chapter 12 Cell Fusion

The key objectives of this book are as follows:

1. Introduces the application of robot-assisted manipulation tools in various cell manipulation tasks, which can potentially diagnose and treat diseases at the single-cell level.
2. Defines many essential concepts in association with the robotic cell manipulation field, including manipulation strategy and manipulation types.
3. Introduces the basic concept and knowledge of various manipulation devices and tasks.
4. Describes some cutting-edge cell manipulation technologies and case studies.

This book systemically introduces robotic cell manipulation technologies and discusses their application prospects in the early diagnosis and treatment of diseases. It covers a wide range of basic concepts, theories, methodologies, experiments, case studies, and potential medical applications. It will enable readers to conduct a systematic review of research and is an essential reference for both new and experienced researchers in this unique field.

Acknowledgments

First, I would like to thank my students listed below. Over the past few years, they have studied for a Ph.D. degree at the City University of Hong Kong under my guidance and have participated in many research developments reported in this book. Without their outstanding contributions and strong support, it would have been impossible for me to complete this book.

Haibo Huang (graduated in 2008)
Haoyao Chen (graduated in 2009)
Yu Xie (graduated in 2010)
Youhua Tan (graduated in 2010)
Songyu Hu (graduated in 2011)
Xiangpeng Li (graduated in 2011)
Yanhua Wu (graduated in 2011)
Xiaolin Wang (graduated in 2012)
Tao Ju (graduated in 2012)
Xiao Yan (graduated in 2013)
Kaiqun Wang (graduated in 2013)
Shuxun Chen (graduated in 2014)
Xue Gou (graduated in 2014)
Hao Yang (graduated in 2015)
Mingyang Xie (graduated in 2016)
Ran Wang (graduated in 2016)
Bill Yu-ting Chow (graduated in 2016)
Weicheng Ma (graduated in 2017)
Zhijie Huan (graduated in 2017)
Xiaojian Li (graduated in 2017)
Fuzhou Niu (graduated in 2017)
Junyang Li (graduated in 2018)
Jundi Hou (graduated in 2018)
Tao Luo (graduated in 2018)
Ke Meng (graduated in 2018)
Dongce Ma (graduated in 2018)
Adnan Shakoor (graduated in 2019)
Pan Liao (graduated in 2019)
Dongfang Li (graduated in 2019)
Wendi Gao (graduated in 2020)

Tanyong Wei (graduated in 2020)
Lei Fan (graduated in 2021)
Fei Pan (graduated in 2021)
Zhangyan Guan (graduated in 2021)
Liuxi Xing (graduated in 2022)

I would also like to thank my research collaborators for their long-term support of my research, especially Professor James K. Mills from the University of Toronto, Canada, Professor Nancy Kwan Man from the University of Hong Kong, Professor Gang Li from the Chinese University of Hong Kong, and Professor Shuk Han Cheng and Professor Raymond Lam from City University of Hong Kong. I would also like to thank Dr. Henry Chu, who was my postdoctoral researcher from 2013 to 2015.

Finally, I am most sincerely grateful to my wife, Sheryl Jiang, for her love, care, and unconditional support.

Introduction

1

1.1 Overview of robot-facilitated cell manipulation

Cells are the smallest functional units of all living organisms. Discovered more than 300 years ago, cells remain a very challenging yet interesting subject for medical and biological researchers. To date, the process of understanding the mechanisms that allow cells to function are still being studied. The functions of cells and organisms are essentially controlled by individual biomolecules and their interactions, whereas cell studies have been limited by the availability of high-resolution technologies.

Cell manipulation refers to a process that can shape and manipulate cells of any type of organism through special technical means, including changing cell functions, which is beneficial to treating and resisting diseases and in aiding cells to rejuvenate. Clinical trials based on cell therapies, such as restoring the vision of a blind patient via stem cell therapy (Science Alert, 2016) and curing an infant's leukemia via gene editing (BBC News, 2015), have been reported. Traditionally, cell manipulation is achieved by chemical methods, such as chemical transfection, to improve the quality of cells. Under certain conditions, physical manipulations, such as optical, mechanical, and electrical techniques, have also been used more frequently in recent years. Recent decades have witnessed transformative developments in the use of various manipulation tools including microneedles, optical tweezers, and electromagnetic devices to achieve single-cell manipulations, such as cell fusion (Chen et al., 2013), optical transfection (Antkowiak et al., 2013), extraction of subcellular organelles (Ando et al., 2008), and cell enucleation (Feng et al., 2013).

Over the past few years, robotics technologies have been demonstrated as proven tools in control, vision, and system intelligence for macro-object manipulations, and they have been further extended to microscale objects successfully by integrating microelectromechanical system (MEMS) technology. The ability to manipulate cells and various biological molecules with high precision and high throughput is essential in many real applications. Combining robotics technology with traditional physical operations has attracted increasing attention because it can achieve high-quality, high-volume, and high-precision automated manipulations at the single-cell level. Currently, robot-assisted cell manipulations rely on the use of microneedles, optical tweezers, electrical and magnetic devices, and microfluidic chip technologies.

1.1.1 Robotic manipulation of biological objects

Robotic manipulation of objects for industrial manufacturing has been sufficiently studied since the 1990s (Sun et al., 1999; Sun and Mills, 2002). In recent decades, there has been a tremendous increase in micro- and nanoscale biological tasks related to

Robotic Cell Manipulation. https://doi.org/10.1016/B978-0-323-85259-3.00010-6

human health and well-being. Examples include injecting pronuclei DNA into cellular embryos (oocytes) to produce transgenic organisms, injecting microRNA into cells and embryos, cell transfection, gene editing, and cell therapy. In these biological processes, the demand for high-precision and high-throughput automated manipulations continues to increase, providing new micro/nanoscale research opportunities in the field of robotics and automation. Although some biomedical processes have been automated, many are conducted manually by highly skilled workers. Given the significant challenge of controlling the position and force applied to biological cells and the variability in human manual control, the success rate of manual operation is relatively low. Therefore, there is a clear need to use robotic devices to automate many micro/nanoscale biological processes.

Benefitting from the great progress of robots in visual servoing, motion and force control, and image processing, robot manipulation of biological objects has made tremendous progress in the past few decades (Sun and Nelson, 2002; Arai et al., 2006; Huang et al., 2009; Chen and Sun, 2012). The manipulation of biological objects requires the ability to observe, locate, and physically transform objects using external forces. For this reason, force sensing and control are often required to enhance these operations to achieve improved manipulation results. In some applications, such as diagnosis based on individual cells, obtaining force information is the main goal (Sun and Nelson, 2002). MEMS-based force-sensing devices have been developed and used to measure microforces encountered in micromanipulation tasks (Mencaissi et al., 2003; Xie et al., 2010). Force control technology has been applied to many micromanipulations, such as PI force feedback (Mencaissi et al., 2004), force-guided assembly of micromirrors (Shen et al., 2003), and dynamic force feedback for automated batch microinjection (Lu et al., 2007).

Visual feedback has been used extensively to perform micro/nano tasks. In the early stages of development, operators used visual feedback through a microscope to manually perform operations. With the improvement of desktop computer capabilities, intense research activities have been carried out using visual feedback to control microscale tasks, such as pick-and-place operations (Kasaya et al., 1999). During microassembly operations, force measurement is important to prevent damage to microparts (Anis et al., 2006). Vision-based feedback has been used to control micromanipulation processes in engineering and biomedical applications (Nelson et al., 1998). Imaging processing is indispensable for successful intracellular microscopy. The identification, positioning, tracking, reconstruction, motion, and orientation control of target specimens and manipulating tools largely depend on the quality of the sampled image.

Computed tomography (CT) and magnetic resonance imaging (MRI) have been widely used to visualize bones, tissues, and organs, but they are not suitable for imaging small specimens such as cells and organelles. Gao et al. (2020) developed an automated intracellular delivery method using a robot-assisted microscope system with 3D reconstruction information. This method uses the movement of the objective lens to optically sample the target cells, and employs wide-field fluorescence microscopy (WFFM) to optically slice the sampled image and store it in the computer. Wei et al. (2020) used photoacoustic imaging technology to visualize the real-time transportation of microrobots in living animals for cell delivery.

1.1.2 Cell microinjection with microneedles

Cell microinjection is a process in which a sharp needle penetrates the cell membrane to transfer biological materials to a specific area of living cells. This method is advantageous because the concentration of the required material can be controlled and injected directly into the cells. Moreover, the required material can be injected into the required area of the cell; for example, DNA can be injected into the cell nucleus. This technique has been widely used in pronuclear DNA injection (Liu et al., 2013), in vitro fertilization (Lassalle et al., 1987), intracytoplasmic sperm injection (van Steirteghem et al., 1993), and drug development (Chamorro et al., 2009).

Cell microinjection techniques can be divided into three categories, namely, manual, semiautomatic, and fully automatic microinjection. Manual microinjection requires the use of a manually controlled micromanipulator to hold the target cells and the use of an injection pipette to inject biological materials while applying positive pressure to the tip. The entire experiment is performed by human hands under a microscope. Operators of this technology should be fully familiar with the operating procedures. Even when operated by a well-trained technician, the productivity of manual operation is usually very low. Semiautomatic microinjection consists of a system with a pipette and a holding pipette, which is mounted on a motorized robotic arm or workbench and controlled by a computer (Sun and Nelson, 2002; Huang et al., 2009). The operator needs to control the robotic arm to manually perform cell injection. However, in this case, the operator does not have to manually control the movement of the pipette, because an electric stage can be used. For the fully automated microinjection system (Pan et al., 2020), the operator only needs to set up the robotic experimental device and locate the target cell. The computer completes the remaining work, that is, aligning the injection pipette with the cell and performing cell injection. The role of the operator is to monitor the process, not to manipulate the stage and pipette. In common computer-assisted cell injection systems, a charge-coupled device (CCD) camera is used to capture real-time video from the microscope and send it to the computer for further processing.

Microinjection has been studied for many years and used in biomedical applications, such as clustered regularly interspaced short palindromic repeat (CRISPR) genome editing using CRISPR-associated protein 9 (Cas9), high-throughput transfection of deoxyribonucleic acid (DNA), and measurement of cell-to-cell communication in gap junctions. Robotic microinjection can accurately deliver a variety of foreign materials to almost all types of cells at the single-cell level and significantly avoid the immunogenicity, chemical toxicity, and high mortality of electroporation caused by virus or chemical-mediated cell transfection.

1.1.3 Cell manipulation with optical tweezers

As one of the most promising tools for manipulating micro/nano-sized objects, optical tweezers have played an increasingly important role in biology since their invention in 1986 (Ashkin et al., 1986). Using low-power laser beams to trap and manipulate particles ranging in size from tens of nanometers to tens of microns, optical tweezers provide a revolutionary solution for the manipulation and characterization of biological materials, especially single biological cells. Several types of cells derived from the body, namely, somatic cells, red blood cells, and nerve cells, as well as gametes (such as human sperm), have been manipulated by optical tweezers. Optical tweezers with multiple laser beam trap capabilities have significant advantages over predecessor optical tweezers with a single laser trap (Rodrigo et al., 2004; Arai et al., 2006).

The increasing demand for high precision and high throughput for cell manipulation has highlighted the need for automated processes by integrating robotics technology into optical tweezers manipulation. Given that optical tweezers can apply force and deformation to micro-objects in the order of micronewtons (pN, 10^{-12} N) and nanometers (nm, 10^{-9} m) in a noncontact manner (Pine and Chow, 2009), the synergy of micromanipulation technology with optical tweezers will produce new and exciting solutions to achieve advanced biological cell manipulation. Such advancements will enable many biomedical applications that have not been possible thus far. In the past few years, optical tweezers have been widely used in single-molecule and cell research due to their flexible and precise control capabilities. Some studies include cell membrane or DNA stretching (Wang et al., 2013), cell sorting (Wang et al., 2011), cell transport (Chen and Sun, 2012), cell fusion (Chen et al., 2013), cell adhesion (Hu et al., 2013), and cell migration (Gou et al., 2014). Various cell types have been manipulated by optical tweezers, including red blood cells, nerve cells, and stem cells. Using holographic technology, multiple optical tweezers can generate multiple traps on the focal plane at the same time, which shows more advantages than a single optical trap.

1.1.4 Dielectrophoresis-based cell manipulation

The dielectrophoresis (DEP) method (Cui et al., 2009) utilizes a nonuniform electric field to polarize and deform cells through a pair of electrodes, and the hardware setup is relatively simple. The majority of DEP-based cell manipulations have been performed using microfluidic chips (Pethig, 2010) as a platform for sorting (Hu et al., 2005), trapping (Rosenthal and Voldman, 2005), and transporting (Hawkin et al., 2009) different biological cells. In cell sorting, the DEP method can be used to separate cells of similar size based on differences in dielectric properties, such as human mesenchymal stem cells (MSCs) and their differentiated progeny (osteoblasts) (Song et al., 2015). Most reported DEP separators require sheath flow or well-designed electrodes to actively prefocus the input cell mixture to the side/center of the microfluidic channel before the input cell mixture enters the DEP separation zone. Luo et al. (2018) proposed a method of combining gravity-based precipitation-based sheathless prefocusing and DEP separation in a simple microfluidic device for continuous cell separation based on size and dielectric properties. In cell stretching, the DEP method can be combined with microfluidic chip technology to provide greater stretching force than optical stretching. To characterize the elastic modulus of diseased cells through the DEP-based deformability test, Zhang et al. (2015) developed a DEP-based microfluidic device to quickly characterize the biomechanical properties of drug-treated cells. Bai et al. (2017) developed a DEP-based method that further combines actin skeleton modeling to characterize the mechanical properties of leukemia NB4 cells. In cell patterning, DEP technology can be used to polarize cells to build 3D cell patterns on multilayer structures with high cell density (Chu et al., 2015). A 3D porous structure called an engineered scaffold is usually used to provide a template for cells to adhere to and gradually proliferate into functional tissues. Scaffolds fabricated by conventional microfabrication techniques such as particle leaching, gas foaming, and electrospinning can achieve high levels of porosity, but the pore size, pore distribution, and interconnection between pores are not easy to control (Levenberg et al., 2005). Advanced 3D manufacturing technologies, such as rapid prototyping, laser cutting, and micromolding technologies, can provide a high degree of controllability (Moutos et al., 2007), but these stents usually have low dimensional resolution. The density of cells seeded on these scaffolds should be increased. The DEP method can be successfully used to polarize cells to construct 3D cell patterns on multilayer structures with high cell density (Chu et al., 2015).

1.1.5 Cell transport with magnetic microrobots

Clinical cell therapy has experienced 20 years of development, and is currently facing a major challenge of how to accurately and quantitatively deliver therapeutic cells to the target site in vivo. Existing blood circulation methods for cell delivery can only ensure that a small percentage of cells reaches their target sites. Therefore, a large number of cells must be used, which may lead to overproduction of cytokines and excessive immune responses. This problem can be solved by developing degradable microrobots that can accurately carry and transport cells into the body. To reduce invasiveness, the design size of the microrobot is smaller than millimeters, thereby solving the problem that traditional medical equipment cannot enter the unprecedented narrow spaces of the body. By using magnetic, acoustic, optical, chemical, and other biological hybrid drive technologies, various actuation methods have been developed to drive the microrobots (Li et al., 2017). Among these methods, the magnetic drive method is the most commonly used method, because this method has a series of unique advantages, including precise controllability, strong drive capability, and good operational safety in the in vivo environment (Sitti et al., 2015; Chen et al., 2017; Alapan et al., 2020). The magneto-dynamic microrobot provides a miniature 3D scaffold through which cells can attach, migrate, proliferate, differentiate, and form 3D living microtissues. These microrobots can be transported magnetically in vitro, and cells can be attached to microrobot structures with good biocompatibility (Steager et al., 2013; Hollister et al., 2005).

To design a microrobot that can fully meet the needs of clinical operations in a minimally invasive manner, manufacturing and material issues are among the most important considerations. In 2012, a 3D printing technology called direct laser writing (NanoScript) was applied to manufacture helical microrobots from polymer materials (Tottori et al., 2012). NanoScript is a 3D direct laser writing tool that provides great flexibility in the process of microrobot design and structural optimization. This tool can achieve a printing resolution of ~200 nm and manufacture microrobots from 5 to 1000 μm. In addition, a variety of structural designs can be easily implemented, so that direct laser writing can be used to manufacture spherical microrobots and many other microstructures, such as brackets, fixtures, and microlenses. In recent years, hydrogel has become an increasingly important smart material in the field of biomedicine, and it has been used as a delivery vehicle for therapeutic proteins and genes. Combined with the hydrogel delivery system, mobile microrobots show great potential by providing high capacity/surface for drug loading and tissue-specific ligand binding, protecting cargo, and releasing low off-target therapeutic agents spatiotemporally (Erkoc et al., 2019). Microrobots made of biodegradable hydrogel composite materials show unique advantages in accurately transporting biological samples in the body (Wei et al., 2020). If magnetic materials (such as Fe_3O_4) and other functional materials are further coated on the surface of the microrobot, the microrobot can be driven and controlled by an external magnetic field to reach inaccessible locations in the body. Therefore, microrobots can be used to achieve targeted cell delivery and other types of micromanipulations, promoting precision and regenerative medicine.

1.1.6 Microfluidic chips used for cell manipulation

Microfluidics is a technology that can accurately manipulate fluids at the picoliter (pL) to microliter (μL) scale (Cole et al., 2017). It is an interdisciplinary technology based on analytical chemistry, microelectronics, micromechanics, bioengineering, and nanotechnology. The basic principle is to integrate operations related to the fields of chemistry and biology, such as sample preparation, reaction, separation, and detection, as well as cell culture, sorting, and lysis, on a chip of a few square centimeters or less. These on-chip functions can be connected through a microchannel network, in which fluid flow can be accurately controlled. Microfluidics can replace various functional units in traditional chemical or biological laboratories; therefore, it is also called the micro total analysis system (microTAS) or lab-on-chip (Svendsen, 2015). The development of soft lithography technology and improvement of the on-chip integration level have enabled the microfluidic technology to be gradually more functional and diversified. Microfluidics technology is used in various fields, including precision medicine, chemical synthesis and analysis, biology, information, and optics. In particular, the cell-based microfluidics technology used in research into biological cell systems has become a research hotspot.

Currently, cell manipulation methods based on microfluidics are divided into two types: active and passive. Active methods refer to the use of external forces to actively control fluids and cells. They include valve-based (Unger et al., 2000), droplet-based (Mazutis et al., 2013), electricity (Thomas et al., 2009; Chow et al., 2018), magnetism (Adams et al., 2008), optical (Wang et al., 2011; Chiu et al., 2018), and acoustic manipulation (Ding et al., 2012; Li et al., 2014). At the same time, the passive method uses the interaction between channel structure and fluid, cell and fluid, and cell and structure, that is, the principle of fluid dynamics, to precisely control the movement of fluid and cells in the microchannel (Carlo, 2009; Choi et al., 2011; Yan et al., 2015; Luo et al., 2018). The passive method is simple and has high throughput.

1.2 Outline of the book

This book introduces a number of robotic systems and technologies to achieve cell manipulation for various biomedical applications. The outline of the book is as follows.

Chapter 2 introduces the technical tools for cell manipulation. The analysis starts with a microneedle or micropipette used to control cell aspiration or achieve cell microinjection. A robotic manipulation system based on optical tweezers is introduced to trap, assemble, transport, and sort cells, which is followed by the introduction of electrokinetic manipulation tools based on dielectrophoresis (DEP) to achieve automatic cell trapping, cell separation, and cell patterning. Next, a magnetic actuation system is introduced, which uses a magnetic field gradient to drive cell-carrying microrobots to achieve targeted delivery in an in vivo environment. Finally, a variety of imaging techniques for intracellular manipulation are introduced, including the state-of-the-art microscopes, such as confocal fluorescence microscopy (CFM), two-photon fluorescence microscopy (TPFM), and light sheet fluorescence microscopy (LSFM), as well as other imaging techniques such as light photoacoustic microscopy (PAM), traditional wide-field fluorescence microscopy (WFFM), advanced structured illumination microscopy (SIM), and stimulated emission loss microscopy (STEDM). The successful development of these tools combined with robotics can greatly support cell manipulation.

Chapter 3 introduces the robotic microinjection of suspension cells and adherent cells. The size of the injected cells ranges from a relatively large size of 500−1000 μm (such as zebrafish embryos) to a small size of 20 μm (such as human cells). The use of robotics technology can realize efficient and accurate automatic injection. The setup and operational strategy of the cell microinjection system are introduced first. The hybrid position and force control for automatic injection of batches of cells are introduced, followed by universal piezoelectric-driven ultrasound cell microinjection, aimed at improving the survival rate of injected cells. Various methods to achieve high performance, high throughput, and high productivity in cell injection are further discussed. Finally, two case studies using robotic microinjection methods for single-cell transfection and cell mechanical characterization are introduced. This chapter illustrates how robotics can help achieve efficient, automated, and precise single-cell injection. Single-cell transfection by robotic microinjection is particularly useful for applications where cell transfection is challenging and requires genetic modification of selected cells.

Chapter 4 discusses cell stretching and deformation using optical tweezers. Various robotic micromanipulation tools are introduced, which can deform cells to characterize cell functions and regulate intracellular transmission. This chapter introduces five methods. First, robotically controlled optical tweezers are used to stretch the cells to explore the mechanobiological characteristics of the cells. Two case studies report on stretching hematopoietic cells to understand the property difference between normal and leukemia conditions, as well as stretching human embryonic stem cells to explore mechanobiological properties in cardiac differentiation. Second, a model of the actin cytoskeleton under optical stretching is established to provide insights into the relationship between cell mechanical behavior and cell function changes. Third, the DEP stretching of individual cells is introduced. Compared with optical stretching, DEP force can provide greater stretching force. Fourth, the method of compressing cells by mechanical restraint is introduced. Compared with optical and DEP stretching methods, mechanical confinement can cause large cell deformations, thereby identifying cell biomechanical properties at different levels. Finally, a unique method is introduced that uses millimeter-sized iron rods or spheres driven by magnetic force to selectively deform cells. This method can be used to achieve in situ intracellular delivery. This chapter demonstrates that robotic cell manipulation techniques combined with different manipulation tools can be successfully used to stretch and compress individual cells, which can play an important role in regulating and characterizing cell functions in biological research and medical treatment.

Chapter 5 discusses automatic cell transfer using the optical tweezers manipulator based on dynamic analysis, motion planning, and controller design. First, the basic theory of using optical tweezers to transport cells is introduced. A controller is developed that can control single and multiple cells in automatic transport without requiring the precise values of the trapping stiffness and drag coefficient. Second, the motion and path planning of automatic cell transportation are introduced. The motion parameters are optimized so that the cells can move effectively while maintaining their position in the laser trap. Several path-planning methods, such as improved A* algorithm, RRT-based path planner, and dynamic path planner, are reported, which can solve the interference problem in the dynamic solution. Third, a unified controller is proposed to simultaneously control cell positioning, cell trapping, and obstacle avoidance, without the need for an additional trajectory planner. The controller is designed based on a geometric coalition model, which aims to confine the cells in the light trap while considering obstacle avoidance. Fourth, a potential field-based controller is introduced, which can drive the two groups of particles into a pair of common arrays while controlling the distance between the pair of particles. Finally, a multistep processing control method is introduced to sequentially transfer a group of cells to a series of task regions, while keeping the cells in an effective trapping area and avoiding conflicts. The controller can simultaneously control cell positions, cell trapping, and collision avoidance in a coordinated manner, and continuously transfer grouping cells to different task areas without interruption. This chapter demonstrates that robotic optical tweezers technology can be successfully used to transfer single and multiple cells, and has the potential to be used in many biomedical applications, such as drug discovery, cell—cell interaction, and tissue engineering.

Chapter 6 introduces the control of cell rotation by the optical tweezers manipulator. After establishing the general dynamic equation of the suspension cell movement, a controller is developed to realize the one-degree-of-freedom in-plane rotation control of the suspension cell, while considering the position control in the plane translation. The automatic control of out-of-plane reorientation is then introduced. On the basis of the general dynamic equation of the trapped cell rotation and the image-processing algorithm to estimate the orientation of the cell, a vision-based adaptive controller is proposed to realize the closed-loop rotation control of the cell out of the image plane. Experiments are performed to illustrate the performance of the in-plane and out-of-plane cell rotation control methods. Successful cell rotation will facilitate single-cell manipulation and enable many cell therapy applications based on cell orientation.

Chapter 7 introduces a 3D image reconstruction method for intracellular surgery using a robot-assisted microscope system. First, a series of optical sections along the vertical direction is obtained by moving the microscope lens. After several process of deconvolution, segmentation, and reconstruction, a 3D reconstruction model of the specimen is established. The experimental results illustrate the effectiveness of the proposed method by using simulated spheres with various noise levels and measuring fluorescent microspheres of specific sizes. Second, a precise intracellular delivery method with 3D image reconstruction information is introduced. The optimal delivery position can be derived from the volume-based model in the geometric analysis. This position guides a robust controller to drive the moving stage and micropipette tip to perform delivery tasks without being affected by external interference. Reconstruction accuracy experiments are performed on the nucleus, and the results are compared with a confocal fluorescence microscope. Intracellular nucleus delivery experiments are further carried out. In summary, the 3D image reconstruction method for intracellular surgery can largely meet the needs of various biomedical applications that require precise delivery.

In Chapter 8, cell sorting and separation are discussed. Two strategies that combine robotic cell manipulation with microfluidic chip technology are introduced. The first strategy is to use a robot-assisted optical tweezers manipulation method to achieve high-precision cell sorting and separation of a small number of cell samples. Using the first strategy, a universal single-cell manipulation tool integrating optical tweezers, microfluidic chips, and imaging-processing technology is developed. Multiple optical traps can be generated at the same time for parallel sorting of multiple cells. This method is ideally suited to the separation and enrichment of rare cells. The second strategy is to combine the sheathless method with the DEP method to separate cells of different sizes or dielectric properties. Sheathless cell focusing can be achieved via gravity sedimentation of the cells in a tubing inserted into the inlet of the microfluidic chip. Efficient separation of cells of interest from cell mixtures is the key to many biomedical applications.

Chapter 9 discusses cell stimulation and migration. This chapter introduces the chemoattractant-induced cell migration model and control based on the stimulus-induced robotic manipulation system. First, a cell migration model that simulates in vivo migration by using optically manipulated chemoattractant-loaded microsources is presented. Using this model, the relationship among protrusion force, cell motility, and chemoattractant gradient can be quantitatively characterized. Experiments on migrating cancer cells show that the ideal migration ability can be achieved by appropriately selecting the chemoattractant gradient and concentration at the front edge of the cell. Second, a potential field function-based controller is developed to enable the optical tweezers to manipulate the microsource beads, thereby stimulating cell migration to the desired area. Here, the chemoattractant-loaded microbeads trapped by the optical tweezers are used to release the stimulus, thereby inducing the target cells to migrate to the desired area. A geometric model is established to confine the microsource beads to the effective trapping area of the optical tweezers and the high-motility area of the cells. Third, the application of electrical stimulation (ES) to stimulate cells is presented, which aims to improve the osteogenic differentiation of MSCs. ES parameters can be optimized depending on the calcium spike pattern of MSCs, which can be used to improve the osteogenic differentiation of MSCs. This method provides a new opportunity for optimizing osteogenic differentiation and can be useful in clinical treatments, such as bone fractures.

Chapter 10 introduces cell patterning. Cell patterning refers to arranging cells in a desired shape at the desired position. The first method used to control a group of cells to form the desired cell pattern is to use robotically controlled optical tweezers based on a multilevel topology design. A potential function-based controller with pattern adjustment control can drive cells to form the required pattern without collision. The second method is to use DEP to manipulate and pattern cells on a multilayer 3D engineering scaffold, which is further applied to automatically seed cells into a multilayer honeycomb pattern for bone tissue engineering applications. Studies have shown that cell pattern technology based on integrated DEP can enhance cell seeding to develop high-quality artificial tissues. The third method is to use the gravitational sedimentation-based approach to realize cell patterning coculture on a microfluidic platform, in which multiple cell types can be patterned simultaneously to form a well-organized cell coculture without complicated hardware settings or sophisticated chip design and fabrication. This method does not require an external field to help the cell arrangement in the microchannel, so it can pattern cells without introducing any stimuli that may affect normal cell behavior.

Chapter 11 introduces the method for manipulating cell adhesion. Cell adhesion is the process by which cells come into contact with each other or with their substratum through specialized protein complexes. This process can be performed using optical tweezers and is helpful for the study of cell—cell interactions. The adhesion of leukemia cancer cells to bone marrow stromal cells is especially studied, and the fluorescence intensity is used as a marker to study the Wnt signaling pathway of leukemia cells. On the basis of the adhesion characteristics of leukemia cells to stromal cells, different adhesion types of tight adhesion, loose adhesion, and free suspension can be clarified. Cell adhesion manipulations will provide a new opportunity to study otherwise inaccessible mechanisms of cell—cell interactions.

Chapter 12 discusses another interesting topic of cell fusion. Cell fusion is the cellular process of combining two or more cells to form a single entity. This chapter introduces cell engineering fusion using robotic manipulation with optical tweezers. The basic working principle is introduced based on the fusion of human embryonic stem cells (hESCs), in which the cells are manipulated by optical tweezers and fused under pulsed ultraviolet (UV) laser irradiation. By using a microwell array-based microfluidic chip, fusion with high selectivity and controllability can be achieved. Finally, a case study of artificial fusion of stem cells and liver cancer cells to isolate fused cell lines is reported. The results of genetic analysis show that the fusion of cancer cells and stem cells results in cancer cells having stronger tumorigenicity and higher chemoresistance. The results also show that the fusion cells are highly similar to tumor-initiating cells in biological processes or cell compartments. The successful development of this laser-induced single-cell fusion technology will provide a unique method for many important studies that facilitate cell differentiation, maturation, and reprogramming.

Chapter 13 discusses the in vivo transport of cells using microrobot technology. This process is particularly useful for precision medicine, such as targeted cancer therapy. First, the manipulation technology based on robotic optical tweezers is used to transport single cells in blood vessels. An enhanced disturbance compensation controller is introduced to minimize the influence of fluid on cells. Simulation and experimental results show that the proposed controller can effectively and automatically transfer a single cell to the desired position. This research is potentially useful for many precision medicine applications, such as metastasis study and drug delivery. Second, a microrobot designed with a burr-like porous spherical structure is proposed to carry and deliver cells in vivo under the driving mechanism of a magnetic gradient field. The microrobot is fabricated using 3D laser lithography technology, which provides sufficient flexibility for the microrobot structure design. Experiments have proved that the proposed microrobot design can enhance the magnetic driving ability, improve the cell carrying capacity, and benefit cell viability. Carrying cells can be spontaneously released from the microrobot to the surrounding tissues. The autonavigation of cell culture microrobots is demonstrated in zebrafish embryos. These results support the feasibility of using magnet-driven microrobots to accurately deliver targeted cells in vivo. Third, the magnetic image-guided degradable microrobot is further designed to precisely deliver engineered stem cells for orthotopic liver tumor treatment. The microrobot is made of synthetic composite materials, which can meet the requirements of degradability, mechanical strength, and magnetic actuation capability simultaneously. The microrobot is guided by a unique photoacoustic imaging technology. Preclinical tests have been performed on nude mice to prove that the microrobot transports these cells to the target site and releases loaded cells, and the cells significantly inhibit tumor growth. Preclinical trials have revealed the feasibility of using degradable microrobots to accurately deliver therapeutic cells in vascular tissues, and have proven their efficacy in tumor treatment.

Chapter 14 introduces intracellular-level manipulation technology to achieve organelle biopsy and single-cell gene editing for precision medicine. The chapter has three perspectives. First, a surgical system based on robotic microneedles is introduced to realize automated single-cell biopsy of small cells (diameter <20 μm). The enabling technologies of microfluidic chip device, sliding mode nonlinear controller, and imaging processing are integrated to achieve biopsy of mitochondria and nuclei of human cells. Second, a method for gene delivery to MSCs using high-throughput robotic microinjection is reported. Compared with traditional methods such as polyethyleneimine (PEI), cationic liposomes (cLipo), and calcium phosphate nanoparticles (CaP), robotic microinjection has higher transfection efficiency, lower cell damage, and stronger ability to retain MSC pluripotency and therapeutic gene function. Third, an automatic optical tweezers manipulation method for single-cell mitochondrial transfer is introduced. This method uses a microfluidic cell positioning device to pattern cells and mitochondria and then employs optical tweezers to collect a predetermined number of healthy isolated mitochondria and automatically transport them to the top of the cell. These mitochondria are taken up by the host cells through endocytosis. Compared with the traditional coculture passive transfer method, this method can effectively control the quantity and quality of mitochondria before transfer. A case study on the transfer of mitochondria from fetal MSCs to adult MSCs to improve antiaging and metabolic gene expression demonstrates the potential value of this method in precision medicine and cell therapy for mtDNA-related diseases.

1.3 Conclusions

This chapter aims to provide readers with an overview of robot-assisted cell manipulation. Various types of cell operations and their target applications are introduced. Traditional cell manipulation methods have limitations in accuracy, success rate, proficiency, efficiency, and consistency. Robotics can overcome these challenging problems and promote the practical application of cell manipulation. An outline of the book is presented.

The following is a list of the main contents related to this chapter:

- Cell manipulation concept and its biomedical applications;
- Automating cell manipulation with high efficiency and accuracy using robotics technology;
- Summary of the key manipulation tools including microneedle, optical tweezers, electrical and magnetic device, and microfluidic chip-in-cell manipulations;
- Review of robotic cell manipulations in achieving cell injection, cell stretching, cell transport and rotation, 3D image reconstruction of cells, cell sorting and separation, cell stimulation and migration, cell patterning, cell adhesion, cell fusion, in vivo cell navigation and delivery, single-cell biopsy, and gene editing.

References

Adams, J.D., Kim, U., Soh, H.T., 2008. Multitarget magnetic activated cell sorter. Proc. Natl. Acad. Sci. USA 105 (47), 18165–18170.

Alapan, Y., Bozuyuk, U., Erkoc, P., Karacakol, A.C., Sitti, M., 2020. Multifunctional surface microrollers for targeted cargo delivery in physiological blood flow. Sci. Robot. 5, eaba5726.

Ando, J., Bautista, G., Smith, N., Fujita, K., Daria, V.R., 2008. Optical trapping and surgery of living yeast cells using a single laser. Rev. Sci. Instrum. 79 (10).

Anis, Y.H., Mills, J.K., Cleghorn, W.L., 2006. Vision-based measurement of microassembly forces. J. Micromech. Microeng. 16, 1639–1652.

Antkowiak, M., Torres-Mapa, M.L., Stevenson, D.J., Dholakia, K., Gunn-Moore, F.J., 2013. Femtosecond optical transfection of individual mammalian cells. Nat. Protoc. 8, 1216–1233.

Arai, F., Endo, T., Yamuchi, R., Fukuda, T., 2006. 3D 6DOF manipulation of micro-object using laser trapped microtool. IEEE Int. Conf. Robot. Automat. 1390–1395.

Ashkin, A., Dziedzic, J.M., Bjorkholm, J.E., Chu, S., 1986. Observation of a single-beam gradient force optical trap for dielectric particles. Opt. Lett. 11 (5), 288–290.

Bai, G., Li, Y., Chu, H.K., Wang, K., Tan, Q., Xiong, J., Sun, D., 2017. Characterization of biomechanical properties of cells through dielectrophoresis-based cell stretching and actin cytoskeleton modeling. Biomed. Eng. Online 16 (41).

BBC News, November 6, 2015. Miracle Genetic Therapy Saves Baby with Leukemia.

Carlo, D.D., 2009. Inertial microfluidics. Lab Chip 9 (21), 3038–3046.

Chamorro, P., Levi, R., Rodrguez, F.B., Pinto, R.D., Varona, P., 2009. Real-time activity-dependent drug microinjection. BMC Neurosci. 10 (1), 296.

Chen, H., Sun, D., 2012. Moving groups of microparticles into array with a robot-tweezers manipulation system. IEEE Trans. Robot. 28, 1069–1080.

Chen, S., Cheng, J., Kong, C.W., Wang, X., Cheng, S.H., Li, R.A., Sun, D., 2013. Laser-induced fusion of human embryonic stem cells with optical tweezers. Appl. Phys. Lett. 103, 033701.

Chen, X., Hoop, M., Mushtaq, F., Siringil, E., Hu, C., Nelson, B.J., Pané, S., 2017. Nanomaterials in biomedical applications. Appl. Mater. Today 9 (37).

Chiu, T., Chao, A., Chou, W., Liao, C., Wang, H., Chang, J., Chen, P., Wu, M., 2018. Optically-induced-dielectrophoresis (ODEP)-based cell manipulation in a microfluidic system for high-purity isolation of integral circulating tumor cell (CTC) clusters based on their size characteristics. Sensor. Actuator. B Chem. 258, 1161–1173.

Choi, S., Ku, T., Song, S., Park, J., 2011. Hydrophoretic high-throughput selection of platelets in physiological shear-stress range. Lab Chip 11 (3), 413–418.

Chow, Y.T., Man, T., Acosta-vélez, G.F., Zhu, X., Wen, X., 2018. Liquid metal-based multi-functional micropipette for 4D single cell manipulation. Adv. Sci. 18 (1), 1700711.

Chu, H.K., Huan, Z., Mills, J.K., Yang, J., Sun, D., 2015. Three-dimensional cell manipulation and patterning using dielectrophoresis via a multi-layer scaffold structure. Lab Chip 15, 920–930.

Cole, R.H., Tang, S., Siltanen, C.A., Shahi, P., Zhang, J.Q., Poust, S., 2017. Printed droplet microfluidics for on demand dispensing of picoliter droplets and cells. Proc. Natl. Acad.Sci. USA 114 (33), 8728–8733.

Cui, H.H., Voldman, J., He, X.F., Lim, K.M., 2009. Separation of particles by pulsed dielectrophoresis. Lab Chip 9 (16), 2306–2312.

Ding, X., Lin, S.S., Kiraly, B., Yue, H., Li, S., Chiang, I., Shi, J., 2012. On-chip manipulation of single microparticles, cells, and organisms using surface acoustic waves. Proc. Natl. Acad. Sci. USA 109 (28), 11105–11109.

Erkoc, P., Yasa, I.C., Ceylan, H., Yasa, O., Alapan, Y., Sitti, M., 2019. Mobile microrobots for active therapeutic delivery. Adv. Therapeut. 2 (1), 1800064.

Feng, L., Hagiwara, M., Ichikawa, A., Arai, F., 2013. On-chip enucleation of bovine oocytes using microrobot-assisted flow-speed control. Micromachines 4 (2), 272–285.

Gao, W., Shakoor, A., Xie, M., Chen, S., Guan, Z., Zhao, L., Jiang, Z., Sun, D., 2020. Precise automated intracellular delivery using a robotic cell microscope system with 3D image reconstruction information. IEEE/ASME Trans. Mechatron. 25 (6), 2870–2881.

Gou, X., Yang, H., Fahmy, T.M., Wang, Y., Sun, D., 2014. Direct measurement of cell protrusion force utilizing a robot-aided cell manipulation system with optical tweezers for cell migration control. Int. J. Robot Res. 33 (14), 1782–1792.

Hawkin, B.G., Gleghorn, J.P., Kirby, B.J., 2009. Dielectrophoresis for cell and particle manipulations. In: Zahn, J.D. (Ed.), Methods in Bioengineering: Biomicrofabrication and Biomicrofluidics. Artech House, Norwood, MA, pp. 133–181.

Hollister, S.J., 2005. Porous scaffold design for tissue engineering. Nat. Mater. 4, 518.

Hu, X., Bessette, P.H., Qian, J., Meinhart, C.D., Daugherty, P.S., Soh, H.T., 2005. Marker-specific sorting of rare cells using dielectrophoresis. Proc. Natl. Acad. Sci. USA 102 (44), 15757–15761.

Hu, S., Gou, X., Han, H., Leung, A.Y.H., Sun, D., 2013. Manipulating cell adhesions with optical tweezers for study of cell-to-cell interactions. J. Biomed. Nanotechnol. 9, 281–285.

Huang, H., Sun, D., Mills, J.K., Cheng, S.H., 2009. Robotics cell injection system with position and force control: towards automatic batch biomanipulation. IEEE Trans. Robot. 25 (3), 727–737.

Kasaya, T., Miyazaki, H., Saito, S., Sato, T., 1999. Micro object handling under SEM by vision-based automatic control. IEEE Int. Conf. Robot. Automat. 2189–2196.

Lassalle, B., Courtot, A., Testart, J., 1987. In vitro fertilization of hamster and human oocytes by microinjection of human sperm. Gamete Res. 16 (1), 69–78.

Levenberg, S., Rouwkema, J., Macdonald, M., Garfein, E.S., Kohane, D.S., Darland, D.C., 2005. Engineering vascularized skeletal muscle tissue. Nat. Biotechnol. 23 (7), 879–884.

Li, S., Guo, F., Chen, Y., Ding, X., Li, P., Wang, L., Cameron, C.E., Huang, T.J., 2014. Standing surface acoustic wave based cell coculture. Anal. Chem. 86 (19), 9853–9859.

Li, J., de Ávila, B.E.F., Gao, W., Zhang, L., Wang, J., 2017. Micro/nanorobots for biomedicine: delivery, surgery, sensing, and detoxification. Sci. Robot. 2, eaam6431.

Liu, C., Xie, W., Gui, C., Du, Y., 2013. Pronuclear microinjection and oviduct transfer procedures for transgenic mouse production. Lipoproteins Cardiovasc. Dis. 217–232.

Lu, Z., Chen, P., Nam, J., Ge, R., Lin, W., 2007. A micromanipulation system with dynamic force-feedback for automatic batch microinjection. J. Micromech. Microeng. 17, 314–321.

Luo, T., Fan, L., Zeng, Y., Liu, Y., Chen, S., Tan, Q., Lam, R.H.W., Sun, D., 2018. A simplified sheathless cell separation approach using combined gravitational-sedimentation-based prefocusing and dielectrophoretic separation. Lab Chip 18 (11), 1521–1532.

Mazutis, L., Gilbert, J., Ung, W.L., Weitz, D.A., Griffiths, A.D., Heyman, J.A., 2013. Single-cell analysis and sorting using droplet-based microfluidics. Nat. Protoc. 8 (5), 54–56.

Mencaissi, A., Eisiberg, A., Carrozza, M.C., Dario, P., 2003. Force sensing microinstrument for measuring tissue properties and pulse in microsurgery. IEEE/ASME Trans. Mechatron. 8 (1), 10–17.

Mencaissi, A., Eisiberg, A., Izzo, I., Dario, P., 2004. From macro to micro manipulation: model and experiments. IEEE/ASME Trans. Mechatron. 9 (2), 311–320.

Moutos, F.T., Freed, L.E., Guilak, F., 2007. A biomimetic three dimensional woven composite scaffold for functional tissue engineering of cartilage. Nat. Mater. 6, 162–167.

Nelson, B., Yu, Z., Vikramaditya, B., 1998. Sensor-based microassembly of hybrid MEMS devices. IEEE Control Syst. Mag. 18 (6), 35–45.

Pan, F., Chen, S., Jiao, Y., Guan, Z., Shakoor, A., Sun, D., 2020. Automated high-productivity microinjection system for adherent cells. IEEE Robot. Automat. Lett. 5 (2), 1167–1174.

Pethig, R., 2010. Review article – Dielectrophoresis: status of the theory, technology, and applications. Biomicrofluidics 4 (2), 02811.

Pine, J., Chow, G., 2009. Moving live dissociated neurons with an optical tweezer. IEEE Trans. Biomed. Eng. 56 (4), 1184–1188.

Rodrigo, P.J., Daria, V.R., Glucksted, J., 2004. Real-time three-dimensional optical micromanipulation of multiple particles and living cells. Opt. Lett. 29 (19), 2270–2272.

Rosenthal, A., Voldman, J., 2005. Dielectrophohoretic traps for single-particle patterning. Biophys. J. 88 (3), 2193–2206.

Science Alert, 2016. A Blind Woman Has Regained Sight Following a Controversial Stem Cell Treatment.

Shen, Y., Xi, N., Li, W., 2003. Force guided assembly of micro-mirrors. In: IEEE/RSJ Int. Conf. Intelligent Robots and Systems Las Vegas, NE, U.S.

Sitti, M., Ceylan, H., Hu, W., Giltinan, J., Turan, M., Yim, S., Diller, E., 2015. Biomedical applications of untethered mobile milli/microrobots. Proc. IEEE 103, 205–224.

Song, H., Rosano, J.M., Wang, Y., Garson, C.J., Prabhakarpandian, B., Pant, K., Klarmann, G.J., Perantoni, A., Alvarez, L.M., Lai, E., 2015. Continuous-flow sorting of stem cells and differentiation products based on dielectrophoresis. Lab Chip 15, 1320–1328.

Steager, E.B., Selman Sakar, M., Magee, C., Kennedy, M., Cowley, A., Kumar, V., 2013. Automated biomanipulation of single cells using magnetic microrobots. Int. J. Robot Res. 32, 346.

Sun, D., Mills, J.K., 2002. Adaptive synchronized control for coordination of multirobot assembly tasks. IEEE Trans. Robot. Automat. 18 (4), 498–510.

Sun, Y., Nelson, B.J., 2002. Biological cell injection using an autonomous microrobotics system. Int. J. Robot Res. 21, 861–868.

Sun, D., Mills, J.K., Liu, Y.H., 1999. Position control of robot manipulators manipulating a flexible payload. Int. J. Robot Res. 18 (3), 319–332.

Svendsen, J.C.W.E., 2015. Lab-on-a-Chip Devices and Micro-total Analysis Systems. Springer International Publishing Switzerland.

Thomas, R.S., Morgan, H., Green, N.G., 2009. Negative DEP traps for single cell immobilisation. Lab Chip 9 (11), 1534–1540.

Tottori, S., Zhang, L., Qiu, F., Krawczyk, K.K., Franco-Obregón, A., Nelson, B.J., 2012. Magnetic helical micromachines: fabrication, controlled swimming, and cargo transport. Adv. Mater. 24, 811.

Unger, M.A., Chou, H., Thorsen, T., Scherer, A., Quake, S.R., 2000. Monolithic microfabricated valves and pumps by multilayer soft lithography. Science 288 (5463), 113–117.

van Steirteghem, A.C., Nagy, Z., Joris, H., Liu, J., Staessen, C., Smitz, J., Wisanto, A., Devroey, P., 1993. High fertilization and implantation rates after intracytoplasmic sperm injection. Hum. Reprod. 8 (7), 1061–1066.

Wang, X., Chen, S., Kong, M., Wang, Z., Costa, K.D., Li, R.A., Sun, D., 2011. Enhanced cell sorting and manipulation with combined optical tweezer and microfluidic chip technologies. Lab Chip 11, 3656–3662.

Wang, K., Cheng, J., Cheng, S.H., Sun, D., 2013. Probing cell biophysical behavior based on actin cytoskeleton modeling and stretching manipulation with optical tweezers. Appl. Phys. Lett. 99, 083702.

Wei, T., Liu, J., Li, D., Chen, S., Zhang, Y., Li, J., Fan, L., Guan, Z., Lo, C.M., Wang, L., Man, K., Sun, D., 2020. Development of magnet-driven and image-guided biodegradable microrobots for the precise delivery of engineered stem cells for cancer therapy. Small 16 (41), 1906908.

Xie, Y., Sun, D., Liu, C., Tse, H.Y., Cheng, S.H., 2010. A force control approach to a robot-assisted cell microinjection system. Int. J. Robot Res. 29 (9), 1222–1232.

Yan, S., Zhang, J., Yuan, Y., Lovrecz, G., Alici, G., Du, H., Zhu, Y., Li, W., 2015. A hybrid dielectrophoretic and hydrophoretic microchip for particle sorting using integrated prefocusing and sorting. Electrophoresis 36 (2), 284–291.

Zhang, X., Chu, H.K., Zhang, Y., Bai, G., Wang, K., Tan, Q., Xiong, J., Sun, D., 2015. Rapid characterization of the biomechanical properties of drug-treated cells in a microfluidic device. J. Micromech. Microeng. 25, 105004.

Cell manipulation tools

2

2.1 Introduction

The micromanipulation of biological cells is playing an increasingly important role in biomedical research and applications. Over the past few decades, a variety of techniques for cell micromanipulation have been developed. These techniques are useful to achieve important functions such as drug discovery, single-cell transfection, cell–cell interactions, and tissue engineering. Various mechanisms and devices have been used to manipulate cells, including micropipette aspiration, optical tweezers, electrokinetics (electrophoresis and dielectrophoresis), magnetic tweezers, atomic force microscopy (AFM), and imaging tools to identify target biological specimens. Combining robotics with these cell manipulation tools to facilitate the automatic and accurate manipulation of cells will overcome the challenges of accuracy, success rate, proficiency, efficiency, and consistency. This chapter outlines the manipulation tools and techniques used to manipulate cells, which include microneedles or micropipettes, optical tweezers, electrokinetic manipulation tools, magnetic manipulator, atomic force microscopy (AFM), and a variety of imaging technologies for intracellular manipulation.

2.2 Microneedle

One of the oldest and most widely used single-cell manipulation methods is microneedle-based manipulation. The microneedle (or micropipette) is fabricated with a glass capillary (Trickey et al., 2000), and its diameter ranges from less than 1 to 10 μm. Microneedles attached to a micromanipulator have been used for multiple cell manipulation tasks, such as cell biopsy (Actis et al., 2012), cell injection (Sun and Nelson, 2002), cell cutting (Yang et al., 2015), patch clamping (Aerts et al., 2014), and organelle removal and transfer (Yu et al., 2014).

Micropipette aspiration is a technique that applies negative pressure to control the aspiration of a desired cell. Positive pressure is used while dispensing the cell. Micropipette aspiration has been used for cell selection, deposition, and patterning. Some studies have also used this tool to characterize the mechanical properties of cells. Robotic manipulation systems equipped with micropipette aspiration have been proposed for automated transportation and positioning of single cells (Anis et al., 2010). Fig. 2.1 shows a typical robotic manipulation system aiming to transport cells automatically, which includes an X–Y motorized stage mounted on an inverted microscope, a micropipette mounted on a micromanipulator, a linear stage for control of picoliters of fluids, and computer vision (Lu et al., 2010). During the cell transport process, the target cells

Robotic Cell Manipulation. https://doi.org/10.1016/B978-0-323-85259-3.00014-3

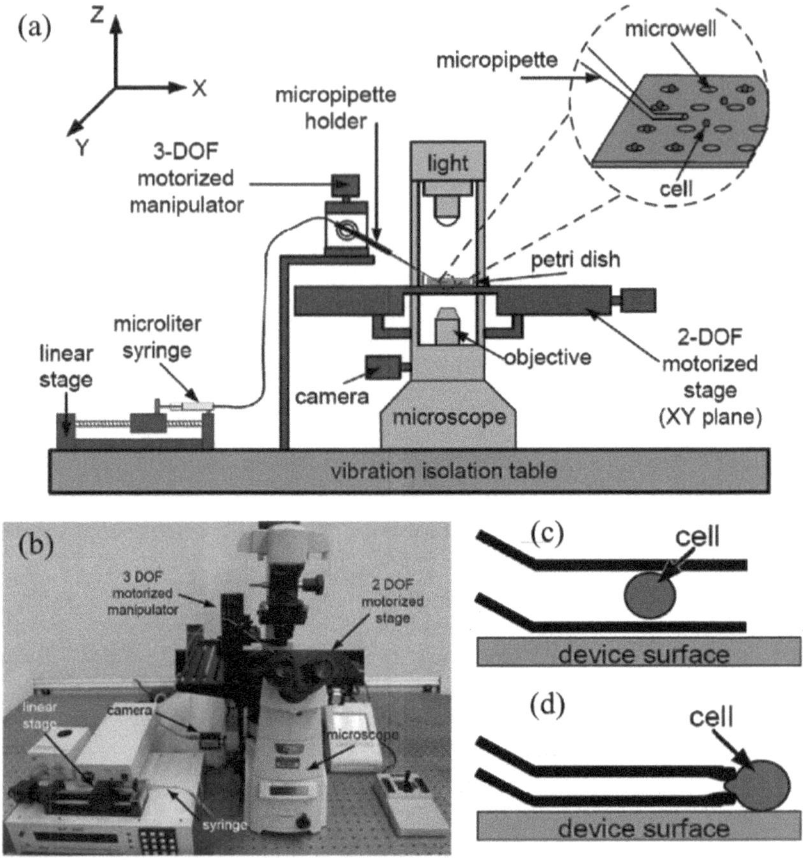

Figure 2.1 Schematic diagram and experimental setup (Lu et al., 2010). (A) Schematic diagram. (B) Experimental setup of the robotic manipulation system. (C) Cell aspiration. (D) partial aspiration techniques used to manipulate single cells.

move close to the micropipette, and suction pressure is applied to suck the cells into the micropipette. The micropipette is then raised from the substrate surface and repositioned, and the cells are dispensed to the desired position.

Microneedles have been used mostly for microinjection of single cells. Microinjection is a common biological practice that delivers biological substances such as RNA, DNA, and mitochondria into cells through a glass capillary. It has become an effective and reproducible method for introducing exogenous material into cells. Fig. 2.2 shows a typical intracytoplasmic sperm injection (ICSI) cell injection process of a mouse's oocyte (diameter: ~100 μm) (Kimura and Yanagimachi, 1995). A microneedle perforates the cell membrane with its small and sharp tip and then injects materials into cells. Fig. 2.3 illustrates a typical automated cell injection system that consists of three main components, namely, a CCD camera, an inverted microscope, and a 3 degrees-of-freedom (3 DOF) microrobot (Sun and Nelson, 2002).

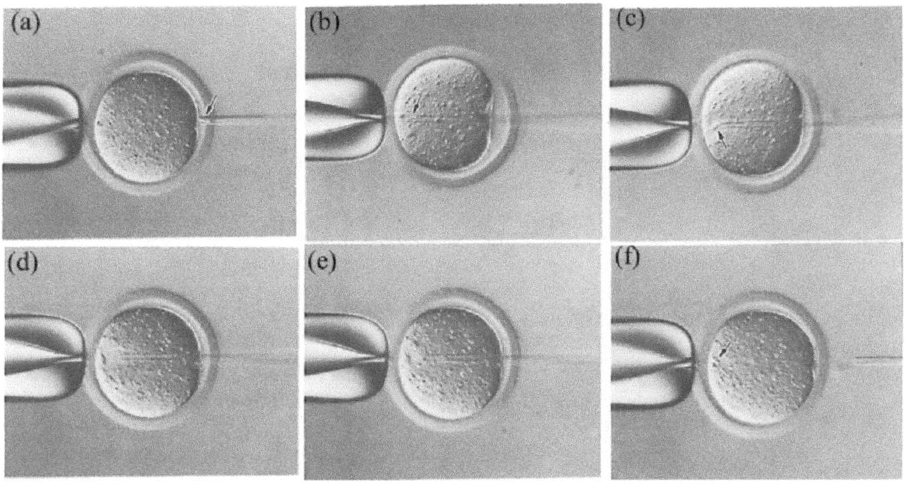

Figure 2.2 A typical ISCI cell injection process using a piezo-driven pipette (Kimura and Yanagimachi, 1995). (A, B) A sperm injection pipette was inserted deeply into an oocyte. (C, D) After the oolemma was broken, the entire spermatozoon was injected. (E) Medium injected with the spermatozoon was retrieved as completely as possible. (F) Withdrawal of the pipette (*arrow* indicates sperm head).

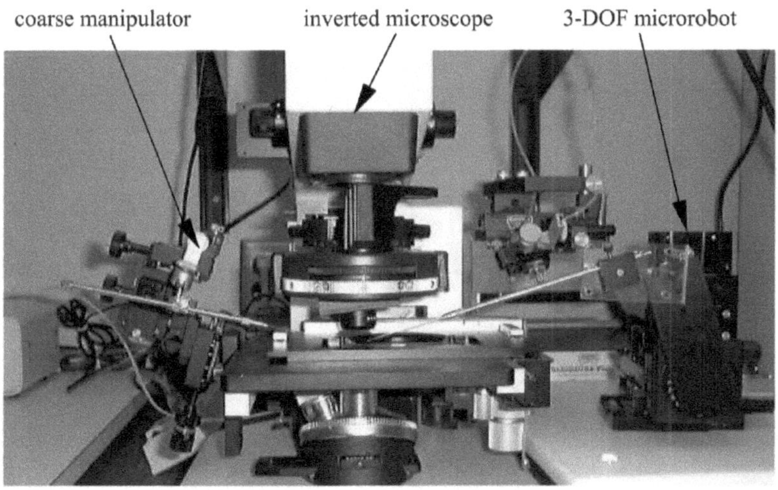

Figure 2.3 An autonomous embryo injection system (Sun and Nelson, 2002).

By integrating robotics, researchers are constantly striving to automate the cell injection process and improve performance. Over the past few decades, many robot-assisted cell injection systems have been developed for suspension cells and adherent cells. Fig. 2.4 shows an experimental setup for automatic out-of-plane injection of large batches of suspension cells (Huang et al., 2009), which uses the hybrid position control in horizontal plane and impedance force control in the z-axis. Fig. 2.5 shows an

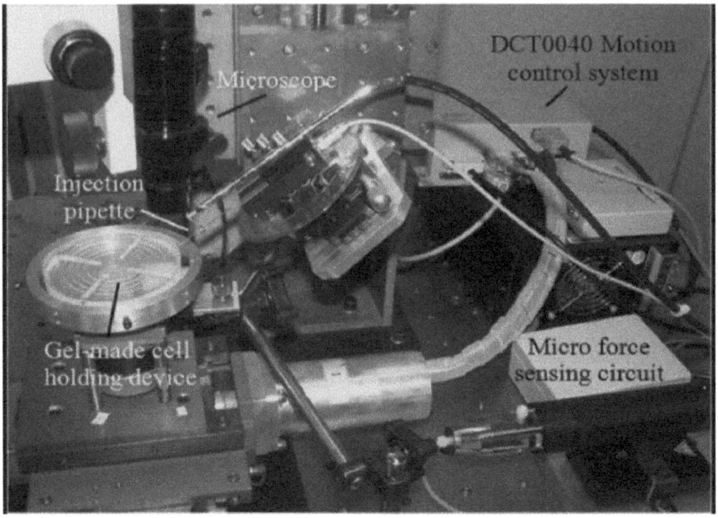

Figure 2.4 An automatic cell-injection system for suspension cells (Huang et al., 2009).

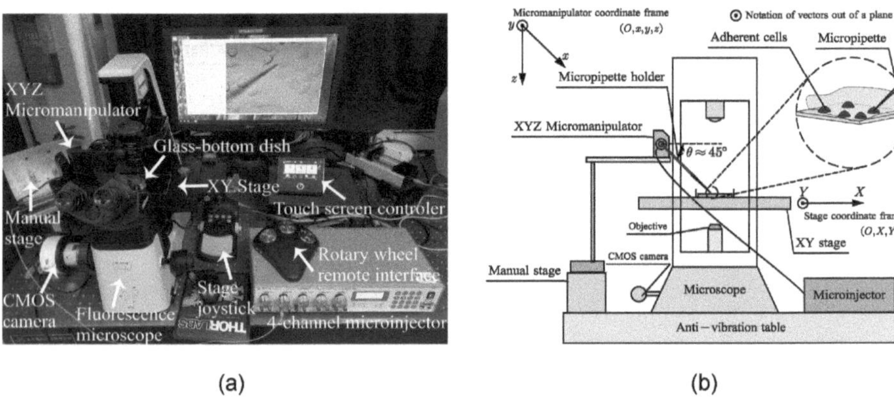

Figure 2.5 A high-productivity robotic microinjection system for adherent cells (Pan et al., 2020). (A) System setup. (B) System schematic diagram.

automated high-productivity system for adherent cell injections. In this system, productivity is improved by automatically detecting cells, quickly optimizing the injection path, adaptively adjusting the penetration depth, and avoiding clogging of micropipettes. These improvements allow the system to inject more than 1500 cells per hour with minimal training and preparation.

Piezo-driven pipettes represent another type of cell-piercing technique. Kimura and Yanagimachi (1995) first reported this method in ICSI, where the injection pipette was driven by a series of piezoelectric pulses with adjustable frequency, amplitude, and duration. Fig. 2.6 illustrates the piezo-driven microinjector mounted on the robotic cell injection system (Huang et al., 2011). The microinjector is properly designed to eliminate unnecessary lateral pipette vibration.

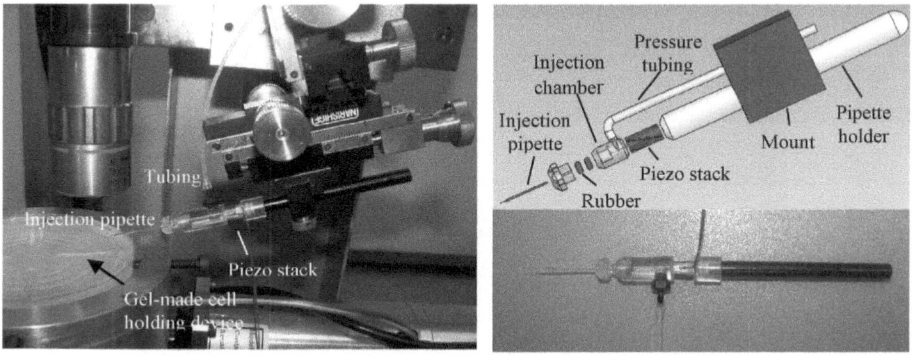

(a) (b)

Figure 2.6 Piezo-driven cell injector (Huang et al., 2011). (A) Close-up view of the injector. (B) Design and prototype of the injector.

Glass microneedles have been used to extract nuclei from individual cells through enucleation by inserting a micropipette inside the cell (Feng et al., 2012). Currently, highly skilled operators use microneedles to mechanically remove cell nuclei and complete this cellular surgery task at the subcellular level. This mechanical enucleation process consists of four basic steps: (1) aligning the position of the glass capillary with respect to the cell nucleus; (2) using the glass capillary to perforate the cell membrane; (3) aspirating the cell nucleus; and (4) removing the glass capillary from the cell. These operations are very cumbersome and time-consuming, and depend on the skill of the operator and the ability to control the position of the glass capillary. To overcome these problems, Shakoor et al. (2019) developed a robotic surgery system that uses microneedles to achieve automated single-cell biopsy of small cells with diameters of less than 20 μm. Fig. 2.7 illustrates this automated single-cell biopsy system.

2.3 Optical tweezers

In 1873, James Clerk Maxwell theoretically proved that light can exert optical force if it reflects off the surface of an object. However, given that the optical power was very weak, it was not demonstrated by experiments. This phenomenon changed after the invention of the laser in the 1960s. In the early 1970s, Ashkin discovered that tightly focused laser beams can draw micron-sized dielectric particles in water and air, and developed a three-dimensional (3D) trap using two counterpropagating laser beams. Ashkin then developed a single-beam optical trap in 1986, called "optical tweezers" (Ashkin et al., 1986).

Optical tweezers use highly focused laser beams to form optical traps to manipulate dielectric spherical particles, which are subjected to two forces, namely, scattering force and gradient force. The scattering force is generated by photons that hit the particle along its propagation direction, and the gradient force is generated by the spatial

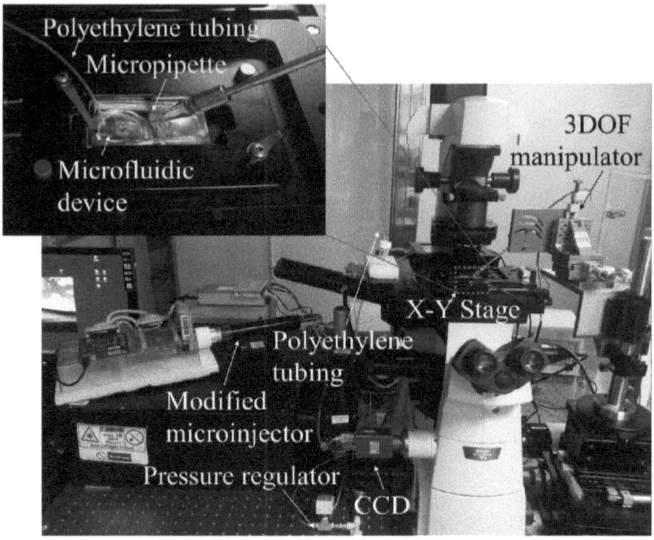

Figure 2.7 Automated single-cell biopsy system (Shakoor et al., 2019).

light gradient. The force exerted on the particle depends on the relationship between the diameter (r) of the trapped particle and the wavelength (λ) of the laser beam (Dholakia et al., 2008; Ramser and Hanstorp, 2010), which can be divided into three states: $r >> \lambda$, $r << \lambda$, and $r \sim \lambda$. $r >> \lambda$. However, the complete theory of optical tweezers is complicated, and only two simplified theoretical models have been developed to calculate the forces on particles (Neuman and Block, 2004). When the particle size is much smaller than the wavelength of the laser beam, the condition of the Rayleigh state is satisfied. When the particle size is much larger than the wavelength of the laser beam, the particle is in the Mie regime.

In most biological applications of optical tweezers, the Mie regime is satisfied. Therefore the discussion here mainly focuses on the Mie regime. The gradient force and the scattering force are produced by the refraction and reflection of light, respectively. The refraction of incident light by a sphere causes a change in the momentum of the light. Given the conservation of momentum, the sphere has an equal and opposite momentum change. When the refractive index of the particle is greater than that of the surrounding medium, the gradient force pushes the particle to the area with the highest light intensity in the direction of the intensity gradient. The scattering force in the light propagation direction comes from the absorption and reflection of light by the trapped sphere. The light must be focused to form a stable trap. In this case, the net force always draws the trapped particle to the focus. If the particle is far from the focus of the beam, the imbalance of the net force will pull it back to the equilibrium position (Fig. 2.8).

The force in the optical trap depends on the size and shape of the trapped object, the refractive index of the trapped object and the surrounding medium, the shape of the laser focus, and the laser power. The trapping force is rarely measured directly, but

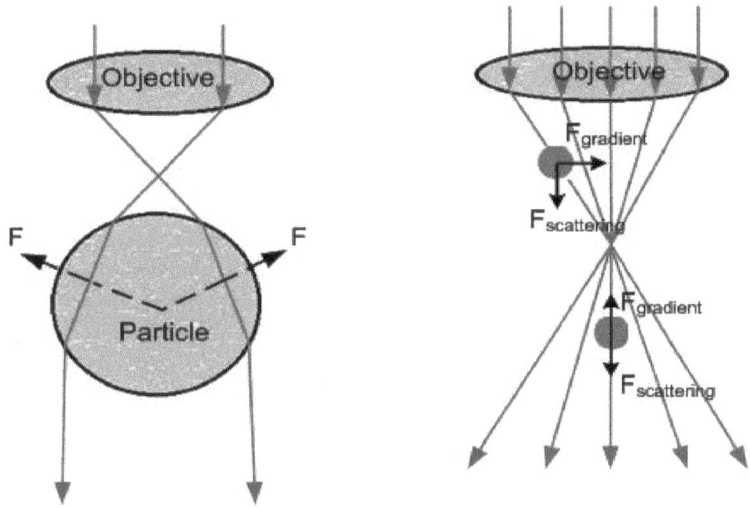

Figure 2.8 Schematic of the trapping force exerted on a particle (Gou, 2014). (A) In a focused laser beam, the trapping force always draws the particle back to focus. (B) Schematic of forces exerted on a particle that is outside the trap.

several methods have been developed to calibrate it. When the radius of the trapped object is known, the power spectrum of the Brownian motion of the trapped object can be used to calibrate the force. The trapping force can be calibrated by studying the thermal fluctuation of the trapped particles. The most widely used calibration method is the viscous drag force method (Svoboda and Block, 1994). For a free particle in the medium, the forces controlling cell movement include the trapping force from the optical trap and the viscous drag force from the medium. Given the critical value of the speed at which the cell escapes the laser trap, the maximum trapping force, which is equal to the viscous drag force, can be calculated.

A typical optical tweezers system consists of several basic components: a laser source, beam expansion, steering optics, a microscope with a high NA objective lens, a chamber holder, a charge-coupled device (CCD) camera, and a computer for observing the trapped sample (Neuman and Block, 2004; Zhang and Liu, 2008). Traditional optical tweezers use a standard Gaussian laser beam. Over the past few decades, attempts have been made to improve the performance of optical tweezers. Non-Gaussian laser beams (Gahagan and Swartzlander, 1998), double beams (Chiou et al., 1997), and multiple traps (Rodrigo et al., 2003) have been used in optical tweezers systems. Complex operations can be achieved by time-sharing a single laser beam among several optical tweezers or by diffractively splitting the beam into multiple traps. Using a mirror driven by an acousto-optic deflector or galvanometer, a single laser beam can be shared among hundreds of optical tweezers in the focal plane, or spread into an extended 1D trap. Specially designed diffractive optical elements can divide a single input beam into hundreds of continuous illumination traps in an arbitrary 3D configuration.

Optical trapping plays an important role in capturing, assembling, transporting, and sorting various particles at the single-cell and single-molecule levels. Many cell biology applications have been studied. Somatic cells (such as mammalian cells, red blood cells, and nerve cells) and gametes (such as human sperm) have been manipulated by optical tweezers. Optical tweezers are also used to manipulate organelles such as chromosomes, globular DNA, and RNA. Cell functions such as mitosis and motility have been studied, and the generation of forces for organelle transport in vivo has been measured. Compared with a single optical tweezers system, the multioptical tweezers configuration has huge advantages and a wide range of applications. On the basis of the mechanism of manipulating biological objects, the application of optical tweezers can be divided into two main categories: direct manipulation and indirect manipulation.

In the first category of direct manipulation, biological objects are trapped and directly manipulated by the laser beam. Applications in this category include cell positioning and transportation, cell assembly, cell sorting, cell fusion, and cell injection. The characteristics of flexible trapping and precise manipulation of optical tweezers allow them to be applied in cell positioning and transportation. An example is the use of optical tweezers to grasp and locate kidney cells (Lucio et al., 2003). The use of optical tweezers has been extended to the manipulation of neuron cells, and it has no significant effect on neuronal capabilities (Winckler et al., 1999). The assembly function of optical tweezers makes it suitable for cell assembly, which can form new structures for tissue engineering (Fig. 2.9) (Jordan et al., 2005). In addition, several groups have applied optical tweezers to cell sorting. Compared

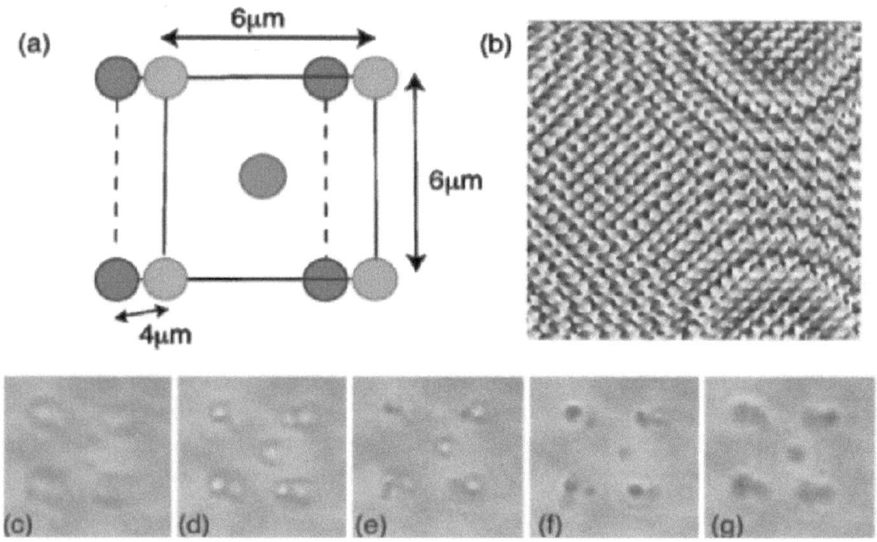

Figure 2.9 Permanently set 3D structures of *E. coli* (Jordan et al., 2005). (A) Schematic of the structure. (B) Hologram used to create the traps. (C–G) Images of the structure at various depths taken on the optical tweezer system.

with traditional fluorescence-activated cell sorting, optical tweezers-based cell sorting shows high purity and recovery when sorting small sample populations (Fig. 2.10) (Wang et al., 2011). Optical tweezers combined with UV or Nd:YAG can be used as scissors to accurately cut objects with submicron resolution. This technology has been applied to cell injection and cell fusion, providing an effective method for injecting biomolecules of interest into cells and fusing target cells, respectively (Fig. 2.11) (Chen et al., 2013).

In the second category of indirect manipulation, the laser beam traps the dielectric components (such as polymers and silica beads) attached to the target object instead of focusing directly on the target object. This method is widely used to manipulate nucleic acids and study the mechanical properties of cells. The ability of optical tweezers to measure displacements with subnanometer precision allows them to study changes in biomolecules. Most research on biomolecules has focused on stretching them to obtain a force–stretch relationship. Tan et al. (2012) probed the biophysical

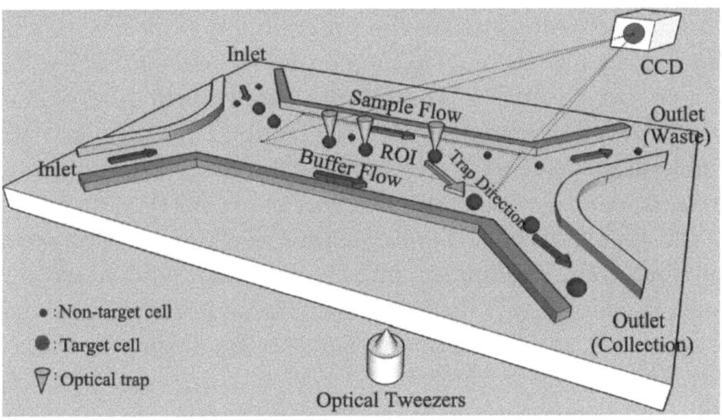

Figure 2.10 Schematic of the cell sorting procedure (Wang et al., 2011).

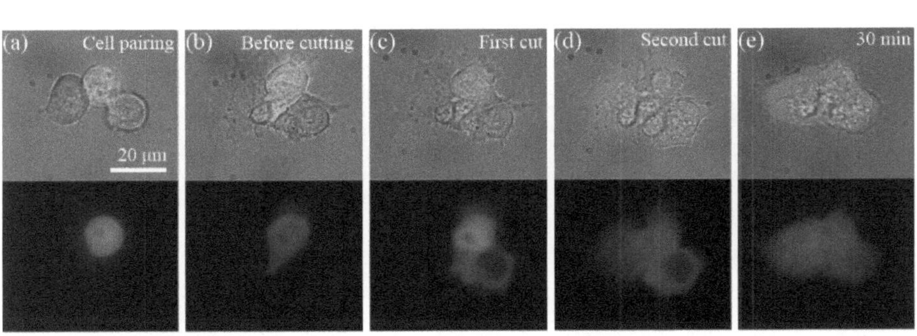

Figure 2.11 Laser-induced cell fusion of three adherent cells (Chen et al., 2013). (A) Three cell form cell pairs. (B) Three cells attach to cover glass in cell pair shape. (C) A GFP-labeled cell (middle) fuse with unlabeled cell (right) after the first cut. (D) The binucleated hESC is then fused with another unlabeled cell (left) by the second cut. (E) Thirty min after laser cutting, three cells become one single cell. Scale bar is 20 μm.

behavior of human embryonic stem cells by stretching them with optical tweezers (Fig. 2.12). Wang et al. (2013) conducted similar experiments on different types of cells. Membrane and cytoskeleton models have been established to explain the mechanical properties of cells, and the experimental results obtained through optical stretching help verify the theoretical model.

By integrating robotics technology, optical tweezers show the advantages of non-invasiveness, flexibility, and precision in various automated cell operations. The application examples include cell transport (Hu and Sun, 2011), cell stretching (Wang et al., 2013), cell mechanical characterization (Tan et al., 2012), cell migration (Gou et al., 2014), and organelle transplantation (Shakoor et al., 2021). Combined with imaging technology, optical tweezers can also be used for in vivo cell manipulation, such as cell transport in mouse (Zhong et al., 2013) and zebrafish (Li et al., 2017).

2.4 Electrokinetics

As micromachining technology makes the patterning of electrodes of arbitrary shapes routine, electrokinetics has become a common technique for manipulating particles. Electrostatic force can be used to control particles with high-resolution electrodes. Since the possibility of operating biological particles by capillary electrophoresis was demonstrated in the late 1980s, electrostatic forces have been used to manipulate viruses, bacteria, cells, and organelles (Kremser et al., 2004). For example, Zhu and Chen (1989) used capillaries coated with fluorinated ethylene–propylene copolymers to study mammalian cells. Red human, pig, chicken, and rabbit blood cells were electrophoresed with hydroxypropyl methylcellulose added to butyl glycidyl ether.

Two commonly used electrokinetic mechanisms are electrophoresis and dielectrophoresis (DEP). Electrophoresis refers to the motion of dispersed particles relative to a fluid caused by a uniform electric field in space (Kremser et al., 2004). In electrophoresis, a uniform electric field is usually applied to sort particles depending on their electrophoretic mobility. Particles with different mobilities can move at varying

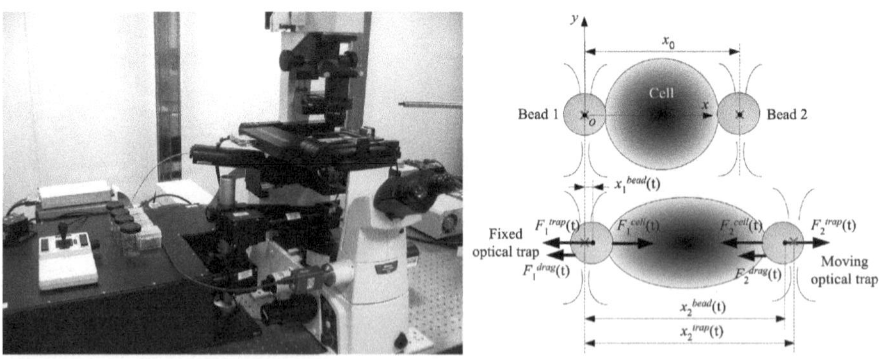

Figure 2.12 Cell stretching system with optical tweezers (Wu et al., 2011; Tan et al., 2012).

speeds. DEP is defined as the motion of particles caused by the application of an external nonuniform electric field (Kadaksham et al., 2004). As a result of the polarization of the neutral particles, the particles receive a force called DEP force and move. This DEP force depends on the electrical properties of the medium and particles, the shape and size of the particles, and the frequency of the electric field. DEP has been used to manipulate biological samples, such as bacteria, viruses, and cells. There are two types of DEP: negative DEP and positive DEP. In negative DEP, the dielectric constant of the particle is smaller than that of the fluid medium, and the particle receives a net force directed to the location where the electric field gradient decreases. The opposite phenomenon occurs in positive DEP. Fig. 2.13 illustrates the working principle of DEP.

The electrokinetic mechanism facilitates parallel and high-throughput cell manipulations. However, to manipulate a single cell, high-resolution and prepatterned electrode pixels are required. To solve the problem of wiring and addressing of these electrodes, complementary metal oxide semiconductor (CMOS) DEP has been proposed, which integrates a DEP actuator and optical sensor. This chip allows the manipulation of more than 10,000 individual cells in parallel (Manaresi et al., 2003). However, CMOS chips are expensive for many applications, especially for disposable devices that prevent cross-contamination. A new type of DEP tweezers was also designed to capture single cells with electric fields. As shown in Fig. 2.14, it uses a sharp glass tip with electrodes on both sides (Hunt and Westervelt, 2006). The glass rod is pulled to the tip of the pipette puller and placed in the high vacuum thermal evaporator to deposit the electrode. Ti and Au evaporate on one side of the pipette, and Ti–Au is deposited on the other side. The pipette is fixed on the micromanipulator mounted on the inverted microscope. The function generator is used to generate voltage for the electrodes. A thorny problem with electromotive force is that it is difficult to use in liquid media with high ion concentrations, which is usually the case for biological cell culture media.

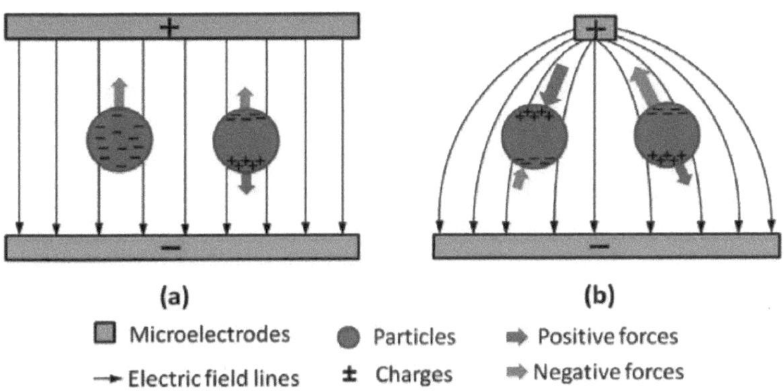

Figure 2.13 Principle of DEP (Huan, 2017). (A) The behavior of particles (charged and neutral) in a uniform electric field. (B) The behavior of neutral particles in a nonuniform electric field, which experience net forces.

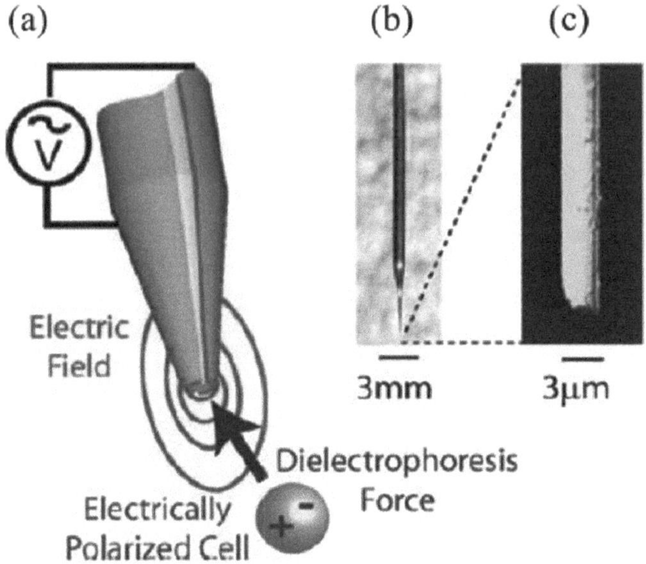

Figure 2.14 Dielectrophoresis tweezers (Hunt and Westervelt, 2006). A voltage across two electrodes on either side of a pipette creates an electric field which polarizes a cell and pulls the cell into the end of the pipette. (A) Schematic of dielectrophoresis tweezers. (B) Photograph of dielectrophoresis tweezers. (C) Scanning electron microscope image of the tweezer tip.

One of the most common applications of DEP is cell separation. The DEP force acting on a cell is generally proportional to the size of the cell. Therefore, the displacement of the cell that deviates from the streamline depends on the cell size. By using this characterization and electro-osmotic flow of DEP in a microfluidic device, heterogeneous biomolecules with a diameter of a few microns to tens of microns can be continuously separated depending on their size (Kang et al., 2008). The microfluidic device integrated with DEP demonstrates the feasibility of using DEP to isolate clinically important cells (such as CTC and malignant cancer cells) from heterogeneous blood samples in a label-free manner (Gascoyne et al., 2009; Vahey and Voldman, 2008). In addition, given that the DEP force depends on the electrical polarization of the cells, the separation of different types of cells based on different DEP responses can be achieved in the microfluidic device. By maximizing the difference in DEP response between live yeast cells (positive DEP response) and inactive (negative DEP response) yeast cells, the patterned electrode in the microfluidic device can be used to separate a mixture of live and inactive yeast cells (Doh and Cho, 2005). To take advantage of the difference in the DEP response of multiple target cells, the amplitude response of the target cell's DEP can be adjusted by labeling the cells with particles with different polarization responses (Hu et al., 2005). Through this method, rare target cells are enriched >200 times in a single microfluidic experiment and separated from the complex mixture in a continuous flow manner.

Another major application of DEP in microfluidics is cell trapping. The dielectric affinity column can be used to trap large cancer cells at the electrode tip through the DEP field, while small blood cells escape. Therefore, cancer cells can be released by turning off the DEP field. With the help of DEP, a microfluidic cytometer was developed in which DEP is used to capture cells to prevent disrupting fluid flow. The microcytometer consists of an array chip, which can be used for noncontact single-cell trapping via DEP (Voldman et al., 2002). The constricted geometry of microchannels made of insulating materials can also be used to generate squeezing electric fields. Electrodeless DEP has many advantages, such as generating high electric fields at low frequencies. DEP force has also been used in cell patterning technology. The position of the cell is fixed by an electric field, and the cell is patterned by a fixing step using a cross-linking agent or cell adhesion protein. By using DEP-based cell patterning technology, 3D microscale tissues were established within the hydrogel (Ramon et al., 2012).

DEP is also used in tissue engineering to create different cell patterns for culture and tissue development. A specific snare electrode array design was proposed for the DEP manipulation of hepatocytes to construct the radial pearl chain pattern of hepatocytes (Ho et al., 2006). The microfluidic chip was used to construct a heterogeneous liver cell model to simulate the lobular morphology of real liver tissue in vivo. A multilayer scaffold with honeycomb pores was designed to simulate the geometry of natural bone tissue (Huan et al., 2017). The cells on the scaffold were automatically patterned into a multilayer honeycomb pattern based on the DEP mechanism to mimic the structure and complexity of natural tissues to improve the performance of tissue culture.

2.5 Magnetic manipulator

Magnetic tweezers are a tool that uses magnetic field gradients to apply and measure forces on magnetic particles. Various settings have been developed for specific experimental purposes. A typical setup includes an electromagnet and a tip-shaped end. The electromagnet generates a magnetic field gradient around the tip, and the magnetic particles within the gradient can be pulled toward the tip. The magnitude of the force depends on the magnitude and gradient of the magnetic field. To control the 3D position of particles in real time, multiple electromagnets can be combined in the system, and a visual feedback system can be integrated (Charlie and Vincent, 2002). When using magnetic tweezers to manipulate cells, magnetic beads (whose surface has been functionalized with antibodies, peptides, or lectins) are attached to the cell membrane, making the cells magnetic. This feature leads to a limitation: the attachment of magnetic beads to cells may affect the intrinsic properties of the target cell, thereby preventing the user from observing the original response.

In recent years, magnetic manipulators have been used to drive particles rather than directly manipulate cells, especially in in vivo biomedical applications. Magnetic actuation has advantages of noninvasiveness and good control ability (Li et al., 2018, 2020), minimal tissue damage (Barnothy, 2013; Ahlbom et al., 2008), and insensitivity to biological substances. Therefore, the electromagnetic control system using electromagnetic coils as the actuator is considered a reliable remote control source, which can provide power for microrobots. As previously reported, different electromagnetic manipulation systems have been developed to drive microrobots in various environments. Magnetic actuation can be achieved by using an array of electromagnetic coils (Kummer et al., 2010; Diller et al., 2016; Niu et al., 2017), which surround a work area called the "driving space." On the basis of rotating magnetic field and gradient magnetic field, two magnetic driving methods are generally adopted. The rotating magnetic field drive method generates a torque on the microrobot to make it rotate. The rotation is converted into driving force through the specially designed shape and structure of the microrobot. In this driving mode, the microrobot must meet the specific requirements in structural design, such as a spiral structure that converts torque into driving force. However, this method may complicate the design of microrobots and reduce their reliability (Ye et al., 2014; Servant et al., 2015). The gradient magnetic field method directly uses magnetic force to drive the microrobot (Niu et al., 2017; Li et al., 2018a,b; Wei et al., 2020). Although this method does not require a special microrobot structure design, it needs a large amount of magnetic gradient, especially when driving the microrobot in an in vivo environment.

Several methods using permanent magnets (Mahoney and Abbott, 2016), Helmholtz and/or Maxwell coil pairs (Xu, 2014), and multiple electromagnets (Diller and Sitti, 2014) have been commonly used to design and construct magnetic manipulation systems, as shown in Fig. 2.15. Helmholtz coils and Maxwell coils can generate uniform magnetic fields and gradient magnetic fields, respectively. However, these coils cannot generate sufficient magnetic field strength and gradient to meet the requirements of manipulating microrobots in complex environments, especially in high-viscosity fluids (Wang et al., 2019). Permanent magnets can provide high magnetic field strength and gradients, but they are difficult to accurately control microrobots (Fountain et al., 2010). Compared with these methods, electromagnetic coils with iron cores can overcome these problems. The intensity and gradient of the magnetic field generated by the electromagnetic coils can be changed by adjusting the energized currents of the coils. The iron core can greatly enhance the magnetic field strength and

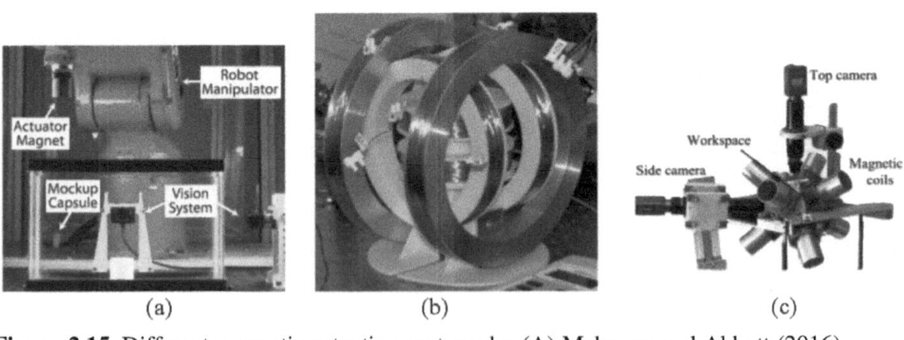

Figure 2.15 Different magnetic actuation systems by (A) Mahoney and Abbott (2016), (B) Xu (2014), and (C) Diller and Sitti (2014).

gradient generated by the electromagnetic control system (Kummer et al., 2010; Diller et al., 2016; Niu et al., 2017). In this way, the microrobot can be easily manipulated in in vitro and in vivo environments.

Kummer et al. (2010) developed an electromagnetic manipulation system called OctoMag, which can effectively perform eye surgery, as shown in Fig. 2.16. The system has a hemispherical working space with a diameter of 130 mm, surrounded by eight electromagnetic coils. Under the control of the manipulation system, the microrobot can be accurately driven in 3D space. However, the system acting on the microrobot does not generate downward force because the eight electromagnetic coils are distributed above the work area. The maximum excitation current of this system is 15 A. In this case, the generated magnetic field strength and gradient can reach 15 mT and 200 mT/m, respectively. Pawashe et al. (2009) developed an electromagnetic manipulation system called Mag-μBot, as shown in Fig. 2.17. Compared with OctoMag, the working space of this system is surrounded by six orthogonally distributed electromagnetic coils. The electromagnetic control system powered by 3 A current can generate a magnetic field strength and gradient of 6.5 mT and 149 mT/m, respectively. However, the working space of these two systems is relatively small. The resulting magnetic field strength and gradient may not be sufficient to drive microrobots in complex environments. To overcome this problem, Niu et al. (2017) developed an electromagnetic manipulation system that optimizes the coil and magnetic field distribution, as shown in Fig. 2.18. The radius of the working space is 65 mm. When the maximum current is applied to the coil, the magnetic field strength and gradient can reach 40 mT and 250 mT/m, respectively. Li et al. (2020) further optimized the core shape of the electromagnetic coils in developing a magnetic gradient field-based actuation system, as shown in Fig. 2.19. On the basis of the mathematical model established by the finite-element method, the shape of the iron core and the size of the probe were optimized so that the gradient of the focused area could be greatly increased. A thin disc is attached to the end of the iron core to reduce the waste of magnetic field energy. With this design, the magnetic field generated by the electromagnetic actuation system can be greatly enhanced to propel the microrobot in the in vivo environment.

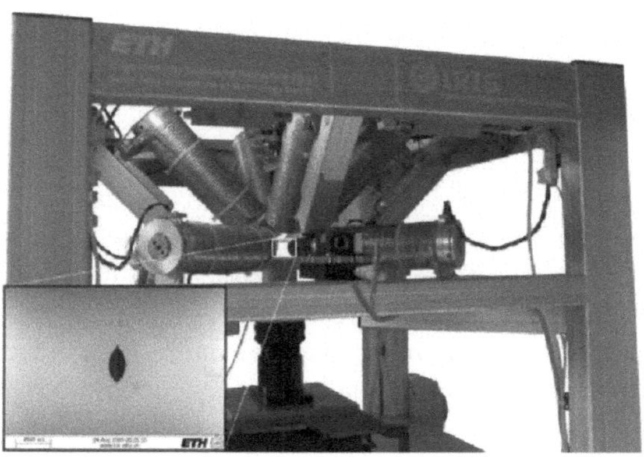

Figure 2.16 The OctoMag prototype system (Kummer et al., 2010).

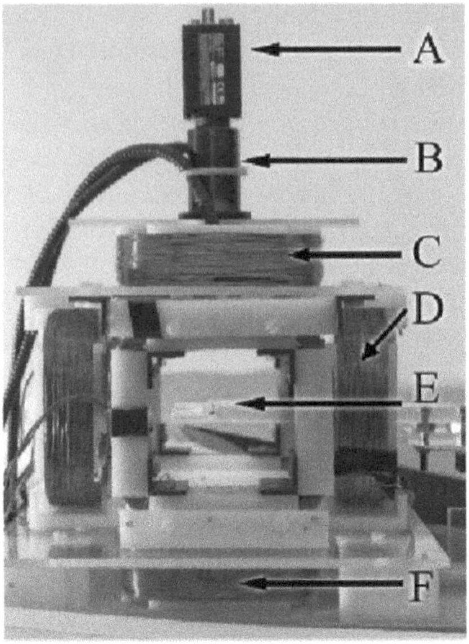

Figure 2.17 Mag-μBot prototype system (Pawashe et al., 2009). (A) CCD camera. (B) Microscope. (C, D, F) Electromagnets. (E) workspace.

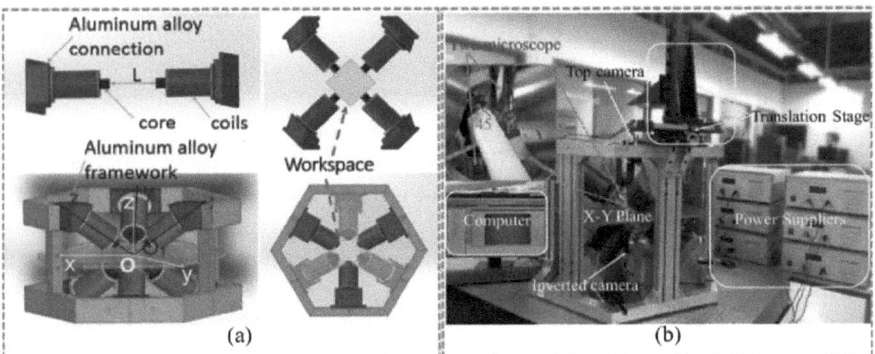

Figure 2.18 A large-space electromagnetic manipulation system (Niu et al., 2017). (A) Schematic. (B) System setup.

2.6 Atomic force microscopy

Atomic force microscopy (AFM) is a type of scanning probe microscopy, which uses a sharp tip mounted on the end of a flexible cantilever to scan (Alessandrini and Facci, 2005). When the tip is close to the cell surface, the cantilever will deflect, and the tip–sample interaction can be monitored by using a laser beam irradiated on the back of the cantilever. The laser beam is then reflected to the split photodetector and detected. The detection force can then be calculated as the product of the deflection and the stiffness of the cantilever. Fig. 2.20 shows the AFM scheme of a typical configuration for biological applications.

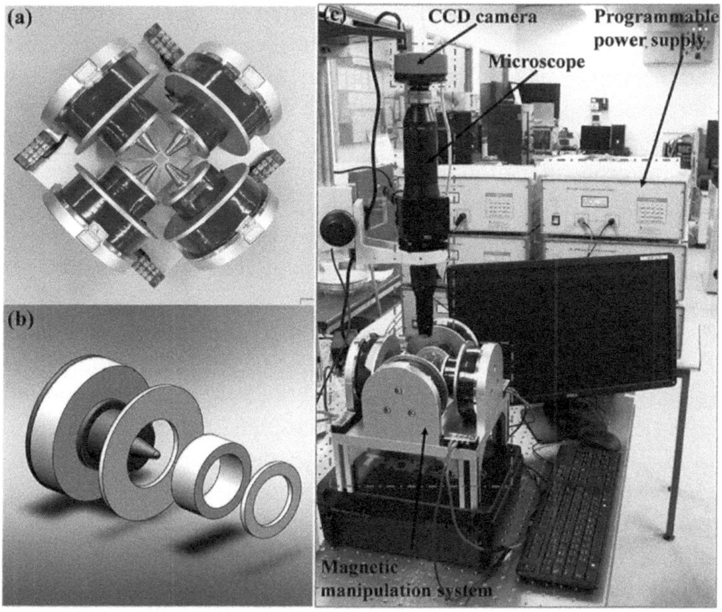

Figure 2.19 A gradient-enhanced magnetic manipulation system (Li et al., 2020). (A) Electromagnetic manipulation platform with four designed coils. (B) Internal structure of a single coil. (C) Electromagnetic manipulation system with four coils, CCD camera, programmable power supplies, and the PC-based user interface.

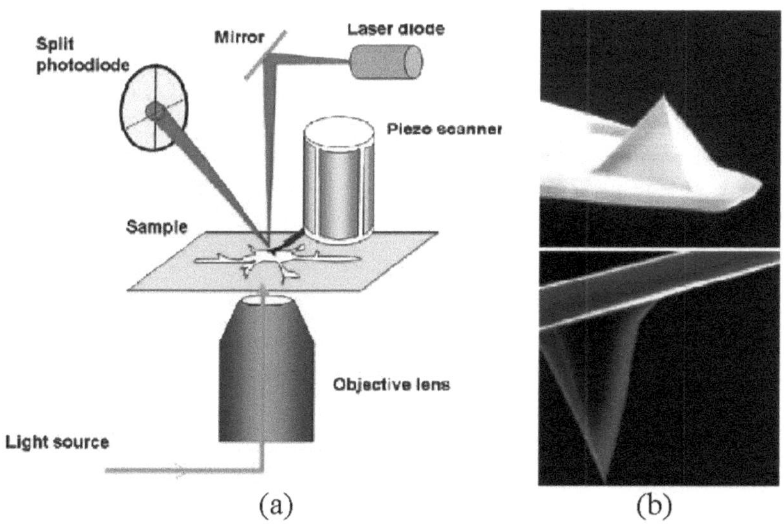

Figure 2.20 Schematic of AFM (Alessandrini and Facci 2005). (A) Scheme of AFM coupled with an inverted microscope. (B) Scanning electron microscope images of AFM cantilevers and tips.

AFM has three major abilities: force measurement, topographic imaging, and manipulation. In force measurement, AFM can be used to measure the forces between the probe and the sample as a function of their mutual separation. This can be applied to perform force spectroscopy and to measure the mechanical properties of the sample, such as the sample's Young's modulus, which is a measure of stiffness. For imaging, the reaction of the probe to the forces that the sample imposes on it can be used to form an image of 3D shape (topography) of a sample surface at a high resolution. In manipulation, the forces between tip and sample can also be used to change the properties of the sample in a controlled way. Examples of this include atomic manipulation, scanning probe lithography, and local stimulation of cells.

AFM has been widely used to study cell biomechanics, especially adherent cells, including osteoblasts, chondrocytes, adipocytes (Darling et al., 2008), and kidney epithelial cells (Rabinovich et al., 2005). AFM has also been used for suspension cells, such as red blood cells (RBCs) (Lekka et al., 2005), neutrophils (Rosenbluth et al., 2006), and even viruses (Kol et al., 2007). Fig. 2.21 illustrates the compression of a single cell by AFM. The indentation force–displacement profile of these cells can be quantitatively obtained by AFM to analyze the mechanical properties of the cells, such as stiffness or viscosity. AFM has several limitations. First, the cantilever of AFM is large and highly stiff, which limits the range of effective force, especially in aqueous conditions. Second, the interaction between the AFM tip and the target molecule is difficult to distinguish from the nonspecific contact of the same molecule (Neuman and Nagy, 2008).

AFM was originally developed to overcome scanning tunneling microscope imaging of nonconductive samples. Often used as a microscope, AFM can be used for other tasks such as surface modification, spectroscopic analysis, and particle manipulation (Alessandrini and Facci, 2005). Automation that can provide real-time visual display, and force feedback during operation has been considered one of the most important goals in AFM operation research. An automated system for patterning nanoparticles using AFM has been developed (Mokaberi et al., 2007). The planner is used to determine the path after the desired particle mode is given. The planner can output a series of commands for positioning and pushing operations.

With the AFM probe, simple 2D tasks can be realized, such as pushing, pulling, cutting, and indenting. However, multiple probes or chemically activated and controlled probes are required for more complex manipulation tasks, such as

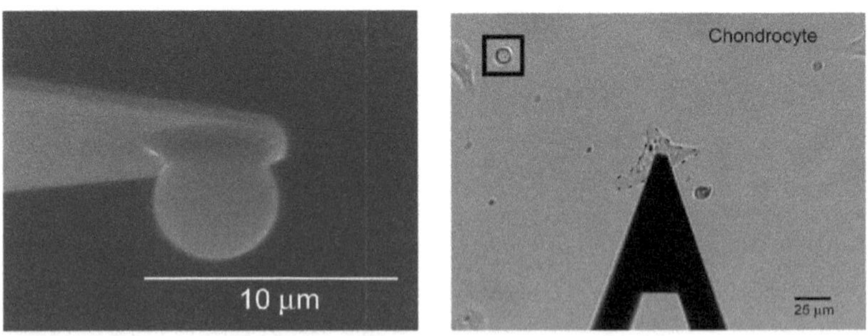

Figure 2.21 Single-cell compression by AFM (Darling et al., 2008).

transportation and positioning. Moreover, although AFM systems can image biological samples with high (nanoscale) spatial resolution, they usually have low temporal resolution (Sitti, 2001). If the characteristics of the sample change rapidly, the AFM image will be significantly distorted. Therefore, it is difficult to use current AFM to study biological processes that occur within a few seconds, such as the rapid movement of cells.

2.7 Imaging for intracellular manipulation

The complexity of the intracellular environment and the culture medium inevitably leads to difficulty in positioning the operating position in cell manipulation. The identification of target biological specimens is susceptible to interference from the unavoidable environment in the imaging field, such as corresponding cells and auxiliary operating tools. The morphological characteristics of most organelles are similar to their intracellular neighbors; therefore, they become indistinguishable under optical observation (Iešmantas et al., 2020). According to Gao et al. (2020), various advanced biological imaging technologies have been studied at the cellular or subcellular level in the past few decades, such as the state-of-the-art microscopes on the market, including confocal fluorescence microscopy (CFM), two-photon fluorescence microscopy (TPFM), and light sheet fluorescence microscopy (LSFM). Other advanced microscopes include laboratory-made photoacoustic microscopy (PAM), traditional wide-field fluorescence microscopy (WFFM), advanced structured illumination microscopy (SIM), and stimulated emission depletion microscopy (STEDM). These imaging devices are described below.

2.7.1 *State-of-the-art microscopes*

CFM has become a routine imaging tool in biology and biomedical sciences. Claxton et al. (2006) expressed the basic concept of confocal microscopy, as shown in Fig. 2.22A. In short, the pinhole aperture placed in front of the microscope's photodetector can focus the illuminating light on the specimen, thereby eliminating most of the out-of-focus blur during the observation process. As a commercial instrument, CFM is widely used to image live cells, intracellular organelles, and components. Fig. 2.22B shows a recording of HeLa cells and porous $CaCO_3$ particles with CFM, which reveals the number of internalized vaterite particles and their crystal structure (Abalymov et al., 2018). Given that it can control the imaging depth of the field and reduce the background blur away from the focal plane, CFM can be used to measure the 3D structure of a specimen. However, CFM has the disadvantages of slow scanning speed (Jonkman and Brown, 2015) and high-intensity light (Tang and Han, 2019), which may lead to short fluorescence lifetime and phototoxicity in living cells (Shaw, 2006). Therefore, the imaging time should be strictly controlled during CFM operation.

The principle of TPFM is based on the phenomenon of two-photon absorption and excitation, that is, the combined energy of two quasi-simultaneously absorbed photons is sufficient to match the energy gap between the ground state and the excited state (Vo-Dinh, 2003). Fig. 2.22C shows the typical structure of TPFM (Lefort, 2017).

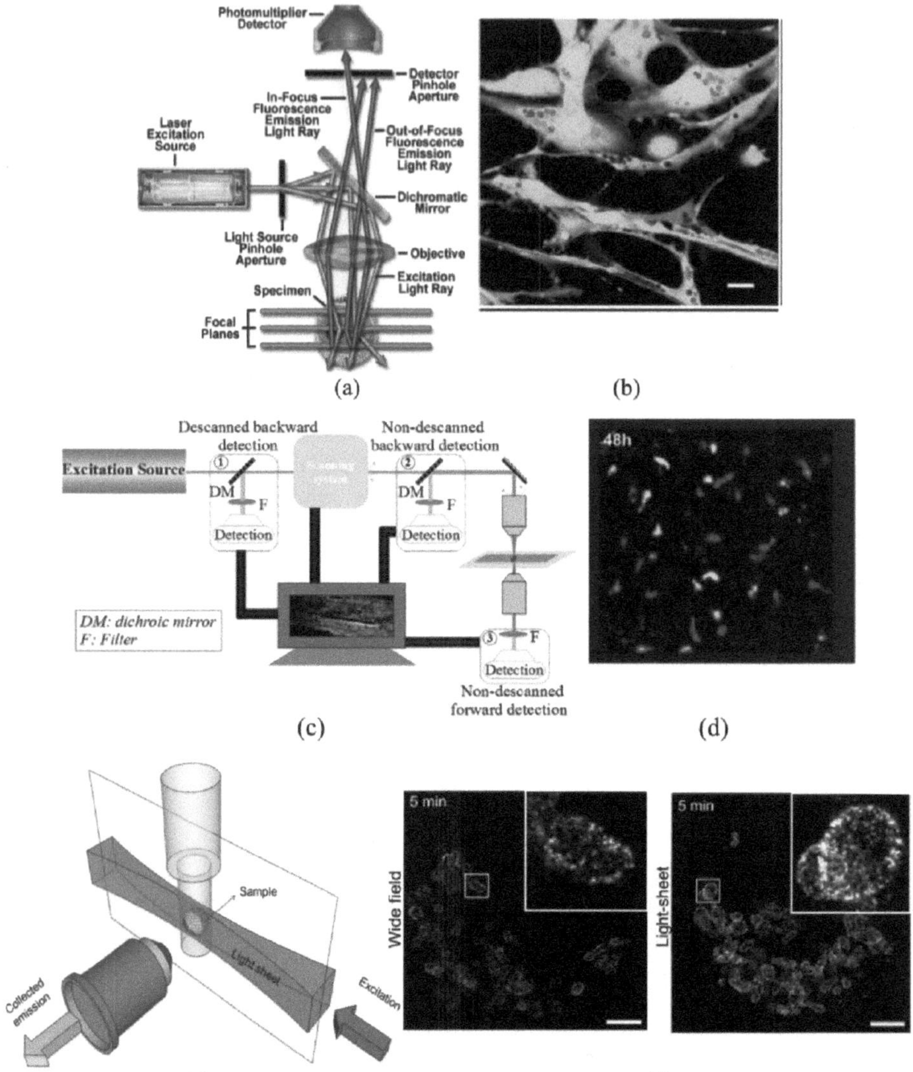

Figure 2.22 State-of-the-art microscopes and their applications in biological imaging (Gao et al., 2020). (A) Schematic of CFM (Claxton et al., 2006). (B) CFM-sampled images of HeLa cells and porous $CaCO_3$ particles (Abalymov et al., 2018). (C) Schematic of a typical TPFM (Lefort, 2017). (D) Long-term motility measurement of transferred T cells with TPFM (Kobezda et al., 2012). (E) Basic schematic of LSFM (Olarte et al., 2018) (reprinted with permission from Olarte el al. 2018© Optica Publishing Group). (F) Comparison of mitochondria visualization between LSFM and WFFM (Meddens et al., 2016) (reprinted with permission from Meddens et al. 2016© Optica Publishing Group).

With the reduction of the photo-bleaching effect, TPFM has become a powerful tool for long-term measurement (Ricard et al., 2018). For example, TPFM can be used to monitor the movement of T-cells transferred in mice within 48 h (Kobezda et al.,

2012), as shown in Fig. 2.22D. TPFM is not susceptible to interference from fluorescence concentration and light source. TPFM can be used to accurately detect fluorescent probes to track the dynamic changes of hydrogen peroxide (H_2O_2) and adenosine triphosphate (ATP) in neurons (Wu et al., 2020). In addition, TPFM can perform tomography to measure samples at different optical depths.

LSFM is another instrument with long-term measurement capability. The light sheet produced by the thin laser sampling beam is focused on only a part of the sample, and the fluorescence is collected perpendicularly from the illumination axis (Olarte et al., 2018), as shown in Fig. 2.22E. Compared with CFM and TPFM, the efficient excitation and collection scheme ensures that the phototoxicity and photobleaching effects of LSFM are minimized (Santi, 2011). Therefore, LSFM is suitable for applications that require long-term measurement and careful exposure. Notably, the sampled images of LSFM are not affected by out-of-focus blur, and they can display more detailed features than ordinary wide-field microscopes (Silvestri et al., 2012). Fig. 2.22F shows the mitochondrial visualization of HeLa cells labeled with the mitochondrial import receptor subunit TOM-20 via LSFM (Meddens et al., 2016). This image shows that the contrast of LSFM is better than that of wide-field illumination. LSFM has a lateral resolution comparable to CFM, but its axial resolution is not as good as CFM, which usually does not exceed 1 μm (Power and Huisken, 2017). Complex sample preparation is a problem with LSFM because its orthogonal configuration hinders sample preservation in standard petri dishes and multiwell plates (Sapoznik et al., 2020). In such a narrow space, the integration of LSFM with other manipulation tools is a huge challenge. Therefore, its applicability in intracellular micromanipulation is greatly restricted.

2.7.2 Photoacoustic microscopy (PAM)

Photoacoustic imaging is inspired by the photoacoustic effect that converts light energy into measurable pressure waves. When the sample is irradiated with a modulated laser source, this effect is triggered, resulting in thermoelastic expansion and photoacoustic wave formation corresponding to the geometric characteristics of specimens (Strohm et al., 2016). Fig. 2.23A shows the two main configurations of photoacoustic microscopy (PAM) in terms of imaging modes. One is the optical resolution (OR) mode, in which a focused laser is irradiated on the specimen. The optical area of OR-PAM is limited, but its lateral resolution is improved. The other is the acoustic resolution (AR) mode with uniform illumination. Unfocused light can achieve deeper penetration, but will produce lower resolution (Steinberg et al., 2019).

Photoacoustic imaging technology is suitable for deep imaging. Given that sound waves can penetrate soft tissues and skin, high-resolution imaging can be achieved at depths far beyond the limit of light diffusion. Photoacoustic imaging technology has been widely used to navigate microrobots in the body. Fig. 2.23B shows that under the guidance of photoacoustic imaging, the migration of the capsule micromotor is controlled to move to the target area in the intestine (Wu et al., 2019). PAM also has the advantages of label-free imaging and defocus blur suppression, and therefore it has become an ideal technology for nontoxic biological imaging. Many subcellular practices have been imaged with enhanced contrast. The instrument can achieve a high lateral resolution of 250 nm. Fig. 2.23C illustrates the sampling image of lipids, proteins,

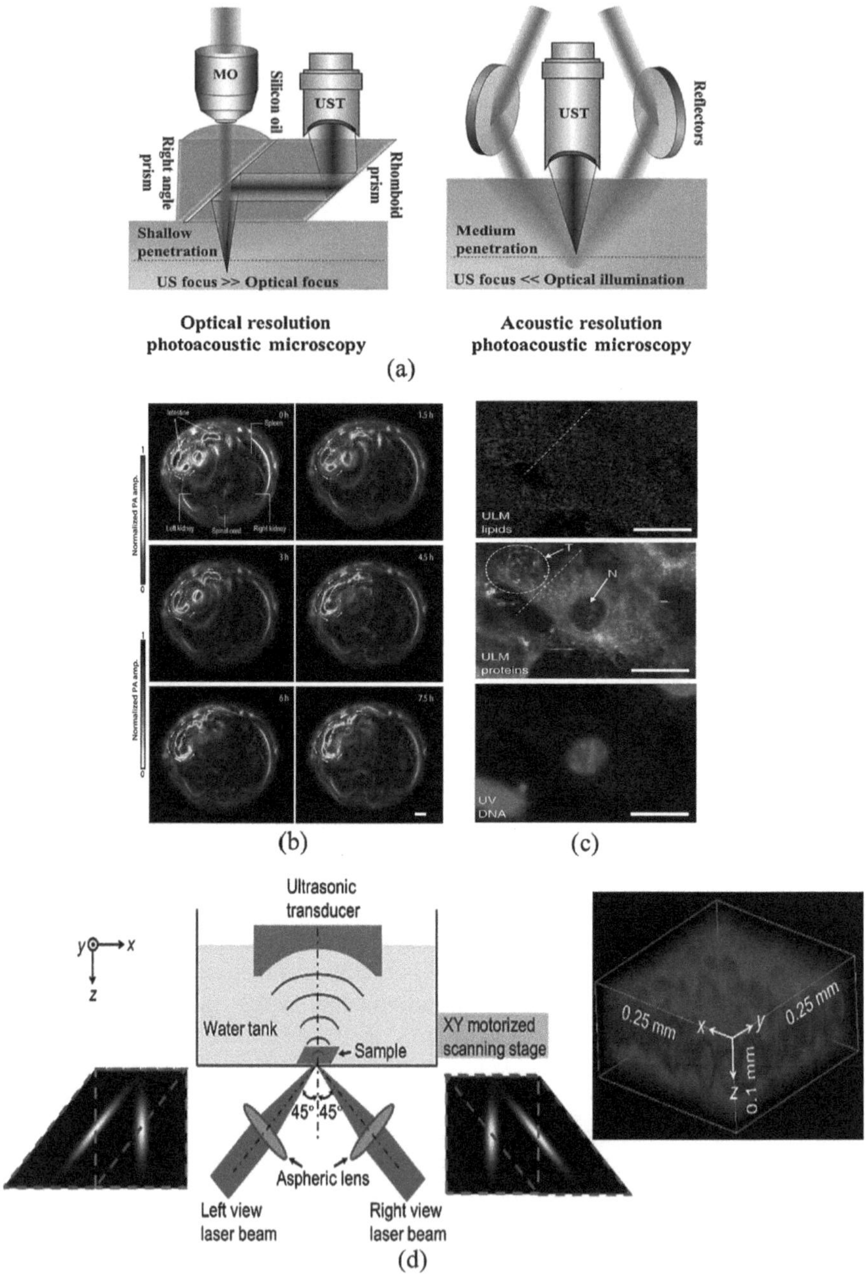

Figure 2.23 Photoacoustic imaging (Gao et al., 2020). (A) Two operation modes of PAM (Steinberg et al., 2019). (B) Time-lapse PAM measurement of microrobot movement in the intestine (Wu et al., 2019). (C) Ultraviolet-localized mid-infrared PAM sampled images of lipids, proteins, and nucleic acids in fibroblast cells (Shi et al., 2019). (D) Dual-view PAM scheme and its sampled images of a mouse brain slice (Cai et al., 2018) (reprinted with permission from Cai et al. 2018© Optica Publishing Group).

and nucleic acids in fibroblasts via mid-infrared PAM positioned by ultraviolet light (Shi et al., 2019). However, it lacks optical sectioning capabilities. Theoretically, the axial resolution of PAM is controlled by the bandwidth of the photoacoustic signal and the center frequency of the ultrasonic transducer (Jeon et al., 2019). Research has been conducted to improve the axial resolution of PAM without losing its lateral accuracy. For example, with Grueneisen relaxation photoacoustic microscopy (GR-PAM) that provides two identical laser pulses, the axial resolution can be increased to 2.3 μm and the lateral resolution to 410 nm (Wang et al., 2014). Dong et al. (2015) developed an isometric PAM based on a transparent microring resonator ultrasonic detector with an axial resolution of 2.12 μm. Cai et al. (2018) further improved the axial resolution to 1.8 μm based on the configuration modification. Fig. 2.23D shows the dual-view PAM and sampled images of a mouse brain slice. The two split lasers are focused on the sample, and the photoacoustic waves are collected by an ultrasonic transducer. In general, due to its relatively low axial resolution, PAM is more commonly used to measure the specimen profile in a 2D sampling plane rather than in a 3D space.

PAM has other limitations that hinder its application in bioimaging. One is its low sampling speed. There is a trade-off between resolution and sampling speed, that is, it takes several minutes to measure an area of 1 m × 1 m with an acceptable optical resolution using OR-PAM (Yao and Wang, 2013). Second, PAM requires complex optical configurations and few commercial tools are available, which limits the accessibility of researchers without expertise in the field. Finally, the potential damage from deposited laser energy is another problem that will affect high-resolution imaging (Liu et al., 2018).

2.7.3 Wide-field fluorescence microscopy (WFFM)

WFFM is popular in bioimaging due to its low purchase cost and high accessibility. Fig. 2.24A shows the WFFM observation results of a burr-like porous spherical microrobot loaded with MC3T3-E1 fibroblasts and the measured movement of the microrobot for automated control in the zebrafish embryo egg yolk (Li et al., 2018a,b). Similar to CFM, WFFM also has a diffraction barrier. Even for a WFFM with a high numerical aperture objective lens, its resolution is difficult to reach 230 nm laterally and 800 nm axially, because the visible light wavelength changes from 390 to 780 nm (Stemmer et al., 2008). During the WFFM operation, the entire specimen is illuminated by the emitted light. The sampled image contains in-plane features, out-of-focus blur, and noise of adjacent depth projections, which will undoubtedly reduce image quality, especially for depth projections far from the focused plane (Preza and Conchello, 2004). This optical behavior can be modeled as a convolution process between the point spread function (PSF) and the measurement sample. To restore the sampled images of WFFM, many methods for numerical inversion of the blur process based on the deconvolution algorithm have been proposed, such as Landweber method (Landweber, 1951), Tikhonov–Miller gradient descent method (Tikhonov, 1963), and Richardson–Lucy maximum likelihood method (Richardson, 1972; Luck, 1974). Fig. 2.24B shows unfocused sampled images of *Caenorhabditis elegans* and deconvoluted images using different deconvolution methods (Sage et al., 2017). The processed image shows clearer features and more details than the original image, providing more accurate information for intracellular micromanipulation tasks. By moving the focal

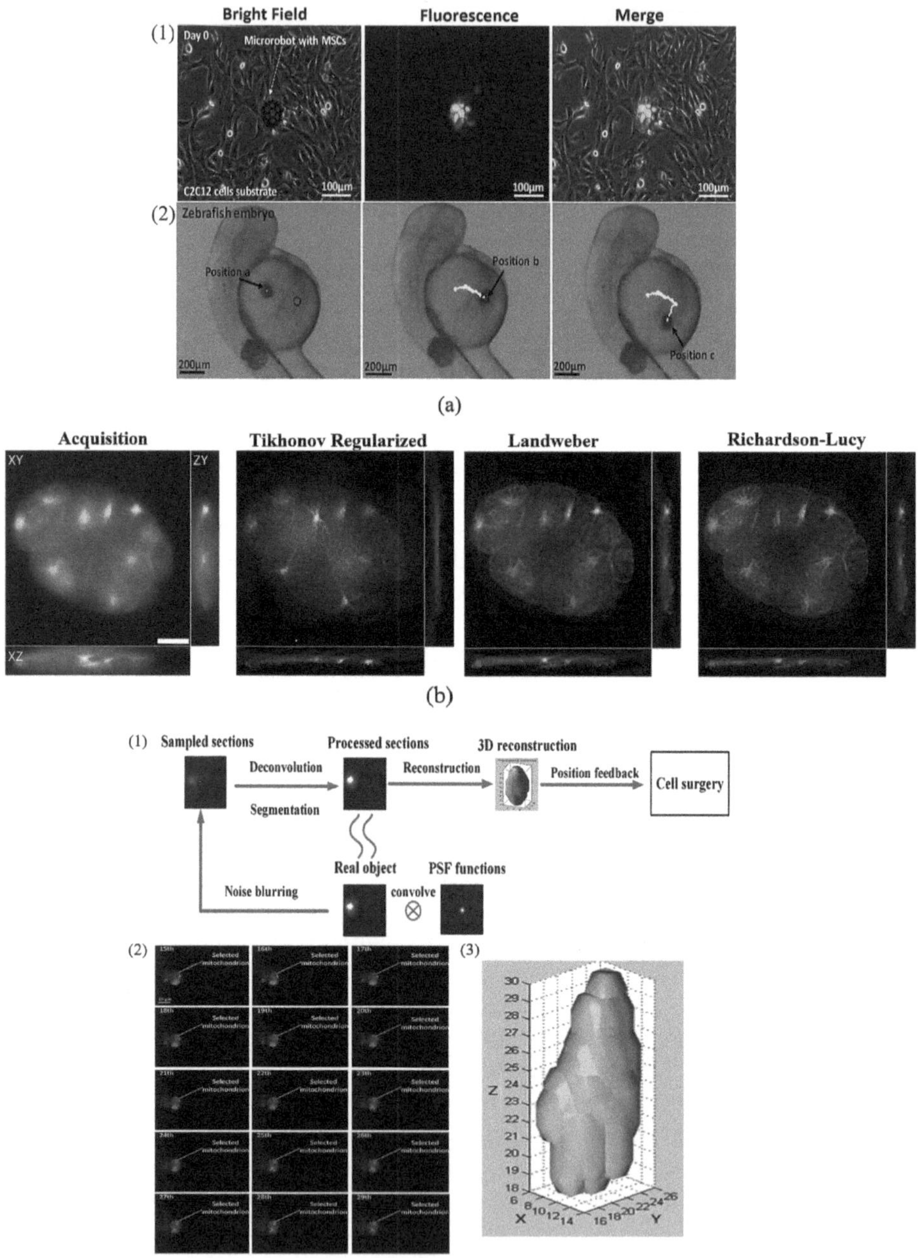

Figure 2.24 Intracellular imaging practices with WFFM (Gao et al., 2020). (A) WFFM observations of a burr-like porous spherical microrobot (Li et al., 2018). (1) A microrobot loaded with MC3T3-E1 fibroblasts. (2) The microrobot moving inside the yolk of a zebrafish embryo. (B) Blurred sampled image of *Caenorhabditis elegans* and restored images with different deconvolution methods (Sage et al., 2017). (C) 3D reconstruction method based on a WFFM (Gao et al., 2018). (1) The reconstruction process. (2) The fluorescence image series of the selected mitochondrion (orange). (3) The reconstructed 3D model of the mitochondrion.

plane, the entire specimen can be scanned, and the sampled image can be optically sliced through WFFM and stored in the computer. After the restoration process of deconvolution, segmentation, and reconstruction, the sampled image can also be reconstructed as a 3D model (Gao et al., 2018). Fig. 2.24C shows the sampled image series of mitochondria in THP-1 cells and their 3D reconstruction models.

WFFM is widely used to visualize micro-objects such as cells, intracellular organelles, and microrobots due to its excellent compatibility, controllability, and programmability. The size of the measurement specimen is usually larger than 1 μm, because the WFFM resolution will be limited even if the restoration algorithm is implemented. The robot-assisted manipulation tool is easy to integrate with WFFM due to its simple configuration and large operating space. Therefore, WFFM is often used in intracellular micromanipulation.

2.7.4 Super-resolution microscopy

In recent years, several super-resolution microscopy techniques have been developed to break the diffraction limit of optical microscopy. Fig. 2.25A illustrates the configuration of structured illumination microscopy (SIM) whose spatial pattern excitation light can be generated by multiple laser beams (Saxena et al., 2015). SIM can be used for super-resolution observation. The optical cross-section can be sampled by generating gratings or fringe patterns on the conjugate plane of the sample. Fig. 2.25B shows a sampled image of the cytoskeleton and nuclear components in endometrial epithelial cells (Allen et al., 2014). Specifically, the resolution of SIM can reach approximately less than 100 nm in the lateral direction and 300 nm in the axial direction. Compared with the image sampled by WFFM, the image obtained using SIM has better shrinkage and resolution. However, the high-resolution sampling of SIM is prone to small position shifts and intensity changes. Therefore, in the case of poor signal-to-noise ratio, the specimen should be fixed during SIM measurement (Carlton, 2008), which will reduce the application of SIM in intracellular microscopy.

Another exciting phenomenon of super-resolution microscopy is stimulated emission, through which the PSF is reduced to the sub-diffraction level (Hell and Wichmann, 1994). Fig. 2.25C shows a typical configuration of an STEDM, in which excited state electrons can return to their ground state by interacting with a depleted laser beam of a specific frequency (Klar et al., 2000). For most commercial systems, the lateral resolution of STEDM can reach 30−80 nm, while the axial resolution of STEDM is less than 100 nm. This can be achieved through a dedicated depletion scheme (Donnert et al., 2006). Fig. 2.25D illustrates an STEDM sampled image of a live hippocampal primary neuron; the enlarged view proves that it can provide nanometer resolution better than CFM (Blom and Widengren, 2017). However, stimulated emission is obtained by using high-power depletion lasers. Although higher laser density leads to higher sampling resolution, it also leads to a non-negligible photobleaching problem (Li et al., 2018a,b).

Super-resolution microscopy technology is advanced in observing small-scale intracellular components (such as proteins, lysosomes, and bacteria). However, SIM and STEDM are seldom used for micromanipulation, because current robot-assisted manipulation tools can only handle objects as small as submicrometers. With the rapid development of microfabrication and information technology, super-resolution microscopes will play a more important role in the future.

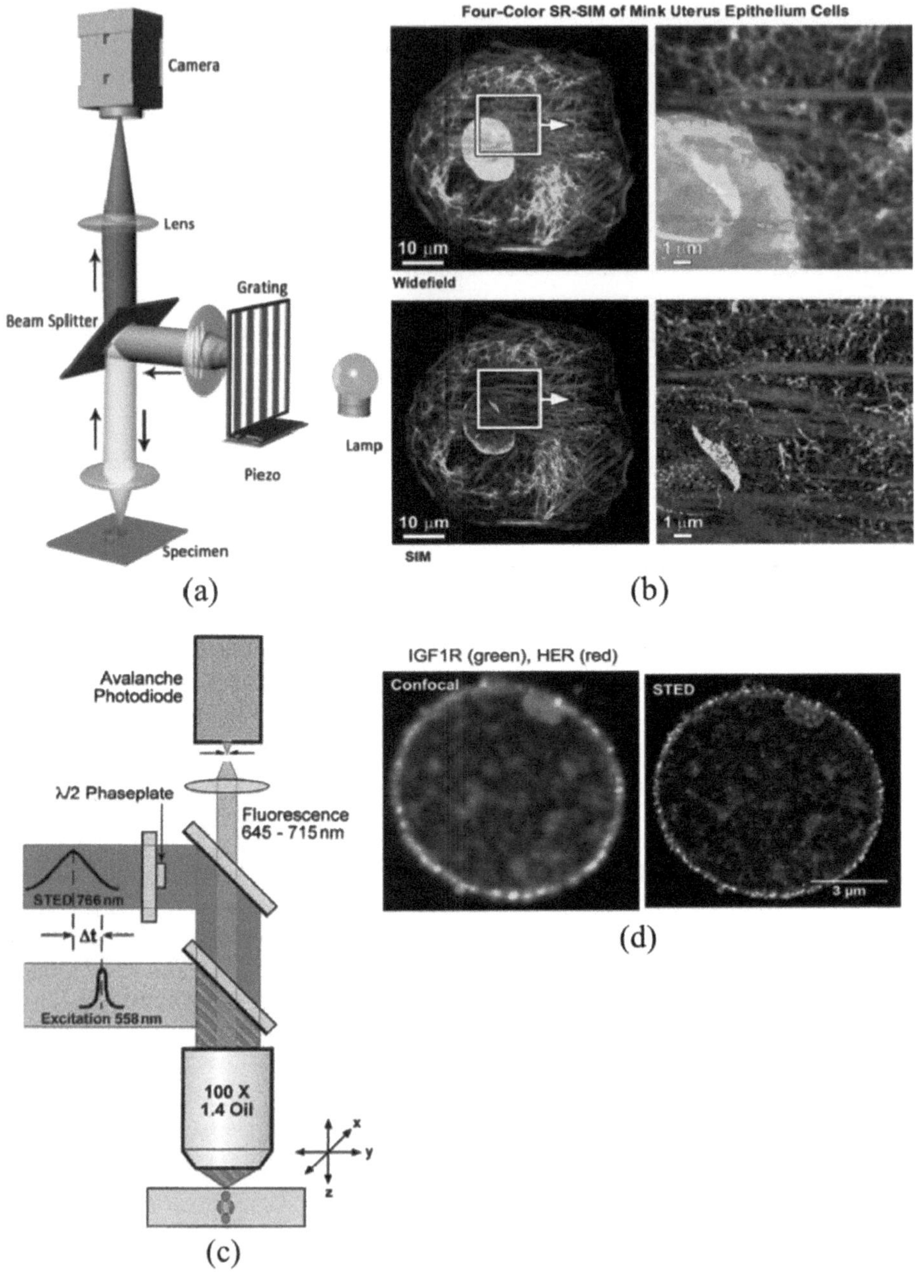

Figure 2.25 Super-resolution microscopy (Gao et al. 2020). (A) Configuration of a typical structured illumination microscope (SIM) (Saxena et al. 2015) (reprinted with permission from Saxena et al. 2015@ Optica Publishing Group). (B) Imaging comparison of cytoskeletal and nuclear components between SIM and WFFM (Allen et al. 2014). (C) Schematic of a stimulated emission depletion microscope (STEDM) (Klar et al. 2000). (Copyright (2000) National Academy of Sciences, U.S.A.) (D) Imaging comparison of living hippocampal primary neurons between STEDM and CFM (Blom and Widengren 2017).

2.8 Conclusions

This chapter reviews the main manipulation tools and technologies used to manipulate cells. First, the use of a microneedle or micropipette to control the aspiration of target cells or achieve microinjection of single cells is introduced. Microinjection systems based on robot-controlled microneedles have become the main technological trend aimed at efficient and precise manipulation of cell transfection and biopsy. Second, an optical tweezers manipulation tool is introduced, which uses a highly focused laser beam to form an optical trap to manipulate cells with high precision. By using holographic technology, multiple optical traps can be generated simultaneously to manipulate multiple cells. Combined with robot technology, the manipulation system based on robot-assisted optical tweezers plays an increasingly important role in trapping, assembly, transportation, and sorting of various particles at the single-cell and single-molecule levels. Third, the electrokinetic manipulation tools based on electrophoresis or dielectrophoresis (DEP) are introduced. DEP-based manipulation tools have been widely used to manipulate biological samples, such as bacteria, viruses, and cells. Currently, DEP has become the main technology for automatic cell trapping, cell separation, and cell patterning. Fourth, magnetic manipulators are introduced, which use magnetic field gradients to apply and measure forces on magnetic particles. Magnetic manipulators have exhibited significant advantages in driving microparticles or microrobots in an in vivo environment to achieve precise targeted delivery (such as drugs or cells). Fifth, AFM is introduced, which has been widely used in the study of cell biomechanics. Automatic AFM can also provide real-time visual display and force feedback during manipulation tasks. Finally, the imaging technologies used for intracellular manipulation are introduced from several perspectives. The first perspective introduces the state-of-the-art microscopes on the market, including CFM, TPFM, and LSFM. Subsequently, other imaging technologies are introduced, such as PAM, traditional WFFM, SIM, and STEDM. These tools, combined with the advanced robotics technology, have greatly supported the rapid development of cell manipulation in the past few decades.

References

Abalymov, A.A., Verkhovskii, R.A., Novoselova, M.V., Parakhonskiy, B.V., Gorin, D.A., Yashchenok, A.M., Sukhorukov, G.B., 2018. Live-cell imaging by confocal Raman and fluorescence microscopy recognizes the crystal structure of calcium carbonate particles in HeLa cells. Biotechnol. J. 13, 1–8.

Actis, P., Kan, S.Y., Penfold, C., Vilozny, B., Pourmand, N., 2012. Single-cell biopsy using nanopipettes. Biophys. J. 102 (3), 188a.

Aerts, J.T., Louis, K.R., Crandall, S.R., Govindaiah, G., Cox, C.L., Sweedler, J.V., 2014. Patch clamp electrophysiology and capillary electrophoresis-mass spectrometry metabolomics for single cell characterization. Anal. Chem. 86 (6), 3203–3208.

Ahlbom, A., Bridges, J., de Seze, R., Hillert, L., Juutilainen, J., Mattsson, M.O., Neubauer, G., Schüz, J., Simko, M., Bromen, K., 2008. Possible effects of electromagnetic fields (EMF) on human health-opinion of the scientific committee on emerging and newly identified health risks (SCENIHR). Toxicology 246, 248–250.

Alessandrini, A., Facci, P., 2005. AFM: a versatile tool in biophysics. Meas. Sci. Technol. 16, R65–R92.

Allen, J.R., Ross, S.T., Davidson, M.W., 2014. Structured illumination microscopy for super-resolution. ChemPhysChem 15, 566–576.

Anis, Y.H., Holl, M.P., Meldrum, D.R., 2010. Automated selection and placement of single cell using vision-based feedback control. IEEE Trans. Autom. Sci. Eng. 7 (3), 598–606.

Ashkin, A., Dziedzic, J.M., Bjorkholm, J.E., Chu, S., 1986. Observation of a single-beam gradient force optical trap for dielectric particles. Optic. Lett. 11 (5), 288–290.

Barnothy, M.F., 2013. Biological Effects of Magnetic Fields. Springer.

Blom, H., Widengren, J., 2017. Stimulated emission depletion microscopy. Chem. Rev. 117, 7377–7427.

Cai, D., Wong, T.T.W., Zhu, L., Shi, J., Chen, S.L., Wang, L.V., 2018. Dual-view photoacoustic microscopy for quantitative cell nuclear imaging. Optic. Lett. 43, 4875–4878.

Carlton, P.M., 2008. Three-dimensional structured illumination microscopy and its application to chromosome structure. Chromosome Res. 16, 351–365.

Charlie, G., Vincent, C., 2002. Magnetic tweezers: micromanipulation and force measurement at the molecular level. Biophys. J. 82, 3314–3329.

Chen, S., Cheng, J., Kong, C.W., Wang, X., Cheng, S.H., Li, R.A., Sun, D., 2013. Laser-induced fusion of human embryonic stem cells with optical tweezers. Appl. Phys. Lett. 103, 033701.

Chiou, A.E., Wang, W., Sonek, G.J., Hong, J., Berns, M.W., 1997. Interferometric optical tweezers. Optic. Commun. 133, 7–10.

Claxton, N.S., Fellers, T.J., Davidson, M.W., 2006. Microscopy, confocal. In: Webster, J.G. (Ed.), Encyclopedia of Medical Devices and Instrumentation. John Wiley and Sons, Inc., Hoboken, NJ, USA.

Darling, E.M., Topel, M., Zauscher, S., Vail, T.P., Guilak, F., 2008. Viscoelastic properties of human mesenchymally-derived stem cells and primary osteoblasts, chondrocytes, and adipocytes. J. Biomech. 41 (2), 454–464.

Dholakia, K., Reece, P., Gu, M., 2008. Optical manipulation. Chem. Soc. Rev. 37, 42–55.

Diller, E., Sitti, M., 2014. Three-dimensional programmable assembly by untethered magnetic robotic micro-grippers. Adv. Funct. Mater. 24, 4397–4404.

Diller, E., Giltinan, J., Lum, G.Z., Ye, Z., Sitti, M., 2016. Six-degree-of-freedom magnetic actuation for wireless microrobotics. Int. J. Robot Res. 35, 114–128.

Doh, I., Cho, Y.H., 2005. A continuous cell separation chip using hydrodynamic dielectrophoresis (DEP) process. Sensor. Actuator. 121, 59–65.

Dong, B., Li, H., Zhang, Z., Zhang, K., Chen, S., Sun, C., Zhang, H.F., 2015. Isometric multimodal photoacoustic microscopy based on optically transparent micro-ring ultrasonic detection. Optica 2, 169–176.

Donnert, G., Keller, J., Medda, R., Andrei, M.A., Rizzoli, S.O., Lührmann, R., Jahn, R., Eggeling, C., Hell, S.W., 2006. Macromolecular-scale resolution in biological fluorescence microscopy. Proc. Natl. Acad. Sci. U.S.A. 103, 11440–11445.

Feng, F., Hagiwara, M., Ichikawa, A., Kawahara, T., Arai, F., 2012. Smooth enucleation of bovine oocyte by microrobot with local flow speed control in microchannel. Proc. IEEE/RSJ Int. Conf. Intell. Rob. Syst. 944–949.

Fountain, T.W.R., Kailat, P.V., Abbott, J.J., 2010. Wireless control of magnetic helical microrobots using a rotating-permanent-magnet manipulator. In: Proc. of IEEE Int. Conf. Robotics and Automation, pp. 576–581.

Gahagan, K.T., Swartzlander, G.A., 1998. Trapping of low-index microparticles in an optical vortex. J. Optic. Soc. Am. B Optic. Phys. 15, 524–534.

Gao, W., Shakoor, A., Zhao, L., Jiang, Z., Sun, D., 2018. 3D image reconstruction of biological organelles with a robot-aided microscopy system for intracellular surgery. IEEE Robot. Automat. Lett. 4, 231–238.

Gao, W., Zhao, L., Jiang, Z., Sun, D., 2020. Advanced biological imaging for intracellular micromanipulation: methods and applications. Appl. Sci. 10, 7308.

Gascoyne, P.R.C., Noshari, J., Anderson, T.J., Becker, F.F., 2009. Isolation of rare cells from cell mixtures by dielectrophoresis. Electrophoresis 30, 1388–1398.

Gou, X., 2014. Probing the Functional Mechanism of Cell-To-Cell Interaction and Cell Migration with Optical Tweezer-Based Cell Manipulation Tool (Ph.D. thesis). City University of Hong Kong.

Gou, X., Yang, H., Fahmy, T.M., Wang, Y., Sun, D., 2014. Direct measurement of cell protrusion force utilizing a robot-aided cell manipulation system with optical tweezers for cell migration control. Int. J. Robot. Res. 33 (14), 1782–1792.

Hell, S.W., Wichmann, J., 1994. Breaking the diffraction resolution limit by stimulated emission: stimulated-emission-depletion fluorescence microscopy. Optic. Lett. 19, 780–782.

Ho, C.T., Lin, R.Z., Chang, W.Y., Chang, H.Y., Liu, C.H., 2006. Rapid heterogeneous liver-cell on-chip patterning via the enhanced field-induced dielectrophoresis trap. Lab Chip 6, 724–734.

Hu, S., Sun, D., 2011. Automatic transportation of biological cells with a robot-tweezer manipulation system. Int. J. Robot Res. 30 (14), 1681–1694.

Hu, X., Bessette, P.H., Qian, J., Meinhart, C.D., Daugherty, P.S., Soh, H.T., 2005. Marker-specific sorting of rare cells using dielectrophoresis. Proc. Natl. Acad. Sci. U.S.A. 102, 15757.

Huan, Z., 2017. Automation of Batched Spatial Manipulation and Assembly of Cells through Dielectrophoresis for Tissue Engineering (Ph.D. thesis). City University of Hong Kong.

Huan, Z., Chu, H.K., Yang, J., Sun, D., 2017. Characterization of a honeycomb-like scaffold with dielectrophoresis-based patterning for tissue engineering. IEEE Trans. Biomed. Eng. 64 (4), 755–764.

Huang, H., Sun, D., Mills, J.K., Cheng, S.H., 2009. Robotics cell injection system with position and force control: towards automatic batch biomanipulation. IEEE Trans. Robot. 25 (3), 727–737.

Huang, H., Mills, J.K., Lu, C., Sun, D., 2011. A universal piezo-driven ultrasonic cell microinjection system. Biomed. Microdevices 13 (4), 743–752.

Hunt, T.P., Westervelt, R.M., 2006. Dielectrophoresis tweezers for single cell manipulation. Biomed. Microdevices 8 (3), 227–230.

Iešmantas, T., Taraseviciene, A., Sutiene, K., 2020. Enhancing multi-tissue and multi-scale cell nuclei segmentation with deep metric learning. Appl. Sci. 10, 615.

Jeon, S., Kim, J., Lee, D., Baik, J.W., Kim, C., 2019. Review on practical photoacoustic microscopy. Photoacoustics 15, 100141.

Jonkman, J., Brown, C.M., 2015. Any way you slice it – a comparison of confocal microscopy techniques. J. Biomol. Tech. 26, 54–65.

Jordan, P., Leach, J., Padgett, M., Blackburn, P., Isaacs, N., Goksor, M., Hanstorp, D., Wright, A., Girkin, J., Cooper, J., 2005. Creating permanent 3D arrangements of isolated cells using holographic optical tweezers. Lab Chip 5, 1224–1228.

Kadaksham, A.T.J., Singh, P., Aubry, N., 2004. Dielectrophoresis of nanoparticles. Electrophoresis 52, 3625–3632.

Kang, Y., Li, D., Kalams, S.A., Eid, J.E., 2008. DC-dielectrophoretic separation of biological cells by size Biomed. Microdevices 10, 243–249.

Kimura, Y., Yanagimachi, R., 1995. Intracytoplasmic sperm injection in the mouse. Biol. Reprod. 52, 709–720.

Klar, T.A., Jakobs, S., Dyba, M., Egner, A., Hell, S.W., 2000. Fluorescence microscopy with diffraction resolution barrier broken by stimulated emission. Proc. Natl. Acad. Sci. U.S.A. 97, 8206–8210.

Kobezda, T., Ghassemi-Nejad, S., Glant, T.T., Mikecz, K., 2012. In vivo two-photon imaging of T cell motility in joint-draining lymph nodes in a mouse model of rheumatoid arthritis. Cell. Immunol. 278, 158–165.

Kol, N., Shi, Y., Tsvitov, M., Barlam, D., Shneck, R.Z., Kay, M.S., Rousso, I., 2007. A stiffness switch in human immunodeficiency virus. Biophys. J. 92 (5), 1777–1783.

Kremser, L., Blaas, D., Kenndler, E., 2004. Capillary electrophoresis of biological particles: viruses, bacteria, and eukaryotic cells. Electrophoresis 25, 2282–2291.

Kummer, M.P., Abbott, J.J., Kratochvil, B.E., Borer, R., Sengul, A., Nelson, B.J., 2010. OctoMag: an electromagnetic system for 5-DOF wireless micromanipulation. IEEE Trans. Robot. 26, 1006–1017.

Landweber, L., 1951. An iteration formula for fredholm integral equations of the first kind. Am. J. Math. 73, 615–624.

Lefort, C., 2017. A review of biomedical multiphoton microscopy and its laser sources. J. Phys. D Appl. Phys. 50, 423001.

Lekka, M., Fornal, M., Pyka-Fosciak, G., Lebed, K., Wizner, B., Grodzicki, T., Styczen, J., 2005. Erythrocyte stiffness probed using atomic force microscope. Biorheology 42 (4), 307–317.

Li, X., Liu, C., Chen, S., Wang, Y., Cheng, S.H., Sun, D., 2017. In vivo manipulation of single biological cells with an optical tweezers-based manipulator and a disturbance compensation controller. IEEE Trans. Robot. 33 (5), 1200–1212.

Li, C., Liu, S., Wang, W., Liu, W., Kuang, C., Liu, X., 2018. Recent research on stimulated emission depletion microscopy for reducing photobleaching. J. Microsc. 271, 4–16.

Li, J., Li, X., Luo, T., Wang, R., Liu, C., Chen, S., Li, D., Yue, J., Cheng, S., Sun, D., 2018. Development of a magnetic microrobot for carrying and delivering targeted cells. Sci. Robot. 3, eaat8829.

Li, D., Niu, F., Li, J., Li, X., Sun, D., 2020. Gradient-enhanced electromagnetic actuation system with a new core shape design for microrobot manipulation. IEEE/ASME Trans. Mechatronics 67 (6), 4700–4710.

Liu, X., Wong, T.T.W., Shi, J., Ma, J., Yang, Q., Wang, L.V., 2018. Label-free cell nuclear imaging by Grüneisen relaxation photoacoustic microscopy. Optic. Lett. 43, 947–950.

Lu, Z., Moraes, C., Ye, G., Simmons, C.A., Sun, Y., 2010. Single cell deposition and patterning with a robotic system. PLoS One 5 (10), e13542.

Lucio, A.D., Santos, R.A.S., Mesquita, O.N., 2003. Measurements and modeling of water transport and osmoregulation in a single kidney cell using optical tweezers and videomicroscopy. Phys. Rev. 68.

Lucy, L.B., 1974. An iterative technique for the rectification of observed distributions. Astron. J. 79, 745.

Mahoney, A.W., Abbott, J.J., 2016. Five-degree-of-freedom manipulation of an untethered magnetic device in fluid using a single permanent magnet with application in stomach capsule endoscopy. Int. J. Robot Res. 35, 129–147.

Manaresi, N., Romani, A., Medoro, G., Altomare, L., Leonardi, A., Tartagni, M., Guerrieri, R., 2003. A CMOS chip for individual cell manipulation and detection. IEEE J. Solid State Circ. 38 (12), 2003.

Meddens, M.B.M., Liu, S., Finnegan, P.S., Edwards, T.L., James, C.D., Lidke, K.A., 2016. Single objective light-sheet microscopy for high-speed whole-cell 3D super-resolution. Biomed. Optic. Express 7, 2219–2236.

Mokaberi, B., Yun, J., Wang, M., Requicha, A., 2007. Automated nanomanipulation with atomic force microscopes. In: Proc. of the IEEE Int. Conf. Robotics and Automation Rome, Italy, pp. 1406–1412.

Neuman, K.C., Block, S.M., 2004. Optical trapping. Rev. Sci. Instrum. 75, 2787–2809.

Neuman, K.C., Nagy, A., 2008. Single-molecule force spectroscopy: optical tweezers, magnetic tweezers and atomic force microscopy. Nat. Methods 5 (6), 491 ~ 505.

Niu, F., Li, J., Ma, W., Yang, J., Sun, D., 2017. Development of an enhanced electromagnetic actuation system with enlarged workspace. IEEE/ASME Trans. Mechatronics 22, 2265–2276.

Olarte, O.E., Andilla, J., Gualda, E.J., Loza-Alvarez, P., 2018. Light-sheet microscopy: a tutorial. Adv. Optic. Photon. 10, 111–179.

Pan, F., Chen, S., Jiao, Y., Guan, Z., Shakoor, A., Sun, D., 2020. Automated high-productivity microinjection system for adherent cells. IEEE Robot. Automat. Lett. 5 (2), 1167–1174.

Pawashe, C., Floyd, S., Sitti, M., 2009. Modeling and experimental characterization of an untethered magnetic micro-robot. Int. J. Robot Res. 28, 1077–1094.

Power, R.M., Huisken, J., 2017. A guide to light-sheet fluorescence microscopy for multiscale imaging. Nat. Methods 14, 360–373.

Preza, C., Conchello, J.A., 2004. Depth-variant maximum-likelihood restoration for three-dimensional fluorescence microscopy. J. Optic. Soc. Am. A 21, 1593–1601.

Rabinovich, Y., Esayanur, M., Daosukho, S., Byer, K., El-Shall, H., Khan, S., 2005. Atomic force microscopy measurement of the elastic properties of the kidney epithelial cells. J. Colloid Interface Sci. 285 (1), 125–135.

Ramon, J., Ahadian, S., Obregon, R., Camci-Unal, G., Ostrovidov, S., Hosseini, V., Kaji, H., Ino, K., Shiku, H., Khademhosseini, A., 2012. Gelatin methacrylate as a promising hydrogel for 3D microscale organization and proliferation of dielectrophoretically patterned cells. Lab Chip 12, 2959–2969.

Ramser, K., Hanstorp, D., 2010. Optical manipulation for single-cell studies. J. Biophot. 3, 187–206.

Ricard, C., Arroyo, E.D., He, C.X., Portera-Cailliau, C., Lepousez, G., Canepari, M., Fiole, D., 2018. Two-photon probes for in vivo multicolor microscopy of the structure and signals of brain cells. Brain Struct. Funct. 223, 3011–3043.

Richardson, W.H., 1972. Bayesian-based iterative method of image restoration. J. Optic. Soc. Am. 62, 55–59.

Rodrigo, P.J., Eriksen, R.L., Daria, V.R., Gluckstad, J., 2003. Shack-Hartmann multiple-beam optical tweezers. Optic. Express 11, 208–214.

Rosenbluth, M.J., Lam, W.A., Fletcher, D.A., 2006. Force microscopy of nonadherent cells: a comparison of leukemia cell deformability. Biophys. J. 90 (8), 2994–3003.

Sage, D., Donati, L., Soulez, F., Fortun, D., Schmit, G., Seitz, A., Guiet, R., Vonesch, C., Unser, M., 2017. DeconvolutionLab2: an open-source software for deconvolution microscopy. Methods 115, 28–41.

Santi, P.A., 2011. Light sheet fluorescence microscopy: a review. J. Histochem. Cytochem. 59, 129–138.

Sapoznik, E., Chang, B.J., Ju, R.J., Welf, E.S., Broadbent, D., Carisey, A.F., Stehbens, S.J., Lee, K.M., Marín, A., Hanker, A.B., Schmidt, J.C., Arteaga, C.L., Yang, B., Kruithoff, R., Shepherd, D.P., Millett-Sikking, A., York, A.G., Dean, K.M., Fiolka, R., 2020. A single-objective light-sheet microscope with 200 nm-scale resolution. BioRxiv 1–40.

Saxena, M., Eluru, G., Gorthi, S.S., 2015. Structured illumination microscopy. Adv. Optic. Photon. 7, 241–275.

Servant, A., Qiu, F., Mazza, M., Kostarelos, K., Nelson, B.J., 2015. Controlled in vivo swimming of a swarm of bacteria-like microrobotic flagella. Adv. Mater. 27, 2981–2988.

Shakoor, A., Xie, M., Luo, T., Hou, J., Shen, Y., Mills, J.K., Sun, D., 2019. Achieving automated organelle biopsy on small single cells using a cell surgery robotic system. IEEE Trans. Biomed. Eng. 66 (8), 2210–2222.

Shakoor, A., Wang, B., Fan, L., Kong, L., Gao, W., Sun, J., Man, K., Li, G., Sun, D., 2021. Automated optical tweezers manipulation to transfer mitochondria from fetal to adult MSCs to improve anti-aging gene expressions. Small 17 (2103086).

Shaw, P.J., 2006. Comparison of widefield/deconvolution and confocal microscopy for three-dimensional imaging. In: Pawley, J.B. (Ed.), Handbook of Biological Confocal Microscopy. Springer, Boston, MA, USA, pp. 453–467.

Shi, J., Wong, T.T.W., He, Y., Li, L., Zhang, R., Yung, C.S., Hwang, J., Maslov, K., Wang, L.V., 2019. High-resolution, high-contrast mid-infrared imaging of fresh biological samples with ultraviolet-localized photoacoustic microscopy. Nat. Photonics 13, 609–615.

Silvestri, L., Bria, A., Sacconi, L., Iannello, G., Pavone, F.S., 2012. Confocal light sheet microscopy: micron-scale neuroanatomy of the entire mouse brain. Optic. Express 20, 20582–20598.

Sitti, M., 2001. Survey of nanomanipulation system. In: Proc. of the 1st IEEE Conf. Nanotechnology Maui, Hawaii, pp. 75–80.

Steinberg, I., Huland, D.M., Vermesh, O., Frostig, H.E., Tummers, W.S., Gambhir, S.S., 2019. Photoacoustic clinical imaging. Photoacoustics 14, 77–98.

Stemmer, A., Beck, M., Fiolka, R., 2008. Widefield fluorescence microscopy with extended resolution. Histochem. Cell Biol. 130, 807–817.

Strohm, E.M., Moore, M.J., Kolios, M.C., 2016. Single cell photoacoustic microscopy: a review. IEEE J. Sel. Top. Quant. Electron. 22, 137–151.

Sun, Y., Nelson, B.J., 2002. Biological cell injection using an autonomous microrobotics system. Int. J. Robot Res. 21, 861–868.

Svoboda, K., Block, S.M., 1994. Biological application of optical forces. Annu. Rev. Biophys. Biomol. Struct. 23, 247–285.

Tan, Y., Kong, C.W., Chen, S., Cheng, S.H., Li, R.A., Sun, D., 2012. Probing the mechanobiological properties of human embryonic stem cells in cardiac differentiation by optical tweezers. J. Biomech. 45 (1), 123–128.

Tang, J., Han, K.Y., 2019. Low-photobleaching line-scanning confocal microscopy using dual inclined beams. J. Biophoton. 12, e201900075.

Tikhonov, A.N., 1963. On the solution of incorrectly put problems and the regularisation method. Outl. Jt. Symp. Partial. Differ. Eq. 4, 261–265.

Trickey, W.R., Lee, G.M., Guilak, F., 2000. Viscoelastic properties of chondrocytes from normal and osteoarthritic human cartilage. J. Orthop. Res. 18, 891–898.

Vahey, M., Voldman, J., 2008. An equilibrium method for continuous-flow cell sorting using dielectrophoresis. Anal. Chem. 80, 3135–3143.

Vo-Dinh, T., 2003. Biomedical Photonics: Handbook. CRC Press, Boca Raton, FL, USA, ISBN 9780203008997.

Voldman, J., Gray, M.L., Toner, M., Schmidt, M.A., 2002. A microfabrication-based dynamic array cytometer. Anal. Chem. 74, 3984–3990.
Wang, X., Chen, S., Kong, M., Wang, Z., Costa, K.D., Li, R.A., Sun, D., 2011. Enhanced cell sorting and manipulation with combined optical tweezer and microfluidic chip technologies. Lab Chip 11, 3656–3662.
Wang, K., Cheng, J., Cheng, S.H., Sun, D., 2013. Probing cell biophysical behavior based on actin cytoskeleton modeling and stretching manipulation with optical tweezers. Appl. Phys. Lett. 99, 083702.
Wang, L., Zhang, C., Wang, L.V., 2014. Grueneisen relaxation photoacoustic microscopy. Phys. Rev. Lett. 113, 174301.
Wang, X., Chen, X.Z., Alcântara, C.C.J., Sevim, S., Hoop, M., Terzopoulou, A., de Marco, C., Hu, C., de Mello, A.J., Falcaro, P., Furukawa, S., Nelson, B.J., Puigmarti-Luis, J., Pane, S., 2019. MOFBOTS: metal-organic-framework-based biomedical microrobots. Adv. Mater. e1901592.
Wei, T., Liu, J., Li, D., Chen, S., Zhang, Y., Li, J., Fan, L., Guan, Z., Lo, C.M., Wang, L., Man, K., Sun, D., 2020. Development of magnet-driven and image-guided biodegradable microrobots for the precise delivery of engineered stem cells for cancer therapy. Small 16 (41), 1906908.
Winckler, B., Forscher, P., Mellman, I., 1999. A diffusion barrier maintains distribution of membrane proteins in polarized neurons. Nature 397, 698–701.
Wu, Z., Li, L., Yang, Y., Hu, P., Li, Y., Yang, S.Y., Wang, L.V., Gao, W., 2019. A microrobotic system guided by photoacoustic computed tomography for targeted navigation in intestines in vivo. Sci. Robot. 4, eaax0613.
Wu, Z., Liu, M., Liu, Z., Tian, Y., 2020. Real-time imaging and simultaneous quantification of mitochondrial H_2O_2 and ATP in neurons with a single two-photon fluorescence-lifetime-based probe. J. Am. Chem. Soc. 142, 7532–7541.
Xu, T., 2014. Propulsion Characteristics and Visual Servo Control of Scaled-up Helical Microswimmers (Ph.D. Thesis). The Université Pierre et Marie Curie-Paris VI, Paris, France.
Yang, R., Song, B., Sun, Z., Lai, K.W.C., Fung, C.K.M., Patterson, K.C., Seiffert-Sinha, K., Sinha, A.A., Xi, N., 2015. Cellular level robotic surgery: nanodissection of intermediate filaments in live keratinocytes. Nanomed. Nanotechnol. Biol. Med. 11 (1), 137–145.
Yao, J., Wang, L.V., 2013. Photoacoustic microscopy. Laser Photon. Rev. 7, 758–778.
Ye, Z., Régnier, S., Sitti, M., 2014. Rotating magnetic miniature swimming robots with multiple flexible flagella. IEEE Trans. Robot. 30, 3–13.
Yu, J., Zhao, Q., Cui, M., Sun, M., Zhao, X., 2014. Robotic donor cell injection in somatic cell nuclear transfer (SCNT). In: Proceeding of the 11th World Congress on Intelligent Control and Automation, pp. 2821–2825.
Zhang, H., Liu, K.K., 2008. Optical tweezers for single cells. J. R. Soc. Interface 5, 671–690.
Zhong, M.C., Wei, X.B., Zhou, J.H., Wang, Z.Q., Li, Y.M., 2013. Trapping red blood cells in living animals using optical tweezers. Nat. Commun. 4, 1768.
Zhu, A., Chen, Y., 1989. High-voltage capillary zone electrophoresis if red blood cells. J. Chromatogr. 470, 251–260.

Robotic cell injection

3

3.1 Introduction

Microinjection is a technique in which a glass micropipette is inserted and small amounts of macromolecules or nanoparticles are pushed into cells. Microinjection has been widely used in biomedical studies to deepen the understanding of cellular functions, such as viral-mediated delivery, chemical-mediated delivery, and physical delivery (Stewart et al., 2018). Currently, cell injection has been widely used for stem cell therapy in precision and regenerative medicine (Newland et al., 2013). The primary advantage of this technique is delivering a large variety of foreign materials to almost every type of cell (Tiefenboeck et al., 2018). Traditionally, microinjections are conducted manually by skilled personnel using microscopic manipulators. During these processes, the operator must simultaneously control the micromanipulator, microinjector, and microscope stage, which is tedious and time consuming. Since 2000, robot-assisted microinjection technologies have been gradually used to automate this complex task. Sun and Nelson (2002) developed a system for autonomously injecting mouse embryos held by another micropipette. Schnizler et al. (2003) developed a system that can automatically inject *Xenopus* oocytes trapped in a standard 96-well plate. Huang et al. (2009a,b) and Xie et al. (2010) developed position and force control methods to improve the performance of microinjection on suspended cells. To enhance the productivity of cell injection, Pan et al. (2020) increased the injection speed through automatic cell detection and optimized injection path and adaptive adjustment of penetration depth. In all these robot-assisted cell injection methods, there are usually automatically controlled end-effectors (such as microinjectors or microneedles) installed on a motorized platform, image-processing systems for automatic detection of cells and instruments, sensing equipment, cell-holding devices for handling a large number of cells, and intelligent control algorithms to ensure high operating efficiency, success rate, and productivity.

Microinjection technology can be used for suspended cells or adherent cells, which vary in size. Many reported studies have focused on the injection of relatively large-scale suspended cells, usually 50 μm−1 mm in size. Examples include *Xenopus* oocyte (~1 mm) (Hogg et al., 2008), zebrafish oocyte (~500 μm) (Wang et al., 2007; Huang et al. 2009a,b, 2011; Xie et al., 2010, 2011; Lu et al., 2007), and mouse embryo (~55 μm) (Liu and Sun, 2009; Sun and Nelson, 2007). These methods utilized robotics technology to achieve efficient automatic injection, while overcoming inherent problems of human fatigue and poor repeatability in manual operations (Wang et al., 2009). Extensive research was also conducted on microinjection of adherent cells that are usually small in size. The injection of small adherent cells places higher demands on the automatic microinjection system. Examples include the

Robotic Cell Manipulation. https://doi.org/10.1016/B978-0-323-85259-3.00001-5

motorized micromanipulator for adherent cell injection (Viigipuu and Kallio, 2004), the dual micromanipulator microinjection system for rice protoplasts and mouse embryonic stem cells (Matsuoka et al., 2004), the dual camera microinjection system (Youoku et al., 2007), the impedance-based microinjection system (Kallio et al., 2007), and several other high-speed semiautomatic microinjection systems (Wang et al., 2008; Becattini et al., 2013; Liu et al., 2015; Chow et al., 2016a). The automatic microinjection system developed by Pan et al. (2020) exhibited high productivity on small adherent cells.

Many advanced cell injection control methods have been proposed. Sun and Nelson (2002) used a visual position control to inject pronuclei DNA into mouse embryo, and then used an image-processing methodology to detect the target position of the end-effector. Wang et al. (2007) developed a robotic system for microinjection of zebrafish embryos, where the cytoplasm center was chosen as the target position by computer vision, and then a PID controller was used for injection. Matsuoka et al. (2006) developed an automatic microinjector for mouse ES cells and rice protoplasts, where a potential sensor was used to measure the intracellular potential change and generate a stop signal to a pulse motor-driven positioning system. Lu et al. (2007) used position control augmented with force feedback to inject zebrafish embryos, where a piezoresistive force sensor was used to monitor the injection process. Huang et al. (2009a) used vision and force feedback to realize three-dimensional (3D) cell microinjection, where an impedance control algorithm was utilized to control the depth movement of the injector. Huang et al. (2009b) further developed a visual-based impedance control for cell injection, where the actual force was used in the controller as a feedback. To regulate the penetration force to follow a desired force trajectory when the microneedle is inserted into the deformable cell, Xie et al. (2010) proposed a force control framework on the robot-assisted cell injection system. When the microneedle approached the cell, an impedance control was used in the inner control loop; after the microneedle touched the cell, the control was shifted to a force tracking nonlinear control in the outer control loop. Microforce sensors have been also developed in the past decades for real-time force sensing in the cell injection process. These developments included a polyvinylidene fluoride (PVDF) sensor (Pillarisetti et al., 2007; Shen et al., 2006), microelectromechanical system (MEMS)-based two-axis cellular force sensor (Sun et al., 2003), micrograting-based injection force sensor (Zhang et al., 2004), and micro-triaxial force sensor (Arai et al., 1999), to name a few.

Microinjection has shown great potential in many biomedical applications such as direct injection of nucleic acids into the cytoplasm or nucleus (Ittner et al., 2007; Tesson et al., 2011). By integrating with robotics, microinjection can achieve higher transfection efficiency than manual operation. Robotic microinjection shows unique advantages in the single-cell transfection process, including cost savings by controlling the amount of injected substance delivered, applicability to different cell types and injected substances, and improved safety due to its virus-free characteristics. Single-cell transfection requires a high degree of quantitative control of the substance delivered, which requires the support of robotics technology. Although manual quantitative microinjection has been applied to large mouse embryos and zygotes to assess the effect of compounds on embryonic development (Eroglu et al., 2003), delivery is neither automated nor reproducible, and the process usually cannot be applied to human cells with a small size of 7–20 μm. To create genetically modified cells with predictable functions, a reliable and high-throughput quantitative microinjection technique that allows precise delivery of a small amount of injection materials into a batch of human cells is needed. Chow et al. (2016a,b) developed a quantitatively controlled microinjection technique to achieve single-cell transfection using an automated micropipette-based microinjection platform. The platform employed a microfluidic chip to pattern the suspended cells in an array for easy injection and measurement. To prove the effective control of the delivered substances, different amounts of synthetically modified mRNA (modRNA) or plasmid mixtures were delivered to human foreskin fibroblast (HFF) cells at different concentration ratios by Chow et al. (2016a,b).

Characterizing the biomechanical properties of cells represents another promising application of microinjection, which plays an important role in regulating cell function. In cell biology, it is important to know how cells respond to mechanical forces and how mechanical responses regulate cellular functions, both of which critically depend on the mechanical properties (Vaziri and Gopinath, 2008). The connection between cell mechanics and cellular functions, such as locomotion, cell division, proliferation, mechanotransduction, and cell death, has been extensively investigated by many researchers including Suresh et al. (2005), Darling et al. (2007), Faria et al. (2008), Cross et al. (2007), Glenister et al. (2002), and Kol et al. (2006). Due to the advantages of low cost, easy operation, and good controllability, Tan et al. (2010) demonstrated that robotic cell injection technology can be an efficient tool for characterizing the biomechanical properties of cells. This approach included the establishment of a mechanical model, incorporation of various constitutive materials into the developed model to present the deformation behaviors of different kinds of cells, verification of the model through finite element analysis (FEA) and microinjection experiments, and demonstration of the modeling approach with various constitutive materials.

The remainder of this chapter provides a detailed introduction to several key topics in robotic cell injection, including the robot-assisted cell microinjection system settings and operating strategies, position and force control in automatic cell injection, and multiple methodologies to achieve high performance, high throughput, and high productivity of cell injection. Finally, two case studies which apply the microinjection methods to single-cell transfection and cell biomechanical characterization are introduced.

3.2 Robot-assisted cell microinjection system with microneedles

3.2.1 Cell injection process and system setup

A robotic manipulation process to achieve automatic injection of cells is introduced first. Fig. 3.1A illustrates a generalized out-of-plane cell injection process with a robotically controlled microneedle (Huang et al., 2009b). Prior to initiation of the process,

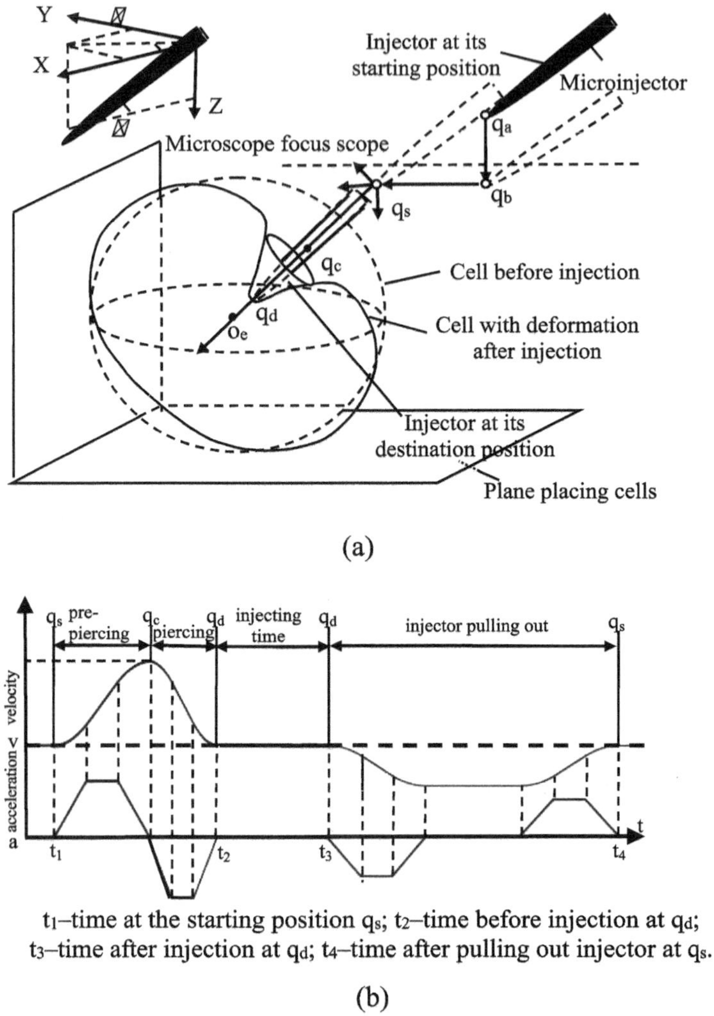

Figure 3.1 Schematic of an out-of-plane cell injection (Huang et al., 2009b). (A) Injection process. (B) Velocity and acceleration profiles of the injector during the injection process.

the injector is located at a Z coordinate position so that it is observed using a microscope. Then, the injector moves in the Z-axis direction to permit the injector to be imaged by the microscope. Let q_a be defined as the vertical displacement of the injector tip before it touches the cell. The injector tip is first translated to the predetermined injection Z coordinate that places the injector tip within the focal range of the microscope, and then the vertical displacement q_b guided by a visual servoing approach. The movement of the injector and deformation of the cell membrane in the $X-Y$ plane can now be observed by the microscope. Under a visual servo control, the injector tip is translated to the starting injection position q_s, and then accelerated toward the embryo in a prepiercing step. Note that the motion of the pipette should be directed along the longitudinal axis of the pipette, and also toward the center of the cell, denoted by o_e. To achieve this motion, the *X*-, *Y*-, and *Z*-axes must move in a coordinated manner. In order to piece the cell membrane successfully, the velocity of the injector tip is designed to be at its highest value when the tip reaches the cell membrane, which occurs when the injector reaches position q_c. The injector is then decelerated to allow the smooth approach to the desired injection position q_d where the material is injected into the cell. Thereafter, the injector is accelerated in the opposite direction, removing the injector from the interior of the cell and exiting the cell membrane. The velocity and acceleration profiles of the injector, starting from the prepiercing step at q_s and terminating at the same coordinate q_s, are shown in Fig. 3.1B.

Fig. 3.1 illustrates the basic operational strategy of robotic cell microinjection, where cells are either suspended or adherent to substrate. In order to achieve high productivity, the injection system must allow a large number of suspended cells to be injected automatically. For this purpose, the operation must follow a required sequence and repeat the same process, which is called batch microinjection. Fig. 3.2A illustrates an example of using the robotic manipulation system for automatic injection of large batches of suspended cells (Huang et al., 2009a). Fig. 3.2B illustrates a cell-holding device fixed on the actuated rotary plate, which permits batches of cells to be transported one by one into the field of view of the microscope for injection. The injection system contains three modules for execution, sensing, and control. The executive module consists of a $X - Y - \theta$ positioning table with the injector mounted on the Z -axis. The cells to be injected are placed on a specially designed cell-holding device. Mounted on the positioning table, the cell holder center is coincident with the θ rotation axis. The coordinated motion of the $X - Y - \theta$ table and the Z -axis is required to perform the cell injection task. The position of the injection pipette is precisely adjusted with a 4 degree of freedom (DOF) ($X - Y - \phi - \beta$) manual positioning table mounted on the $Z-$ axis, where ϕ is the tilt angle of the injector, β is the angle between the injector and the X -axis, and both ϕ and β are fixed as shown in Fig. 3.1A. A hydraulic microinjector pipette is driven by a stepper motor, permitting a minimum volume resolution to be delivered into the cell. The sensory module contains a vision

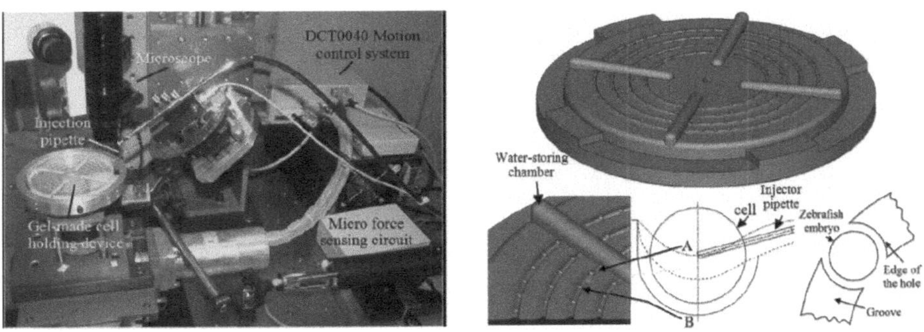

(a) (b)

Figure 3.2 A robot-assisted manipulation system for automated cell injection (Huang et al., 2009a). (A) Injection system setup. (B) The cell-holding device.

system that includes an optical microscope, lighting system, CCD camera, image capture and processing card, and image-processing computer. The lighting system is suitable for observing transparent biotechnology objects. The working plate is made of glass. A very thin chip LED backlights provides illumination of the working area from behind to create a silhouette image. The control module consists of a host computer and a motion control/drive system.

3.2.2 Cell-holding device

The design of the cell-holding device is based on the idea of a hemispherical hole-shaped cell scaffold (Fujisato et al., 1998) and a groove-shaped cell scaffold (Lu et al., 2007). The hole array can readily immobilize the cells, while the groove makes the embryo pick-and-place process easier to implement. It is important for the micropipette to maintain a certain angle of attack with the horizontal plane; otherwise, the injection pipette will only brush the cells out of the holding device and cannot penetrate the cell wall. To avoid the tedious work of placing cells in individual holes for batch injection, the holding device is designed as a semicircular groove, as shown in Fig. 3.2B. The hole array is located on a circular contour groove centered on the geometric center of the holder. The diameter of the hole varies according to different applications. For example, it is 1.4 mm for injection of fish embryos (Huang et al., 2009a). As shown in Fig. 3.2B, the dash-dot line A and solid line B represent the cross-section profiles of edge of groove and edge of the hole, respectively.

The main advantages of the above design are threefold. First, the groove makes the process of picking and placing embryos easier. Multiple embryos can be placed in the groove and rolled into the holes one by one along the groove. Second, the hole array can easily fix the cells so that injections can be made from all directions. Third, with the help of the edge of each groove, fluid stays in the groove during injection to keep the cells moist, and excess fluid flows through the edge of the groove into the water storage chamber. In addition, the image quality is good.

The cell-holding device is made of low-melting agarose gel, a material commonly used in biological research. Agarose gel has soft, hydrous, and transparent characteristics, which are very suitable for fabricating the proposed cell holder. To make this cell-holding device, the gel with 5% agarose in a Petri dish is made by dissolving and heating it in a microwave oven, and then, the designed mold is pressed on the surface of the gel and taken out after the agarose gel is cooled.

3.2.3 Image processing

The automatic cell injection process starts with the use of image-processing technology to identify the positions of the manipulated cell and the injection pipette. Considerable work on image-processing and image-recognition algorithms for detecting the cell and the pipette has been reported in the literature. Fig. 3.3 illustrates an example of imaging zebrafish embryos. With a specially designed cell-holding device, as introduced in Fig. 3.2B, only the cell embryo and the injection pipette need to be identified, as shown in Fig. 3.3A, which greatly simplifies the visual processing.

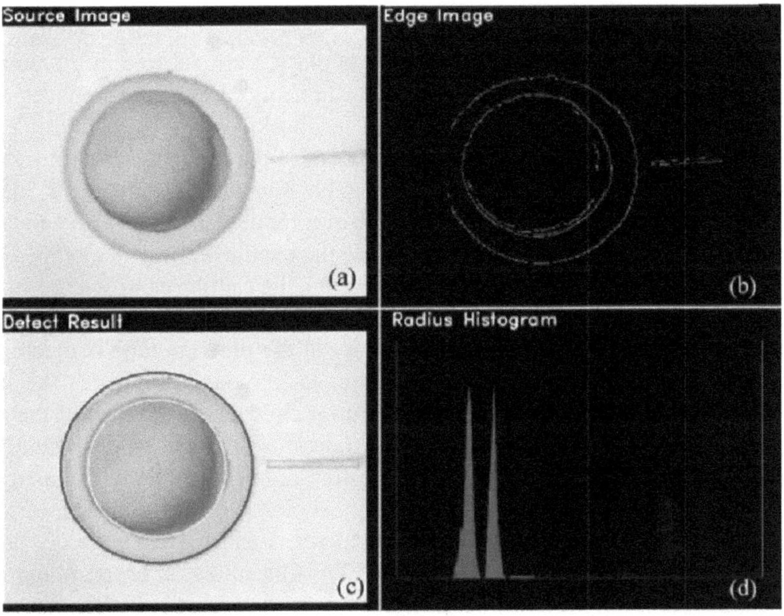

Figure 3.3 A typical image grabbed and processed by a vision system (Huang et al., 2009a). (A) Source image of zebrafish embryo. (B) Edge detection. (C) Detection result. (D) Radius histogram of zebrafish embryos.

The procedure for image processing is as follows. First, preprocessing is conducted to obtain relatively noise-free binary images. The image is first convolved with a low-pass Gaussian filter for noise suppression. Then, the gray-level image is filtered to find the edge of the cell chorion, cytoplasm, and pipette by using the Canny edge detection algorithm, as shown in Fig. 3.3B. The traditional Hough transform has the limitation of long calculation time and relatively low precision to track the movement of cell embryos. Qu (2005) proposed a faster and more precise method, the chord midpoint Hough transform (CMHT), to improve the efficiency and accuracy of ellipse detection in an image. The position of the injection pipette can be determined by using the correlation-based pattern-matching method. Fig. 3.3C shows the image-processing result. Fig. 3.3D shows the radius histogram of zebrafish embryos with and without chorion.

The image-processing technology is used to detect cell diameters, such as chorionic diameter, yolk diameter, and extracellular, and then guide the injection pipette to the desired starting position through visual servoing. When the pipette touches the cell and starts the injection, the position feedback (rather than image feedback) obtained by the motor encoder will be used for the position control to improve the processing speed and accuracy.

3.2.4 Force sensing

Similar to image processing, force sensing also plays a critical role in the automatic robot-assisted microinjection on a batch of cells. In many cases, force feedback control can be more effective than the visual position feedback control, as direct force information reflects the changes to the physical behavior of the cell, such as deformation or extent of penetration, more quickly and accurately (Sun and Nelson, 2002). Many reported microforce sensors are based on the use of a cantilever beam, where the needle is bonded to the free end of the cantilever while the cantilever base is mounted on the manipulator. However, in actual cell microinjection, the cantilever structure is difficult to transfer the solution from the pressure tube to the needle. In addition, when the needle is connected to the pressure tube, the gravity of the pressure tube is much greater than the penetrating force on the micro-Newton scale, which dominates the sensing signal. Another problem in the design of microforce sensors is the lack of theoretical investigation. In the current model, the linear relationship between penetration force and sensor output is based on experimental testing rather than theoretical analysis.

PVDF (polyvinylidene fluoride) film is a typical piezoelectric material used to measure deformation caused by applied mechanical stress and has been widely used for decades (Sun and Mills, 2002; Yi, 2008). PVDF film allows a broad range of frequency bandwidth from 0.001 to 10^9 Hz. Successful design of a PVDF force sensor for microinjection requires the design of a mechanical transducer and an electrical transducer. Xie et al. (2010) proposed a mechanical transducer that contains a simply supported beam used to sense the penetration force applied on the cell embryo, and a PVDF film that is adhesively bonded to the supporting beam, as shown in Fig. 3.4A. The electrical transducer includes a charge amplifier and a low-pass amplifier, which is used to convert the charge output from the PVDF film to a voltage signal. A simplified diagram of the proposed force sensor is illustrated in Fig. 3.4B. As the processing speed is relatively slow during injection, the injection process can be treated as a quasistatic process. According to Newton's law, the cell penetration force equals the force applied on the PVDF film, which is the charge source. A charge amplifier is needed to convert the charge output from the PVDF film into a voltage signal while removing the influence from the cable capacitance. Following the charge amplifier, a low-pass

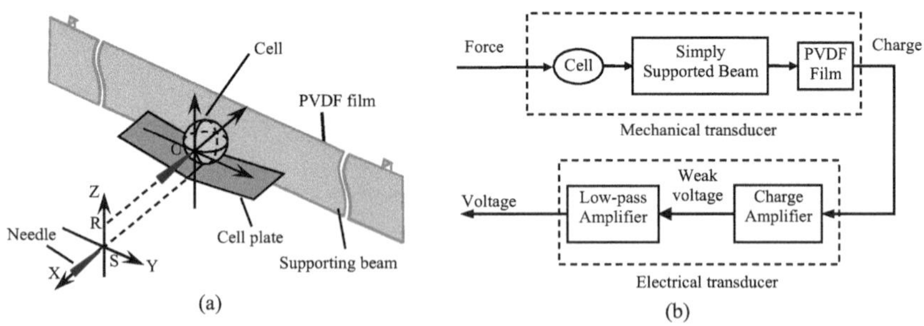

Figure 3.4 A PVDF force-sensing system. (A) Force-based cell injection and sensing scheme (Xie et al., 2010). (B) Sensing mechanism (Xie et al., 2011).

amplifier with a cutoff frequency (e.g., 70 Hz) is added to remove the noise from the circuit and amplify the weak voltage signal. An analog-to-digital converter (ADC) then feeds the force signal to the control loop. In addition to the low-pass filters, shielding techniques can also be used to prevent electromagnetic interference (EMI) from noise.

3.2.5 System modeling

A brief introduction to the modeling of the cell microinjection system is given here. Fig. 3.5 illustrates the configuration of the basic microinjection system. Define $O-XYZ$ as the coordinate frame whose origin O is located at the center of the working plate. A microscope mounted on the visual servoing system is positioned on a positioning table. The optical axis of the microscope coincides with the Z-axis, as shown in Fig. 3.5. Define $O_c - X_cY_cZ_c$ as the camera coordinate frame, where the origin O_c is located at the center of the camera, and Z_c coincides with the optical axis of the microscope. Define $O_i - uv$ as the coordinate frame in the image plane, with three coordinates u, v and the rotary angle θ_i. The origin O_i is located in the optical axis, and the u and v axes are within the camera image plane perpendicular to the optical axis.

The relationship between the image coordinates $[u,\quad v,\quad Z,\quad \theta_i]^T$ and the positioning table coordinates $[X,\quad Y,\quad Z,\quad \theta]^T$ is given as

$$\begin{bmatrix} u \\ v \\ Z \\ \theta_i \end{bmatrix} = T \begin{bmatrix} X \\ Y \\ Z \\ \theta \end{bmatrix} + \begin{bmatrix} f_X d_X \\ f_Y d_Y \\ 0 \\ 0 \end{bmatrix}, \tag{3.1}$$

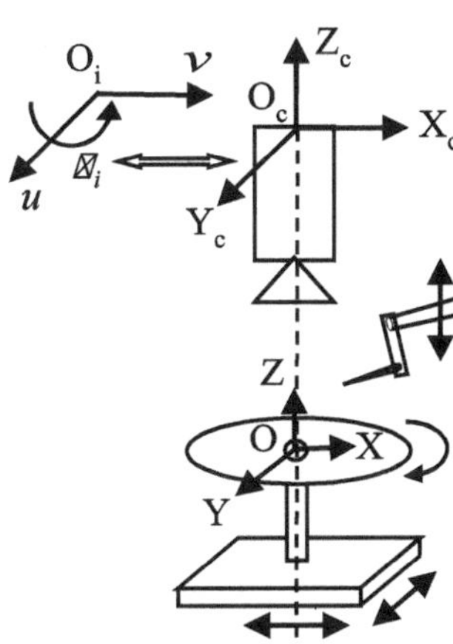

Figure 3.5 Configuration of the cell injection system (Huang et al., 2009a).

where $T \in \Re^{4\times4}$ is the transformation matrix between the image frame and the positioning table frame. Since both frames are fixed, T is time-invariant. f_X and f_Y are the display resolutions of the vision system in X and Y coordinate directions, respectively, and d_X and d_Y are distances between the two frames in the two directions, respectively.

Using Lagrange's equation of the motion, the dynamics of the four DOF motion stage is given as

$$M\begin{bmatrix}\ddot{X}\\ \ddot{Y}\\ \ddot{Z}\\ \ddot{\theta}\end{bmatrix}+N\begin{bmatrix}\dot{X}\\ \dot{Y}\\ \dot{Z}\\ \dot{\theta}\end{bmatrix}+\begin{bmatrix}0\\ 0\\ G_z\\ 0\end{bmatrix}=\tau-\begin{bmatrix}J^Tf_e\\ 0\end{bmatrix}, \tag{3.2}$$

where $M=\begin{bmatrix}m_X+m_Y+m_p & 0 & 0 & 0\\ 0 & m_Y+m_p & 0 & 0\\ 0 & 0 & m_Z & 0\\ 0 & 0 & 0 & I\end{bmatrix}$ denotes the inertia matrix of the system, and m_X, m_Y, and m_Z are masses of the X, Y, and Z positioning tables, m_p is the mass of the working plate, and I is the inertia of the rotational axis and the working plate. N denotes the system damping and viscous friction effects. $G_Z=-m_Zg$ is the gravitational force vector. $\tau=\begin{bmatrix}\tau_X, & \tau_Y, & \tau_Z, & \tau_r\end{bmatrix}^T$ denotes the torque inputs to the driving motors. $J=\mathrm{diag}\{J_X, J_Y, J_Z\}$ is the Jacobian matrix related to task and joint coordinates. $f_e=\begin{bmatrix}f_{eX}, & f_{eY}, & f_{eZ}\end{bmatrix}^T$ is the external force applied to motors, and $f_e=0$ if the injection pipette does not touch the cells.

Define $q=\begin{bmatrix}u, & v, & Z, & \theta_i\end{bmatrix}^T$ as the generalized coordinate. Then, the following dynamic equation is obtained based on the coordinate q:

$$MT^{-1}\ddot{q}+NT^{-1}\dot{q}+G=\tau-\begin{bmatrix}J^Tf_e\\ 0\end{bmatrix}. \tag{3.3}$$

3.3 Hybrid position and force control for automated batch injection of cells

3.3.1 Controller design

During the out-of-plane cell injection, the depth motion of the injection pipette cannot be observed by the microscope. Therefore, a force control in the Z-axis direction is utilized to implicitly control the depth motion. Based on the force feedback from the microforce sensor and the position feedback from the motor encoder, a hybrid position and force control methodology can be developed.

The relationship between cell membrane deformation and cell injection force can be derived from the calibration of the cell injection task in the $X-Y$ plane ($\phi = 0$), where the injection pipette and the focal plane of the microscope are on the same plane. This geometry is chosen so that the pipette pierces the cell at its vertical midpoint and the $X-Y$ plane deflection observed by the camera is correct. Assuming that the batch of cells has roughly the same membrane dynamics, a similar injection force trajectory will be obtained when the pipette injects into the cells with the desired velocity and acceleration curve, as shown in Fig. 3.1B. After calibration, the empirical relationship between the desired cell injection force F^d and the desired pipette trajectory ρ^d can be obtained as follows:

$$F^d = U\left(\rho^d\right). \tag{3.4}$$

In out-of-plane injection, the desired injection force corresponding to the desired position trajectory can be estimated from the cell membrane deformation in the $X-Y$ plane and the known angle ϕ of the injection pipette relative to the $X-Y$ plane, leading to Eq. (3.4). This desired injection force will be the input of the force controller designed later.

The out-of-plane cell injection can be decoupled into two relatively independent control processes: position control in the horizontal ($X-Y$) plane and force control in depth (Z axis). In this way, the position of the injector in the $X-Y$ plane, which can be observed with the microscope, and the injection force using the force sensor in the Z-axis direction, in which depth information cannot be known, can be controlled simultaneously. As indicated above, there exists an empirical relationship between the desired cell injection force and trajectory. As a result, the depth movement of the pipette can be indirectly controlled via a force control.

During the cell injection process, the motion planning of the pipette can be simplified if the moving coordinates are expressed in the spherical polar coordinate system. Define $o_e - \rho\phi\beta$ as the spherical polar coordinate frame whose origin o_e is located at the center of the cell, as shown in Fig. 3.1A. The desired trajectory of the pipette is then expressed as

$$\begin{bmatrix} X^d \\ Y^d \\ Z^d \end{bmatrix} = \begin{bmatrix} \rho^d \sin\phi \cos\beta \\ \rho^d \sin\phi \sin\beta \\ \rho^d \cos\phi \end{bmatrix}, \tag{3.5}$$

where ρ^d denotes the desired trajectory of the injection pipette, and neither β nor ϕ change during the injection process.

The dynamics Eq. (3.2) can be partitioned into two distinct equations of motion during the injection process, namely

$$\begin{cases} \tau_{XY} = M_{XY}\begin{bmatrix} \ddot{X} \\ \ddot{Y} \end{bmatrix} + N_{XY}\begin{bmatrix} \dot{X} \\ \dot{Y} \end{bmatrix} + \begin{bmatrix} J_X^T f_{eX} \\ J_Y^T f_{eY} \end{bmatrix}, \\ \tau_Z = M_Z\ddot{Z} + N_Z\dot{Z} + G_Z + J_Z^T f_{eZ} \end{cases} \tag{3.6}$$

where τ_{XY} and τ_Z are the torque distributions in the $X-Y$ plane and the Z axis, respectively, M_{XY} and N_{XY} are submatrices of M and N in the X and Y axes, M_Z, N_Z, and G_Z are submatrices of M, N, and G in the Z axis, and f_{eX}, f_{eY}, and f_{eZ} are the actual external forces along the three axes, measured by the PVDF force sensor.

The position error in the $X-Y$ plane is defined as $e_{XY} = \rho^d \sin\phi\begin{bmatrix} \cos\beta \\ \sin\beta \end{bmatrix} - \begin{bmatrix} X \\ Y \end{bmatrix}$. A computed torque controller with measured force compensation is designed for position control in the $X-Y$ plane, expressed as

$$\tau_{XY} = M_{XY}\left(\begin{bmatrix} \ddot{X}^d \\ \ddot{Y}^d \end{bmatrix} + k_v\dot{e}_{XY} + k_p e_{XY}\right) + N_{XY}\begin{bmatrix} \dot{X} \\ \dot{Y} \end{bmatrix} + \begin{bmatrix} J_X^T f_{eX} \\ J_Y^T f_{eY} \end{bmatrix}\phi, \tag{3.7}$$

Where k_v and k_p are positive control gain matrices. The controller Eq. (3.7) leads to the closed-loop dynamics $\ddot{e}_{XY} + k_{v1}\dot{e}_{XY} + k_{p1}e_{XY} = 0$, which implies $e_{XY} = 0$.

As for the depth movement of the pipette, the impedance control is utilized to directly control the pipette's position in the Z axis. The control law is given as:

$$m\ddot{e}_Z + b\dot{e}_Z + ke_Z = \Delta f_{eZ}, \tag{3.8}$$

where m, b, and k are the desired impedance parameters, and $e_z = Z^d - Z = \rho^d\cos\phi - Z$, representing the position error of the pipette in the Z axis. The actual position Z can be obtained from the encoder of the drive motor. $\Delta f_{ez} = f_{eZ}^d - f_{eZ}$ is the force error in the Z axis. The desired force f_{eZ}^d can be obtained based on the actual position of the pipette in the $X-Y$ plane and the calibrated relationship between the injection position and the force. This indicates that f_{eZ}^d is closely related to Z^d. $f_{eZ} = f_e\cos\phi$ is the projection of the cell injection force in the Z axis, which can be measured by the PVDF force sensor.

By solving Eq. (3.8), $\ddot{Z}$ can be derived as follows:

$$\ddot{Z} = m^{-1}\left(m\ddot{Z}^d + b\dot{e}_Z + ke_Z - \Delta f_{eZ}\right). \tag{3.9}$$

Substituting Eq. (3.9) into Eq. (3.6) yields the Z-axis torque controller as follows:

$$\tau_Z = M_Z(\ddot{Z}^d + m^{-1}(b\dot{e}_Z + ke_Z - \Delta f_{eZ})) + N_Z\dot{Z} + G_Z + J_Z^T f_{eZ}. \quad (3.10)$$

Under Eq. (3.10), the cell injection force can be regulated to meet the desired impedance requirement. Since the desired force has an empirical relationship to the desired position trajectory, the pipette position in the Z axis is controlled indirectly.

3.3.2 Experiments

To verify the effectiveness of the above cell injection control approach, experiments were performed using the setup shown in Fig. 3.2A. The modeling parameters of the system are determined as follows. The rotation angle between the image frame and the stage frame during the injection is set to zero ($\theta = 0$ degree) for simplicity. The displacement between origins of the two frames is $d = [0, \ 0, \ 30\,\text{mm}]^T$. The magnification factor of the microscope objective is $\lambda = 30$. After system calibration, the inertia matrix is determined as $M_{xy} = \begin{bmatrix} 0.022180 & 0 \\ 0 & 0.011386 \end{bmatrix}$ Kg$\cdot$ m^2, and the system damping and viscous frictional matrix is $N_{xy} = \begin{bmatrix} \frac{1.146}{\dot{X}} + (2.465e-003)\dot{X} - 0.04749 & 0 \\ 0 & \frac{0.172}{\dot{Y}} - (1.473e-003)\dot{Y} + 0.04023 \end{bmatrix}$ Kg$\cdot$m^2/s. The angles between the injection pipette and the X and Z axes are $\beta = 45$ degree and $\phi = 35$ degree, respectively.

The cells chosen for injection are zebrafish embryos. Zebrafish embryos are commonly used as animal models in biological manipulation due to their genetic similarity with higher vertebrates, easy availability, short generation time, external fertilization, and translucent embryos. The diameter of the zebrafish egg is approximately 1.15–1.25 mm (including the chorion). The radius of the injector pipette is 7.5 μm. To ensure the consistency of the cell membrane characteristics used in different experiments, all cells were collected according to standard embryo preparation procedures, and all cells were placed at room temperature (22–24°C) for 2 h after fertilization (blastocyst stage) before injection.

Calibration was first performed to obtain the empirical relationship between the desired cell injection force and the desired pipette trajectory p^d. The same pipette radius and the same velocity and acceleration profiles were used in the calibration test. During the prepiercing period, the pipette was accelerated to reach the maximum velocity when it contacted the cell membrane. During the next piercing period, the pipette was decelerated and pierced the cell membrane, moving a certain distance within the cell. Then, it stopped for a few seconds at the destination to inject the genetic materials into the cell. Finally, the injector pipette was extracted from the cell, using a lower speed than during the piercing period. Due to changes in cell characteristics, the force threshold for cell membrane penetration varies from embryo to embryo. This difference in penetrating force is not enough to affect the sensitivity of the microforce sensor, so it will not have a great impact on the injection. After calibration experiments, the relationship between the desired cell injection force F^d and the desired pipette trajectory ρ^d can be determined. In the report of Huang et al. (2009a), the desired force F^d and trajectory ρ^d have the following relationship:

$$\begin{aligned} &F^d = 0.0001694 \cdot \left(r - \rho^d\right)^2 + 0.3987 \cdot \left(r - \rho^d\right) - 8.389 \\ &r - 317.5\mu\text{m} < \rho^d < r \end{aligned} \tag{3.11}$$

where r is the radius of the injected cell.

Fig. 3.6 illustrates the injection procedures. The computed torque control gains are $k_v = \text{diag}\{21.645,\ 28.87,\ 31.75\} \times 10^3 \text{s}^{-1}$, $k_p = \text{diag}\{27.42,\ 43.4,\ 66.4\} \times 10^6 \text{s}^{-2}$. The impedance control gains are $m = \text{diag}\{0.330,\ 0.165,\ 0.1635\} \text{N} \cdot \text{s}^2/\text{m}$, $b = \text{diag}\{7.143,\ 4.763,\ 5.191\} \times 10^3 \text{N} \cdot \text{s}/\text{m}$, and $k = \text{diag}\{9.049,\ 7.144,\ 10.855\} \times 10^6 \text{N}/\text{m}$.

Fig. 3.7A and B illustrate position tracking results in the X axis and Y axis, respectively. It can be seen that the actual position follows the desired position very well, and the maximum position tracking error in each axis is about 1.5 μm only. This indicates that the position control algorithm exhibits satisfactory tracking performance for micromanipulation. The good performance of the $X-Y$ plane position control ensures that the force control in the Z axis is successful, because the desired force in the Z axis is based on the actual position feedback in the $X-Y$ plane. Fig. 3.7C illustrates the

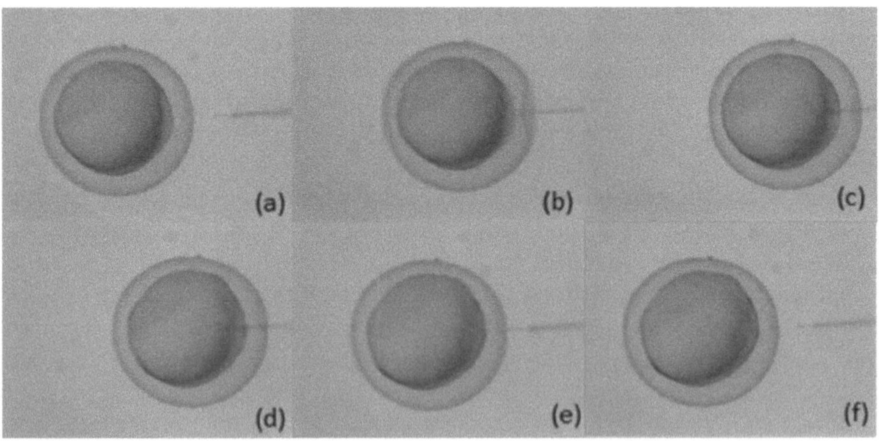

Figure 3.6 Out-of-plane cell injection process with position and force control (Huang et al., 2009a). (A) Prepiercing. (B) Piercing. (C) Arrival of the desired injection position. (D) Stage of injecting material. (E and F) Pulling out the pipette from the cell.

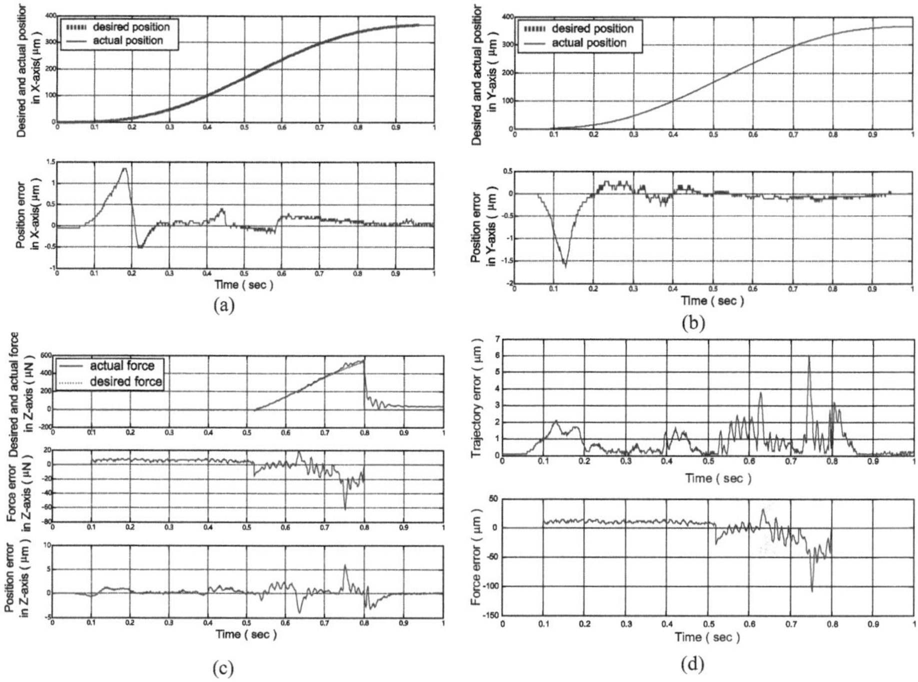

Figure 3.7 Cell injection experimental results (Huang et al., 2009a). (A) Position tracking results in the X axis. (B) Position tracking results in the Y axis. (C) Injection force control results in the Z axis and depth motion error. (D) Combined position and force tracking errors.

impedance control result in the Z axis and the depth motion error. During the prepiercing period ($0 \text{ s} < t < 0.5 \text{ s}$), the injection force is zero because the pipette does not touch the cell. When the pipette touches the cell after 0.5 s of movement, the injection force that can be measured by the force sensor starts to increase. The desired force is determined based on the actual position in the $X-Y$ plane and the calibration relationship in Eq. (3.11). The maximum force error along the Z axis is approximately 60 μN. The maximum position error in the Z axis is about 6 μm, which is greater than the position error in the $X-Y$ plane because it is controlled indirectly through the impedance control. Fig. 3.7D shows the position and force tracking errors that combine the results in all three axes. The position error denotes the difference between the actual and desired positions in 3D, calculated based on the desired pipette trajectory ρ^d and the fixed angles β and ϕ. The force error is detected along the pipette axis by the installed PVDF force sensor. It is seen that the maximum position error corresponds to the maximum force error. This is because that the depth control follows the force control in the Z axis, and the force control performance has great influence on the depth control and subsequently the whole position control performance.

The same experiment was repeated to simulate out-of-plane cell injection of a batch of 20 zebrafish embryos. Fig. 3.8 shows the maximum force error and the largest position tracking error of these 20 embryos. The maximum force error standard deviation

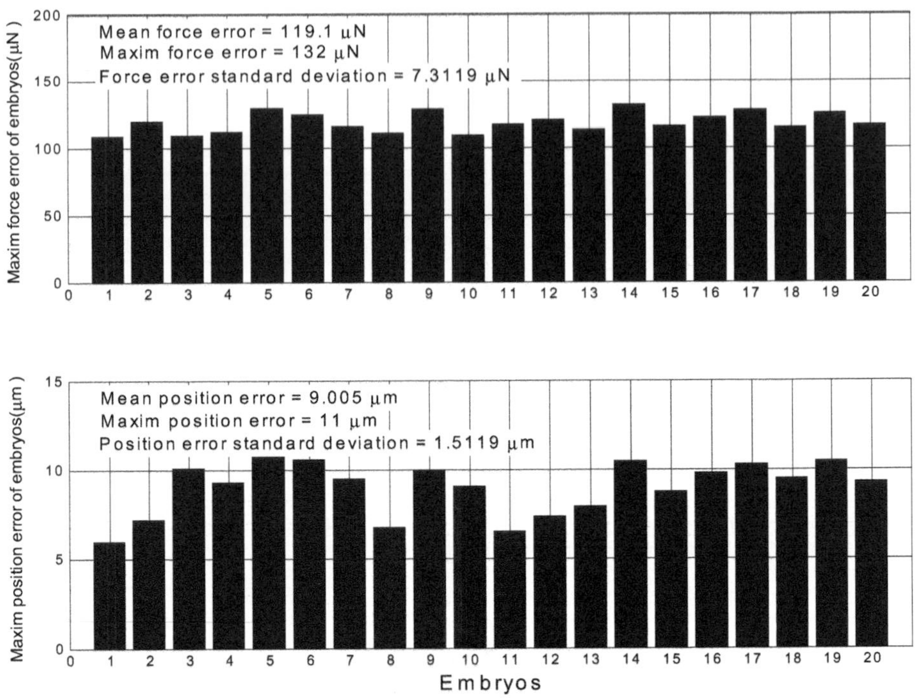

Figure 3.8 Evaluation of batch injection performance (Huang et al., 2009a).

and maximum position error standard deviation are 7.3119 μN and 1.5119 μm, respectively. The results of mean error, standard deviation, and maximum error are all satisfied, indicating that the control method exhibits stable and consistent repeatable performance. The injection speed of these tests is about 10 embryos (with chorion) per minute, and the overall success rate in all trials is approximately 98%. This demonstrates that the automatic cell injection system is capable of repeatedly piecing the zebrafish embryos with a relatively high success rate.

3.4 Universal piezo-driven ultrasonic cell microinjection

Piezoelectric-driven pipettes can also be used to pierce cells during cell injection, and have been successfully used for intracytoplasmic sperm injection (ICSI) in many mammals. Kimura and Yanagimachi (1995) proposed a piezo-driven ICSI method, in which the injection pipette is driven by a series of piezoelectric pulses with adjustable frequency, amplitude, and duration. Using the piezoelectric ICSI method, sperm-injected mouse oocytes can achieve a survival rate of 80%, of which 70% can successfully develop into blastocysts (Huang et al., 2011). Piezoelectric drills have been widely used in the ICSI process of human, mouse, and bovine embryos, with satisfactory performance. The researchers also found that a very small mercury column in the injection pipette can significantly increase the success rate of piezoelectric ICSI (Katayose et al., 1999). However, due to the high-frequency vibration of the piezo-driven pipette, the pipette tip may undergo undesirable lateral movement. Lateral oscillation can cause large deformation of cells or embryonic membranes before puncturing the membranes and cause substantial damage to the cells. Considerable research has been conducted to investigate the effect of the mercury column on the zona-piercing mechanism in piezoelectric ICSI. Fan et al. (2006) used the finite element method to study the influence of the liquid around the pipette tip and found that the use of mercury can reduce the amplitude of pipette oscillation. Ediz and Olgac (2005) and Gan et al. (2008) found that the presence of mercury easily reduces the amplitude of pipette tip oscillations, so mercury may help reduce physical damage to oocytes. As for the zona-piercing mechanism in piezoelectric ICSI, Kimura and Yanagimachi (1995) and Fan et al. (2006) pointed out that the movement of the axial pipette can promote the penetration of the zona pellucida in mice. Huang et al. (2011) proposed a universal piezo-driven ultrasonic cell injection technique for automatic batch injection of suspended cells. This method used a piezoelectric stack to concentrate the piezoelectric oscillation power on the injection pipette, thereby eliminating the vibration of other parts of the manipulator. Because no mercury column is required, the lateral oscillation of the pipette is greatly reduced, and the damage to the injected cells is also minimized. The method is ideally suitable for precision injection.

Fig. 3.9A shows the design of a piezo-driven cell injector installed on the robotic cell injection system, which aims to eliminate the lateral vibration of the pipette (Huang et al., 2011). The piezo stack is assembled at the distal end of the piezo-driven injector to minimize the load on the piezo stack. All other parts are placed on the fixed end. The immovable components are made of low-density material (acrylic). As shown in Fig. 3.9A, the injection pipette can be easily replaced and fixed with a rubber ring. The soft plastic pressure tube can inject the solution into the cells. Fig. 3.9B shows the prototype of a piezo-driven cell injector designed by Huang et al. (2011). The drive system of the injector is composed of a signal wave generator and an

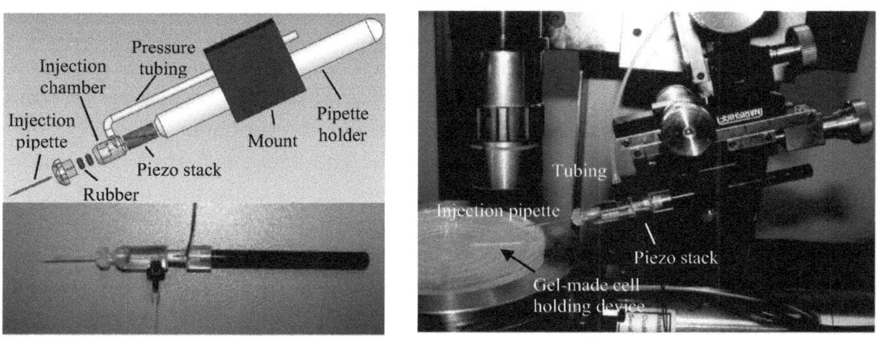

(a) (b)

Figure 3.9 Piezo-driven cell injector (Huang et al., 2011). (A) Schematic of the injector design. (B) Injector prototype.

amplifier. For simplicity, a commercial function generator is used to generate sine, square, triangular, pulse, and ramp signals of 0.5 Hz–5 MHz, 0–20 V, and input to the piezoelectric actuator amplifier. To drive the piezoelectric stack, a power amplifier circuit should also be designed.

Most piezoelectric drilling systems use adjustable duty cycle voltage pulses to drive the piezoelectric actuator to perforate the cell. The three parameters of amplitude, frequency, and duty cycle are adjusted for specific control tasks. The harmful lateral tip oscillation depends on the frequency of the excitation signal. Because the frequency spectrum of the triangular pulse is very wide, including the frequency close to the lateral resonance of the injector, high oscillation will occur at the tip of the pipette. Therefore, the single-frequency sine wave voltage signal can be used for piezo-driven cell injection. During the injection process, the tip of the glass pipette oscillates at an ultrasonic frequency to transmit ultrasonic energy to the cell membrane. Under the action of ultrasound, the cell membrane particles around the oscillating pipette tip will vibrate at the same frequency and amplitude. As the vibration energy propagates, the internal particles of the cell membrane also vibrate. When the piezo-driven injector vibrates with a pure sinusoidal input signal, the vibration and acceleration will produce ultrasonic intensity expressed as (Sun et al., 2006):

$$I = \frac{1}{2}\rho v(2\pi f)^2 \varepsilon_m^2, \tag{3.12}$$

where ρ is the cell membrane density, v is the velocity of ultrasonic wave transmission in the medium, and f and ε_m are the vibration frequency and amplitude.

Taking into account the number of cell membrane layers, each particle layer in the cell membrane is alternately compressed and stretched by ultrasonic waves. This is the so-called ultrasonic mechanical effect. Due to the high frequency, the mechanical action of ultrasound can produce huge force and instantaneous acceleration on local tissues. Due to the large alternately applied ultrasonic force, some small deformations appear in the internal tissue medium. The stress is highly concentrated in these microdeformations.

When the ultrasonic intensity is high, the cell membrane ruptures as the stress exceeds its compression or tensile elastic limit. As can be seen from Sun et al. (2006) and Eq. (3.12), the particle acceleration of the cell membrane and square root of sound intensity are directly proportional to the vibration amplitude of the particle. When the ultrasonic energy is above the ultrasonic cavitation threshold, ultrasonic cavitation will occur, which will damage the injected cells and cause cell wall perforation to spread. Small vacuum bubbles or voids will grow in the cells, and the injected cell wall will rupture. Therefore, cavitation contributes to the perforation of the cell wall.

To verify the effectiveness of the piezo-driven cell injection method, experiments were performed on injection of zebrafish embryos using the setup shown in Fig. 3.9. The radius of the injection pipette was 7.5 μm. A series of sine wave signals (frequency 0.5 Hz–40 kHz, amplitude 10 V) were used as excitation signals for piezoelectric actuators. When the piezoelectric actuator vibrated, the injection pipette also vibrated laterally, which may damage the cells. Fig. 3.10 illustrates the vibration responses when the pipette tip was in the air and water during the piercing of zebrafish

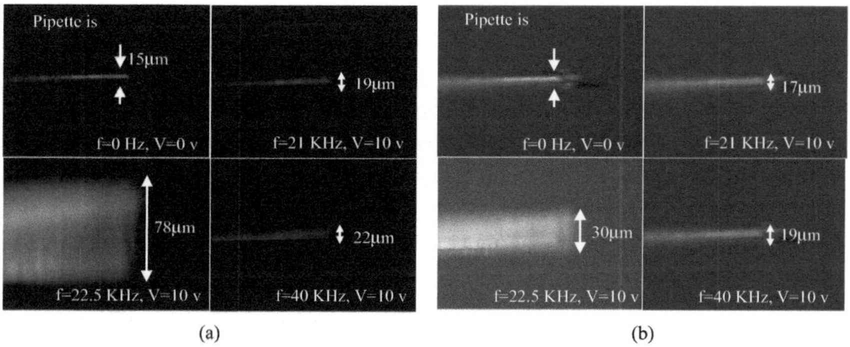

Figure 3.10 The inspiring pulse signals for piezo-driven cell injection (Huang et al., 2011). (A) Lateral vibration of pipette tip in the air. (B) Lateral vibration of pipette immersed in water.

embryos. From these tests, the ideal parameters were determined to be 21 kHz and 10 V, since the oscillating amplitude under these parameters was the lowest (i.e., 17 μm). The lateral oscillation of the pipette tip means that the size of the injected cells cannot be arbitrarily small. In addition, thicker cell walls move with the lateral vibration of the injection pipette, which may cause greater cell damage. Therefore, cells with relatively thin cell walls (such as zebrafish cells) are more suitable for piezoelectric-driven injection.

In the cell injection experiments of Huang et al. (2011), a robotic microinjection system continuously injected ntl-MO (no-tailed morpholino oligonucleotide) into a total of 200 embryos to simulate typical injection materials used in zebrafish research. The injected ntl-MO chemicals led to the development of tailless zebrafish. To quantitatively evaluate the performance of the piezo-driven injection system, two indicators were used. The first indicator is survival rate, which is defined as the ratio of the number of injected embryos that can develop into larvae to the total number of injected embryos, representing the severity of cell damage after injection. If the injection causes less cell damage, the embryo is more likely to survive and develop normally. Based on 200 injected zebrafish embryos, an overall survival rate of 96% was achieved when using the developed piezo-driven cell injection system. The second indicator is the success rate. This measure is defined as the ratio between the number of embryos with material successfully deposited in the cytoplasmic center and the total number of embryos injected. In essence, this measure represents the reliability and repeatability of the system. It differs from the survival rate in that it assesses the correctness of the required deposition destination. The experimental results showed that the overall success rate can reach 80.7%, showing a high degree of repeatability of the piezo-driven cell injection system.

3.5 Automated microinjection for small human cells

The research described above focuses on the injection of large-scale cells (such as zebrafish embryos), usually 50 μm–1 mm in size. Most human cells are smaller, for example, smaller than 20 μm. The automated injection of small cells, especially small adherent cells, encounters many challenges. First, the shape of adherent cells is irregular, which makes it difficult to automate the cell recognition process robustly, especially when the cells are very small. Second, the height of the cells adhering to the substrate is only a few microns, which requires high precision when manipulating the needle and the cells at the same time. Third, the injection of small (<20 μm) adherent cells requires a much smaller micropipette. Chow et al. (2016a) developed an automated high-throughput cell injection system for small cells. Through this research, a vacuum-based microfluidic chip was designed, which can be used as a cell holder to position each single cell in a regular-shaped channel. Regularly shaped channels can fix cells in a one-dimensional (1D) array, which greatly simplifies the cell search process during microinjection.

Fig. 3.11A illustrates a schematic of an injection system that consists of an injection module, control module, and vision module. The injection module is composed of an $X-Y$ stage, a Z-axis linear stage, a micropipette, a microfluidic cell-holding device, and a pressure-based microinjector. The microfluidic cell holder is placed inside a Petri dish, which is fixed in the $X-Y$ stage with two clamps. A glass micropipette, with an outer diameter of 1.0 mm and an inner diameter of 0.5 mm, is heated and pulled using a laser-based micropipette puller. The micropipette is mounted on the Z-axis linear stage and connected to the microinjector via a pressure tube. The diameter of the micropipette tip is approximately 0.5 μm. The microinjector is connected to the outlet cell holder and provides negative pressure. The control module is composed of a computer and a motion controller. The vision module consists of a CCD camera and an objective lens, which are installed at the two ends of the observation tube. The light source provides illumination. Images are captured and displayed using image-processing technology. Both the injection module and the vision module are placed in a PMMA chamber, which is installed on an antivibration table. Fig. 3.11B illustrates the use of a bent micropipette to inject cells on a specially designed microfluidic-based cell holder. The cell holder contains many regularly shaped channels, and each channel allows a cell to be docked.

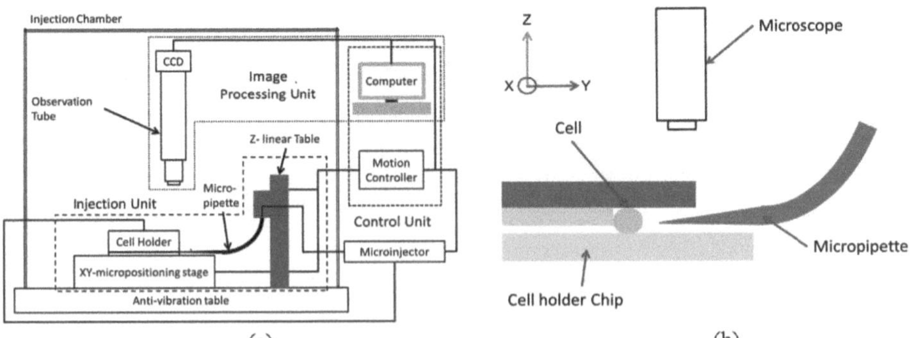

Figure 3.11 Microinjection system for small adherent cells (Chow et al., 2016a). (A) Schematic of a microinjection system. (B) Use of a bent micropipette to inject cells located in a cell holder.

The cell holder chip adopts a biequivalent tree-like symmetric structure, which can capture and dock cells to form a 1D array of 256 cells. The chip is made of polydimethylsiloxane (PDMS), which is a biocompatible material. It is designed in two layers, a thin layer (3−5 μm) and a thick layer (10−15 μm). Fig. 3.12A shows the two-layer structure forming the hydrodynamic cell capture channel. The size of the capture channel (including thin and thick layers) can be adjusted according to the size of the injected cells. The size should be equal to or slightly smaller than the cell size (for example, 80%−100% of the cell diameter), so it can generate greater friction to firmly hold the cell during the injection process. Too small a channel may put a lot of pressure on the cells, thereby reducing cell viability. The design of the thin channel allows cells to be sucked through the capture zone. Because the adherent cell is very soft, it is easy to squeeze out of the thin channel if the height of the thin channel is not low enough. Therefore, the height of the thin channel can be designed to be 25% or less of the cell diameter. The negative pressure provided by the microinjector generates a current, which flows from the cell docking area to the outlet of the chip. Cells move toward the channel with the fluid, but cannot pass through the channel due to size limitations. The above-mentioned microfluidic chip design has three advantages. First, the cell holder can use different sizes for each channel to capture cells of different sizes. In the study of Chow et al. (2016a), the cell holder was used to capture human cells with diameters of 10−25 μm. Second, the cell holder can capture cells and form a 1D cell array, which simplifies the cell recognition process and improves throughput. Third, the combination of the cell holder design and the bent micropipette can simplify the injection process of uniaxial motion. Fig. 3.12B shows the cell holder prototype.

A visual-guided position control scheme, as shown in Fig. 3.13, can be used to automate the cell injection process. Initially, the micropipette and the cell holder are aligned with the Z-axis direction to stay in the focused plane of the CCD camera. After alignment, the positions of the micropipette and the cell holder in the Z axis remain unchanged throughout the injection process, and the automated injection is accomplished in the X−Y plane only (see Fig. 3.11B). The control scheme includes the

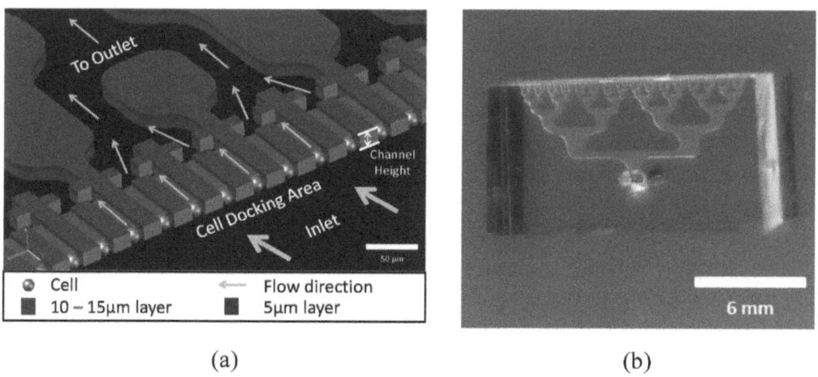

Figure 3.12 Cell-holder chip (Chow et al., 2016a). (A) Current flow diagram when negative pressure is applied to the cell holder outlet. (B) Cell holder prototype.

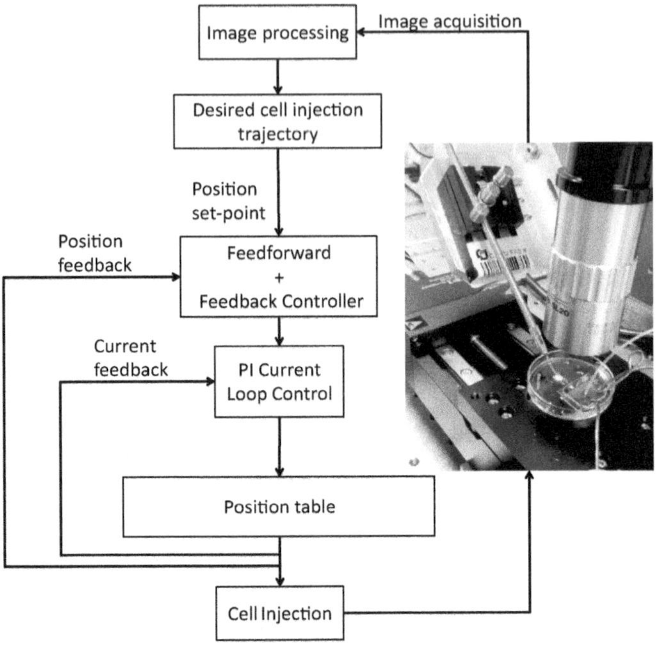

Figure 3.13 A visual-based feedback control scheme (Chow et al., 2016a).

identification of cell position using image-processing technology and the control of the $X-Y$ stage to drive the cell holder to complete the injection process. Considering that the frame rate of the CCD camera is relatively low, the use of visual feedback in the controller reduces the sampling frequency and degrades injection performance. To solve this problem, a motor encoder can be mounted on the $X-Y$ stage to measure positions with high sampling frequency (e.g., 1000 Hz). The images acquired by the CCD camera are used to locate the cells and determine the destination of the injection motion. The information is then used to guide the $X-Y$ stage toward the micropipette. The control algorithm for each motion axis employs a feedforward plus PID (proportional-integral-derivative) feedback control.

The cell holder design shown in Fig. 3.12 can greatly simplify the process of identifying target cells. The morphology of human cells is irregular, so common image-processing techniques such as Hough transform may not work effectively. Using the cell holder as shown in Fig. 3.12, irregular cells can be captured into a regular-shaped structure, which greatly simplifies the recognition process. In this way, the cell-tracking problem is changed to determine whether the cell channel is filled up by the cell. When a channel is occupied by a cell, there will be an extra semicircular edge in the image (see Fig. 3.14), while an empty channel has no such edge. Therefore, the identification problem is reduced to edge detection. Fig. 3.14A shows a template image used by the system. Fig. 3.14B shows the captured image preprocessed with a low-pass Gaussian filter, and the edge information is extracted using the Sobel edge detector. The extracted contours are further smoothened by a

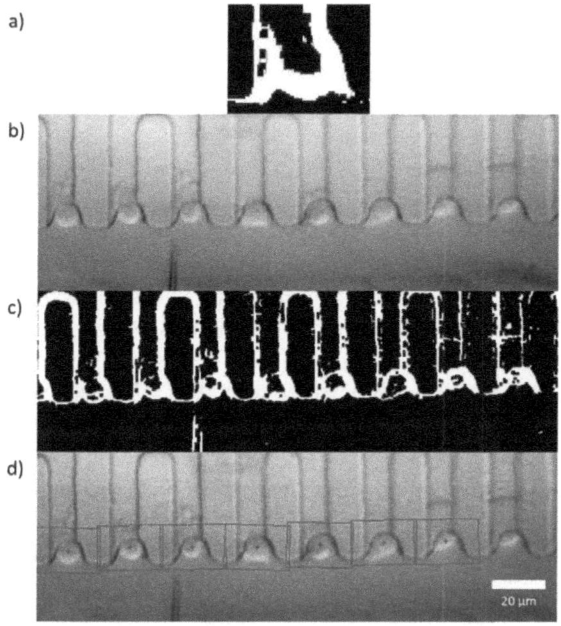

Figure 3.14 Cell-recognizing process (Chow et al., 2016a). (A) Template image. (B) Original image. (C) Preprocessed image. (D) Recognition result after applying edge template matching algorithm.

morphological operation, as shown in Fig. 3.14C. By applying the edge-matching algorithm, the correlation between the actual image and the template image can be obtained. If the correlation is large enough, the center of the template is accepted as the position of the cell center, as shown in Fig. 3.14D. The image-processing algorithm can be evaluated according to five criteria: true positive (TP), false positive (FP), true negative (TN), false negative (FN), and accuracy (ACC), which are defined as follows:

TP = no. of occupied cell channels recognized as targets;
FP = no. of empty cell channels recognized as valid targets;
TN = no. of empty cell channels ignored;
FN = no. of occupied cell channels ignored;

$$ACC = \frac{TP + TN}{\text{no.of total cell channels}}.$$

With the above method, injection experiments on human foreskin fibroblasts (HFFs) and human embryonic stem cell-derived vascular cardiomyocytes (hESC-VCMs) were performed by Chow et al. (2016a). Before the experiments, the cells were enzymatically detached from the cell culture plate and isolated to single cells. The cells were then suspended in the stated culture medium. The microfluidic cell holder was sterilized by flowing 70% ethanol through the channel for 10 min. The channels were rinsed by flowing DMEM for 10 min. The chip was then exposed to UV for 30 min and filled with cell culture medium by connecting its outlet to a 1-mL syringe (BD Falcon). The chip was vacuumed and fixed in a Petri dish filled with the cell culture medium. Negative pressure was applied to the chip by connecting the outlet to the microinjector through polyethylene tubing. In the experiment, the cell was aligned with the micropipette, and the cell holder moved toward the micropipette and then stopped for injection. After injection, the cell holder moved back to the original position and moved horizontally so that the next target cell was aligned with the cell micropipette. The process was repeated until all the trapped cells were injected. The total injection process for a single cell, including recognizing the trapped cell in channel, moving the cell holder mounted on the position table, and performing injection, took approximately 1.7 s.

To verify the cell recognition efficiency, a total of 377 cells were processed in the experiment. The cell recognition results are: TP (340), TN (9), FP (23), FN (5). The accuracy of the cell recognition algorithm was 92.6%, indicating that the system can recognize the occupied cell channels as targets and skip the empty cell channels efficiently. The recognition system only incorrectly treated 7.4% of the examined cell channels. TN, FN, and FP were rare because most of the cell channels were occupied. In the above dataset, the correlation threshold was set as 70%. Table 3.1 provides a summary of the trapping efficiency. The trapping efficiency is defined as the ratio of the number of filled cell channels to the number of total cell channels. The measured efficiency was 82.2% for hESC-VCM and 82.7% for HFF in the experiments. Notably, a high cell trapping efficiency can help reduce false positives (FPs) in the recognition results. When most of the cell channels were occupied by cells, the chance of miscounting empty cell channels decreased.

To further examine the injection effect, the injected cells were analyzed using a fluorescent microscope. The injected cell showed red fluorescence if the dye was successfully injected into the cell. Fig. 3.15A shows the images of HFF before and after injection of TRITC-dextran, and Fig. 3.15B shows the images of HESC-VCM after injection of TRITC-dextran. The summary of the cell injection performance is given in Table 3.2. The injection efficiency is defined as the ratio of the number of the fluorescent cells to the number of total injected cells, namely,

$$\text{Injection efficiency} = \frac{\text{no. of fluroscent cells}}{\text{no. of injected cells}}$$

Table 3.1 Cell trapping results (Chow et al., 2016a).

Cell type	Cell channel width (μm)	No. of channels observed	No. of trapped cells	Trapping efficiency (%)
hESC-VCM	20	714	587	82.2
HFF	20	735	608	82.7

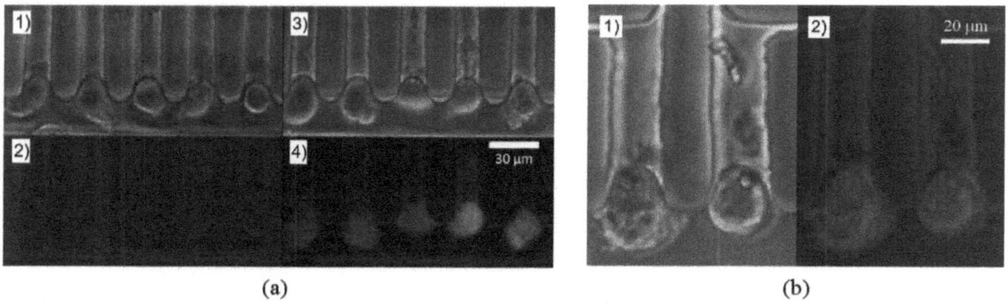

Figure 3.15 Injected cells analyzed by fluorescent microscope (Chow et al., 2016a). (A) Images of HFF before and after injection TRITC-dextran: (1) brightfield, (2) fluorescent overlaid image of cell before injection, (3) brightfield, and (4) fluorescent overlaid image of cells after injection. (B) Images of HESC-VCMs after injection of TRITC-dextran: (1) brightfield image and (2) fluorescent overlaid image.

Table 3.2 Cell injection results (Chow et al., 2016a).

Cell type	No. of injected cells	No. of fluorescent cells	Injection efficiency (%)
hESC-VCM	400	234	58.5
HFF	657	581	88.4

The overall injection efficiencies were 58.5% and 88% for hESC-VCM and HFF, respectively. After cell injection, the injected cells were incubated for 24 h to examine the cell survival rate. The survival rate is defined as

$$\text{Survival rate} = \frac{\text{no. of fluroscent cells after 24 hrs of injection}}{\text{no. of fluroscent cells right after injection}}$$

The survival rates for HFF and hESC-VCM were 81.5% and 63.5%, respectively. Fig. 3.16 shows images of the cells 24 h after injection. The survived cells exhibited normal morphology and were attached to the chip bottom (see Fig. 3.16A and B), showing that cell damage caused by injection was minimal. Fig. 3.16C and D illustrate the dead cells, which became round and were detached from the chip bottom.

3.6 Automated high-productivity microinjection for adherent cells

There is an increasing demand for high-productivity microinjection. Table 3.3 shows a comparison of existing microinjection systems for adherent cells based on injection throughput. It can be seen that most of the systems still cannot process large quantities

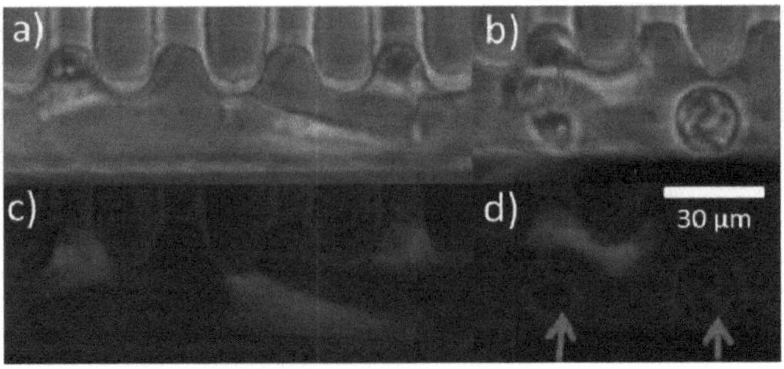

Figure 3.16 Images of HFF after injection of TRITC-dextran and incubation for 24 h (Chow et al., 2016a). (A and C) Brightfield images (B and D) Fluorescent overlaid images. The arrows indicate the dead cells.

of adherent cells in microinjection. Considering that the demand for adherent cell injection is much higher than that of suspended cells, the automated high-productivity microinjection system for adherent cells is very important to bring robot-assisted microinjection technology into practical applications. Since microinjection productivity can be expressed by multiplying the effective injection time by the injection speed, the productivity can be improved by increasing the injection speed while extending the effective injection time. On the one hand, the injection speed can be accelerated by automatically detecting cells, thereby quickly optimizing the injection path and adaptively adjusting the penetration depth. On the other hand, the effective injection time can be prolonged by using constant-outflow injection, thereby avoiding frequent clogging and replacement of the micropipette. Pan et al. (2020) proposed four approaches to increase productivity in the microinjection of cells. First, the cells to be injected are selected automatically, not manually. Second, the cell injection path is optimized quickly to save time. Third, the penetration depth is adjusted adaptively according to the movement plane of the dish holder plate. Finally, injection based on constant outflow is used to minimize clogging. The first three approaches aim to improve the injection speed, and the last one aims to extend the use time of micropipettes. Large-scale injection experiments were performed on MC3T3-E1 cells to evaluate cell detection efficiency, injection speed, success rate, and survival rate. The results confirmed that the proposed injection method can inject more than 1500 cells in 1 h without extensive manpower training and material preparation.

3.6.1 A high-productivity microinjection system

Fig. 3.17A shows a schematic of the high-productivity microinjection system developed by Pan et al. (2020), which is composed of two subsystems: computer vision and motion control. The computer vision subsystem consists of an inverted fluorescence microscope and an attached CMOS camera. Dozens of cells can be observed simultaneously in the field of view. As seen in Fig. 3.17B, the pixel coordinate frame (O_p-AB) is associated with the images, where A represents the image columns and B represents the image rows. The motion control system is composed of a motorized

Table 3.3 Comparison of microinjection systems for adherent cells (Pan et al., 2020).

Works	System type	Cell line	Injection number	Injection duration	Injection speed
Viigipuu and Kallio (2004)	Semiautomated	Retinal pigment epithelial cells; human breast cancer cell line; SH-SY5Y human neuroblastoma cells	137 cells	Unknown	Unknown
Matsuoka et al. (2004)	Semiautomated	Mouse embryonic stem cell	Unknown	Unknown	120–140 cells/h
Sakai et al. (2005)	Automated	PC-12 cells	100 cells	Unknown	Unknown
Youoku et al. (2007)	Automated	Human embryonic kidney 293 cells	131 cells	Unknown	500 cells/h
Kallio et al. (2007)	Semiautomated	Human breast cancer cell line	55 cells	Unknown	Unknown
Wang et al. (2008)	Semiautomated	Primary porcine aortic endothelial cells	1012 cells	Unknown	25 cells/min
Becattini et al. (2013)	Semiautomated	Human embryonic kidney cells; Chinese hamster ovarian cells	301 cells	Unknown	5.71 cells/min
Liu et al. (2015)	Semiautomated	HeLa cells; Human embryonic kidney 293 cells; HL-1 cardiac muscle cells	4465 cells	191 min	22.7 cells/min
Chow et al. (2016a)	Automated	Human embryonic stem cell-derived vascular cardiomyocytes; human foreskin fibroblasts	1057 cells	Unknown	35.3 cells/min
Pan et al. (2020)	Automated	MC3T3-E1 mouse fibroblast cells	6015 cells	3 h	33.4 cells/min

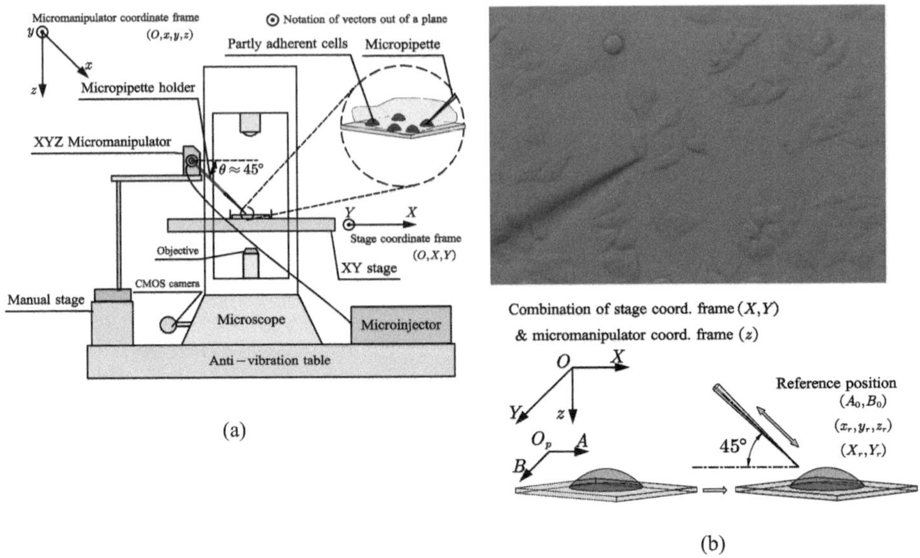

Figure 3.17 Automated microinjection system for adherent cells (Pan et al., 2020). (A) System schematic. (B) Graphical user interface and the pixel coordinate frame during cell injection.

$X-Y$ stage and a motorized $X-Y-Z$ micromanipulator fixed on a manual $X-Y-Z$ rotation stage. A stainless-steel micropipette holder holding a glass micropipette is attached to the X axis of the micromanipulator. The injection pressure is provided by a multichannel microinjector. The micromanipulator is driven by a touchscreen controller connected to the rotary wheel interface and the host computer. Cells are cultured and injected into a glass-bottomed dish, which is placed onto a hollow acrylic plate throughout the experiment. The stage is driven and tuned by an external controller commanded either by the program or by an interactive joystick. All the electromechanical components are placed on an antivibration table. The coordinate frame associated with the micromanipulator is denoted by O-xyz, and the coordinate frame related to the stage is denoted by O-XY. Most image-processing operations and movements of the motorized devices are handled by computer programs.

As shown in Fig. 3.17, the X axis of the micromanipulator is tilted to 45 degrees relative to the horizontal level. Before injection, the reference position of the micropipette tip, including (A_0, B_0), (x_r, y_r, z_r), (X_r, Y_r) as shown in Fig. 3.17B, is recorded when the tip touches the dish bottom. Here, (A_0, B_0) denotes the tip position in the pixel coordinate frame, (x_r, y_r, z_r) denotes the reference position of the tip, and (X_r, Y_r) denotes the reference position of the stage. During the cell injection, the X axis of the micromanipulator is withdrawn back 20 μm $(x_r - 20, y_r, z_r)$, and then the target cell moves to the reference position (X_r, Y_r). Finally, the X axis of the micromanipulator pushes the micropipette forward to the reference position (x_r, y_r, z_r) to pierce the cell.

3.6.2 Approaches to enhance productivity

3.6.2.1 Cell detection

Automatic selection of injected cells largely depends on cell detection and injection location positioning. In the study of Pan et al. (2020), cell nuclei were stained with DNA-binding bisbenzimide fluorochrome Hoechst 33,342 (4 μg/mL) and emitted 461 nm blue-cyan fluorescent light under 350 nm ultraviolet light irradiation, as shown in Fig. 3.18A. As shown in Algorithm 1, the cell detection procedure includes the following steps. First, the source color images I with a size of $M \times N (M > N)$ are blurred by a Gaussian function $H^{G,\sigma}(x,y) = e^{-(x^2+y^2)/2\sigma^2} / 2\pi\sigma^2$ to reduce image noises, where σ is the standard deviation of the Gaussian distribution. Second, the blurred images $\bar{I}$ are converted to grayscale images I_{gs}. Third, the grayscale images I_{gs} are changed to binary images I_{bin} using the Otsu's binarization method; the white areas in Fig. 3.18B are cell nuclei. Fourth, due to the nonuniformity of cell nuclei staining, the binary images I_{bin} are closed morphologically (denoted by $\widetilde{I}_{\text{bin}}$) to fill in holes. The transition from Fig. 3.18B−C shows the improvement of the image quality. Fifth, the OpenCV function *findContours* is used to find contours of cell nuclei and return a contour sequence Seq_i (the subscript i denotes the ith contour). Sixth, the detected contours Seq_i are approximated by polygonal curves $\overline{\text{Seq}_i}$ with the OpenCV function *approxPolyDP*. Seventh, the OpenCV function *boundingRect* is used to calculate minimal up-right bounding rectangles $\widetilde{\text{Seq}_i}$ for polygonal curves $\overline{\text{Seq}_i}$. Eighth, the bounding rectangles smaller than a lower limit a_{lo} are not used, and only those larger

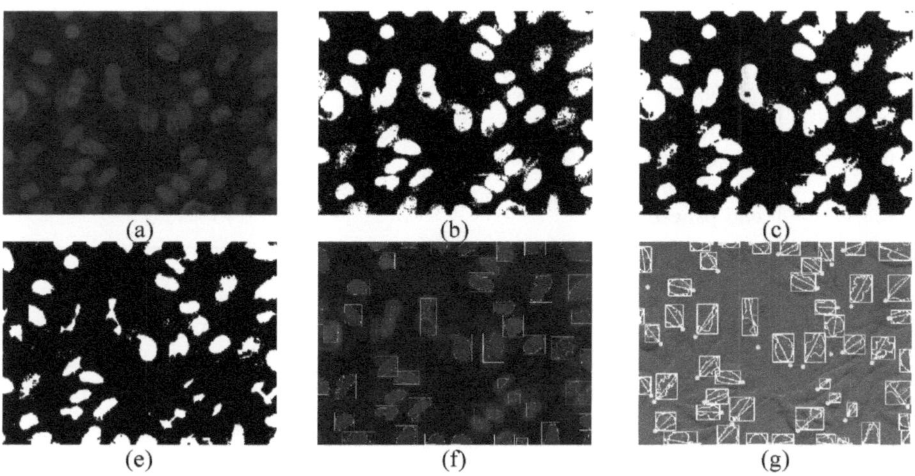

Figure 3.18 Cell detection under 40X magnification (Pan et al., 2020). (A) Stained cell nuclei. (B) Initial adaptive thresholding. (C) Binary image after close operations. (D) Binary image after erosion operations. (E) Contours found and overlaid on the fluorescent image. (F) Injection locations overlaid on the original differential interference contrast (DIC) image.

than an upper limit a_{up} are chosen to enter into a *while* loop, in which the region of interest of every rectangle is eroded and examined by functions *findContours*, *approxPolyDP*, and *boundingRect* until every bounding rectangle is smaller than a_{up}. Fig. 3.18D and E show the processing results. Finally, the function CalculateGradient is used to determine the injection position as the cell position for each detected boundary rectangle, which is a pixel ζ that is off-center along the longitudinal direction of the corresponding contour. ζ is proportional to the area of the bounding rectangle. Fig. 3.18F displays an overlay of polygonal curves, bounding rectangles, and injection sites. The sequence of cell positions $\text{Seq}_{\text{loc}} : (A_i, B_i)_{i=1,\ldots,n}$ is returned to coordinate the stage and the micromanipulator.

Algorithm 1 Cell detection algorithm

procedure AUTOMATIC CELL DETECTION(I, a_{lo}, a_{up})	
$\bar{I} \leftarrow I * H^{G,\sigma}$	$\triangleright O(6 \times M \times N \times k_G)$
$I_{gs} \leftarrow \bar{I}$	$\triangleright O(3 \times M \times N)$
$I_{bin} \leftarrow$ OtsuThresh(I_{gs})	$\triangleright O(M \times N)$
$\widetilde{I_{bin}} \leftarrow$ Close(I_{bin})	$\triangleright O(4 \times M \times N \times k_c)$
$Seq_i \leftarrow$ findContours($\widetilde{I_{bin}}$)	$\triangleright O(M \times N)$
$\overline{Seq_i} \leftarrow$ approxPolyDP(Seq_i)	$\triangleright O(nlogn)$
$\widetilde{Seq_i} \leftarrow$ boundingRect($\overline{Seq_i}$)	$\triangleright O(M_p \times N_p)$
$\widetilde{I'_{bin}} \leftarrow$ Filter($\widetilde{Seq_i}, a_{lo}$)	$\triangleright O(1)$
while $\exists$ Rectangle of which area $\geq a_{up}$ **do**	
ErodeROI(I'_{bin})	$\triangleright O\left(2M_j^p N_j^p k_c\right)$
$Seq'_i \leftarrow$ findContours($\widetilde{I'_{bin}}$)	$\triangleright O\left(M_j^p N_j^p\right)$
$\overline{Seq'_i} \leftarrow$ approxPolyDP(Seq'_i)	$\triangleright O\left(n_j logn_j\right)$
$\widetilde{Seq'_i} \leftarrow$ boundingRect($\overline{Seq'_i}$)	$\triangleright O\left(M_j^p N_j^p\right)$
end while	
$Seq_{loc} \leftarrow$ CalculateGradient(Seq_i)	$\triangleright O\left(fn_f^2\right)$
return $Seq_{loc} : (A_i, B_i)_{i=1,\ldots,n}$	
end procedure	

Several parameters and assumptions are clarified here. The source image is an 8-bit three-channel color image. The kernel size of the Gaussian filter is $k_G \times k_G$, and the kernel size of the close operation is $k_c \times k_c$. Before the *while* loop, c contours are found, among which the longest one has n nodes. In the *while* loop, the rectangular area containing the largest polygon is $M_p \times N_p$. Find most c_j contours in the jth loop, where the longest contour has n_j nodes. The rectangular area containing the largest polygon is $M_j^p \times N_j^p$. At the final stage, find f contours (polygons or bounding rectangles), where the longest contour has n_f nodes. The computational complexity of each step is shown in Algorithm 1. In the worst case, the overall complexity is $O\left((M \times N \times k_c)^{(M-2)}\right)$.

3.6.2.2 Injection path optimization

The productivity of cell injection can be improved by optimizing the injection path. The injection starts with the cell closest to the tip of the micropipette until the farthest one in the shortest path. This process is an asymmetric TSP problem ($n + 1$ nodes), which must be converted to a symmetric TSP problem ($2n + 2$ nodes) before it can be solved by the Concorde symmetric TSP Solver.

The position of the micropipette tip in the pixel coordinate frame is denoted by (A_0, B_0). The positions of n cells are denoted by $(A_i, B_i)_{i=1,\ldots,n}$. Let $D_{(n+1)\times(n+1)}$ be the distance matrix of the sequence of nodes (cells) $(A_i, B_i)_{i=0,\ldots,n}$, where $d_{ij} = \sqrt{(A_i - A_j)^2 + (B_i - B_j)^2}$. $D_{(n+1)\times(n+1)}$ is symmetric and non-negative.

To ensure the optimal path starting from (A_0, B_0), all the distances to node 0 are set to zero, so $D_{(n+1)\times(n+1)}$ becomes $\widetilde{D}_{(n+1)\times(n+1)}$. Define $\widetilde{d}_{\max} = \max\widetilde{d}_{ij}$ and transform $\widetilde{D}_{(n+1)\times(n+1)}$ to $D'_{(n+1)\times(n+1)}$ as follows:

$$d'_{ij} = \begin{cases} 0 & \text{if } i = j \\ \widetilde{d}_{ij} + 3\widetilde{d}_{\max} + \varepsilon & \text{otherwise,} \end{cases} \tag{3.13}$$

where $\varepsilon > 0$ is a small positive number.

Using the asymmetric distance matrix $D'_{(n+1)\times(n+1)}$, a symmetric distance matrix $\overline{D}_{(2n+2)\times(2n+2)}$ can be constructed as follows

$$\overline{D} = \begin{bmatrix} \infty & (D')^{\mathrm{T}} \\ D' & \infty \end{bmatrix}_{(2n+2)\times(2n+2)}, \tag{3.14}$$

where ∞ can be replaced by a large positive matrix.

The Concorde TSP Solver can be used to solve the matrix $\overline{D}$ and obtain the optimal injection path. The mapping between the nth and $(n-1)^{\text{th}}$ cells is $(A_n - A_{n-1} + A_0, B_n - B_{n-1} + B_0)$. The optimization process only takes about 0.1 s. Fig. 3.19 shows an example of optimizing the injection path under 20× magnification.

3.6.2.3 Adaptive adjustment of the penetration depth

Because the dish holder plate and the installation of the motorized stage are not strictly horizontal, the penetration depth must be adjusted according to the height variation of the moving plane of the dish holder plate. As shown in Fig. 3.20A, the stage is moved to three or more noncollinear positions to collect the stage position $(X_i, Y_i)_{i=1,\ldots,m}$ and the depth of the tip $(z_i)_{i=1,\ldots,m}$ when the tip touches the bottom of the dish, and the data

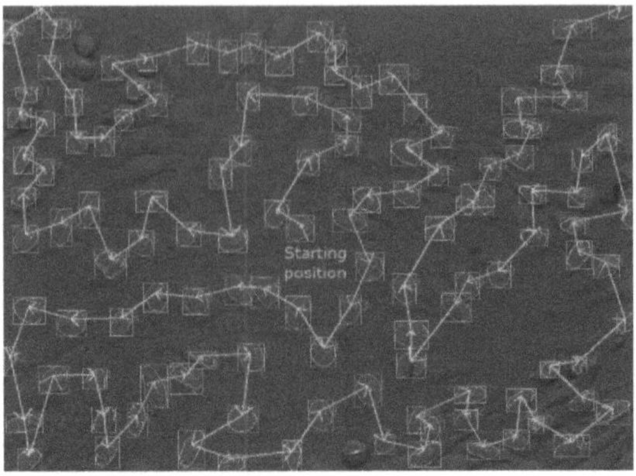

Figure 3.19 Example of generating an optimal injection path under 20X magnification (Pan et al., 2020).

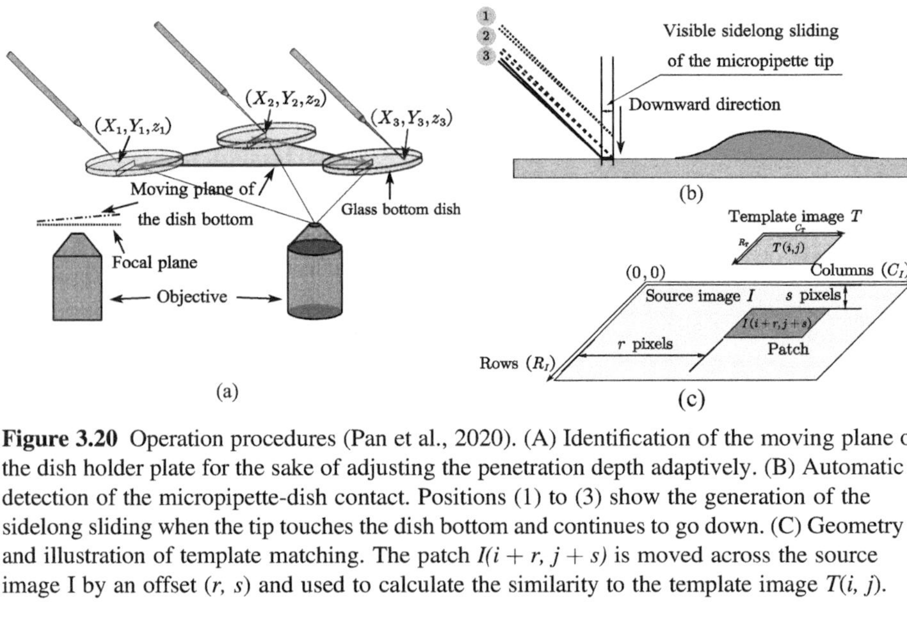

Figure 3.20 Operation procedures (Pan et al., 2020). (A) Identification of the moving plane of the dish holder plate for the sake of adjusting the penetration depth adaptively. (B) Automatic detection of the micropipette-dish contact. Positions (1) to (3) show the generation of the sidelong sliding when the tip touches the dish bottom and continues to go down. (C) Geometry and illustration of template matching. The patch $I(i + r, j + s)$ is moved across the source image I by an offset (r, s) and used to calculate the similarity to the template image $T(i, j)$.

are used to determine the moving plane. A common method to determine the tip depth is to manually lower the micropipette until the tip touches the bottom of the dish and deforms to produce a significant lateral displacement, as shown in Fig. 3.20B. This operation is time-consuming and error-prone, causing damage to the micropipette. To solve this problem, we can recursively match the template image and the source image in four steps.

First, the template image T of the tip in focus is collected. Second, the source image I is compared with the template image T to find a match. The OpenCV function *matchTemplate* with the matching method "*CV_TM_SQDIFF*" and function minMaxLoc can be used to identify the matching area. As shown in Fig. 3.20C, function *matchTemplate* selects a patch at every location in a source image and calculates the similarity between the patch and the template image, and then stores the similarity in a result matrix $d_E(r,s)$. The similarity is calculated by adding the squared difference between the pixel intensity of the template image $T(i,j)$ and the pixel intensity of the patch at each position in the source image $I(i+r, j+s)$, expressed as

$$d_E(r,s) = \sum_{i=0}^{C_T} \sum_{j=0}^{R_T} [I(i+r, j+s) - T(i,j)]^2, \tag{3.15}$$

where (r,s) is in the range $[0, C_I) \times [0, R_I)$. After obtaining the result matrix, the function minMaxLoc searches for the best similarity and finds its position as the position of the micropipette tip in the pixel coordinate system. Temporarily record these matching positions, and then compare every other position of the matching result (every frames 1 and 3) to determine whether the tip touches the bottom. Third, the micropipette is low down at a constant speed of 1 μm/s. Finally, the micropipette is retracted immediately once the position difference in the second step exceeds the threshold; at the same time, the positions of the tip and the stage are determined.

The least-square method can be used to identify the moving plane based on stage positions $(X_i, Y_i)_{i=1,\dots,m}$ and tip depths $(z_i)_{i=1,\dots,m}$. The formula of the moving plane is $z = PX + QY + R$, where P, Q, and R are unknown scalars to be determined. To avoid ill-conditioned numerical calculations, the averages $\overline{X} = \sum_{i=1}^{m} X_i/m$, $\overline{Y} = \sum_{i=1}^{m} \frac{Y_i}{m}$ and $\overline{z} = \sum_{i=1}^{m} \frac{z_i}{m}$ are calculated first and substituted into the original plane formula to form a new plane formula $\widehat{z} = P\widehat{X} + Q\widehat{Y} + \widehat{R}$, where $\widehat{z} = z - \overline{x}$, $\widehat{X} = X - \overline{X}$, $\widehat{Y} = Y - \overline{Y}$, and $\widehat{R} = R + P\overline{X} + Q\overline{Y} - \overline{z}$.

The best fit only occurs when the sum of the squared error between the depth $\widehat{z}_i$ and plane value $P\widehat{X}_i + Q\widehat{Y}_i + \widehat{R}$ is the smallest. The sum (the error function) is written as

$$e(P, Q, \widehat{R}) = \sum\nolimits_{i=1}^{m} \left[\left(P\widehat{X}_i + Q\widehat{Y}_i + \widehat{R} \right) - \widehat{z}_i \right]^2. \tag{3.16}$$

Eq. (3.16) is non-negative and reaches its minimum only when all partial derivatives evaluated at $P_{\text{best}}, Q_{\text{best}}, \widehat{R}_{\text{best}}$ are zero, that is, $\frac{\partial e}{\partial P|_{P=P_{\text{best}}}} = 0$, $\frac{\partial e}{\partial Q|_{Q=Q_{\text{best}}}} = 0$, $\frac{\partial e}{\partial \widehat{R}|_{\widehat{R}=\widehat{R}_{\text{best}}}} = 0$. The detailed calculation is presented in Pan et al. (2020).

3.6.2.4 *Constant outflow-based injection*

Clogging of micropipettes is a frequent problem that considerably impedes long-time injection and requires micropipettes to be changed from time to time. In most injection systems, such as those of Xie et al. (2010), Viigipuu and Kallio (2004), Kallio et al. (2007), Becattini et al. (2013), Liu et al. (2015), and Chow et al. (2016a), the cell is first penetrated by the micropipette and then filled by a pressure pulse of about 100 ms. The main negative effect of this method is that the inverse flow brings cell debris into the micropipette tip after the pressure pulse vanishes, which gradually accumulates to complete clogging after injecting 50–100 cells (Liu et al., 2015). To avoid the inverse flow problem, the injection sample can be pushed out of the micropipette tip constantly (Pan et al., 2020). The cell is filled as soon as the micropipette tip pierces the cell membrane. The injection volume is determined by the duration of the micropipette tip staying inside the cell. This solution not only avoids clogging but also adjusts the injection volume easily. As a result, the usage time of a micropipette in an experiment is extended, and the productivity is increased.

3.6.3 Experiments

Experiments were performed to demonstrate the following characteristics: the number of injected cells, the percentage of cells correctly detected, the percentage of cells successfully injected, and the rate of cells alive after injection. The performance of the cell detection methodology refers to its hit ratio and error rate. The hit ratio is the percentage of the number of single cells correctly detected over the total cell number, and the error rate is the portion of the number of falsely detected cells over the total cell number. Errors fall into two categories: detection of cytoplasm and detection of multiple cells. Sometimes injections in the cytoplasm or the middle of multiple cells may be successful, but only the hit ratio is considered to ensure the quality of statistical data. In a similar way to Becattini et al. (2013), the results of performance evaluation are quantified in terms of true-positive rate (TPR) and false-positive rate (FPR), which are defined as follows:

$$\mathrm{TPR} = \frac{\mathrm{TP}}{\mathrm{TP} + \mathrm{FN}}, \tag{3.17}$$

$$\mathrm{FPR} = \frac{\mathrm{FP}}{\mathrm{TP} + \mathrm{FN}}, \tag{3.18}$$

where TP (true positive) is the number of single cells correctly detected, FN (false negative) is the number of cells undetected, and FP (false positive) is the number of detection errors. Ideally, every cell is detected correctly, and cytoplasm or multiple cells are not detected (i.e., TPR = 100% and FPR = 0%). As summarized in Table 3.4, 90 images containing 3065 cells were generated and evaluated. A total of 3560 possible cells were detected, of which 2757 were true positives, 803 were false positives, and 308 were false negatives. The TPR was 89.95%, and the FPR was 26.20%.

To evaluate the success and survival rate of injections, MC3T3-E1 fibroblast cells were injected with fluorescein isothiocyanate (FITC). The cell density was retained at approximately 20–30 cells per field of view under 40× magnification. The injection sample was 0.5 mg/mL FITC. The typical balance pressure for injection was 0.5 psi,

Table 3.4 Cell detection results (Pan et al., 2020).

Image number	Cell number	Detection number	TP	FP	FN	TPR	FPR
90	3065	3560	2757	803	308	89.95%	26.20%

and the insertion duration was 100 ms. Only injected cells can emit green fluorescent light (518 nm) because FITC is impermeable to cell membranes and dissolves quickly in the medium. All cells were subcultured onto a glass-bottomed dish a day before experiments by the standard protocol. The time interval between two injections was set to 1.7 s, and the interval between two fields of view was set to 3 s. The duration for every experiment was set to 1 h, including cell detection and microinjections. Experimental results showed that a 1-h experiment contained about 50 fields of view and over 1500 cells. Fifteen minutes were used to detect cells and optimize the path, while the remaining 45 min were used to inject cells. Once an experiment was finished, cells were washed with fresh medium and then returned to the incubator. After 30 min, cells were stained with PI to examine their survival rate. PI can only stain dead cells whose membranes have turned permeable and emit 617 nm red light for visual inspection. As summarized in Table 3.5, in total 6015 injection trials were made, of which 2623 cells were successfully injected, and 114 cells died later. The success rate was 43.75%, and the survival rate was 95.74%.

3.7 Single-cell transfection through precise microinjection with quantitatively controlled injection volumes

This section will introduce a case study of the application of robotic microinjection technology to cell transfection. Cell transfection is a process wherein foreign genetic substances (e.g., nucleic acids) are delivered into cells to produce genetically modified cells. Genetic materials or gene products are usually delivered to enhance or inhibit specific gene expressions in cells so that the functions of the genes of interest can

Table 3.5 Cell microinjection results (Pan et al., 2020).

Experiment number	Injection number	Injected cells	Survived cells	Success rate (%)	Survival rate (%)
#1	1950	1058	1004	54.26	94.89
#2	2035	784	781	38.53	99.62
#3	2030	781	724	38.47	92.70
Total	6015	2623	2509	43.75	95.74

be studied. Many cell transfection methods involve batch gene transfection, which requires a large number of expression vectors for each cell and relies on a random process to provide an average dose. Because the function of a cell changes according to its location and time, the single-cell resolution of gene expression is important for elucidating gene function. Therefore, the design of a highly quantitative method to deliver precise amount of genetic modification substance into single cells is necessary.

Cell transfection can be achieved by biological, chemical, or physical methods. Biological methods employ viral vectors to achieve gene transfer, but they suffer from safety issues, such as promotion of immune responses or genetic mutations (Woods et al., 2003). Chemical methods, such as lipofection reagents, have the advantages of safety, large-scale production, and the capacity to deliver large gene fragments. However, the transfection efficiency of the chemical methods is largely affected by the cell type, reagent formulation, and DNA/reagent ratio, among others (Cortesi et al., 1996). Physical methods can achieve bulk transfection or single-cell transfection by utilizing diverse physical tools for delivering genetic substances. Some physical methods, such as ultrasound-based sonoporation (Delalande et al., 2015), magnetic field-based magnetofection (Schillinger et al., 2005), and electric field-based electroporation (Takahashi et al., 2015), can transfect a large number of cells by creating transient holes in the cell membrane to allow the passage of nucleic acids. Other methods using laser irradiation (Antkowiak et al., 2013), mechanical constriction (Sharei et al., 2013), or micropipette penetration (Ittner and Gotz 2007) can also achieve transfection for specific cell types or subcellular regions. Although most of these physical methods can achieve specific delivery, they rely on a random process to deliver an average dose, and the controllability of the delivered substance is relatively low.

Microinjection has unique advantages in processing single-cell transfection, including cost savings by controlling the amount of injected material delivered, applicability to different cell types and injected materials, and improved safety due to its virus-free nature. As introduced earlier, several microinjection systems have been integrated with robotics technology to enable automated injection with high transfection efficiency. Most robotic microinjection methods focus on automating the injection process to overcome problems that inherently exist during manual operation, such as human fatigue and poor reproducibility. To create genetically modified cells with predictable functions, a more reliable and high-throughput quantitative microinjection technique is essential, which allows a small amount of injected material to be accurately delivered to a batch of human cells. Chow et al. (2016b) presented a robotic microinjection technology that can quantitatively control the delivered substance for single-cell transfection, using the automated microinjection system, as reported in Section 3.5. The experiments and results are described as follows.

Injection volume calibration: The first experiment aimed to demonstrate that injection volume control can be achieved by adjusting the injection pressure and time. First, the micropipette was calibrated with different injection parameters, and the injection volume was measured by checking the volume change of the water drop before and after the microinjection. The water droplets were dispersed in mineral oil before injection. After several injections, the volume of the water droplets increased first and then increased linearly with the increase of injection pressure and time. Based on these calibration results, the cells were injected with an injection time of 100 ms and an injection pressure of 21 kPa to achieve the required injection volume. The operation process can be computer-controlled to ensure its repeatability and consistency. To verify the accuracy of the calibration results, tetramethylrhodamine isothiocyanate (TRITC)-dextran was injected into the water droplets dispensed in the cell-trapping channel of a cell holder chip. Fig. 3.21A shows the change of fluorescence intensity with the concentration of TRITC-dextran, which indicates that there is a strong linear correlation between the measured fluorescence intensity and the concentration of TRITC-dextran. The fluorescence intensity—TRITC concentration curve was obtained by dispensing a known concentration of TRITC-dextran solution to form TRITC-dextran droplets in oil, and then measuring the fluorescence intensity of each TRITC-dextran droplet. This curve can be used as a standard curve for calculating the concentration of TRITC-dextran in water droplets after quantitative microinjection. As shown in Fig. 3.21B, the injected water droplets show similar fluorescence intensity, for example, SD (standard deviation)-to-mean ratio = 0.124 (n = 26), indicating that the precise injection volume is reproducible. Fig. 3.21C shows that the fluorescence intensity curve obtained based on the increased injection volume of TRITC-dextran is linear, similar to the standard curve, with a maximum error of 20.3%. Similar results can be obtained after injecting TRICT-dextran into HFF cells. These results confirm that the robotic microinjection technology can deliver accurate volumes to target cells.

modRNA injection: The second experiment aimed to demonstrate quantitative injection of modRNA encoding nuclear eGFP into HFF cells. About 420 fL of modRNA of different concentrations (5, 20, and 100 ng/μL) were separately injected into HFF cells. Fluorescence signals were checked 18 h after injection. Fig. 3.22A shows HFF cells with different eGFP intensities, indicating that these cells received different amounts of modRNA. As the amount of the injected modRNA increased, HFF cells showed increased eGFP intensity, which meant that more eGFP protein was synthesized in the cell. Fig. 3.22B shows that the fluorescence intensity changed linearly with the increase of modRNA injection volume. The amount of mRNA can determine

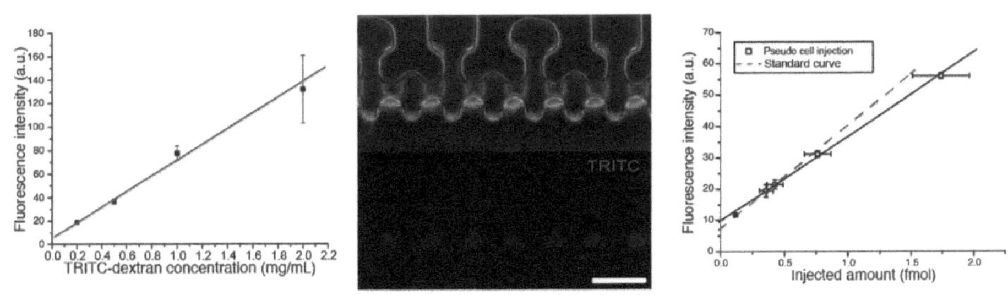

(a) (b) (c)

Figure 3.21 Pseudo cell injection (Chow et al., 2016b). (A) Fluorescence intensity as a function of TRITC-dextran concentration ($R^2 = 0.993$, $y = 5.05 + 66.9x$, $n = 5$). (B) Droplets after TRITC-dextran injection. Scale bar, 50 μm. (C) Fluorescence intensity of pseudo cells after quantitative microinjection ($R^2 = 0.999$, $y = 9.66 + 26.9x$).

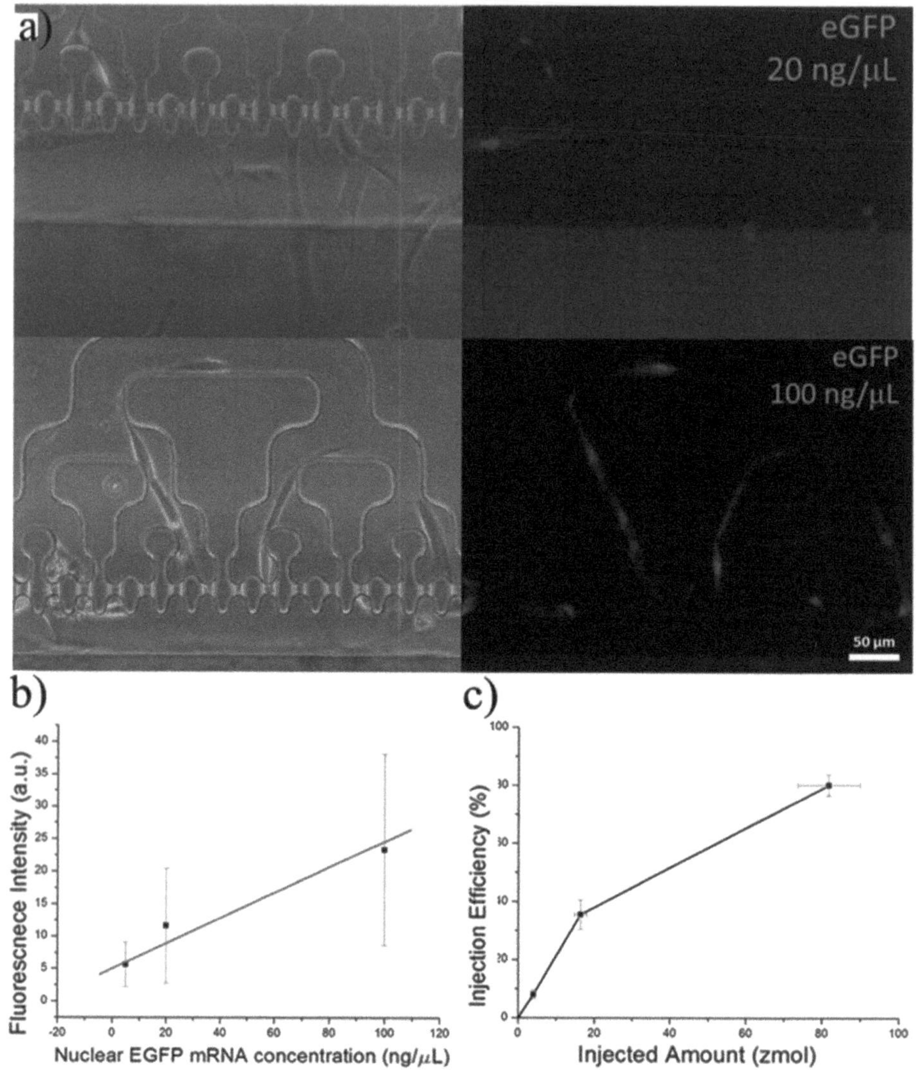

Figure 3.22 Delivery of different concentrations of modRNA encoding nuclear eGFP (Chow et al., 2016b). (A) HFF cells injected with different concentrations of nuclear eGFP encoding modRNA. (B) Linear change in fluorescence intensity with increasing amount of injected modRNA ($R^2 = 0.966$, $y = 5.03 + 0.195x$). Each measurement represents the mean ± SD of at least 46 cells. (C) Transfection efficiency of injection of different concentrations of modRNA. Each measurement represents the mean ± SD of at least three independent experiments.

the expression level of protein in a cell, which indicated that the amount of protein synthesized in living cells can be controlled by quantitative microinjection of microRNA. The transfection efficiency of delivering different amounts of modRNA to HFF cells can be further measured. Transfection efficiency is defined as the ratio of the number of cells with nuclear eGFP to the number of cells injected. Fig. 3.22C shows that as the amount of modRNA injected increased, the transfection efficiency increased. After 100 ng/μL modRNA was injected into the cells, the transfection efficiency could reach 80%. Cell viability can also be studied by incubating cells with 0.5 μM SYTOX Orange dye (Molecular Probes) in the medium for 10 min. According to Chow et al. (2016b), after 1 h of incubation, about 82% of the cells injected with FITC-dextran were alive (checked by SYTOX Orange dye) and adhered to the cell holder chip, while 97.5% of the cells without injection were alive.

Plasmid cocktail injection: The third experiment aimed to show that DNA can be delivered to cells, which represents an important strategy in a great deal of cell biology research. Cellular heterogeneity exhibits different cellular behaviors between cells and plays a vital role in the study of single-cell biology. Chow et al. (2016b) performed experiments on 14 plasmid mixtures; in each experiment, the mixture of plasmid encoding eGFP and plasmid encoding mCherry was injected into HFF cells at different ratios. Fig. 3.23A and B show HFF cells 48 h after injection of eGFP and mCherry plasmids at ratios of 1:1 and 9:1, respectively. It can be seen that $11.8\% \pm 0.807\%$ (mean ± SD) of positive cells show a single eGFP expression, $4.10\% \pm 0.68\%$ (mean ± SD) of positive cells show a single mCherry expression, and $82.8\% \pm 2.99\%$ (mean ± SD) of positive cells show coexpression of eGFP and mCherry. The intensity of eGFP and mCherry is related to the concentration of plasmid injected into the cell. Fig. 3.23C shows HFF cell without injection. Fig. 3.23D shows that the intensity ratio between eGFP and mCherry has a linear relationship with the injected plasmid ratio. These results indicate that the proportion of target protein synthesized can be controlled by quantitatively injecting appropriate proportions of plasmids into single cells.

The above experimental results have demonstrated well single-cell transfection using microneedle-based microinjection based on quantitatively controlled injection volume. The calibration substance can be used to quantify the delivery volume of the injected substance based on the injection pressure and time. In the calibration study, the injection volume is measured by the volume change of the water droplets in the mineral oil. Pseudo-cell injection experiments have proved that this method can achieve precise delivery of a small amount of fluorescent dye to the target droplet, and the delivery amount is linearly related to the fluorescence intensity. Compared with other transfection methods such as electroporation and lipofection, the robotic microinjection method can achieve single-cell transfection, regardless of the cell type or delivered substance. By injecting a mixture of modRNA and plasmid into HFF cells, the effectiveness of the proposed technology is further proved. The results indicate that a higher modRNA concentration can lead to higher transfection efficiency before reaching saturation, which implies that the amount of substance entering the cell is a key factor in improving modRNA transfection efficiency. The technology also allows for the microinjection of multiple components into a single cell. The experimental results of delivering the plasmid mixture into HFF cells have proved that different ratios of eGFP and mCherry plasmid mixture can affect the amount of synthesized protein.

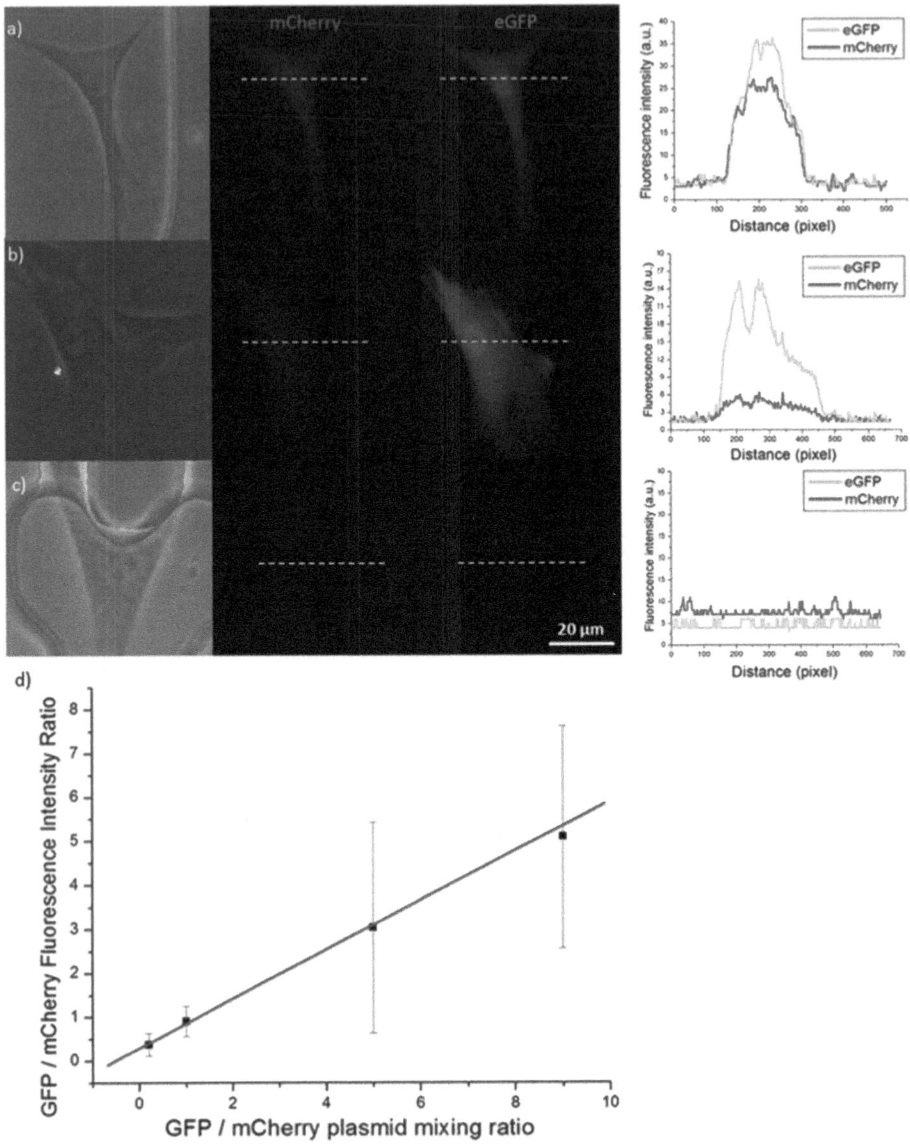

Figure 3.23 eGFP and mCherry plasmid cocktail injection (Chow et al., 2016b). (A) HFF cell injected with a mixture of eGFP and mCherry plasmids at a 1:1 ratio. (B) HFF cells injected with a mixture of eGFP and mCherry plasmids at a 9:1 ratio. (C) HFF cell without injection. Scale bar, 20 μm. (D) Ratio of eGFP/mCherry fluorescence intensity in relation to the ratio of the eGPF/mCherry plasmids ($R^2 = 0.998$, $y = 0.368 + 0.514x$). Each measurement represents the mean ± SD of at least 50 cells.

Quantitative microinjection technology can be used to study the response of cells to different doses of foreign DNA or RNA. In gene therapy applications, modRNA delivery has several advantages over plasmid DNA delivery (Leonhardt et al., 2014). Synthetic modified mRNA (modRNA) is a new type of reprogramming tool that is commonly used to control intracellular targeting and in situ logical evaluation of disease-related conditions (Warren et al., 2010). Precise microinjection methods can clarify single-cell gene expression by precisely controlling the delivery of modRNA, including the number of RNA complexes delivered and the number of proteins expressed. RNA interference has gradually become a powerful tool to knock out specific genes (Fire et al., 1998). Robotic microinjection technology can be used as a more effective and reliable tool to automatically and effectively deliver small inhibitory RNA (siRNA) in clinical applications. This method can be applied to a wide range of cell types, especially those that are difficult to treat with traditional methods. The robotic microinjection system can be used as a powerful research tool because it can deliver virus-free DNA and RNA to transfect challenging primary cells such as postmitotic neurons (Karra and Dahm 2010) and MSCs (Newland et al., 2013). Through the development of microfluidic-based cell holder chips, high-throughput and multiprocessing modules can be further realized.

3.8 Characterization of mechanical properties of cells through microinjection

Another case study using a cell microinjection technique to characterize mechanical properties of cells is discussed in this section. Cell mechanics plays an important role in regulating cellular function (Vaziri and Gopinath, 2008). How the cell responds to mechanical forces and how the mechanical response regulates cell function have become significant problems in cell biology. The link between cell mechanics and cell functions (such as locomotion, cell division, proliferation, mechanotransduction, and cell death) has been extensively studied in recent years. It has been reported in the literature that alterations to cell mechanical properties may be associated with the onset and progression of some diseases. For example, the transformed human chondrosarcoma cells with decreasing malignancy show a decrease in cell modulus and viscosity (Darling et al., 2007). Three prostate cancer cells with different metastatic potentials are distinguished by their distinct Young's moduli (Faria et al., 2008). The cell stiffness of metastatic cancer cells is much less than that of their benign counterparts (Cross et al., 2007). Red blood cells parasitized by *Plasmodium falciparum* become rigid and poorly deformable, and show abnormal circulatory behavior (Glenister et al., 2002). The Young's modulus of the virus shell in the mature form is fourfold higher than that of the immature form (Kol et al., 2006). These researches have suggested that cell mechanical properties may be regarded as indicators of the pathogenesis of certain diseases. For advantages of low cost, easy operation, and good controllability, robotic cell injection can be an effective tool to characterize the mechanical properties of cells. The characterization includes three main processes: establishment of the cell mechanical model (Tan et al., 2008), analysis of constituent materials for the model, and model verification and property characterization (Tan et al., 2010). The following introduces the characterization from these three perspectives.

3.8.1 Mechanical model of cells

Before introducing the cell mechanical model in microinjection, some assumptions on theoretical analysis are listed below:

(1) The cells are spherical, and the contribution of intracellular fluid (i.e., cytoplasm) to cell deformation is considered to be the uniform hydrostatic pressure on the membrane.
(2) The biomembrane is composed of incompressible homogeneous and isotropic material, and its thickness before deformation is constant.
(3) The cytoplasm is not compressible, so the cell volume remains constant.

As with most continuum models, it is further assumed that biomembrane is incompressible, homogeneous, isotropic, and elastic. The main purpose of this assumption is to make complex problems mathematically easy to handle. Take the membrane of teleost fish as an example. It has a three-layer thick structure. The outer layer is covered with protrusions. In the middle and inner layers, many nano-sized holes are uniformly distributed. Since the inner layer (75%–80% of the membrane volume) is much thicker than the middle and outer layers, the mechanical properties of the membrane are determined by the incompressible homogeneous and isotropic inner layer.

It is well known that the bending rigidity or the flexural rigidity is related to the cubic power of the membrane thickness in the elastic deformation of plates and shells. When the membrane thickness is very small, the contribution of the bending rigidity is negligible compared to the extensional rigidity. Therefore, the response force contributed by the bending rigidity can be neglected.

The nonlinear Mooney–Rivlin material is adopted to model the membrane, and its strain energy function is expressed as

$$W = C_1(I_1 - 3) + C_2(I_2 - 3) = C_1[(I_1 - 3) + \vartheta(I_2 - 3)], \tag{3.19}$$

where C_1 and C_2 are material constants with the dimension of stress $\vartheta = C_2/C_1$. For homogeneous and isotropic modeling, incompressible elastic material C_1 is equal to $\frac{E}{6(1+\vartheta)}$, where E is the elastic modulus. I_1 and I_2 are strain invariants related to the principal stretch ratios λ_1 and λ_2, which are expressed as

$$I_1 = {\lambda_1}^2 + {\lambda_2}^2 + \frac{1}{{\lambda_1}^2{\lambda_2}^2}, \tag{3.20}$$

$$I_2 = {\lambda_1}^2{\lambda_2}^2 + \frac{1}{{\lambda_1}^2} + \frac{1}{{\lambda_2}^2}, \tag{3.21}$$

$$\lambda_1 = \frac{\sqrt{\rho'^2 + \eta'^2}}{r_0}, \tag{3.22}$$

$$\lambda_2 = \frac{\rho}{r_0 \sin\psi}, \tag{3.23}$$

where r_0 is the initial radius of the cell, ρ and η are the horizontal and vertical ordinates of the deformed cell shape, respectively, and subscripts 1 and 2 refer to the meridian and circumferential directions of the deformed membrane, respectively. The co-ordinates are defined in Fig. 3.24. The spherical coordinates (r, Θ, ψ) are used to describe the cell membrane before microinjection, and the cylindrical coordinates (ρ, Θ, η) are used to describe the cell membrane after injection.

The principal stresses σ_i and tensions T_i of the biomembrane can be derived from the strain energy function as

$$\sigma_i = \lambda_i \frac{\partial W}{\partial \lambda_i}, (i = 1, 2), \tag{3.24}$$

$$T_i = \frac{h}{\lambda_1 \lambda_2}\sigma_i, (i = 1, 2), \tag{3.25}$$

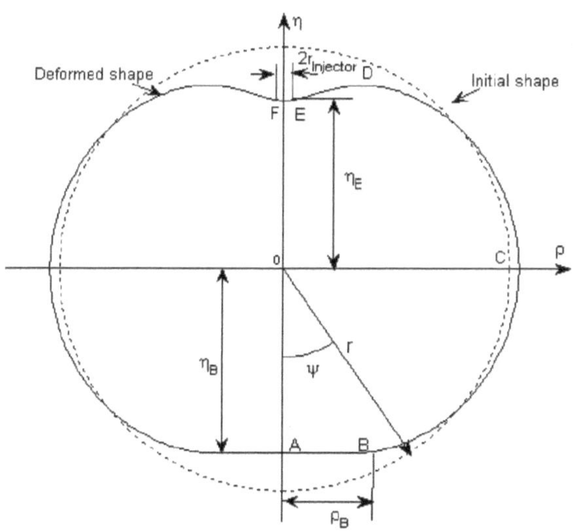

Figure 3.24 Cell shapes before and after microinjection (Tan et al., 2008).

where h is the membrane thickness. To model the deformed shape of cells, the quasistatic equilibrium equations in the meridian tangential and normal directions of the biomembrane are utilized, that is,

$$\frac{\partial T_1}{\partial \lambda_1}{\lambda_1}' + \frac{\partial T_1}{\partial \lambda_2}{\lambda_2}' = \frac{\rho'}{\rho}(T_2 - T_1), \tag{3.26}$$

$$K_1 T_1 + K_2 T_2 = P, \tag{3.27}$$

where P is the external pressure acting on the biomembrane in the normal direction, and K_1, K_2 are the principal curvatures. The prime in the foregoing and subsequent equations denotes the derivatives with respect to ψ (see Fig. 3.24).

As the first step in the mechanical model, certain material should be chosen to model the deformation behavior of the biomembrane. According to Eqs. (3.24) or (3.25), the principal tensions in the governing equations are derived. Since all the parameters of K_1, K_2, and ρ can be expressed as functions of λ_1 and λ_2, the left unknown quantities in the governing Eqs. (3.26) and (3.27) are λ_1, λ_2, and ψ. Given appropriate constraints and boundary conditions, the governing equations can be solved by using the Runge–Kutta method (Fausett, 2003). Then the cell deformation and the injection force can be calculated, and subsequently, the force–deformation relationship is established.

3.8.2 Constitutive materials of cell mechanical model

Constitutive laws define the relationship between membrane tension and strain. Several constitutive materials have been used to model the membrane behaviors of cells.

3.8.2.1 Mooney–Rivlin material

Mooney–Rivlin material has been used to model the cell behaviors (Caille et al., 2002). In the Mooney–Rivlin law, the strain energy function takes the form of Eq. (3.19). The membrane tensions can be obtained according to Eq. (3.25).

$$\begin{cases} T_1 = 2hC_1 \cdot \left(\dfrac{\lambda_1}{\lambda_2} - \dfrac{1}{(\lambda_1\lambda_2)^3}\right) \cdot \left(1 + \vartheta {\lambda_2}^2\right) \\ T_2 = 2hC_1 \cdot \left(\dfrac{\lambda_2}{\lambda_1} - \dfrac{1}{(\lambda_1\lambda_2)^3}\right) \cdot \left(1 + \vartheta {\lambda_1}^2\right) \end{cases} . \tag{3.28}$$

3.8.2.2 Neo-Hookean material

In the Mooney–Rivlin law, if α is assumed to be zero, the Mooney–Rivlin material is simplified to neo-Hookean material, and the strain energy function is expressed as

$$W = C_1(I_1 - 3). \tag{3.29}$$

By following Eq. (3.25), the tensions are then expressed as follows

$$\begin{cases} T_1 = 2hC_1 \cdot \left(\dfrac{\lambda_1}{\lambda_2} - \dfrac{1}{(\lambda_1\lambda_2)^3}\right) \\ T_2 = 2hC_1 \cdot \left(\dfrac{\lambda_2}{\lambda_1} - \dfrac{1}{(\lambda_1\lambda_2)^3}\right) \end{cases}. \tag{3.30}$$

3.8.2.3 Yeoh material

Yeoh (1993) proposed a new type of model using higher-order terms of I_1, expressed by

$$W = C_1(I_1 - 3) + C_2(I_1 - 3)^2 + C_3(I_1 - 3)^3. \tag{3.31}$$

The tension resultants are then calculated with Eq. (3.25) as follows:

$$\begin{cases} T_1 = \dfrac{2h}{\lambda_1\lambda_2} \cdot \left(\lambda_1^2 - \dfrac{1}{(\lambda_1\lambda_2)^2}\right) \cdot \left[C_1 + 2C_2(I_1 - 3) + 3C_3(I_1 - 3)^2\right] \\ T_2 = \dfrac{2h}{\lambda_1\lambda_2} \cdot \left(\lambda_2^2 - \dfrac{1}{(\lambda_1\lambda_2)^2}\right) \cdot \left[C_1 + 2C_2(I_1 - 3) + 3C_3(I_1 - 3)^2\right] \end{cases}. \tag{3.32}$$

3.8.2.4 STZC material (Skalak, Tozeren, Zarda, and Chien material)

Skalak et al. (1973) proposed using a strain energy function to describe the deformation of red blood cells, which is formulated as

$$W(\lambda_1, \lambda_2) = \frac{B}{4}\left(\frac{1}{2}I_1^2 + I_1 - I_2\right) + \frac{C}{8}I_2^2, \tag{3.33}$$

where $I_1 = \lambda_1^2 + \lambda_2^2 - 2$, and $I_2 = (\lambda_1\lambda_2)^2 - 1$. The principal tensions are then given by

$$\begin{cases} T_1 = \frac{C}{2}\cdot\frac{\lambda_1}{\lambda_2}\left[\gamma({\lambda_1}^2 - 1) + {\lambda_2}^2\cdot I_2\right] \\ T_2 = \frac{C}{2}\cdot\frac{\lambda_2}{\lambda_1}\left[\gamma({\lambda_2}^2 - 1) + {\lambda_1}^2\cdot I_2\right] \end{cases}, \tag{3.34}$$

where $\gamma = B/C$.

3.8.2.5 ES material (Evans and Skalak material)

Evans and Skalak (1980) introduced a constitutive law to model the behavior of red blood cells, expressed by

$$W(\lambda_1, \lambda_2) = \frac{1}{2}k\alpha^2 + \mu\beta, \tag{3.35}$$

where $\alpha = \lambda_1\lambda_2 - 1$, and $\beta = \frac{\lambda_1^2+\lambda_2^2}{2\lambda_1\lambda_2} - 1$. The principal tensions are calculated as follows:

$$\begin{cases} T_1 = k(\lambda_1\lambda_2 - 1) + \mu\frac{{\lambda_1}^2 - {\lambda_2}^2}{2(\lambda_1\lambda_2)^2} \\ T_2 = k(\lambda_1\lambda_2 - 1) + \mu\frac{{\lambda_2}^2 - {\lambda_1}^2}{2(\lambda_1\lambda_2)^2} \end{cases}. \tag{3.36}$$

3.8.2.6 Cheng material

Cheng (1987) expressed the generalized Hooke's law strain energy function as follows:

$$W(\lambda_1, \lambda_2) = \frac{Eh}{2(1-\nu^2)}\left[(\lambda_1 - 1)^2 + (\lambda_2 - 1)^2 + 2\nu(\lambda_1 - 1)(\lambda_2 - 1)\right],$$

where ν is the Poisson ratio. The principal tensions can then be calculated as

$$\begin{cases} T_1 = \frac{Eh}{(1-p_o^2)}\cdot\frac{1}{\lambda_2}\cdot[(\lambda_1 - 1) + \nu(\lambda_2 - 1)] \\ T_2 = \frac{Eh}{(1-p_o^2)}\cdot\frac{1}{\lambda_1}\cdot[(\lambda_2 - 1) + \nu(\lambda_1 - 1)] \end{cases}.$$

Of the above materials, the Mooney–Rivlin, neo-Hookean, and Yeoh laws are classified as the 3D constitutive laws, and the others are the 2D constitutive laws. All parameters regarding these materials in the constitutive laws must be chosen appropriately to ensure that the modeling results can match the experimental data. To this end, a deviation parameter δ can be utilized to quantitatively measure the fitness between cell modeling and experiment (Caille et al., 2002; Tan et al., 2010). δ is defined as

$$\delta = \frac{1}{n}\sum_{i=1}^{n}\left[\frac{F_e(i) - F_s(i)}{F_e(i)}\right]^2,$$

where n is the number of the sampled experimental results, $F_e(i)$ is the ith experimental force, and $F_s(i)$ is the corresponding modeling force. Given the material parameters, the value of δ can be calculated with the constitutive law. When δ is minimized by adjusting the parameters, the best fitness can be realized, and then, the cell mechanical properties can be identified.

3.8.3 Model verification and property characterization

The above modeling approach can be verified by finite element analysis (FEA) and microinjection experiments. The zebrafish embryo was used in the verification experiment, which was modeled as a spherical shape before being deformed in the commercial FEA software ANSYS (ANSYS 8.0, Canonsburg, PA). Due to the axis symmetry, a quarter of the cell was analyzed, as shown in Fig. 3.25A, where half of the cell is shown for ease of expression. The injector and substrate are represented as the upper and lower rigid half-cylinders. Hyperelastic materials, such as Mooney–Rivlin, neo-Hookean, and Yeoh materials, were used to describe the mechanical behavior of the biomembrane. The shell 41 incompressible membrane element was adopted to discretize the computational domain of the cell model. The spacing ratio of the cell size in the contact and noncontact areas was set to 1/6 to obtain high-precision injection force at a relatively low computational cost. The mesh density was carefully chosen to make sure that the solution process was converged and the accuracy of the analysis results was acceptable. To implement the FEA correctly, appropriate constraints and boundary conditions must be selected (see Fig. 3.25A). The interaction between the injector and the cell has no friction, that is, the tangential force is zero. Since the volume inside the biomembrane is assumed to be constant, the expansion pressure should be adjusted to meet this constraint under different deformations. The experimental results in Fig. 3.25B illustrate the nonlinear relationship between injection force and cell deformation, especially under large deformations. Fig. 3.25C shows the deformed cell shapes obtained from FEA and cell injection experiments, suggesting the similarity of these two cell shapes. The FEA modeling results at different developmental stages of zebrafish are shown in Fig. 3.25D.

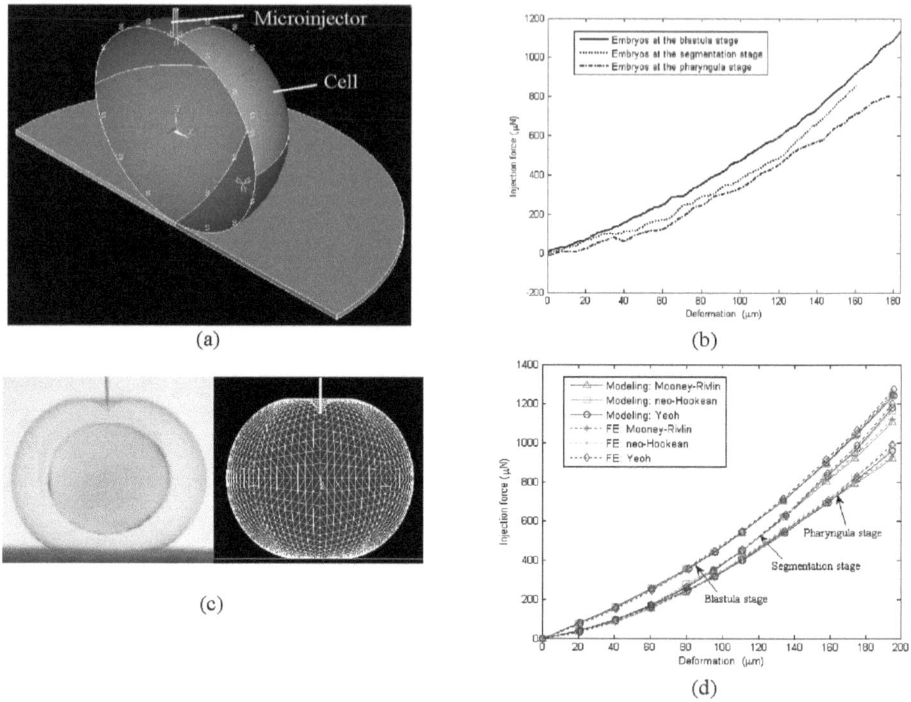

Figure 3.25 Simulation and experimental results (Tan et al., 2010). (A) FEA model for microinjection analysis: the internal pressure acts normally on the membrane (denoted by *arrows*) and appropriate boundary conditions are imposed. (B Experimental results of zebrafish embryos at different developmental stages. (C) The deformed cell shapes in the microinjection experiments (left) and the finite element analysis (right). (D) Comparisons of FE analysis and mechanical modeling results of zebrafish embryos at different developmental stages.

Mooney–Rivlin, neo-Hookean, and Yeoh materials are chosen for FEA. With the same material parameters, FEA results coincide with the counterparts obtained from the modeling approach, which demonstrates the validity of our developed model.

The model was also verified by the microinjection experiments. Fig. 3.26 shows the comparison between the experimental and modeling results. The constitutive laws were used to model the deformations of zebrafish embryos at different developmental stages by adjusting the material parameters. Based on the different constitutive materials, various mechanical properties were obtained, such as elastic modulus, shear elasticity modulus, area compressibility modulus, and other material properties, and these parameters are listed in Table 3.6. It can be seen that the values of the material parameters in Table 3.6 decrease from the blastula stage to the pharyngula stage for all the constitutive materials, indicating that the zebrafish embryo became soft. The elastic moduli obtained from the three-dimensional constitutive materials are different, where the values acquired from Mooney–Rivlin material are the largest, followed by neo-

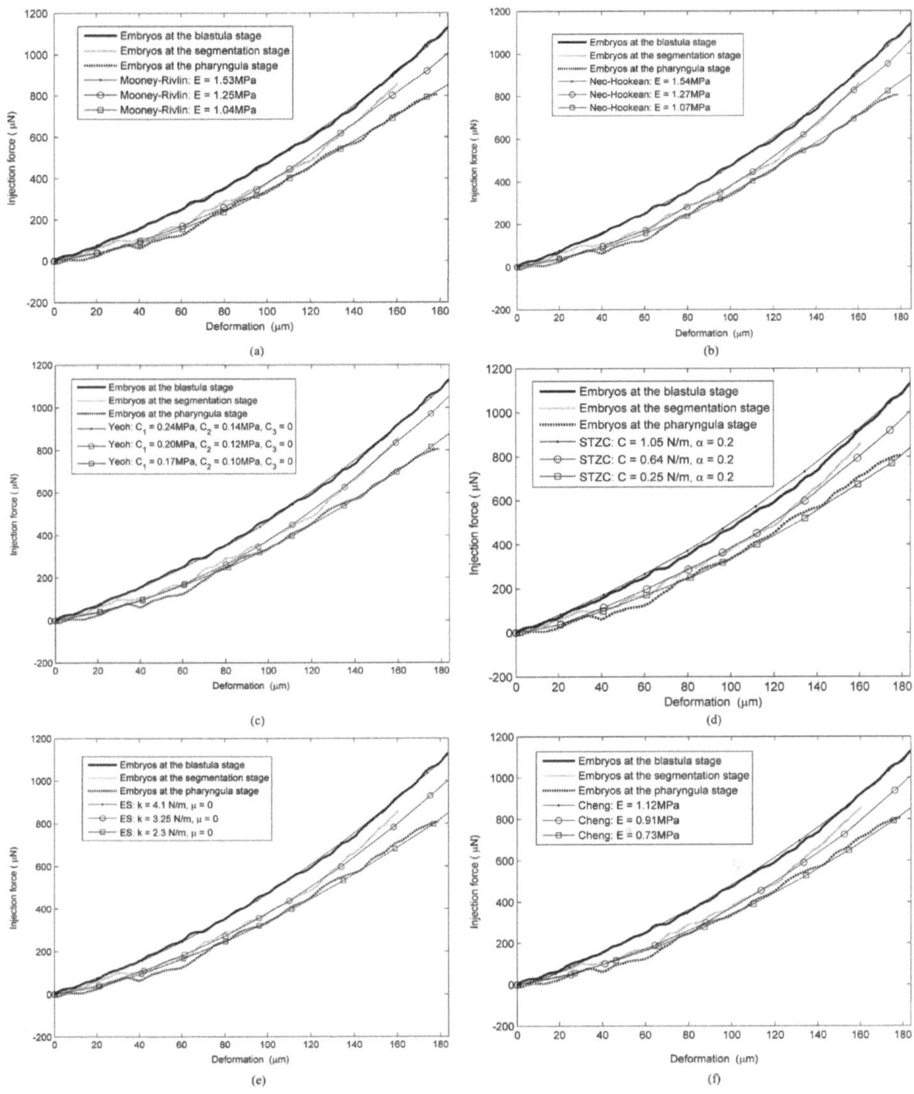

Figure 3.26 Comparisons of the experimental results and mechanical modeling results of zebrafish embryos at different developmental stages based on various constitutive materials (Tan et al., 2010). (A) Mooney–Rivlin material. (B) Neo-Hookean material. (C) Yeoh material. (D) STZC material. (E) ES material. (F) Cheng material.

Hookean material, and the elastic moduli from Yeoh material are the smallest. The elasticity modulus calculated from STZC material contributes to the mechanical responses in both shearing deformation and area change, which is much higher than that of red blood cells. Moreover, the area compressibility modulus obtained from ES material is significantly larger than that of red blood cells, suggesting that the

Table 3.6 Modeling parameters for different constitutive materials (Tan et al., 2010).

Stage / Material	Blastula	Segmentation	Pharyngula
Mooney–Rivlin	$C_1 = 0.2125 \pm 0.0012$, $\vartheta = 0.2$	$C_1 = 0.1736 \pm 0.0025$, $\vartheta = 0.2$	$C_1 = 0.1444 \pm 0.0014$, $\vartheta = 0.2$
Neo-Hookean	$C_1 = 0.2567 \pm 0.0026$	$C_1 = 0.2167 \pm 0.0034$	$C_1 = 0.1750 \pm 0.0017$
Yeoh	$C_1 = 0.240 \pm 0.008$, $C_2 = 0.140 \pm 0.005$, $C_3 = 0$	$C_1 = 0.200 \pm 0.010$, $C_2 = 0.120 \pm 0.007$, $C_3 = 0$	$C_1 = 0.170 \pm 0.007$, $C_2 = 0.100 \pm 0.011$, $C_3 = 0$
STZC	$B = 0.21 \pm 0.02$, $C = 1.05 \pm 0.03$	$B = 0.13 \pm 0.01$, $C = 0.64 \pm 0.03$	$B = 0.05 \pm 0.03$, $C = 0.25 \pm 0.05$
ES	$k = 4.10 \pm 0.03$, $\mu = 0$	$k = 3.25 \pm 0.02$, $\mu = 0$	$k = 2.30 \pm 0.04$, $\mu = 0$
Cheng	$E = 1.12 \pm 0.03$	$E = 0.91 \pm 0.02$	$E = 0.73 \pm 0.02$
FE: Mooney–Rivlin	$C_1 = 0.2125 \pm 0.0014$, $\vartheta = 0.2$	$C_1 = 0.1738 \pm 0.0030$, $\vartheta = 0.2$	$C_1 = 0.1445 \pm 0.0022$, $\vartheta = 0.2$
FE: neo-Hookean	$C_1 = 0.2570 \pm 0.0031$	$C_1 = 0.2169 \pm 0.0028$	$C_1 = 0.1784 \pm 0.0022$
FE: Yeoh	$C_1 = 0.240 \pm 0.010$, $C_2 = 0.120 \pm 0.008$, $C_3 = 0$	$C_1 = 0.210 \pm 0.009$, $C_2 = 0.110 \pm 0.011$, $C_3 = 0$	$C_1 = 0.180 \pm 0.011$, $C_2 = 0.120 \pm 0.007$, $C_3 = 0$

Units for C_1, C_2, C_3, and E are MPa, and units for B, C, k, and μ are N/m. θ is a dimensionless quantity. The standard deviations are also given in the table.

membrane of zebrafish embryos is much stiffer than that of red blood cells. These results indicate that the reported modeling method provides an alternative way to characterize the mechanical properties of cells. Modeling methods can use a variety of constitutive materials, and different materials may be suitable for different cells.

3.9 Conclusions

This chapter introduced various robot-assisted microinjection methods on single cells. These methods are introduced from the following aspects. First, the microneedle-based microinjection system is introduced, including system settings, system modeling, image processing, force sensing, and operating strategies. Second, the hybrid position and force control for automatic injection of batches of cells is introduced. Third, the universal piezoelectric-driven ultrasonic cell microinjection is introduced, which aims to improve the survival rate of the injected cells. Then, the focus is shifted from automatic injection of relatively large-scale cells (such as zebrafish embryos of 500 μm−1 mm) to small-scale cells (such as most human cells which are smaller than 25 μm) with high throughput. The injection efficiency and cell survival rate are discussed also. Fifth, automated high-productivity microinjection technology for adherent cells is introduced. The results confirm that the technology can be used to inject thousands of cells in 1 h, without the need for excessive training or prior preparation. Finally, two case studies using robotic cell microinjection technology are introduced. One is single-cell transfection with quantitative control of injection volume. The unique quantitative microinjection technology can be used to study the response of cells to different doses of foreign DNA or RNA. The other is characterizing mechanical properties of cells through microinjection, which helps to identify the link between cell mechanics and cell functions, such as movement, cell division, proliferation, mechanical transduction, and cell death. This chapter demonstrates that robotic microinjection technology can effectively deepen the understanding of cell functions and has great potential in promoting precision cell therapy and regenerative medicine.

References

Antkowiak, M., Torres-Mapa, M.L., Stevenson, D.J., Dholakia, K., Gunn-Moore, F.J., 2013. Femtosecond optical transfection of individual mammalian cells. Nat. Protoc. 8, 1216−1233.

Arai, F., Sugiyama, Fukuda, T., Iwata, H., Itoigawa, K., 1999. Micro triaxial force sensor for 3D bio-manipulation. In: Proceedings of the IEEE International Conference on Robotics and Automation, pp. 2744−2749.

Becattini, G., Mattos, L.S., Caldwell, D.G., 2013. A fully automated system for adherent cells microinjection. IEEE J. Biomed. Health Inform. 18 (1), 83−93.

Caille, N., Thoumine, O., Tardy, Y., Meister, J.J., 2002. Contribution of the nucleus to the mechanical properties of endothelial cells. J. Biomech. 35, 177−187.

Cheng, L.Y., 1987. Deformation analyses in cell and developmental biology part II—mechanical experiments on cells. J. Biomech. Eng. Trans. ASME 109, 18–24.

Chow, Y.T., Chen, S., Liu, C., Liu, C.C., Li, L., Kong, C.W., Cheng, S.H., Li, R.A., Sun, D., 2016a. A high throughput automated microinjection system for human cells with small size. IEEE/ASME Trans. Mechatron. 21 (2), 838–850.

Chow, Y.T., Chen, S., Wang, R., Liu, C.C., Kong, C.W., Li, R.A., Cheng, S.H., Sun, D., 2016b. Single cell transfection through precise microinjection with quantitatively controlled injection volumes. Sci. Rep. 6, 24127.

Cortesi, R., Esposito, E., Menegatti, E., Gambari, R., Nastruzzi, C., 1996. Effect of cationic liposome composition on in vitro cytotoxicity and protective effect on carried DNA. Int. J. Pharm. 139, 69–78.

Cross, S.E., Jin, Y.S., Rao, J.Y., Gimzewski, J.K., 2007. Nanomechanical analysis of cells from cancer patients. Nat. Nanotechnol. 2, 780–783.

Darling, E.M., Zauscher, S., Block, J.A., Guilak, F., 2007. A thin-layer model for viscoelastic, stress-relaxation testing of cells using atomic force microscopy: do cell properties reflect metastatic potential. Biophys. J. 92, 1784–1791.

Delalande, A., Leduc, C., Midoux, P., Postema, M., Pichon, C., 2015. Efficient gene delivery by sonoporation is associated with microbubble entry into cells and the clathrin-dependent endocytosis pathway. Ultrasound Med. Biol. 41, 1913–1926.

Eroglu, A., Lawitts, J.A., Toner, M., Toth, T.L., 2003. Quantitative microinjection of trehalose into mouse oocytes and zygotes, and its effect on development. Cryobiology 46, 121–134.

Ediz, K., Olgac, N., 2005. Effect of mercury columan on the microdynamics of the piezo-driven pipettes. J. Biomech. Eng. 127, 531–535.

Evans, E.A., Skalak, R., 1980. Mechanics and Thermodynamics of Biomembranes. CRC, Boca Raton, FL.

Fan, M., Feng, Z.C., Agca, Y., Critser, J.K., 2006. Vibration study of piezodriven pipettes immersed in viscous liquids. J. Appl. Phys. 100 (7), 074701–074708.

Faria, E.C., Ma, N., Gazi, E., Gardner, P., Brown, M., Clarke, N.W., Snook, R.D., 2008. Measurement of elastic properties of prostate cancer cells using AFM. Analyst 133, 1498–1500.

Fausett, L., 2003. Numerical Methods: Algorithms and Applications. Prentice-Hall, Englewood Cliffs, NJ.

Fire, A., Xu, S., Montgomery, M.K., Kostas, S.A., Driver, S.E., Mello, C.C., 1998. Potent and specific genetic interference by double-stranded RNA in *Caenorhabditis elegans*. Nature 391 (6669), 806–811.

Fujisato, T., Abe, S., Tsuji, T., Sada, M., Miyawaki, F., Ohba, K., 1998. The development of an OVA holding device made of microporous glass plate for genetic engineering. In: Proceedings of the 20th Annual International Conference of the IEEE Engineering in Medicine and Biology Society, vol. 20, pp. 2981–2982.

Gan, Y., Chen, Z., 2008. A Study of the zona piercing process in piezodriven intracytoplasmic sperm injection. J. Appl. Phys. 104, 044702.

Glenister, F.K., Coppel, R.L., Cowman, A.F., Mohands, N., Cooke, B.M., 2002. Contribution of parasite proteins to altered mechanical properties of malaria-infected red blood cells. Blood 99, 1060–1063.

Hogg, R.C., Bandelier, F., Benoit, A., Dosch, R., Bertrand, D., 2008. An automated system for intracellular and intranuclear injection. J. Neurosci. Methods 169 (1), 65–75.

Huang, H., Sun, D., Mills, J.K., Cheng, S.H., 2009a. Robotics cell injection system with position and force control: towards automatic batch biomanipulation. IEEE Trans. Robot. 25 (3), 727–737.

Huang, H., Sun, D., Mills, J.K., Li, W.J., Cheng, S.H., 2009b. Visual-based impedance control of out-of-plane cell injection systems. IEEE Trans. Autom. Sci. Eng. 6 (3), 565–571.
Huang, H., Mills, J.K., Lu, C., Sun, D., 2011. A universal piezo-driven ultrasonic cell microinjection system. Biomed. Microdev. 13 (4), 743–752.
Ittner, L.M., Gotz, J., 2007. Pronuclear injection for the production of transgenic mice. Nat. Protoc. 2, 1206–1215.
Kallio, P., Ritala, T., Lukkari, M., Kuikka, S., 2007. Injection guidance system for cellular microinjections. Int. J. Robot Res. 26 (11/12), 1303–1313.
Karra, D., Dahm, R., 2010. Transfection techniques for neuronal cells. J. Neurosci. 30, 6171–6177.
Katayose, H., Yanagida, K., Shinoki, T., Kawahara, T., Horiuchi, T., Sato, A., 1999. Efficient injection of bull spermatozoa into oocytes using a piezo-driven pipette. Theriogenology 52, 1215–1224.
Kimura, Y., Yanagimachi, R., 1995. Intracytoplasmic sperm injection in the mouse. Biol. Reprod. 52 (4), 709–720.
Kol, N., Gladnikoff, M., Barlam, D., Shneck, R.Z., Rein, A., Rousso, I., 2006. Mechanical properties of murine leukemia virus particles: effect of maturation. Biophys. J. 91, 767–774.
Liu, J., Siragam, V., Gong, Z., Chen, J., Fridman, M.D., Leung, C., Lu, Z., Ru, C., Xie, S., Luo, J., Hamilton, R.M., Sun, Y., 2015. Robotic adherent cell injection for characterizing cell-cell communication. IEEE Trans. Biomed. Eng. 62 (1), 119–125.
Liu, X., Sun, Y., 2009. Automated mouse embryo injection moves toward practical use. In: Proceedings of the IEEE International Conference on Robotics and Automation, pp. 526–531.
Leonhardt, C., Schwake, G., Stögbauer, T.R., Rappl, S., Kuhr, J.T., Ligon, T.S., Rädler, J.O., 2014. Single-cell mRNA transfection studies: delivery, kinetics and statistics by numbers. Nanomedicine 10 (4), 679–688.
Lu, Z., Chen, P.C., Nam, J., Ge, R., Lin, W., 2007. A micromanipulation system with dynamic force-feedback for automatic batch microinjection. J. Micromech. Microeng. 17 (2), 314–321.
Matsuoka, H., Komazaki, T., Mukai, Y., Shibusawa, M., Akane, H., Chaki, A., 2004. High throughput easy microinjection with a single-cell manipulation supporting robot. J. Biotechnol. 116 (2), 185–194.
Matsuoka, H., Shimoda, S., Miwa, Y., Saito, M., 2006. Automatic positioning of a microinjector in mouse ES cells and rice protoplasts. J. Biochem. 69, 187–192.
Newland, B., Dowd, E., Pandit, A., 2013. Biomaterial approaches to gene therapies for neurodegenerative disorders of the CNS. Biomater. Sci. 1, 556.
Pan, F., Chen, S., Jiao, Y., Guan, Z., Shakoor, A., Sun, D., 2020. Automated high-productivity microinjection system for adherent cells. IEEE Robot. Autom Lett. 5 (2), 1167–1174.
Pillarisetti, A., Pekarev, M., Brooks, A.D., Desai, J.P., 2007. Evaluating the effect of force feedback in cell injection. IEEE Trans. Autom. Sci. Eng. 4 (3), 322–331.
Qu, W.T., 2005. Chord midpoint Hough transform based ellipse detection method. J. Zhejiang Univ. (Eng. Sci.) 39 (8), 1132–1135.
Sakai, S., Youoku, S., Suto, Y., Ando, M., Ito, A., 2005. Automated high-throughput microinjection system for floating cells. In: Imaging, Manipulation, and Analysis of Biomolecules and Cells: Fundamentals and Applications III, San Jose, California, vol. 5699, pp. 59–66.
Schillinger, U., Brill, T., Rudolph, C., Huth, S., 2005. Advances in magnetofection - magnetically guided nucleic acid delivery. J. Magn. Magn Mater. 293 (1), 501–508.

Suresh, S., Spatz, J., Mills, J.P., Micoulet, A., Dao, M., Lim, C.T., Beil, M., Seufferlein, T., 2005. Connections between single-cell biomechanics and human disease states: gastrointestinal cancer and malaria. Acta Biomater 1, 15–30.

Schnizler, K., Küster, M., Methfessel, C., Fejtl, M., 2003. The roboocyte: automated cDNA/mRNA injection and subsequent TEVC recording on xenopus oocytes in 96-well microtiter plates. Recept. Channel 9 (1), 41–48.

Sharei, A., Zoldan, J., Adamo, A., Sim, W.Y., Cho, N., Jackson, E., Mao, S., Schneider, S., Han, M.J., Lytton-Jean, A., Basto, P.A., Jhunjhunwala, S., Lee, J., Heller, D.A., Kang, J.W., Hartoularos, G.C., Kim, K.-S., Anderson, D.G., Langer, R., Jensen, K.F., 2013. A vector-free microfluidic platform for intracellular delivery. Proc. Natl. Acad. Sci. USA 110 (6), 2082–2087.

Shen, Y.T., Wejinya, U.C., Xi, N., Pomeroy, C.A., 2006. Forcemeasurement and mechanical characterization of living drosophila embryos for human medical study. J. Eng. Med. 220, 99–112.

Skalak, R., Tozeren, A., Zarda, R.P., Chien, S., 1973. Strain energy function of red blood cell membranes. Biophys. J. 13, 245–264.

Sun, D., Mills, J.K., 2002. Control of a rotating cantilever beam using a torque actuator and a distributed piezoelectric polymer actuator. Appl. Acoust. 63 (7), 885–899.

Sun, L.N., Wang, H.X., Chen, L.G., Liu, Y.X., 2006. A novel ultrasonic Microdissection technique for biomedicine. Ultrasonics 44, 255–260.

Sun, Y., Nelson, B.J., 2002. Biological cell injection using an autonomous microrobotics system. Int. J. Robot Res. 21, 861–868.

Sun, Y., Wan, K.T., Roberts, K.P., Bischof, J.C., Nelson, B.J., 2003. Mechanical property characterization of mouse zona pellucida. IEEE Trans. Nanobioscience 2 (4), 279–286.

Sun, Y., Bradley, B.J., 2007. Biological cell injection using an autonomous microrobotic system. Int. J. Robot Res. 21 (10/11), 861–868.

Stewart, M.P., Langer, R., Jensen, K.F., 2018. Intracellular delivery by membrane disruption: mechanisms, strategies, and concepts. Chem. Rev. 118 (16), 7409–7531.

Takahashi, M., Kikkawa, T., Osumi, N., 2015. Electroporation Methods in Neuroscience, Chapter 11. Springer, New York, pp. 141–157.

Tan, Y., Sun, D., Huang, W., Cheng, S.H., 2008. Mechanical modeling of biological cells in microinjection. IEEE Trans. Nanobioscience 7 (4), 257–266.

Tan, Y., Sun, D., Huang, W., Cheng, S.H., 2010. Characterizing mechanical properties of biological cells by microinjection. IEEE Trans. Nanobioscience 9 (3), 171–180.

Tesson, L., Usal, C., Ménoret, S., Leung, E., Niles, B.J., Remy, S., Santiago, Y., Vincent, A.I., Meng, X., Zhang, L., Gregory, P.D., Angegon, I., Cost, G.J., 2011. Knockout rats generated by embryo microinjection of TALENs. Nat. Biotechnol. 29, 695–696.

Tiefenboeck, P., Kim, J.A., Leroux, J.C., 2018. Intracellular delivery of colloids: past and future contributions from microinjection. Adv. Drug Deliv. Rev. 132, 3–15.

Vaziri, A., Gopinath, A., 2008. Cell and biomolecular mechanics in silico. Nat. Mater. 7, 15–22.

Viigipuu, K., Kallio, P., 2004. Microinjection of living adherent cells by using a semi-automatic microinjection system. Altern. Lab. Anim. 32 (4), 417–423.

Wang, W., Liu, X., Gelinas, D., Ciruna, B., Sun, Y., 2007. A fully automated robotic system formicroinjection of zebrafish embryos. PLoS One 2 (9) e862-1–e862-7.

Wang, W., Sun, Y., Zhang, M., Anderson, R., Langille, L., Chan, W., 2008. A system for high-speed microinjection of adherent cells. Rev. Sci. Instrum. 79 (10), 104302.

Wang, W.H., Liu, X.Y., Sun, Y., 2009. High-throughput automated injection of individual biological cells. IEEE Trans. Autom. Sci. Eng. 6, 209–219.

Warren, L., Manos, P.D., Ahfeldt, T., Loh, Y.H., Li, H., Lau, F., Ebina, W., Mandal, P.K., Smith, Z.D., Meissner, A., Daley, G.Q., Brack, A.S., Collins, J.J., Cowan, C., Schlaeger, T.M., Rossi, D.J., 2010. Highly efficient reprogramming to pluripotency and directed differentiation of human cells with synthetic modified mRNA. Cell Stem Cell 7 (5), 618−630.

Woods, N.B., Woods, N.B., Muessig, A., Schmidt, M., Flygare, J., Olsson, K., Salmon, P., Trono, D., Kalle, C., Karlsson, S., 2003. Lentiviral vector transduction of NOD/SCID repopulating cells results in multiple vector integrations per transduced cell: risk of insertional mutagenesis. Blood 101 (4), 1284−1289.

Xie, Y., Sun, D., Liu, C., Tse, H.Y., Cheng, S.H., 2010. A force control approach to a robot-assisted cell microinjection system. Int. J. Robot Res. 29 (9), 1222−1232.

Xie, Y., Sun, D., Liu, C., Tse, H.Y., Cheng, S.H., 2011. Force sensing and manipulation strategy in robot-assisted microinjection on zebrafish embryos. IEEE/ASME Trans. Mechatronics 16, 1002−1010.

Yeoh, O.H., 1993. Some forms of the strain energy function for rubber. Rubber Chem. Technol. 66, 754−771.

Yi, J., 2008. A Piezo-sensor-based ‘smart tire’ system for mobile robots and vehicles. IEEE/ASME Trans. Mechatron. 13 (1), 95−103.

Youoku, S., Suto, Y., Ando, M., Popp, A., 2007. Automated Microinjection System for Adherent Cells. Biophotonics 2007: Optics in Life Science, Munich, Germany, 6633_27.

Zhang, X.J., Zappe, S., Bernstein, R.W., Chen, C.C., Sahin, O., Fish, M., Scott, M.P., Solgaard, O., 2004. Micromachined silicon force sensor based on diffractive optical encoders for characterization of microinjection. Sens. Actuators, A 114 (2/3), 197−203.

Cell stretching and compression

4

4.1 Introduction

The deformation of cells by stretching or compression is a typical cell manipulation operation. The purpose of such operations includes characterizing the biophysical properties of cells, regulating cell functions (such as cell migration and differentiation), and in situ intracellular delivery. Through integrating robotics with manipulation tools such as optical tweezers, dielectrophoresis (DEP), microfluidic channels, and magnetic manipulators, cell deformation can be automatically realized with high throughput and accuracy. This chapter introduces the use of robot-assisted micromanipulation tools to achieve cell stretching and compression operations and their biomedical applications.

Cell biomechanics is closely related to various critical cellular processes, such as cell division, differentiation, growth, motility, and apoptosis (Bao and Suresh, 2003; Chowdhury et al., 2010). Changes in cell mechanics may have important effects on cell functions and mechanical transduction. The destabilization of cellular structure can lead to abnormal cell mechanics and further lead to the development of many diseases. A great deal of evidence has shown that the mechanical properties of cells may be related to the onset and development of diseases. For example, the stiffness of metastatic cancer cells is much less than that of benign cells (Cross et al., 2007), while the mechanical stiffness of differentiated human embryonic stem cell (hESC)-derived cardiomyocytes (hESC-CMs) increases after cardiac differentiation (Tan et al., 2012). Normal and leukemia hematopoietic cell populations with unique primitive properties show different deformabilities, indicating that their biophysical properties may be related to the ability of stem cells or leukemia initiating cells (LIC) (Tan et al., 2011). The mechanical stiffness largely depends on the reorganization of F-actin, which is the basis for the functional properties of Jurkat and K562 cells treated with DOX (Wang et al., 2013). Through these studies, a deeper understanding of the relationship between cell mechanics and diseases has been gained.

A variety of techniques can be used to assess the biomechanical properties of cells, including micropipette aspiration (Rosenbluth et al., 2006), mechanical probing (Warnat et al., 2015), and structure-induced deformation (Hou et al., 2009). Micropipette aspiration technology applies suction pressure (ranging from 10 pN to 10 μN) to deform the cells and pull them into the pipette. By monitoring the deformation of the cells in the pipette, different parameters can be measured to estimate the elastic modulus of the cells. Using this method, a force of 10 pN to 10 μN can be applied to the cells, but the accuracy of this contact-based method depends largely on the experience of the operator and the experimental device that minimizes the evaporation of the medium (Hochmuth et al., 2000). Mechanical probing using atomic force microscopy (AFM) is another contact-based method that uses tools to directly characterize

Robotic Cell Manipulation. https://doi.org/10.1016/B978-0-323-85259-3.00006-4

cells. This technique can accurately quantify the force exerted on the cells, but suffers from limitations such as low throughput and the requirement for specific microwells for nonadherent cell trapping (Lam and Fletcher, 2011). In addition to direct probing of cells, cell deformation can also be induced by squeezing cells through narrow channels or other structures. Using this structure induction technology, parameters such as cell volume and adhesion between the cell membrane and the channel wall are coupled to the deformability of the cell. Therefore, differences between cell types, especially sticky cells, may cause measurement errors (Zhang et al., 2013).

Noncontact cell deformation techniques have been proposed to evaluate and analyze cell characteristics, such as optical stretchers (Wu et al., 2011), magnetic twisting cytometry (Mijailovich et al., 2002), and dielectrophoresis (Chen et al., 2014). These techniques have the advantage of minimizing invasiveness and potential bacterial contamination of cells. The optical stretcher uses two unfocused laser beams to trap target cells, and deformation of the cells is achieved by the induced surface force from the beams. However, the key limitation of the optical stretcher is the relatively weak force generated, which limits the types of cells to be examined (Hou et al., 2009). The magnetic twisting cytometry uses magnetic beads attached to the cell surface to twist the cells. This method is to used arbitrarily attach the beads to the cells, so the deviation of the position of the beads between different cells may cause differences in the measured values (Mijailovich et al., 2002). Dielectrophoresis uses a nonuniform electric field through electrode pairs to polarize and deform cells, and the hardware setup is relatively simple. High throughput can be achieved using microwell arrays or longer electrode pairs. With the advancement of microfabrication technology, microchips with different integrated microelectrode designs have been studied to characterize the mechanical properties of various cells through dielectrophoretic stretching.

Cell deformation also has the ability to transport multiple substances to multiple cell types through rupture of the cell membrane. Living cells can deform to produce instantaneous damage to the cell membrane, allowing surrounding macromolecules to passively diffuse into the cytoplasm. This idea has become a promising alternative to intracellular delivery in recent years. However, the inherent limitations of this method include potential membrane damage and poor throughput. For example, membrane disruption induced by a single nanoneedle was used to deliver plasmid DNA, but the yield was low (Han et al., 2005). With the development of nanotechnology and microfluidic technology, cell membranes have achieved high-throughput delivery of various biomolecules through the penetration of a series of nanowires (Shalek et al., 2010) or nanoneedles (Wang et al., 2014). Membrane deformation caused by narrow microfluidic channels was used to transport a variety of materials (Ding et al., 2017). Ultrasonic cavitation can permeabilize cell membranes for intracellular molecular delivery (Keyhani et al., 2001). Electroporation was used to deliver various biomolecules (Xie et al., 2013). However, all these methods cannot selectively deliver materials to target cells in situ. Microinjection (Chow et al., 2016) and optical transfection (Antkowiak et al., 2013) can achieve highly selective delivery, but at the cost of low throughput. Wang et al. (2018) reported a carrier-free method that uses millimeter-sized iron rods or spheres driven by magnetic force to selectively deform target cells, thereby causing instantaneous destruction of cell membranes and allowing foreign bodies to be delivered to the cytoplasm in situ.

The remainder of this chapter introduces numerous methods of using robot-assisted micromanipulation tools, including optical tweezers, DEP, microfluidic channels, and magnetic devices to stretch or compress individual cells. These cell manipulations can be used to characterize the biophysical properties of cell or achieve in situ intracellular delivery.

4.2 Cell stretching with optical tweezers

Optical tweezers use highly focused low-power laser beams to trap and move micron-sized suspended objects (Ashkin et al., 1986). Specifically, the amount of force (in piconewtons) applied to the cell and its degree of deformation (in nanometers) can provide information about its mechanical flexibility. The beads are attached to the cell surface and used as a handle. Cell stretching is achieved by using light traps to move the beads and gradually increasing the distance between them. Through force calibration and image processing, the relationship between the tensile force and the induced cell deformation can be established, and the biomechanical properties of the cells can be characterized based on the computational model. Using this technique, several research groups have studied the deformability of cells in physiological and pathological states (Suresh et al., 2005; Khan et al., 2009; Tan et al., 2012), and their findings provided insights into the cellular mechanics of cells.

4.2.1 Optical stretching models

Wu et al. (2011) reported a multitrap optical tweezers system for stretching a single biological cell (Fig. 4.1). The system consists of a continuous-wave laser source with a wavelength of 1064 nm, an inverted microscope, a holographic optical trap (HOT) device, a motorized stage, and CCD camera. This system can simultaneously

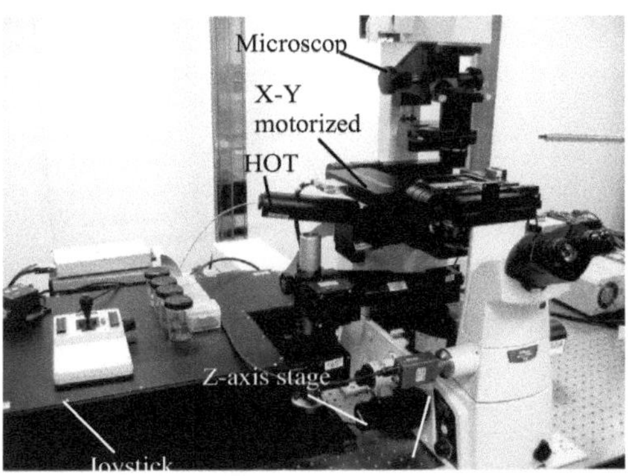

Figure 4.1 Cell stretching system with optical tweezers (Wu et al., 2011).

create multiple optical traps for many biomedical applications (Hu and Sun, 2011). The operation is conducted in an environmentally controlled room, where the temperature and CO_2 concentration are adjusted to 37°C and 5%. The optical trap is used as a micromanipulator to manipulate a single cell, and two beads are attached to the opposite sides of the diameter of the cell. One bead is held in place by one trap, while the other bead uses another trap to move along the joining line of the centroids of the two beads, as shown in Fig. 4.2. By gradually extending the distance between the beads, increased membrane tension can be applied to the cells. The cell is stretched until one of the beads escapes the trap. After the beads are released, the cells gradually return to their original shape. The instantaneous centroid of the beads during the cell-stretching process can be determined by image processing technology.

The following introduces two theoretical models in dynamic and static states to represent the mechanical behavior of cells during optical stretching.

4.2.1.1 Dynamic model of cells in optical stretching

The mechanical response of the cells can be evaluated by analyzing the dynamics of the captured beads. The force exerted on the beads includes the viscous drag force exerted by the surrounding medium, the optical trapping force, and the cell recovery force caused by elongation. According to Stokes' law, the viscous drag force is calculated as

$$F_{\text{drag}} = \frac{6\pi r_b \eta V}{1 - 9/16(r_b/h) + 1/8(r_b/h)^3 - 45/256(r_b/h)^4 - 1/16(r_b/h)^5} = \beta V, \tag{4.1}$$

where β is the drag coefficient, r_b denotes the radius of the trapped bead, η is the fluid viscosity, V represents the velocity of the bead, and h is the separation depth between the beads and the surface of the chamber right below the bead (Tan et al., 2010; Wu et al., 2011).

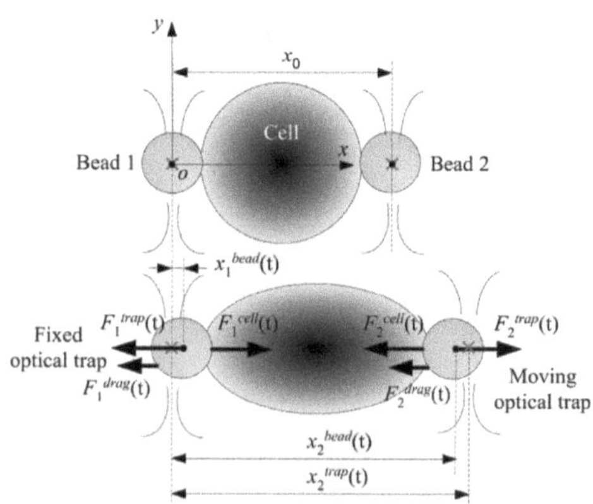

Figure 4.2 Schematic of cell stretching, where $x_1^{\text{bead}}(t)$, $x_2^{\text{bead}}(t)$, and $x_2^{\text{trap}}(t)$ are the positions of beads 1, 2, and the moving optical trap, and x_0 is the initial distance between the two beads. The dots and crosses denote the centroids of the beads and centers of the traps (Tan et al., 2012).

The optical force on the trapped bead is approximately expressed as (Neuman and Block, 2004):

$$F_{\text{trap}} = k_{\text{trap}}(t)\varepsilon = \begin{cases} k\varepsilon, & |\varepsilon| \le \varepsilon_0 \\ k\varepsilon \cdot e^{-\lambda(|\varepsilon|-\varepsilon_0)/\varepsilon_0}, & |\varepsilon| > \varepsilon_0 \end{cases}, \tag{4.2}$$

where k is the trapping stiffness, ε denotes the derivation of the bead relative to the laser focus, and ε_0 is the critical deviation, beyond which the trapping force will decay as an exponential function of the coefficient λ. The critical deviation ε_0 can be measured experimentally, and the coefficient λ can be determined by fitting the numerical results (Simmons et al., 1996) with an exponential function.

Through force balance analysis, the dynamics of the two beads are expressed as follows:

$$m_1\ddot{x}_1^{\text{bead}}(t) = F_1^{\text{cell}} - F_1^{\text{trap}} - F_1^{\text{drag}}, \tag{4.3}$$

$$m_2\ddot{x}_2^{\text{bead}}(t) = F_2^{\text{trap}} - F_2^{\text{cell}} - F_2^{\text{drag}}, \tag{4.4}$$

where subscripts 1 and 2 represent the corresponding responses of beads 1 and 2, m is the mass of the beads, $x_i^{\text{bead}}(t)$ denotes the instantaneous position of the beads, and F_i^{cell} denotes the cell restoration force, which is the mechanical response of the cells.

Using Eqs. (4.1) and (4.2), Eqs. (4.3) and (4.4) can be rewritten as follows:

$$F_1^{\text{cell}} = m_1\ddot{x}_1^{\text{bead}}(t) + k_1^{\text{trap}}(t)x_1^{\text{bead}}(t) + \beta_1\dot{x}_1^{\text{bead}}(t), \tag{4.5}$$

$$F_2^{\text{cell}} = k_2^{\text{trap}}\left(x_2^{\text{trap}}(t) - x_2^{\text{bead}}(t)\right) - m_2\ddot{x}_2^{\text{bead}}(t) - \beta_2\dot{x}_2^{\text{bead}}(t), \tag{4.6}$$

where $x_2^{\text{trap}}(t)$ denotes the position of the moving optical trap. The instantaneous positions of the beads and optical trap can be determined experimentally. Therefore, cell mechanical responses can be calculated using Eqs. (4.5) and (4.6).

Maxwell material can be used to model the dynamic behavior of cells. The relationship between stress σ and strain γ is governed by the following equation (Levinson, 1970):

$$\frac{d\gamma}{dt} = \frac{\sigma}{\eta} + \frac{1}{E}\frac{d\sigma}{dt}, \tag{4.7}$$

where E is the elastic modulus. The strain rate $d\gamma/dt$ is expressed as $d\delta(t)/\,(r_0 dt)$, where r_0 is the initial radius of the cell, $\delta(t)$ is the deformation of the cell over time, expressed as $\delta(t) = \left(x_2^{\text{bead}}(t) - x_1^{\text{bead}}(t) - x_0\right)/2$, and x_0 is the initial distance between two beads (Fig. 4.2). In addition, $\sigma = F^{\text{cell}}/\left(\pi r_{\text{con}}^2\right)$, where r_{con} denotes the contact radius between the cell and the bead. Then, the relationship between cell restoration force and deformation can be established, and therefore, the mechanical properties E and η can be characterized.

4.2.1.2 Static model of cells in optical stretching

Since the applied force and cell shape have dual rotational symmetry, the mechanical model is simplified to a two-dimensional problem. Chapter 3 uses membrane theory to simulate the deformation behavior of cells during micromanipulation. The equilibrium equations used to express the force balance of the cell membrane are expressed as follows (Tan et al., 2010):

$$\frac{\partial T_m}{\partial \lambda_m}\lambda_m' + \frac{\partial T_m}{\partial \lambda_c}\lambda_c' = \frac{r'}{r}(T_c - T_m), \tag{4.8}$$

$$K_m T_m + K_c T_c = \sigma_n, \tag{4.9}$$

where λ_m and λ_c are the principal stretch ratios, T_m and T_c are the principal tensions, and K_m and K_c are the principal curvatures. The indices m and c refer to the corresponding component in the meridian and circumferential directions of the deformed membrane, respectively. The prime denotes the derivative with respect to a specific angle. σ_n and σ_t are the applied optical stress in the normal and tangential directions of the deformed cell surface, respectively. The detailed definitions of all the quantities can be found in Tan et al. (2010).

The constitutive material proposed by Evans and Skalak (1980) is used to represent the deformation characteristics of the cell membrane. Ignoring the contribution of shear stiffness and diaphragm tension, the following result can be obtained:

$$T_m = T_c = k_\alpha \alpha, \tag{4.10}$$

where k_α is the elastic area compressibility modulus, and α is the area dilation ratio.

Given the elasticity modulus k_α, the equilibrium Eqs. (4.8) and (4.9) can be solved numerically (Tan et al., 2010), based on which the stretching force and cell deformation can be calculated. Then, the deformation−force relationship is established.

4.2.2 Stretching force calibration

4.2.2.1 Method

The following steps are used to calibrate the force on living cells (Wu et al., 2011).

Step 1 Calibrate the trapping force on the micropolystyrene bead

Micropolystyrene (PWM) or silicone beads are often used as the "handle" for force measurement. Since the force is usually generated in the lateral direction, calibration of the viscous force in the lateral direction is more important than that in the vertical direction. The trapping force on an individual bead can be calibrated in the low Reynolds (Re) number region by the so-called static drag force measurement method

(Hu et al., 2005). When the fluid passes through the polystyrene bead trapped by a laser beam, it has a deviation of x from the center of the trap. When the bead is in a state of force balance (e.g., moving at a constant speed), the trapping force $F_{\text{trap-bead}}(x)$ is equal to the drag force $F_{\text{drag-bead}}(V)$ applied to the bead:

$$F_{\text{trap-bead}}(x) = F_{\text{drag-bead}}(V). \tag{4.11}$$

Using Eqs. (4.1) and (4.11), the trapping force $F_{\text{trap-bead}}(x)$ on the bead can be calculated.

It is also noted that the trapping force on the bead is approximately proportional to the deviation x (Neuman et al., 2004), namely

$$F_{\text{trap-bead}}(x) = kx \; |x| < x_0, \tag{4.12}$$

where k denotes the trapping stiffness that relates to the laser power, and x_0 is the critical deviation when the trapping force starts to decrease.

Step 2 Calibrate the drag force on the cell

As shown in Fig. 4.3, the bead is bound to the cell, and the bead is only trapped by the optical tweezers. Note that the diameter of the laser beam is half the diameter of the bead, so the radiation on the cell can be ignored. Under the drag force, the deviation of the cell and the bead from the original position is the same. Considering the turbulence between the bead and the cell, there is the following relationship:

$$F_{\text{drag}}(V) = \alpha F_{\text{drag-bead}}(V) + \beta F_{\text{drag-cell}}(V), \tag{4.13}$$

where $F_{\text{drag}}(V)$ is the total drag force on the cell–bead mixture at the moving speed V, $F_{\text{drag-cell}}(V)$ and $F_{\text{drag-bead}}(V)$ are the drag forces exerted on the cell and the bead when they move separately, and α and β are parameters for the turbulence. The Reynolds number of the bead is depicted by (Oertel, 2004)

$$\text{Re} = \rho VD/\mu. \tag{4.14}$$

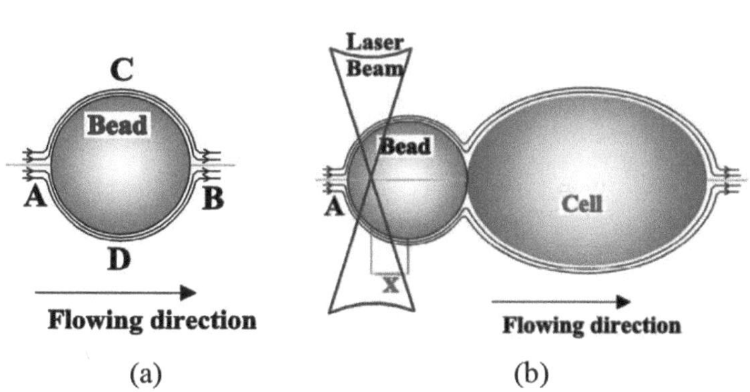

Figure 4.3 Sketch map of stream lines in the low Reynolds number flow (Wu et al., 2011). (A) Passing the single bead. (B) Passing the bead–cell mixture.

In the case study of Wu et al. (2011), the density is $\rho = 10^3 \text{kg/m}^3$, the bead diameter is $D = 3.1$ μm, and the fluid viscosity coefficient is $\mu = 10^{-3}$Pa s. When V is less than 100 μm/s, Re $< 10^{-4} << 1$, which indicates that the flow is a laminar flow with an ultralow Reynolds number. The microscale fluid dynamics, in which the flow velocity is on the order of μm/s, is very different from the macroscale fluid dynamics, where the macroscale surface tension plays a major role. In this situation, there is no turbulence, any induced vortex disappears, and there is no flow separation, as shown in Fig. 4.3. The viscous drag force is only caused by friction in the interface. Many studies have shown that the separation between the flow and the object becomes more unconscious as the Re number decreases, even when the flow passes through two tangent spheres with low Re number (Re $= 10^{-2}$). Therefore, a reasonable conclusion is that when the Re number is very low, the total drag force on the cell—bead mixture is approximately equal to the sum of the drag forces applied to the bead and the cell. As a result, α and β in Eq. (4.13) can be regarded as 1.

In the force balance state, since the radiation on the cell can be ignored as described above, the trapping force acting on the bead is equal to the drag force in Eq. (4.13), namely,

$$F_{\text{drag}}(V) = F_{\text{trap-bead}}(x). \tag{4.15}$$

Substituting Eq. (4.15) into Eq. (4.13) and considering $\alpha = \beta = 1$, the following drag force on the cell can be obtained

$$F_{\text{drag-cell}}(V) = F_{\text{trap-bead}}(x) - F_{\text{drag-bead}}(V). \tag{4.16}$$

Using Eq. (4.16), the drag force can be determined by the velocity of the cell.

Step 3 Calibrate the trapping force on the cell

In a similar way to step 1, the trapping force on the cell is then calibrated, which is equal to the drag force when the cell is in force equilibrium, namely,

$$F_{\text{trap-cell}}(x) = F_{\text{drag-cell}}(V). \tag{4.17}$$

Therefore, both the trapping and drag forces applied on the cell can be obtained.

Note that the stiffness of the trap is considered a constant for spherical particles (Neuman et al., 2004). In addition to uniform spheres, numerical modeling and analysis of biconcaves (Grover et al., 2001), cylinders (Gauthier, 1997), ellipsoids (Yan et al., 2007), and even multilayer spheres (Chang et al., 2005) show that the trap stiffness can also be regarded as a constant. As a result, based on Eq. (4.12), the transverse trapping force on the cells having these shapes can be linearly fitted by the deviation of the cells from the center of the optical trap.

4.2.2.2 Experiments

Wu et al. (2011) performed the calibration experiments on PWM beads, yeast cells, and CD34+ cells. Fig. 4.4A illustrates the result calculated by the numerical method

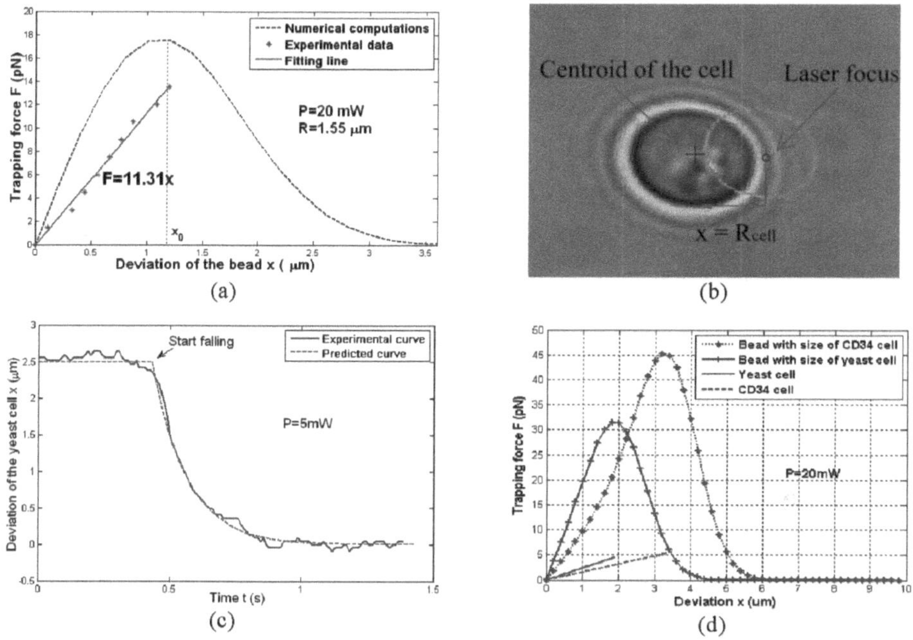

Figure 4.4 Calibration results (Wu et al. 2011). (A) The trapping force on the PWM bead. (B) Calibration experiment on the yeast cell. (C) Experimental and predicted deviations of the yeast cell falling into the optical trap. (D) Comparison of trapping forces among the yeast cell, CD34 cell, and isometric PWM beads.

(Simmons et al., 1996), the experimental data, and the fitting curve of the experimental data, with a laser power of 20 mW. It can be seen that the trapping force acting on the bead increased as the deviation increased. When the deviation was greater than the critical deviation $x_0 = 1.2\mu m$, the trapping force decreased. Therefore, force characterization should be ideally performed within the increased range ($x < x_0$). Using the obtained experimental data, the trap stiffness was fitted by the least square method. The trap stiffness of the beads obtained through experiments was about $k = (11.31 \pm 0.79)$ pN/mm. In the numerical calculation based on the ray-optic model, the stiffness was determined by the slope of the numerical curve when $x < x_0$ in Fig. 4.4A. Due to the uncertainty of the parameters used in the numerical calculation, especially when the beads are coated with protein, the refractive index may change greatly, so the numerical results are different from the experimental data. Table 4.1 summarizes

Table 4.1 Force parameters of the yeast cell with different laser powers (Wu et al., 2011).

Laser power (mW)	**20**	**30**	**40**
Trap stiffness *k*	2.52	3.62	5.01
Drag coefficient *b*	0.081	0.076	0.084

the trap stiffness under different laser powers. From the experiment, the relationship between the average stiffness of the bead and the laser power can be obtained, expressed by $k = (0.51 \pm 0.03)P$, where P is the laser power.

The drag force on the yeast cell was then calibrated. The average radius of the yeast cells was $r_c = 2.5\ \mu m$. According to the procedure introduced in step 2, after calibrating the total drag force of the bead–cell mixture, the relationship between the drag force and the moving speed of yeast cells was obtained, expressed as $F_{\text{drag-cell}}(V) = 0.081V$. Then, the trapped cell was moved at different moving speeds to obtain the relationship between the deviation x and the moving speed, expressed as $V = 34.06x$, which further yields

$$F_{\text{trap-cell}}(x) = F_{\text{drag-cell}}(V) = 0.081V = 2.52x. \tag{4.18}$$

Table 4.1 provides the calibration results of the trapping and drag forces acting on the yeast cell with different laser powers. It can be seen that the trapping force for yeast cells is approximately proportional to the laser power in the following way:

$$F_{\text{trap-cell}}(x) = kx = (0.12 \pm 0.008)Px,\ x < 2.5\ \mu\text{m}. \tag{4.19}$$

The average drag force under different powers is:

$$F_{\text{drag-cell}}(V) = bV = (0.08 \pm 0.005)V. \tag{4.20}$$

The experiment to verify the above calibration results is described below. At the beginning, when the laser power was turned off, the distance between the yeast cells and the laser focus was $x = r_c = 2.5\mu\text{m}$, as shown in Fig. 4.4B. When the laser power was turned on with a power of 5 mW, the cell fell into the laser focus. In the process of movement, the cell was affected by the trapping force and the viscous drag force simultaneously. The dynamics equation of the cell is:

$$F_{\text{trap-cell}}(x) - F_{\text{drag-cell}}(V) = m\ddot{x}, \tag{4.21}$$

where m is the mass of the cell, which can be ignored when the Re number is very small. Since the specimen stage was fixed, the relative velocity V between the cell and the fluid was the absolute velocity of the cell (namely $\dot{x}$). Then, Eq. (4.21) becomes

$$F_{\text{trap-cell}}(x) = F_{\text{drag-cell}}\left(\dot{x}\right). \tag{4.22}$$

Substituting Eqs. (4.20) and (4.21) into Eq. (4.22) and solving the resultant equation yield:

$$x = r_c e^{-kt/b} = 2.5e^{-7.5t}. \tag{4.23}$$

Fig. 4.4C illustrates the predicted motion based on Eq. (4.23), which is consistent with the actual experimental results. This verifies the correctness of the calibration result in Eqs. (4.19) and (4.20).

Finally, a calibration experiment on CD34+ cells was performed. CD34+ cells are important members of pluripotential hemopoietic stem cells. The calibration procedure of CD34+ cells was the same as that of yeast cells. The following equations were derived:

$$F_{\text{trap-cell}}(x) = kx = (0.081 \pm 0.006)Px, \tag{4.24}$$

$$F_{\text{drag-cell}}(V) = bV = (0.13 \pm 0.91)V. \tag{4.25}$$

Fig. 4.4D compares the trapping force of yeast cells, CD34+ cells, and the isometric PWM beads. It can be seen that through numerical calculation, when the deviation exceeds the sum of the radius of the cell and the bead, the trapping force on the isometric bead becomes smaller or even zero. The trapping force on the cells is less than that on equidistant beads. This explains why radiation on the cells can be ignored in the bead–cell mixture. Table 4.2 summarizes the trapping and drag coefficients of two live cells and the isometric transparent PWM beads. It can be seen that the drag force of the two kinds of living cells is about 1.2 times that of the isometric beads, but the trap stiffness of the living cells is very different from that on the beads. The difference in the trapping force between experimental results and numerical estimates highlights the importance of force calibration for live cells.

4.2.3 Stretching hematopoietic cells from normal and leukemic sources to characterize biophysical property

Hematopoiesis is a highly conserved key process, which is produced and maintained by rare hematopoietic stem cells (HSCs). Abnormal regulation of HSCs and their progenitor cells (HSPCs) leads to diseases including acute myeloid leukemia (AML). Advances in stem cell biology and genomic medicine have provided important insights into the genetic and signaling processes of hematopoiesis and leukemogenesis (Cheung et al., 2008). However, there is limited information on the biophysical

Table 4.2 Comparison of forces between cells and beads (Wu et al., 2011).

Objects	Yeast cell (experiment)	Bead with yeast size (numerical calculation)	CD34+ cell (experiment)	Bead with CD34+ size (numerical calculation)
Trap stiffness k	$(0.12 \pm 0.008)P$	$0.98P$	$(0.081 \pm 0.006)P$	$0.50P$
Drag coefficient b	0.080 ± 0.006	0.065	0.14 ± 0.01	0.11

properties of hematopoietic cells during their early differentiation under normal and leukemic conditions. Tan et al. (2011) stretched the cells with optical tweezers to verify the hypothesis that hematopoietic cells at different stages during normal and leukemia differentiation show distinctive biophysical properties. The details of this case study are described below.

Hematopoietic cells were obtained from the bone marrow (BM) of patients with AML and umbilical cord blood (UCB). Streptavidin-coated microbeads were incubated with biotin conjugated concanavalin A and then added proportionally to cells to create cell—bead attachment. Cells were contained in an environment-controlled chamber and stretched by manipulating the beads attached to the cell surface with optical traps generated by holographic optical tweezers. Cell deformation was measured by image processing with resolution as high as 20 nm. The deformation behaviors of UCB $CD34^+$ (containing HSPC) and $CD34^-$ cells (devoid of HSPC) were first examined in isotonic conditions. Within the range of the applied optical force, all $CD34^+$ cells were unstretchable (n = 6 experiments, total 221 cells), that is, no detectable deformation was found even under the maximum optical force (~42 pN). In contrast, a small percentage (15 ± 3.3%) of CD34_ cells (n = 6 experiments, total 193 cells) were stretchable, underscoring the heterogeneity of this cell population from the biophysical perspective. To increase the dynamic range in which one could evaluate their mechanical compliance, the experiments on UCB $CD34^+CD38^-$ (enriched in HSPC) and $CD34^+CD38^+$ (devoid of HSPC) cells, under hypotonic condition, were repeated. Under isotonic conditions, both populations cannot be stretched with optical tweezers, which was consistent with the results obtained from UCB $CD34^+$ cells. In hypotonic conditions, both $CD34^+CD38^-$ and $CD34^+CD38^+$ populations showed significant cell softening, and a greater percentage of cells became stretchable when the tonicity decreased, particularly in the $CD34^+CD38^-$ cells ($P < .05$), as seen in Fig. 4.5A. Among the stretchable cells, the deformability was significantly higher in the $CD34^+CD38^-$ than the $CD34^+CD38^+$ population, as seen from Fig. 4.5B.

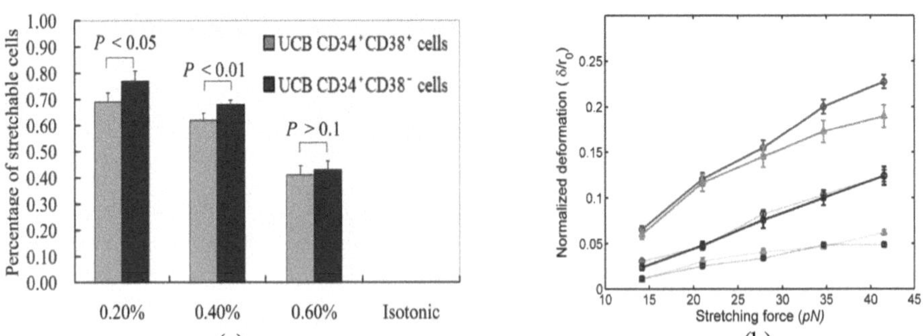

(a) (b)

Figure 4.5 The percentage of immunophenotypically distinct hematopoietic cells from UCB that were stretchable in hypotonic saline and their deformability (Tan et al., 2011). (A, B) The percentage (A) and deformability (B) of $CD34^+CD38^+$ (thin lines) and $CD34^+CD38^-$ cells (thick lines) that were stretchable with optical tweezers (n = 4 experiments, total 61, 52, 49 cells and 65, 57, 60 cells for $CD34^+CD38^+$ and $CD34^+CD38^-$ cells in 0.6%, 0.4%, and 0.2% saline, respectively). δ is cell deformation and r_0 is initial cell radius.

Then, whether the differences in biophysical properties observed in normal hematopoietic cells at different stages can be similarly observed under leukemia conditions was examined. BM $CD33^+CD34^+$ and $CD33^+CD34^-$ myeloblasts were isolated from seven patients with AML. Previous studies have shown that the $CD33^+CD34^+$ population contains primitive leukemia initiating cells (LIC), which are not present in the $CD33^+CD34^-$ population (Bonnet and Dick, 1997). The results in Fig. 4.6A show that the percentage of stretchable cells in the $CD33^+CD34^+$ population was significantly higher ($P < .01$). Among the stretchable cells, $CD33^+CD34^+$ cells also showed higher deformability, as seen in Figs. 4.2B and C.

The biophysical properties of UCB $CD34^+CD38^-$ and $CD34^+CD38^+$ cells and leukemic $CD33^+CD34^+$ and $CD33^+CD34^-$ myeloblasts were further characterized and compared according to the optical stretching model. The tension of the membrane is linearly related to the biophysical parameters of the cell, for example, the compressible modulus k_α of the elastic region. The stiffness distributions of these cell populations under isotonic and hypotonic conditions were all fitted by Gaussian functions. The k_α values of UCB samples are shown in Table 4.3, and the k_α values of AML BM samples are shown in Fig. 4.7. Generally, as the tonicity decreased, the elastic

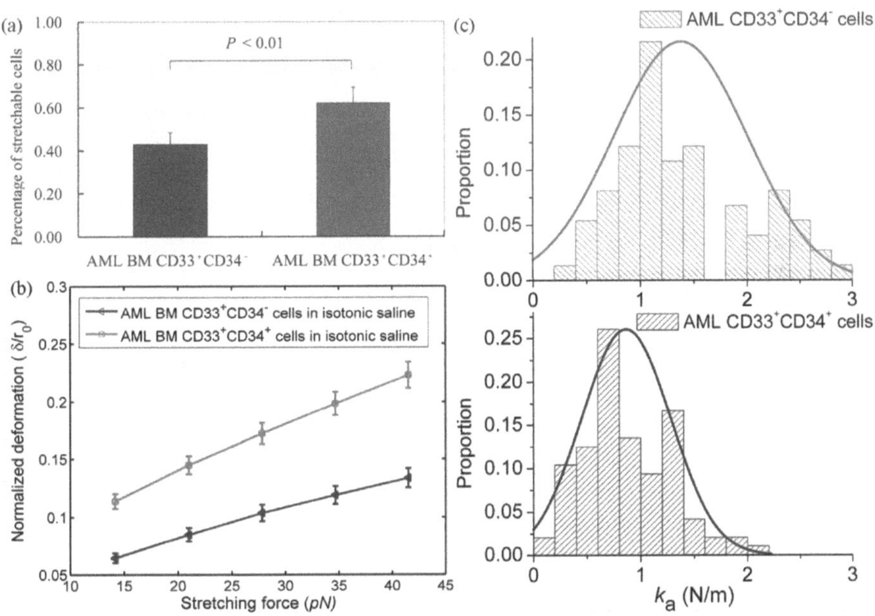

Figure 4.6 The deformation behaviors of $CD33^+CD34^+$ and $CD33^+CD34^-$ cells from BM of AML patients (Tan et al., 2011). (A) The percentage of AML $CD33^+CD34^+$ and $CD33^+CD34^-$ cells that were stretchable with optical tweezers in isotonic saline (n = 14 experiments, total 286 $CD33^+CD34^+$ cells and 254 $CD33^+CD34^-$ cells from seven patients). (B) The deformability of the stretchable AML hematopoietic cells in isotonic saline. (C) Histogram of the elastic area compressibility modulus k_α for seven cytological samples collected from AML patients. The distributions were best fitted by Gaussian functions.

Table 4.3 Biophysical property of primitive hematopoietic cells with distinct immunophenotypes in isotonic and hypotonic saline (Tan et al., 2011).

	Elastic area compressibility modulus k_α (N/m)		
Saline	**UCB $CD34^+CD38^+$**	**UCB $CD34^+CD38^-$**	***P*-value**
0.2%	1.77 ± 0.051	1.05 ± 0.065	$<10^{-5}$
0.4%	2.32 ± 0.14	1.09 ± 0.063	$<10^{-5}$
0.6%	2.54 ± 0.075	1.60 ± 0.086	$<10^{-5}$
Isotonic	NA	NA	NA

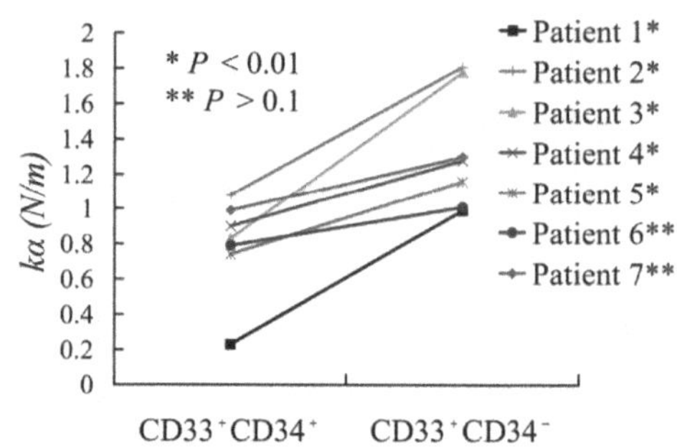

Figure 4.7 The elastic area compressibility modulus k_α of $CD33^+CD34^+$ and $CD33^+CD34^-$ myeloblasts from seven patients with AML (Tan et al., 2011). Each symbol represents an individual AML patient. Statistical analysis indicated that $CD33^+CD34^-$ cells exhibited significantly larger elasticity moduli than $CD33^+CD34^+$ cells for patients 1–5 ($P < .01$) but not for patients 6 and 7 ($P > .1$).

modulus of hematopoietic cells decreased. $CD34^+CD38^-$ cells exhibited much lower mechanical stiffness and were 37%–53% softer than $CD34^+CD38^+$ cells. Among these seven patients, the elastic modulus k_α of leukemia $CD33^+CD34^+$ cells from patients 1–5 was significantly lower than that of $CD33^+CD34^-$ cells ($P < .01$, Fig. 4.3), especially in patient 1 (Fig. 4.7). For patients 6 and 7, there was no significant difference in cell stiffness between $CD33^+CD34^-$ and $CD33^+CD34^+$ myeloblasts.

This case study reported the use of robotically controlled optical tweezers to stretch cells to characterize the biophysical properties of primitive hematopoietic cells derived from normal UCB and leukemia. The results revealed that primitive $CD34^+CD38^-$ UCB cells had higher deformability than the less primitive $CD34^+CD38^+$ cells. This difference was clearly manifested under hypotonic conditions. There are similar reports in chondrocytes (Wozniak et al., 2010), mesenchymal stem cells (Yourek et al., 2007), and mouse and human embryonic stem cells (Chowdhury et al., 2010). In AML, the putatively more primitive $CD33^+CD34^+$ myoblasts also showed higher mechanical compliance than the less primitive $CD33^+CD34^-$ population, which was very similar to the observations in normal HSPC. These observations indicate that there may be a link between early hematopoietic differentiation and changes in biophysical properties under normal and leukemia conditions. The hypothesis is that the higher deformability of the HSPC and LIC populations may give them the ability to enter and exit the BM niche, in which they receive specific survival or differentiation signals (Wilson and Trumpp, 2006). Further interpretation of these observations will require functional and mechanistic studies to correlate deformability with inherent stem cell and LIC capabilities and specific cell signaling pathways that are known to function in these populations. In summary, this work shows that normal and leukemic hematopoietic cell populations with different primitives exhibit different deformability, indicating that the biophysical properties may be related to stem cell or LIC capabilities. These findings also provide a solid foundation for studying normal and leukemia cell signals and their biophysical properties at the single-cell level.

4.2.4 Stretching human embryonic stem cells (hESCs) in cardiac differentiation to probe the mechanobiological properties

Another case study to be reported explores the mechanical and biological properties of hESCs in cardiac differentiation by stretching the cells with optical tweezers. hESCs and hESC-CMs have broad prospects in the treatment of cardiovascular diseases. However, the mechanobiological properties of hESCs and hESC-CMs remain elusive. Mechanobiological properties play an important role in regulating cell behavior, such as maintaining cell integrity, cell division, differentiation, motility, growth, and apoptosis (Bao and Suresh, 2003; Bausch and Kroy, 2006; Lauttenschlager et al., 2009). Any abnormal changes in biomechanics (such as micromechanical properties) may lead to disorders of cell viability and pathological changes (Cross et al., 2007; Suresh et al., 2005). Various evidences have indicated that micromechanical properties are indicators of cell phenotype (Darling et al., 2008), disease (Cross et al., 2007; Suresh et al., 2005), and differentiation potential (Treiser et al., 2010). For example, the viscoelastic modulus of cardiomyocytes is significantly higher than that of skeletal muscle cells (Mathur et al., 2001). Compared with the control group, CMs from diseased mice or under different physiological load conditions show distinct mechanobiological behaviors (Nishimura et al., 2006; Turdi et al., 2009). Recent research into stem cells has revealed the important role of mechanical factors in determining cell fate and differentiation (Chowdhury et al., 2010; Engler et al., 2006). Changes in the cell mechanics of mesenchymal stem cells (MSCs), mouse ESCs, and human ESCs (hESCs) during differentiation have been reported. Tan et al. (2012) explored changes in the micromechanical properties of hESCs through hESC-CMs using optical tweezers stretching at the single-cell level after cardiac differentiation. The results of this research are presented here.

Cell-stretching experiments were performed on hESCs and hESC-CMs, and the diameters were 17.8 ± 2.5 and 18.6 ± 4.3 μm, respectively. A total of 36 hESCs and 29 hESC-CMs were tested, and each measurement was repeated five times to obtain average results. The instantaneous positions of the moving light trap $x_2^{\text{trap}}(t)$ and microbeads $x_1^{\text{bead}}(t)$ in Fig. 4.2 were obtained through image processing. The results in Fig. 4.8A show that the displacement of the attached beads basically followed the movement of the moving optical trap until the beads escaped the trap. According to Eqs. (4.5) and (4.6), the mechanical response on both sides of the cell was calculated (Fig. 4.8B). The results showed that the cell-restoring force on the side of the moving trap (F_2^{cell}) was slightly greater than the restoring force of the cell on the side of the fixed trap (F_1^{cell}), indicating that the mechanical response ($F_2^{\text{cell}} - F_2^{\text{cell}}$) resisted the

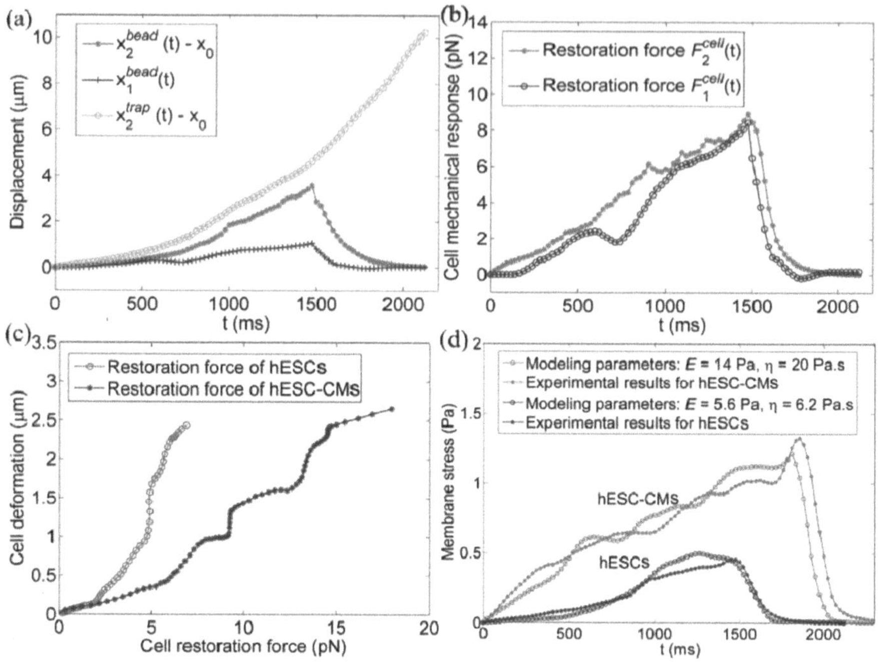

Figure 4.8 Dynamic mechanical responses of cells in optical stretching (Tan et al., 2012). (A) Motion profiles of the optical trap and microbeads. (B) Cell restoration forces, where $k = 7.8$ pN/μm, $\varepsilon_0 = 1.5$μm, and $\lambda = 1.47$. (C) The relationship between the cell restoration force and the deformation of hESCs and hESC-CMs, where the trapping stiffness values were 21.6 and 7.8 pN/μm, respectively. (D) Comparison of modeling mechanical responses and experimental results.

cell stretching caused by light force. Since no significant difference was found between these two mechanical responses, F_2^{cell} was used to establish the relationship between cell deformation and restoring force (Fig. 4.8C). According to Eq. (4.7), the cell membrane stress $[F_2^{\text{cell}}/(\pi r_{\text{con}}^2)]$ from the cell strain $[(x_2^{\text{bead}}(t) - x_1^{\text{bead}}(t) - x_0)/(2r_0)]$ was calculated, as shown in Fig. 4.8D. When the appropriate elastic modulus E and viscosity η were selected, the simulation results were in good agreement with the experimental data (Fig. 4.8D). Then, the mechanical properties of the cells were characterized, as shown in Table 4.4. The results showed that the elastic modulus

Table 4.4 Mechanical properties of hESC and hESC-CM characterized from the dynamic responses (Tan et al., 2012).

Mechanical property **Cell type**	**Elastic modulus** ***E* (Pa)**	**Viscosity** **η (Pa.s)**
hESC	5.6 ± 1.4	6.2 ± 2.4
hESC-CM	14 ± 3.5	20 ± 5.3

and viscosity coefficient of hESC-CMs were greater than for hESCs. These findings indicated that the membrane structure of hESCs became more organized and strengthened after differentiation, and the intracellular inclusion bodies were more viscous. These changes in mechanobiological properties may be related to the loss of pluripotency and the acquisition of unique functional properties (such as contractility during cardiac differentiation) of hESCs.

The mechanical properties of hESCs and hESC-CMs under equilibrium were then examined. The images of the beads escaping from the optical trap were extracted for deformation analysis. The trapping force was obtained from the calibration relationship between the trapping force and the viscous resistance. Fig. 4.9 illustrates the quantitative analysis of the mechanical response of hESCs and hESC-CMs at equilibrium during cell stretching. The results showed that hESCs exhibited much higher deformability than hESC-CMs. In order to extract their mechanical properties, static cell modeling methods were used to reveal the deformation characteristics. The modeling results were in good agreement with the experimental data. As shown in Fig. 4.9, there were some changes in hESCs, which may be caused by the strain hardening effect of constitutive materials in the modeling, especially in a relatively large strain range. The k_α values of hESCs and hESC-CMs were determined to be 0.36 ± 0.12 and 1.89 ± 0.29 N/m (mean $\pm$ standard deviation), respectively. These results indicate that the mechanical stiffness of differentiated hESC-CMs is significantly greater than that of hESCs, which is reminiscent of the observations in dynamic characterization.

The results of this case study indicate that the mechanical stiffness of hESC-CMs, which is characterized by dynamic and static response, is significantly improved compared with undifferentiated hESCs. The biomechanics of cells, especially the micromechanical properties, depend to a large extent on the cytoskeleton network (McCain and Parker, 2011). Changes in mechanical compliance may reflect the progress of cytoskeletal organization. Therefore, the above results are based on the fact that differentiated hESC-CMs have a more pronounced and organized cytoskeleton, which

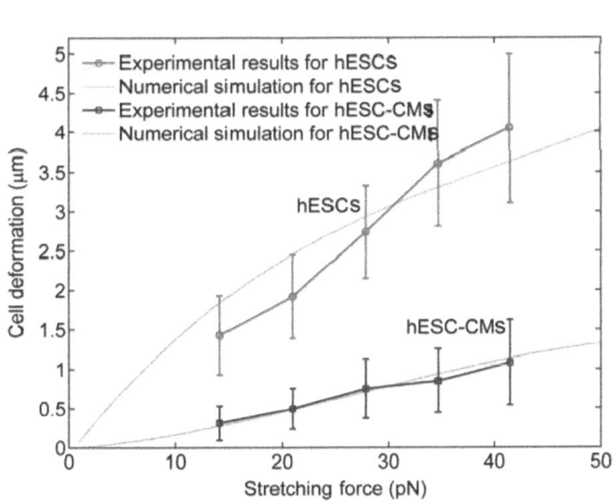

Figure 4.9 Quantitative analysis of the mechanical responses of hESCs and hESC-CMs from both experiments (solid line) and numerical simulation (dashed line) (Tan et al., 2012). The error bar denotes the standard deviation of the results.

can enhance the cell's resistance to external forces. The previously reported changes in the ultrastructural properties of hESC-CMs during early cardiac differentiation further support this finding. As reported, the in vitro differentiation of hESCs to hESC-CMs combines the ultrastructural maturation characterized by the gradual increase in the amount and tissue of myofibrils, that is, early hESCs with irregular and sparse myofibril distribution are gradually developed into more mature CMs with an organized and well-defined sarcomeric pattern (Snir et al., 2003). Densely packed myofibrils may lead to higher mechanical stiffness. Moreover, the myofibril assembly in the in vitro maturation of CMs is similar to that found during myocyte differentiation in vivo. Therefore, the results of this case study indicate that similar biomechanical changes also occur during CM differentiation in vivo. In addition, the cytomechanical changes to hESCs during cardiac differentiation are consistent with the reported results in the literature, such as fibroblasts and dedifferentiated cancer cells (Martin et al., 2006), primitive hematopoietic cells (Tan et al., 2011), mESCs and their differentiated counterparts (Chowdhury et al., 2010), MSCs and MSC-derived chondrocytes, and osteoblasts (Yourek et al., 2007).

Cell mechanics plays an important role in the regulation of various cellular functions. Mechanical stiffening during cardiac differentiation likely correlates with the functional properties of myocytes. Force generation is associated with myofibrils, which consist of contractile proteins including myosin and actin filaments (Ehler and Perriard, 2000). These filaments are spatially organized into sarcomeres in CMs, which endow them with the ability to contract spontaneously and further respond to the heart beating assisted by other heart muscle cells.

CM differentiation recapitulates many processes of early in vivo cardiogenesis. Cell-stretching experiments with optical tweezers have shown that the mechanical stiffness of hESCs increases after cardiac differentiation. This sclerosis may be related to the assembly of myofibrils, which is the basis for the mature functional characteristics of contracted hESC-CMs during cardiac differentiation. These findings suggest that hESC-CMs can be used as a model to study mechanical and contractile defects in heart disease conditions such as Duchenne muscular dystrophy and heart failure.

4.3 Probing cell biophysical behavior based on actin cytoskeleton modeling of cells and stretching manipulation with optical tweezers

Actin filaments (F-actin) are semiflexible, and can significantly promote the mechanical behavior of cells (Lam et al., 2008; Gardel et al., 2004). Structural changes to the actin cytoskeleton during disease progression may lead to changes in cell mechanics. Therefore, cell mechanical properties are considered to be effective biomarkers for distinguishing healthy cells from abnormal cells and monitoring changes in cell physiological or pathological conditions (Cross et al., 2007; Suresh et al., 2005). This section introduces how the optical tweezers' cell-stretching operation based on actin cytoskeleton modeling can help probe the biophysical behavior of cells.

4.3.1 Actin cytoskeleton microstructural model

Wang and Sun (2012) proposed a microstructure model, which is represented by a three-dimensional (3D) random actin cytoskeleton network formed by the Delaunay triangulation method. Considering the highly weighted influence of actin filaments, the effects of microtubules and intermediate filaments are ignored in the modeling. Actin filaments and actin-binding protein (ABP) are used as the basic elements of the actin cytoskeleton network. The MacKintosh-derived wormlike chain (WLC) model is used to reflect the mechanical properties of actin semiflexible polymers. ABP is represented by a linear Hookean spring.

Niederman et al. (1983) observed that the 3D network structure of the actin cytoskeleton could be used to probe the effect of the actin cytoskeleton on the mechanical properties of cells. The actin vertices are randomly distributed between the cell membrane and the nuclear membrane. Those distributed in the outer and inner diameters represent transmembrane and membrane-associated proteins, which anchor the actin network on the cell membrane and nuclear membrane, respectively (Ujihara et al., 2010). Delaunay triangulation is used to connect the vertices of actin to form a closed 3D random actin cytoskeleton network. Each element represents a separate actin filament, and the actin filaments that intersect the inner diameter are deleted. ABP is also integrated into the actin network, represented by a linear spring to randomly connect the ends of any two filaments. Its concentration can be determined by changing the maximum length of ABP.

Actin filaments exhibit semiflexible polymer properties. Compared with flexible polymers, their permanent length is the same order of magnitude as their contour length. This model only focuses on the tightly cross-linked and bound actin cytoskeleton network whose contour length is less than its permanent length. The MacKintosh-derived WLC model describes the force extension behavior of actin filaments, reflecting the semiflexibility of actin (Palmer et al., 2008), as shown below.

$$f_a = \frac{81\ k_B T L_p^2 L_c^2 (\Delta r + \delta r_0)}{\left(L_c^2 - 6L_p\Delta r - 6L_p\delta r_0\right)^2 \left(L_c^2 + 3L_p\Delta r + 3L_p\delta r_0\right)}, \tag{4.26}$$

where f_a is the stretching force, L_c is the contour length, Δr is the extension of the actin filament, δr_0 is the pre-extension of the actin filament caused by prestress, L_p is the persistence length, k_B is the Boltzmann's constant, and T is the absolute temperature.

The contour length of actin filaments is affected by the diameter of F-actin, the concentration of actin, and the concentration of cross-linking, calculated as follows (Gardel et al., 2004; Palmer et al., 2008).

$$L_c = \frac{\rho_c^{0.2} d_{\text{Actin}}}{2}\sqrt{\frac{\pi}{c_{AF}}}, \tag{4.27}$$

where d_{Actin} denotes the diameter of the F-actin, c_{AF} is the actin concentration, and ρ_c is the density of the cross-links, $\rho_c = c_{CL}/c_{AF}$.

As suggested in the literature, the stiffness k_c of the ABPs is set at 100 pN/μm. The actin filaments and actin-binding proteins are immersed in the cytosol. The viscosity η of the cytosol is in the range of 0.001 N/m^2 to 10 N/m^2, which can be set at 10 N/m^2 in the model.

During the stretching process with optical tweezers, the stretching force $\pm F_s$ is applied to the beads attached to the opposite ends of the cell. By denoting S_1 as a set of actin vertices subjected to stretching force F_s, and S_2 as a set of vertices subjected to stretching force $-F_s$, the stretching process of optical tweezers is simulated as shown below, assuming the stretching force is in the z direction.

$$S_1 = \{\ i|x_i^2 + y_i^2 \le r_b^2, r_n < \sqrt{x_i^2 + y_i^2 + z_i^2} \le r_c,\ \ z_i > 0\}, \tag{4.28}$$

$$S_2 = \{\ i|x_i^2 + y_i^2 \le r_b^2,\ r_n < \sqrt{x_i^2 + y_i^2 + z_i^2} \le r_c,\ \ z_i < 0\}, \tag{4.29}$$

where x_i, y_i, and z_i are 3D coordinates of every vertex, r_b denotes the radius of the microbead, and r_c and r_n denote the radii of the cell membrane and the nuclear membrane, respectively. N denotes the total number of vertices in the network, and $i \in 1 \ldots N$.

The number of vertices subject to the stretching force is cardinality of the set, that is, $n_1 = |S_l|$, $n_2 = |S_2|$. Therefore, the stretching forces imposed on the vertices can be described as

$$f_{s1} = \frac{F_s}{n_1}, \cdots f_{s2} = \frac{F_s}{n_2}. \tag{4.30}$$

Force balance is derived using Newtonian equation of motion to follow the position of all actin vertices $r_i = [x_i\ y_i\ z_i]^{\mathrm{T}}$. The actin network is immersed in almost incompressible fluid, so the following volume constraints of the network are considered in the modeling:

$$m_i \ddot{r}_i + \eta \dot{r}_i = F_i, \tag{4.31}$$

where m_i is the fictitious mass of the vertex, and η is the viscosity of the cytoplasm describing the influence of the cytoplasm on the actin network. F_i is the resultant force of vertex i, which is a combination of internal forces of the actin filaments and the ABPs connected to the ith vertex, and the external force f_s, expressed as:

$$F_i = \sum_{i=1}^{n_a} f_{a\_i} + \sum_{i=1}^{n_c} f_{c\_i} + f_s, \tag{4.32}$$

where n_a is the number of the actin filaments, n_c is the number of the ABPs connected to the ith vertex, and f_s is expressed as

$$f_s = \begin{cases} f_{s1} & i \in S_1 \\ f_{s2} & i \in S_2 \\ 0 & i \notin S_1 \text{ and } i \notin S_2 \end{cases} . \tag{4.33}$$

Discretizing Eq. (4.31) gives the instantaneous velocity of each vertex as

$$v_i^{k+1} = \frac{m v_i^k + F_i^k \delta}{m + \eta\delta}, \tag{4.34}$$

where v_i is velocity of the ith actin vertex, k is the index of computational steps, δ is an increment of time, and F_i^k is the resultant force of the ith vertex at the kth step. The new positions of each node are adjusted in the direction of its resultant force and can be derived from

$$r_i^{k+1} = r_i^k + v_i^{k+1}\delta. \tag{4.35}$$

The above process is repeated until all vertices of the network are in equilibrium and the positions of all vertices are r_i^k. As shown in Fig. 4.10, D_b and D_a are defined as the unit cell diameter before and after stretching, respectively. Therefore, the cell deformation ε can be expressed as

$$\varepsilon = D_a - D_b, \tag{4.36}$$

where

$$\begin{cases} D_b = \|r_{u0} - r_{l0}\| \\ D_a = \|r_{uk} - r_{lk}\| \end{cases}, \tag{4.37}$$

$$\begin{cases} r_{u0} = \frac{1}{n_1}\sum_{i \in S_1} r_i^0 r_{l0} = \frac{1}{n_2}\sum_{i \in S_2} r_i^0, \end{cases} \tag{4.38}$$

$$\begin{cases} r_{uk} = \frac{1}{n_1}\sum_{i \in S_1} r_i^k r_{lk} = \frac{1}{n_2}\sum_{i \in S_2} r_i^k. \end{cases} \tag{4.39}$$

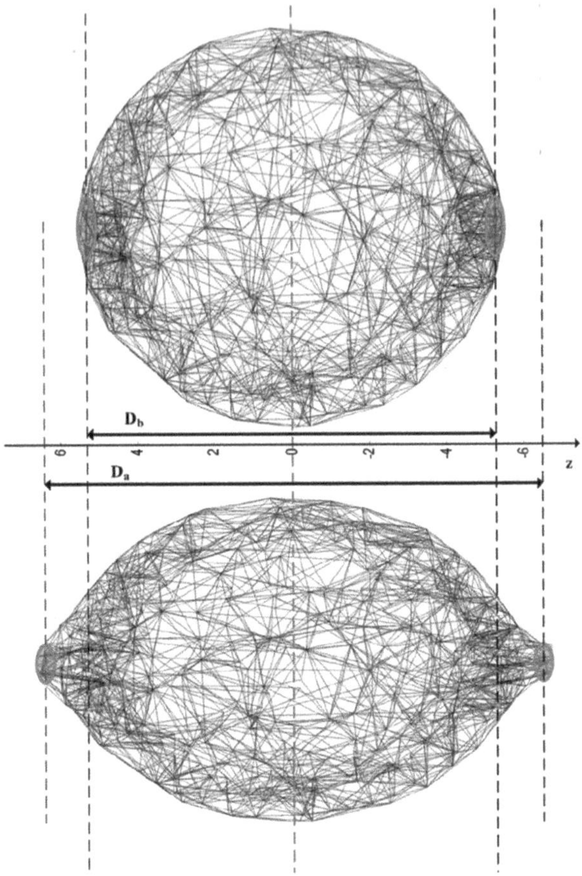

Figure 4.10 Schematic of the cell deformation before and after stretching, with vertices that are subject to the stretching force in the magneta ellipse region (Wang and Sun, 2012).

Further, the stiffness of the cell can be defined as

$$K = \frac{F_s}{\varepsilon}. \tag{4.40}$$

Substituting Eqs. (4.37)–(4.39) into Eqs. (4.36) and (4.40), the cell deformation ε and cell stiffness K can be obtained. In the model, both r_u and r_l are functions of L_c, L_p, δr_0 and k_c. If c_{AF}, ρ_c, δr_0, and k_c are prescribed first, the cell deformation and cell stiffness are derived from the following formulations through numerical calculations:

$$\varepsilon = \varepsilon\left(L_c(c_{AF}, \rho_c),\ L_p(\rho_c),\ \delta r_0, k_c\right), \tag{4.41}$$

$$K = K\left(L_c(c_{AF}, \rho_c),\ L_p(\rho_c),\ \delta r_0, k_c\right). \tag{4.42}$$

The actin cytoskeleton model introduced above has the following unique characteristics.

First, the developed model highlights the influence of the semiflexibility of the actin cytoskeleton on the mechanical properties of cells. Many microstructure models simplify actin filaments into Hookean springs, and some of these models consider the influence of the semiflexibility of the actin cytoskeleton on the mechanical properties of cells. In the above-introduced model, a MacKintosh-derived WLC model is used to reflect the mechanical properties of actin semiflexible polymers.

Second, the proposed model combines the influence of cross-linking density on cell mechanical properties. Some other models only consider the influence of the number of cross-links. A large number of studies have shown that ABP can sensitively mediate the stiffness of F-actin bundles. The link between the stiffness and cross-link density of actin filaments represents a unique characteristic caused by the semiflexibility of actin filaments. This model analyzes the effect of cross-link density on cell mechanical properties by considering the enhanced actin-binding effect.

4.3.2 Probing cell biophysical properties

The actin microstructure model can be used in cell-stretching operations with optical tweezers to quantify the direct role of the actin cytoskeleton in cytomechanical behavior related to changes in cell function. Wang et al. (2013) used leukemia cell lines, Jurkat and K562 cells, as research samples, and changed the cell stage through treatment with the chemotherapy drug doxorubicin (DOX). The study demonstrated an effective method to quantitatively characterize how the actin cytoskeleton remodeling profile reflects the relationship between cell mechanical behavior and cell function changes. The findings can help to provide novel and dynamic information, revealing the mechanisms that drive normal cells to disease states. By analyzing this unique underlying mechanism, it will be possible to study more specific clinical methods from the perspective of biophysics. The probing process includes the following main steps.

First, optical tweezers were used to stretch the DOX-treated Jurkat cells (Jurkat-D) and K562 DOX-resistant cells (K562-DR) for 96 h to study the changes in cell mechanical behavior after treatment. Before stretching the cells with optical tweezers, the streptavidin-coated microbeads were attached to the cell surface as handles. The cell sample was placed in the incubation chamber and stretched by optical tweezers. The stretching operation process was monitored by the CCD detection system, thereby obtaining deformation of the cells.

The deformations of the 106 Jurkat and 73 Jurkat-D cells after optical tweezers stretching were measured in three independent tests (Wang et al., 2013). Within the range of the applied stretching force, the deformation of Jurkat-D cells was less than that of the control group (untreated Jurkat cells). Fig. 4.11 shows the quantitative analysis of the deformation behaviors of Jurkat-D and Jurkat cells. The experimental results were obtained by stretching the cells with optical tweezers, and simulation results were obtained using the actin cytoskeleton model as introduced above (Wang and Sun, 2012). It can be seen that the error bars of the deformation of Jurkat-D cells were smaller than those of the control group, which indicated that Jurkat-D cells have more homogeneous biophysical behavior compared with Jurkat cells. In addition, all the measurement results showed that Jurkat-D cells were harder than the control cells

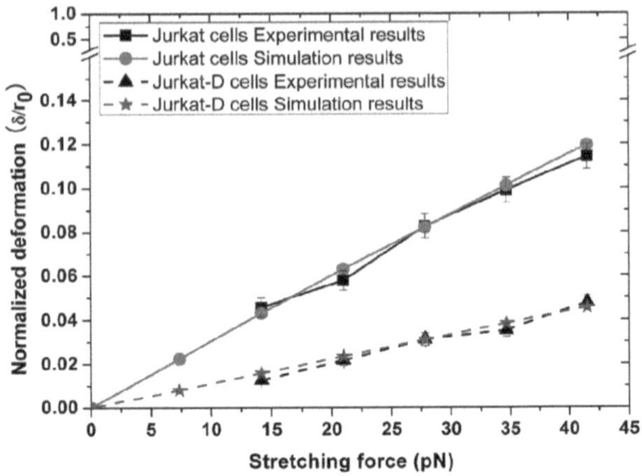

Figure 4.11 Alterations in the deformation behavior of DOX-treated Jurkat cells (δ is the cell deformation, and r_0 is the initial cell radius) (Wang et al., 2013).

under the same stretching force ($P < .01$). These results of changes in the cytomechanical behavior of Jurkat cells under DOX treatment were consistent with previously reported results, such as the results of other leukemia cells treated with different chemotherapy drugs (Lam et al., 2008).

The deformations of 135 K562 and 135 K562-DR cells after optical tweezers stretching were also measured in five independent tests to examine whether the difference in biophysical behavior could be observed in the K562 cells when they became resistant to DOX. The deformation behaviors of K562 and K562-DR cells under the stretching forces are illustrated in Fig. 4.12. Compared with K562-DR cells, the deformation of K562 cells changed in a relatively large range. This indicated that from the viewpoint of cell biomechanics, DOX-treated K562 cells changed toward uniformity of the cell fraction, which was consistent with the results obtained from Jurkat cells. In addition, all measurement results showed that under the same stretching force, K562 cells were softer than DOX-resistant cells ($P < .01$), indicating that the deformability of K562 cells with different DOX sensitivity changed.

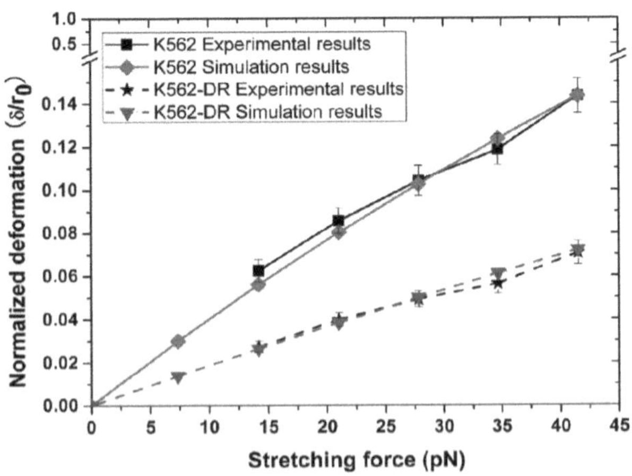

Figure 4.12 Alterations in the deformation behavior of K562-DR cells (Wang et al., 2013).

Second, the effects of F-actin remodeling in relation to above-mentioned changes in cell mechanical behavior were examined using a confocal microscope. It was observed that the changes in the structure of F-actin were related to the changes in the mechanical behavior of Jurkat and K562 cells under DOX treatment. Fig. 4.13 depicts the changes observed in the typical actin cytoskeleton structure of Jurkat cells under DOX treatment. It was found that there were significant differences in the DOX-treated Jurkat cells. F-actin was distributed in a significantly larger periphery, while the density of F-actin in Jurkat-D cells was lower than that of the control group. Fig. 4.14 illustrates the typical actin cytoskeleton structure observed in K562-DR and K562 cells. When K562 cells became resistant to DOX, F-actin was located on the wider edge. In addition, the F-actin density of K562-DR cells was greater than that of K562 cells. These findings revealed the potentially important role of the F-actin remodeling mechanism in regulating the biophysical behavior of DOX-treated Jurkat and K562 cells.

Third, the microstructure model of actin cytoskeleton (Wang and Sun, 2012) was fitted with the data obtained from the stretching experiment to extract the structural parameters of F-actin. These structural parameters facilitate the quantification of the basic F-actin remodeling profile by showing that the mechanical behavior of Jurkat and K562 cells is related to chemotherapy drug treatment. The original structure of the model was developed based on confocal images of Jurkat and K562 samples. The modeling deformations of the Jurkat and K562 samples were in good agreement with the experimental stretching results (Figs. 4.12 and 4.13). The corresponding structural parameters of the actin cytoskeleton network extracted from the model are provided in Tables 4.5 and 4.6. Other parameters used in this model can be found

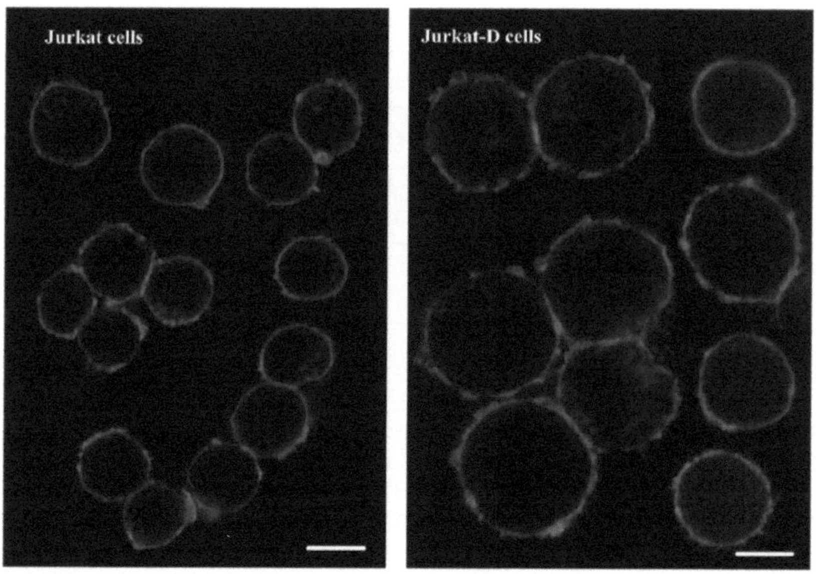

Figure 4.13 Typical confocal images of actin cytoskeleton architecture of Jurkat cells treated with 0.05 μM DOX for 96 h and the control groups (Wang et al., 2013). The scale bar is 10 μm.

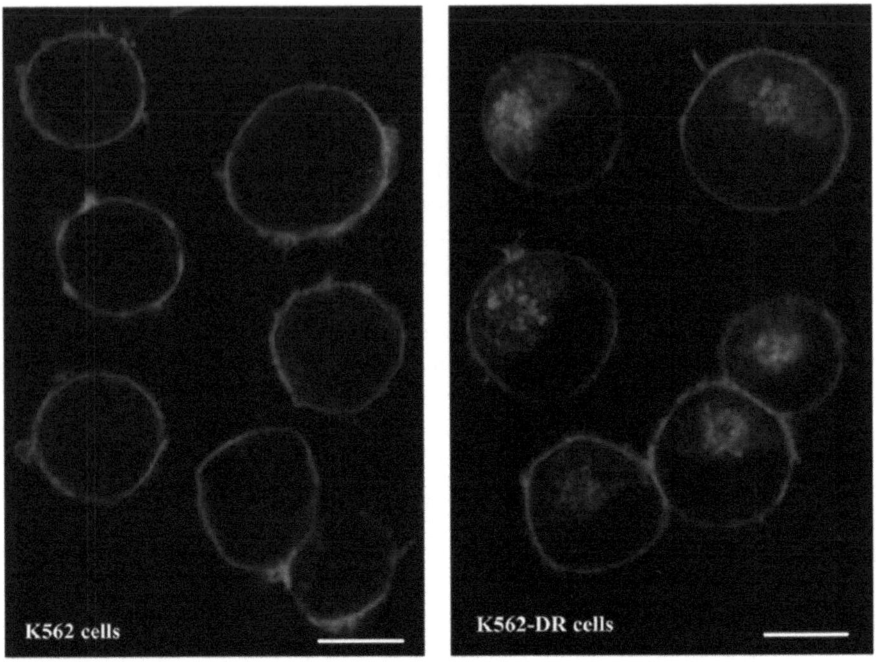

Figure 4.14 Typical confocal images of actin cytoskeleton architecture of K562 and K562-DR cells (Wang et al., 2013). The scale bar is 10 μm.

Table 4.5 Estimation of structural parameters of actin cytoskeleton of DOX-treated Jurkat and Jurkat-D cells extracted based on the model (Wang et al., 2013).

Cell type	R_E (μm)[a]	R_I (μm)[b]	C_A (μM)[c]	N_A[d]	C_c[e]	L_p (μm)[f]
Jurkat cells	7.09	6.31	39.2	8603	0.04	3
Jurkat-D cells	9.78	8.69	37.8	22,187	0.04	3

[a] R_E is the external radius of the actin network.
[b] R_I is the internal radius of the actin network.
[c] C_A is F-actin density.
[d] N_A is the number of F-actin in the network.
[e] C_c is the cross-link density.
[f] L_p is the persistence length of F-actin.

Table 4.6 Estimation of structural parameters of actin cytoskeleton of K562 and K562-DR cells extracted based on the model (Wang et al., 2013).

Cell type	R_E (μm)	R_I (μm)	C_A (μM)	N_A	C_c	L_p (μm)
K562 cells	8.67	7.77	19.6	7500	0.04	3
K562-DR cells	9.14	7.64	21.6	14,326	0.04	3

in Wang and Sun (2012). All parameters used in this model were consistent with previously reported work (Cross et al., 2007).

Finally, it was analyzed how the reorganization of F-actin significantly affects the mechanical behavior of DOX-treated Jurkat and K562 cells. Both the mechanical behavior and the amount of F-actin affect the mechanical behavior of cells to a large extent. The mechanical behavior of F-actin can be determined by persistence length, cross-link density, and F-actin density, as described above (Wang and Sun, 2012). The extracted values of persistence length, cross-link density, and F-actin density (shown in Tables 4.5 and 4.6), based on the MacKintosh-derived WLC model, were used to obtain the force–elongation relationship of Jurkat and K562 cells before and after drug treatment. The number of F-actin in the network was calculated based on the F-actin density and the value of the outer/inner radius of the F-actin network, as shown in Tables 4.5 and 4.6. For Jurkat cells treated with DOX, the distribution of actin became significantly larger and wider (the volume of actin distribution was larger), and the density of actin decreased. It can be seen from Table 4.5 that the number of F-actin in Jurkat-D cells was significantly greater than that in the control group. According to the structural parameters of F-actin extracted from the model, the mechanical behavior of F-actin in DOX-treated Jurkat cells was similar to that of the control group. Therefore, it is hypothesized that the mechanical stiffening of Jurkat-D cells may be due to the significant increase in the number of F-actin, which participates in the dispersion of external stretching force to resist deformation, although the mechanical behavior of Jurkat cell samples has not been found to be obvious before and after drug treatment. For K562-DR cells, the density of actin increased, and the distribution of actin became significantly larger and wider. Therefore, the F-actin of K562-DR cells showed stronger mechanical behavior than K562 cells, and the amount of F-actin of K562-DR cells was significantly increased. Both the hardening behavior and the increase in the amount of F-actin may cause slight deformation of K562-DR cells. Therefore, the actin cytoskeleton model can be used to directly explain the distinct deformation behavior of DOX-treated Jurkat and K562 cells. These results demonstrate the effectiveness of the proposed method in quantitatively detecting the basic mechanism of cell mechanical behavior corresponding to cell function changes.

In summary, this section reports an effective quantitative method to study the cytoskeleton remodeling profile of actin, which reflects the interrelationship between cell mechanical behavior and cell function changes. This study quantitatively explains how F-actin reorganization determines cell stiffening, which is the basis for the functional characteristics of DOX-treated Jurkat and K562 cells. Although only the results of leukemia cell samples (such as Jurkat and K562 cells) are reported here, the method can be used for other cell types. The proposed method can be further used to explain how to change the mechanical behavior of cells for different physiological/pathological states, which may be used in clinical practice. By effectively detecting changes in the mechanical behavior of cells, it is possible to characterize the progress of the physiological/pathological state of cells, and on this basis, targeted treatment options can be studied from the perspective of biophysics.

4.4 Cell stretching with dielectrophoresis technology

Dielectrophoresis (DEP) is considered to be one of the most effective methods for noncontact cell manipulation and characterization. This method uses a relatively simple hardware setup and a nonuniform electric field through electrode pairs to polarize and deform cells. High throughput can be achieved by using microwell arrays or longer electrode pairs. With the advancement of microfabrication technology, microchips with different integrated microelectrode designs have been studied to characterize the mechanical properties of various cells through dielectrophoretic stretching. For example, MacQueen et al. (2010) used planar microelectrode arrays to characterize the mechanical properties of mammalian cells. Different cells were checked and their elastic modulus was calculated through numerical simulation. Guido et al. (2011) studied the deformation response of cancer cells and noncancerous cells, showing that electrodeposition can be used to distinguish two different cell types due to the difference in microtubule structure. Most DEP research focuses on the evaluation of cell deformation (Chen et al., 2011; Doh et al., 2012) and the biophysical properties of cells, such as membrane capacitance and cytoplasmic conductivity (Chen et al., 2012, 2014). To characterize the elastic modulus of diseased cells through DEP-based deformability testing, Zhang et al. (2015) developed a DEP-based microfluidic device that can quickly characterize the biomechanical properties of drug-treated cells. Bai et al. (2017) developed a DEP-based method that can be combined with actin skeleton modeling to characterize the mechanical properties of leukemia NB4 cells. This section introduces the use of DEP technology to stretch cells and clarify the biophysical properties of cells.

4.4.1 DEP-based cell stretching

In the studies of Zhang et al. (2015) and Bai et al. (2017), human acute promyelocytic leukemia NB4 cells were used as cell samples. NB4 cells were cultured in RPMI 1640 medium (Sigma, St. Louis, MO) supplemented with 10% fetal bovine serum (Atlanta Biologicals, GA). To prepare the ATRA stock solution, ATRA was firstly dissolved in absolute ethanol to obtain a concentration of 100 μmol/L, and then the solution was diluted to a final concentration of 1 μmol/L with RPMI medium. Before the experiment, the cells were incubated in two Petri dishes at 37°C and 5% CO_2. For drug treatment, the medium in one of the Petri dishes was replaced with a medium containing ATRA and incubated for 3 days. After 3 days, the cells from the two Petri dishes were centrifuged and the cell pellet was resuspended in isotonic buffer for stretching experiments. The medium contained 8.5% sucrose, 0.3% glucose, and 20 mg/L $CaCl_2$, which can induce positive dielectrophoretic force on cells. The conductivity and relative permittivity of the medium were approximately 10 mS/m and 78, respectively. To ensure that the cells were in a healthy state, experiments were conducted and completed within 1 hour.

4.4.1.1 Cell deformation and elastic modulus estimation through dielectrophoresis

DEP is the movement of dielectric particles in a nonuniform electric field (Pohl, 1951). The strength of the DEP force acting on a lossless dielectric sphere with a permittivity ε_p and radius r is (Jones, 1995):

$$F_{\mathrm{DEP}} = 2\pi\varepsilon_m r^3 \mathrm{Re}[f_{CM}]\nabla E_{rms}^2, \tag{4.43}$$

where f_{CM} is the Clausius–Mossoti factor, ε_m is the permittivity of the suspending medium, Re[f_{CM}] is the real part of the f_{CM}, and E_{rms} is the root-mean-squared strength of the supplied electric field. The Clausius–Mossoti factor, f_{CM}, can be represented as follows:

$$f_{CM} = \frac{\varepsilon_p^* - \varepsilon_m^*}{\varepsilon_p^* - 2\varepsilon_m^*}, \tag{4.44}$$

where ε^* is the complex permittivity, which is calculated by $\varepsilon^* = \varepsilon - j\Omega/\omega$. Ω is the conductivity, and ω is the frequency of electric field. Subscripts p and m denote the particle and medium, respectively. When the particle is more polarizable than the medium, Re[f_{CM}] > 0, the induced force pushes the particle toward the higher density region of the electric field (p-DEP response). In contrast, when the particle is less polarizable than the medium, Re[f_{CM}] < 0, the induced force repels the particle toward the lower density region of the electric field (n-DEP response).

In order to induce the DEP force of cell deformation, two parallel microelectrodes can be used to trap multiple cells and generate the required nonuniform electric field. First, a low-amplitude AC voltage is supplied to the microelectrodes, and the cells are in contact with one of the microelectrodes through p-DEP. Since the input voltage is relatively low, cell deformation is not observed at this stage. In the subsequent steps, the amplitude of the AC voltage is increased and a higher electric field strength is generated from the microelectrodes. Then, the cells begin to deform, changing their shape from spherical to ellipsoidal, along the direction of the electric field.

The DEP force acting on the cell can be calculated using Eq. (4.43). The amount of stress (σ) exerted on the cell can be calculated by dividing the force by the surface area of the hemispherical cell, so the stress equation can be further simplified as MacQueen et al. (2010):

$$\sigma = n\mathrm{Re}[f_{CM}]\ \varepsilon_m E_0^2, \tag{4.45}$$

$$n = \frac{E}{r_c \frac{d|E|}{dx}}, \tag{4.46}$$

where n is the geometric constant, which can be determined by COMSOL simulation.

In order to determine the elastic modulus of the two cell types, the cells can be modeled as a standard linear solid model. Under normal stress, the model assumes that the strain (γ) of the cell behaves like a spring (k_1) in parallel with Maxwell material [a spring (k_2) in series with a damper (κ)]. The compliance function, denoted by $J(t)$, describes the response of the material under pressure, which can be expressed as MacQueen et al. (2010):

$$J(t) = \frac{\gamma}{\sigma} = \frac{1}{k_1}\left[1 - \left(\frac{k_2}{k_1 + k_2}\right)e^{-t/\tau_0}\right], \tag{4.47}$$

where the time constant τ_0 is:

$$\tau_0 = \kappa\frac{(k_1 + k_2)}{k_1 k_2}. \tag{4.48}$$

4.4.1.2 Microfluidic chip

In order to provide a closed experimental environment, a microfluidic chip can be used as a platform to observe cells under a microscope (Zhang et al., 2015). The microfluidic chip is made of PDMS, which is a biocompatible material. Glass slides coated with conductive, optically transparent indium tin oxide (ITO) are used to construct parallel microelectrodes. Fig. 4.15 illustrates the process of manufacturing ITO microelectrodes and PDMS chips using photolithography. First, a positive photoresist (RZJ-304) is spin-coated on the surface of ITO glass (size: 25.4 × 76.2 mm) (Fig. 4.15A). Then, the coated ITO glass is exposed to UV light through a mask aligner, and the parallel micro-electrode pattern on the chrome mask is transferred to the photoresist. A developer solution is used to develop the patterned photoresist, and an ITO etchant is used to etch away unprotected ITO areas. After etching, the photoresist is removed and ITO electrodes are formed (Fig. 4.15B). To fabricate the PDMS layer of the microfluidic chip, a 50 μm thick photoresist (SU-8 2050) is spin-coated on a 2-inch silicon wafer and used to define the microchannel of the chip (Fig. 4.15C). The PDMS is cast into the finished SU-8 mold and cured in an oven at 65°C for 4 h (Fig. 4.15D). The cured PDMS is then peeled off the mold and combined with the ITO glass with microelectrodes using a plasma cleaner (Fig. 4.15E and F). The RF power is adjusted to 30 W, and the vacuum pressure is set to 200 mTorr.

4.4.1.3 Cell trapping and stretching protocol

DEP-based cell stretching and manipulation experiments require an experimental platform consisting of a function generator, positioning table, optical microscope, syringe pump, and computer system. In the cell-trapping experiment, the microfluidic chip with integrated microelectrodes was placed on the positioning table for viewing under an optical microscope. The overall size of the microchannel was 5000 μm by 50 μm, and the cell-containing medium was injected into the channel by a syringe pump. Integrated microelectrodes with a gap width of 20 μm were patterned on a glass slide coated

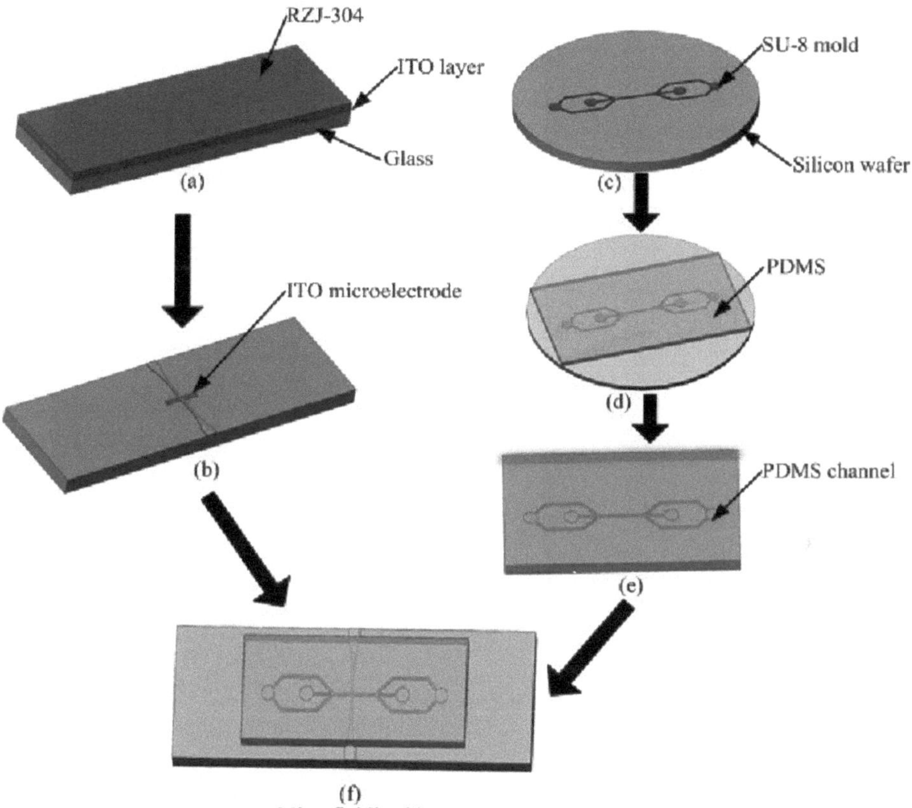

Figure 4.15 Fabrication procedure of ITO microelectrode and PDMS microfluidic chip (Zhang et al., 2015).

with indium tin oxide (ITO) by photolithography. The LabSmith fluid flow control system was used to load the medium containing the cells into the inlet of the microfluidic chip and remove the cells from the chip after the experiment. To stretch the cells, the microfluidic chip was connected to a function generator to generate a sinusoidal signal to the ITO electrode. The frequency of the electric field was chosen so that a net DEP force was applied to the cells to direct them toward the maximum value of the electric field.

The crossover frequency of leukemia cells (such as HL60 and T cells) from negative DEP to positive DEP was about 90 kHz, and experiments with positive DEP were performed at about 100 kHz to 1 MHz. Therefore, a frequency of 500 kHz was used. To start the tensile experiment, the NB4 cell was attracted to one of the electrodes by applying a voltage of 1.15 V_{pp} to the electrodes. At this voltage, no visible deformation on the cells was observed. After successfully trapping a cell, the voltage input increased to 3.5 V_{pp}. Since the higher DEP force was induced on the cell, the unbalanced force between the two halves of the cell caused the cell to stretch along the electric field. An optical microscope with a CCD visual inspection system was used to observe the elongation of the cells. The finite element software COMSOL Multiphysics can also be used to simulate the electric field distribution to calculate the DEP force acting on the cell.

4.4.1.4 DEP force computation

Three different methods can be used to estimate the DEP force acting on the cell. The first method uses the widely used DEP force equation (Jones, 1995), as shown in Eq. (4.43). This method uses the equivalent dipole moment (EDM) to derive the net force induced at the two poles of the polarization cell. The force calculation needs to use the gradient of the square of the electric field, which depends on the geometry of the microelectrode and can be obtained by computer simulation (Du et al., 2014) or analysis using the boundary element method (Rosales and Lim, 2005).

Alternatively, the DEP force can be calculated by integrating the Maxwell stress tensor (MST) on the surface of the cell to generate the force. For the general tip-to-tip electrode configuration, Engelhardt et al. (1984) proposed a simple approximation, assuming that the electric field inside the cell is smaller than the electric field outside, so the force can be estimated as

$$F_{\mathrm{DEP}} = \frac{1}{4}\varepsilon_0 \varepsilon E^2 A, \tag{4.49}$$

where E is the electric field expressed as $E = U/d$, in which U is the applied potential and d is the electrode gap (20 μm), and A is the surface area of the cell. This rough approximation ignored the effect of the applied frequency, which may cause the DEP force to vary between positive and negative at various frequencies. To better estimate power, Wang et al. (1997) used the phasor representation of the electric field ($E = E_0 e^{iwt}$) to determine the DEP force as follows:

$$F_{\mathrm{DEP}} = \frac{1}{4}\varepsilon_0 \varepsilon \int_A \left(EE^* + E^* E - |E|^2 \right) \cdot \hat{n} dA, \tag{4.50}$$

where E^* is the complex conjugate of the electric field, and $\hat{n}$ is the unit vector normal to A.

4.4.2 Experimental validation

4.4.2.1 DEP stretching results

Cell deformation under the DEP force was examined. In each predefined time interval, the CCD camera captured the image of the cell, and the following method was used to evaluate the strain of the cell:

$$\gamma(t) = \frac{L(t) - L_0}{L_0}, \tag{4.51}$$

where L_0 is the original diameter of the cell, $L(t)$ is the diameter of cell after stretching at time t. Image processing software ImageJ was used to measure the diameters of the captured images. Figs. 4.16A–D show images of NB4 cells, and Figs. 4.16E–H show images of NB4 cells treated with drugs at different time intervals. To illustrate the subtle differences in the biophysical properties of the cells, more than 40 cells of each type were tested (N = 42 for NB4 and N = 58 for drug-treated NB4). The strain of the cells from each trial after 3 min was calculated and summarized in Fig. 4.17. The data were grouped into strain intervals of 0.03, which was approximately equal to 0.5 μm elongation of a 14 μm NB4 cell. The results showed that the average strain value of most NB4 cells was about 0.06–0.09, and the maximum strain value was only 0.22. In contrast, for ATRA-NB4 cells, a large number of cells had an average strain value of 0.18 or higher, and some of them (>0.30 category) could even be stretched until they reached the opposite electrode in less than 3 min. According to the results, the strain value of 0.2 can be regarded as the threshold for the microfluidic chip to distinguish between NB4 cells and ATRA-treated NB4 cells. The results also showed that NB4 cells treated with ATRA for 3 days were softer than untreated cells, which was

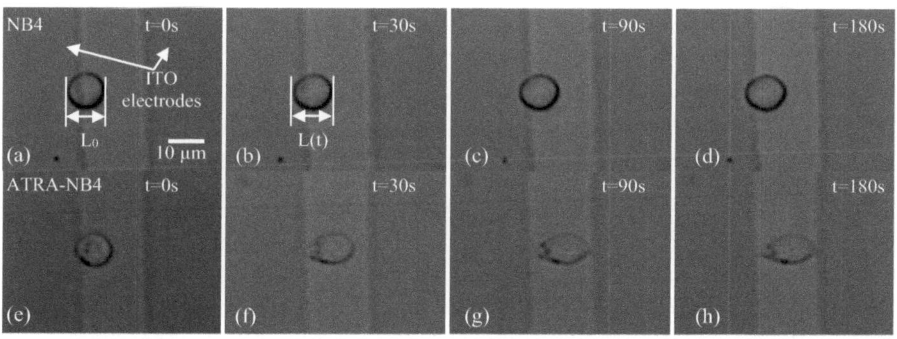

Figure 4.16 Images of an NB4 cell under the stretching experiment at different time intervals of (A) initial time, (B) 30 s, (C) 90 s, and (D) 180 s. Images of an NB4 cell treated with ATRA drug under the stretching experiment at different time intervals of (E) initial time, (F) 30 s, (G) 90 s, and (H) 180 s (Zhang et al., 2015).

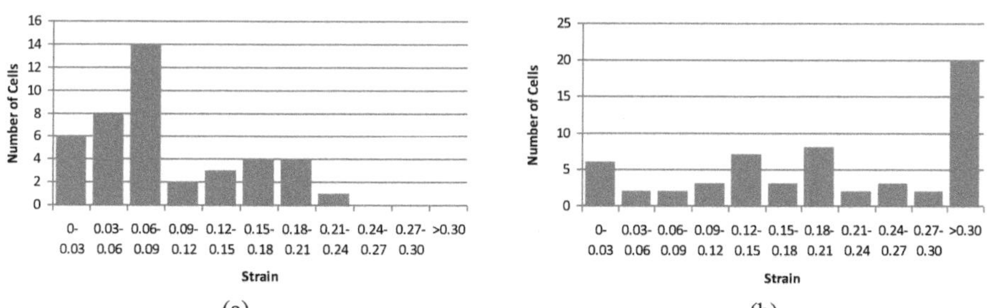

Figure 4.17 The number of cells at different strain values (Zhang et al., 2015). Aa) NB4 cells. (B) ATRA-NB4 cells.

consistent with the study by Lautenschlager et al. (2009). Theoretically, the role of ATRA in leukemia cells is to induce immature promyelocytic cells to differentiate into mature granulocytes, and the stiffness decreases due to remodeling of the actin filament network (Lautenschlager et al., 2009). The strains of the two cell types examined in the study had relatively scattered and plate distribution. The possible reason may be the effects of physiological conditions such as pH and temperature on cell characteristics and different cell life cycle stages, where the cells became more rigid as they entered the later stages of their life cycle.

The above experimental results reveal that the NB4 cells treated with ATRA drugs are more susceptible to deformation, and many of them can be stretched from one electrode to the opposite electrode, which can be intuitively observed from the captured image, as shown in Fig. 4.16. Since the gap distance between the two electrodes was set to 20 μm, the cell was deformed by about 150%. This degree of deformation may damage the cell, and the cell cannot be restored to its original size even when the applied voltage is turned off. In addition, 150% of the elongated cells can form a conductive path between the electrodes to allow current to flow, which will cause the cells to lyse quickly. In order to evaluate the influence of the culture medium on cell viability, the culture medium containing the cells was examined with trypan blue. Fig. 4.18 shows that even if the cells were stored in isotonic medium for 1 h, at least 80% of the cells remained viable.

4.4.2.2 Comparison between DEP stretching and optical tweezers stretching

Bai et al. (2017) compared the performance of the DEP stretching method and the optical tweezers stretching method. First, DEP with different voltage inputs was used to stretch NB4 and NB4-DOX cells, and their deformation was measured using an optical microscope. The corresponding DEP force was calculated using the Maxwell stress tensor (MST) method, and the result is plotted in Fig. 4.19A. The strain of the deformed cell was calculated as $(r-r_0)/r_0$, where r and r_0 represent the current and

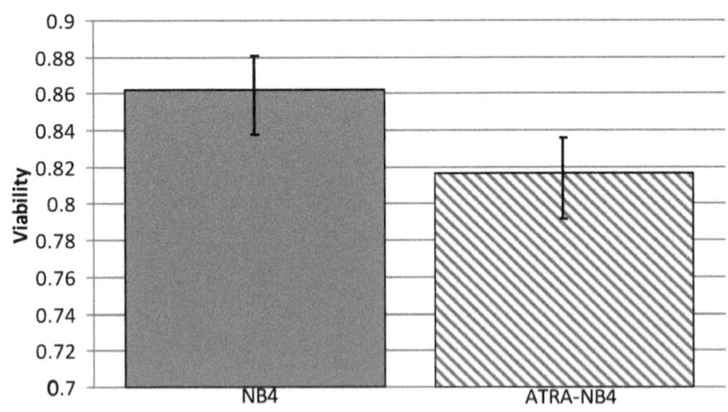

Figure 4.18 Cell viability for NB4 cells and ATRA-NB4 cells in an isotonic medium (Zhang et al., 2015).

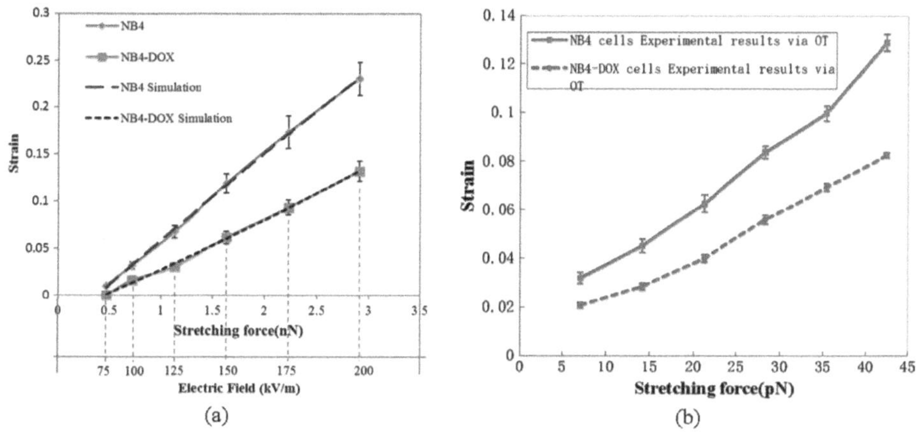

Figure 4.19 Strain—force curves of NB4 and NB4-DOX cells (Bai et al., 2017). (A) Results of DEP stretching (mean ± SE, NB4 cells: n = 54, NB4-DOX cells: n = 55). (B) Results of optical tweezers (OT)-based stretching (mean ± SE, NB4 cells: n = 20, NB4-DOX cells: n = 20).

initial radius of the cell, respectively. To illustrate the subtle differences in cells, more than 50 cells (n > 50) were examined in each group. the experimental results showed that, after DOX treatment, NB4 cells became hard. Under a force input of 2.9 nN, the average strain of NB4 cells was 0.23, and the average strain of NB4-DOX cells was 0.13. The same stretching experiment was repeated using optical tweezers, and the results are plotted in Fig. 4.19B. With a force input of 43 pN, the average strains of NB4 and NB4-DOX units were 0.13 and 0.08, respectively.

The elastic moduli of NB4 and NB4-DOX cells were estimated by relating the stress (force/area) to the deformation using the method of Leung et al. (2016). According to the experimental data, the moduli of the NB4 and NB4-DOX cells from the DEP results were about 36 and 62 Pa, respectively, while the moduli from the optical tweezers results were only 1.2 and 1.8 Pa, respectively. The R^2 value obtained from the two curves was >0.98, indicating that the data were accurate. Similar to the findings reported by Leung et al. (2016) and Urbano and Clyne (2016), the DEP can produce a higher force than other manipulating methods such as AFM.

It is worth noting that the results obtained from these two methods may not be used for direct comparison. Although similar cell deformation behaviors after DOX treatment were observed using the two methods, the range of applied stretching force differed by two orders of magnitude, mainly due to the inherent characteristics of each stretching mechanism. Several research groups have tried various methods to compare the mechanical properties of cells, and significant differences have also been reported. For example, Laurent et al. (2002) compared the elastic modulus of epithelial cells measured using magnetic cytometry and optical tweezers, and the observed difference was up to fivefold. They concluded that bead attachment strongly affects the force exerted on the cells, and the increased stress in magnetic cytometry enhances nonlinearity and cell plasticity. Urbano and Clyne (2016) used the DEP push and AFM indentation method to examine the attached epithelial cells and found that the elastic modulus differed by at least 10-fold. Fortier et al. (2016) used AFM to characterize leukemia cells with two different probes, and found that compared with spherical probes, the modulus of elasticity by conical probes was larger and had a wider distribution.

The loading rate corresponding to the stretching mechanism is another factor affecting cell deformability. Using the optical tweezers method, the cells are gradually stretched through the beads to prevent the beads from escaping the optical trap during the stretching process. In contrast, when using the DEP method, the function generator directly stretches the cell through the applied electric field, and any adjustments to the power supply voltage are immediately applied to the cell. As reported by Efremov et al. (2015), the loading rate and apparent elastic modulus are related, and a higher loading rate can lead to a higher apparent elastic modulus. Therefore, for the same deformation, the DEP method requires a higher stretching force. Other research groups have also examined cell behavior at different loading rates. Pravincumar et al. (2012) reported that the applied pressure or the slow rate of deformation may cause high levels of cortical actin to deform, thereby affecting the mechanical properties or elastic modulus of the tested cells. Nawaz et al. (2012) showed that the elastic modulus of 3T3 cells increased from 140 Pa with a low deformation rate to 330 Pa with a high deformation rate. Therefore, in various methods, subtle changes in factors such as the size of the applied force, the contact area, and the deformation speed may cause a wide range of cell deformation.

The influence of an electric field on NB4 cells may be another factor leading to differences in experimental results. According to Wigge et al. (2010) and Titushikin and Cho (2009), the use of electric fields can change the arrangement of actin filaments in the cytoskeleton structure. When biological cells were exposed to an electric field for 60 min, the elasticity of hMSC cells decreased by 70%, while the elasticity of osteoblasts decreased by only 30%. As cells tend toward cell death, the decrease in cell elasticity may be related to the increase in cell stiffness (Nikolaev et al., 2014).

4.5 Cell compression under mechanical confinement

Cells can also be compressed by mechanical constraints. Many methods have proven that mechanical restriction can be used as a physical cue to modulate intracellular signaling, thereby changing the biophysical properties of cells (Pathak and Kumar, 2012). Although new cell elasticity measurement techniques have been frequently reported in the past 2 decades, most are based on the assumption of small cell deformation and linear elasticity (Cross et al., 2007; Gavara and Chadwick, 2012). Compared with these cell compression methods (such as optical tweezers and DEP), mechanical restriction can cause larger cell deformation. In fact, cells that deform greatly can reflect more representative biomechanical properties. For example, in metastasis, cancer cells exhibit large deformations during invasion and extravasation, in which both nucleus and cytoplasm must deform together. It has been pointed out that the deformability of the nucleus rather than the deformability of the cytoplasm is the rate-limiting factor in the process of metastasis in vivo (Beadle et al., 2008). Therefore, characterizing the elasticity of severely deformed cancer cells can provide a more specific marker for cancer diagnosis.

To date, some techniques have been reported for describing larger deformed cells. Lim et al. (2004) applied hollow-shell hyperelastic theory and a computational finite element model to describe the mechanical properties of red blood cells that deform during capillary obstruction. Bernick et al. (2011) proposed a homogeneous material model to characterize the deformation of neurons over time to study traumatic brain injury (TBI) caused by high physical compression. Hu et al. (2018) revealed the elasticity of largely deformed cells flowing along constrained microchannels. Ma et al. (2018) developed a microfluidic platform to probe the migration characteristics of cancer cells under periodic mechanical constraints. This section introduces two methods to reveal the elasticity of deformed cells and uses closed microchannels to probe the migration characteristics of cancer cells.

4.5.1 Revealing the elasticity of largely deformed cells flowing along confining microchannels

As previously introduced, a variety of measurement techniques based on small deformation of biomechanical cell properties have been developed. However, many of these methods do not support cells whose internal cellular components (such as the nucleus) undergo large or direct deformation. In order to analyze the large deformation of the floating cells, an analytical model extended from the Hertz–Tatara theory, namely the hyperelastic Tatara model, can be used.

Consider a cell moving along a constrained channel, as shown in Fig. 4.20. Cell deformation is caused by the hydraulic dragging force F_{drag} and the geometric limitation of the side wall. The side wall is treated with molecular lubricant (pluoronic F127). The force balance is $F_{\text{compress}} = F_{\text{drag}}/(2 \sin \theta)$.

The Hertz contact model provides a general form for spherical contact under small deformations. The Young's modulus E is

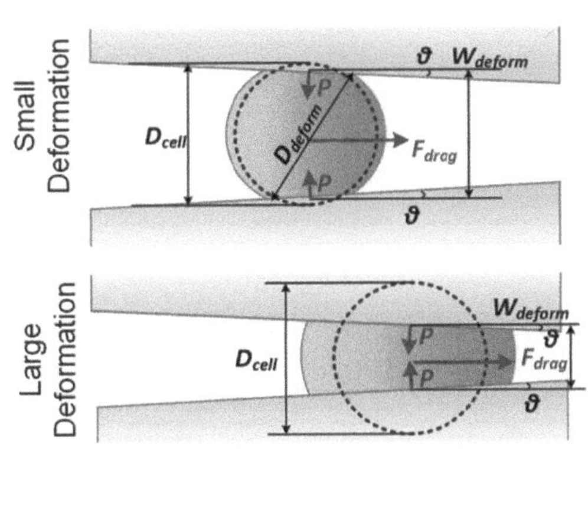

Figure 4.20 Key parameters of small and large deformation of a floating cell squeezing along a confining microchannel (Hu et al., 2018).

$$E = \frac{3(1-\nu^2)F_{\text{compress}}}{\sqrt{D_{\text{cell}}(D_{\text{cell}} - W_{\text{deform}})^3}}, \tag{4.52}$$

where D_{cell} is the cell diameter, D_{deform} is the cell deformed diameter, W_{deform} is the cell deformed width, and $\nu = 0.5$ is the Poisson's ratio of a cell (Fig. 4.20).

The Tatara model extends the description of the Hertz model to a larger deformation range, which takes into account the deformed nonspherical geometry. The Young's modulus E obtained by the Tatara model can be expressed as (Tatara, 1991):

$$E = \frac{3(1-\nu^2)F_{\text{compress}}}{2(D_{\text{cell}} - W_{\text{deform}})a} - \frac{2F_{\text{compress}}}{\pi(D_{\text{cell}} - W_{\text{deform}})f(a)}, \tag{4.53}$$

where a is the contact radius and $f(a)$ is the characteristic length of the nonspherical geometry after deformation, expressed as:

$$a = \frac{1}{2}\left(\sqrt{D_{\text{cell}}^2 - W_{\text{deform}}^2} + D_{\text{defrom}} - D_{\text{cell}}\right), \tag{4.54}$$

$$f(a) = \left[\frac{(1+\nu)D_{\text{cell}}^2}{2(a^2 + D_{\text{cell}}^2)^{3/2}} + \frac{1-\nu^2}{(a^2 + D_{\text{cell}}^2)^{1/2}}\right]^{-1}, \tag{4.55}$$

Hyperelasticity is well known as an intrinsic property of biologic cells. The hyperelastic theory can describe a wide range of cell deformations. For a spherical hyperelastic cell, the hyperelastic Tatara model gives an expression of the Young's modulus E as (Tatara, 1991):

$$E = \frac{3(1-\nu^2)A}{2(D_{\text{cell}} - W_{\text{deform}})}\left(1 + \frac{2Ba^2}{D_{\text{deform}}^2}\right)\frac{F_{\text{compress}}}{a} - \frac{2A}{\pi(D_{\text{cell}} - W_{\text{deform}})}\left(1 + \frac{4Ba^2}{5D_{\text{deform}}^2}\right)\frac{F_{\text{compress}}}{a}, \tag{4.56}$$

where A and B (related to hyperelastic correction) are calculated by:

$$A = \frac{(1-\varepsilon)^2}{1-\varepsilon+\varepsilon^2/3}, \quad B = \frac{1-\varepsilon/3}{1-\varepsilon+\varepsilon^2/3}, \quad \varepsilon = 1 - \frac{W_{\text{deform}}}{D_{\text{cell}}}, \tag{4.57}$$

where ε is the deformation of the cell.

Hu et al. (2018) reported the experiment on a confining channel with inlet width W_{in} (=30 mm), outlet width W_{out} (=4 mm), channel length L_{channel} (=300 mm), and tapering angle θ ($\approx 2.5°$ as $\tan\theta = (W_{\text{in}} - W_{\text{out}})/L_{\text{channel}}$), as shown in Fig. 4.20. Floating cells were injected into the microfluidic device and then trapped in the confined microchannels. When hydraulic pressure pushed the cell forward to the narrower outlet, the cell moved along the channel and deformed until the compression force balanced the hydraulic pressure. Therefore, the different compression force $F_{compress}$ acting on the cell can be adjusted through different inlet pressures. To estimate $F_{compress}$, laminar flow simulation was performed first using COMSOL software, and then the compressive force $F_{compress}$ was calculated by $F_{compress} = F_{drag}/(2 \sin \theta)$ to obtain the hydraulic drag force on cell F_{drag}. The friction coefficient of the microchannel wall treated with Pluronic F-127 was 0.008, so the friction force acting on the unit was less than 10% of the drag force. Therefore, cell deformation was mainly caused by $F_{compress}$. In the experiment, the hydraulic drag force applied to the cell was 1–50 nN, and the compression force was 12–600 nN.

Experiments were performed on a human breast epithelial cell line (MCF-10A) to characterize cell deformation under different inlet pressures (100 Pa, 200 Pa, 300 Pa, and 400 Pa). The cell position L and deformation diameter D_{deform} obtained from the image were analyzed according to the micrograph, as shown in Fig. 4.21A. The deformation width W_{deform} was obtained by $W_{deform} = W_{in} - 2L\tan \theta$. The cell diameter D_{cell} was obtained by the following method:

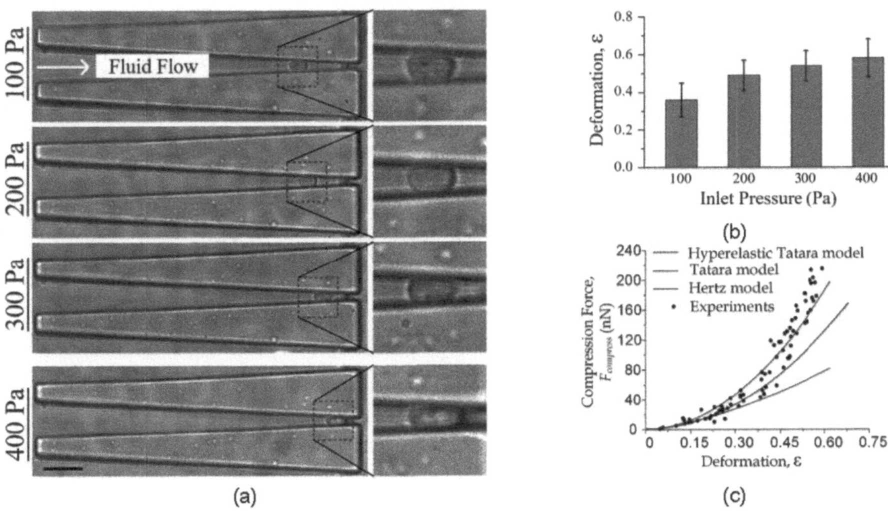

Figure 4.21 Deformation of cells (MCF-10A) as a function of inlet pressure applied at the device inlet (Hu et al., 2018). (A) Cell deformed in a confining channel under different inlet pressure levels (100 Pa, 200 Pa, 300 Pa, and 400 Pa). Scale bar: 30 mm. (B) Statistics of the deformation level against the inlet pressure, n = 31. Error bars represent the standard deviation. (C) Cell deformation properties toward large deformations. The compression force versus cell deformation under 100 and 200 Pa compared with the predictions based on the Hertz model, Tatara model, and hyperelastic Tatara model, respectively. The parameters (Young's modulus and cell diameter) in the predictions were obtained by the measurement results under 100 Pa.

$$D_{\text{cell}} = \frac{4}{3}\pi\left(\frac{D_{\text{cell}}}{2}\right)^3 \approx 2\pi\left(\frac{D_{\text{deform}}}{2}\right)^2\left(\frac{W_{\text{deform}}}{2}\right) - \frac{2}{3}\pi\left(\frac{W_{\text{deform}}}{2}\right)^3. \tag{4.58}$$

The measured diameter of the MCF-10A cell was 14.83 ± SE 0.45 mm. Fig. 4.21B shows that the deformation ε defined by Eq. (4.57) gradually increased as the inlet pressure level increased. Fig. 4.21C shows the transition from small deformation to large deformation (namely, the inlet pressure from 100 to 200 Pa), showing the relationship between compression force and deformation compared with the predictions made by the above three models (three rows).

The physical properties of large cell deformation usually imply genetic and structural deformation (Swaminathan et al., 2011). Hu et al. (2018) tested four types of cells: breast cancer epithelial cells MCF-10A, breast cancer cells MCF-7, more invasive breast cancer cells MDA-MB-231, and prostate cancer cells PC3. Applying a lower inlet pressure (100 Pa) caused less deformation, and then applying a higher inlet pressure (400 Pa) caused greater deformation. Following the same steps described in the previous section for characterizing MCF-10A cells, the initial modulus E_i of 100 Pa and the final modulus E_f of 400 Pa of the four types of cells were calculated by the hyperelastic Tatara model. Under minor deformation, cancer cells (MCF-7, MDAMB-231, and PC3) were significantly softer than normal breast cells MCF-10A (Fig. 4.22A), indicating the disruption of the cytoskeletal fibers in the cytoplasm.

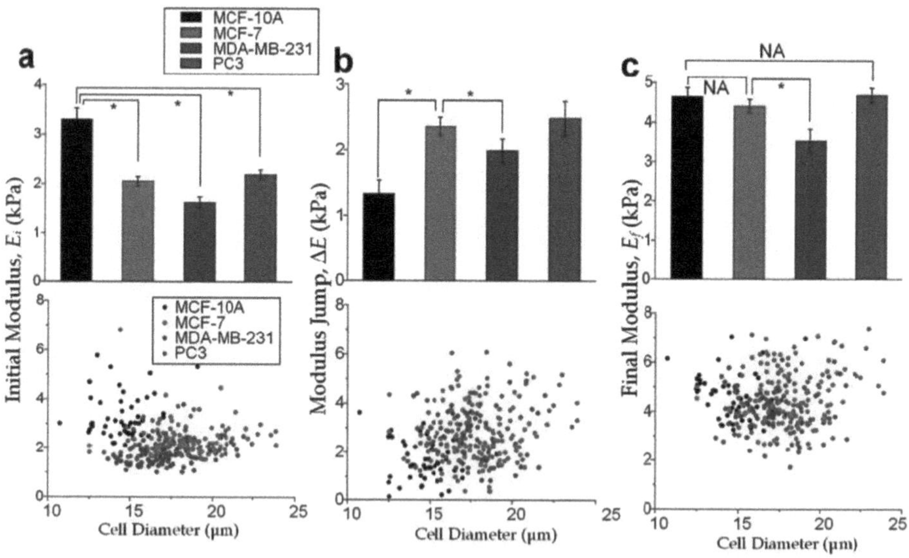

Figure 4.22 Cell mechanical properties under large deformations (Hu et al., 2018). Cell numbers, MCF-10A: n = 53, MCF-7: n = 73, MDA-MB-231: n = 67, PC3: n = 85. Bar charts and scattering plots of (A) the initial modulus E_i at 100 Pa, (B) the modulus jump DE between 100 and 400 Pa, (C) the final modulus E_f at 400 Pa. Error bars are standard errors. * indicates $P < .01$.

However, under large deformation, MCF-7 and PC3 cells did not show the significance of Young's modulus compared with the normal cell type MCF-10A (Fig. 4.22C). This transition meant that the nuclei of MCF-7 and PC3 cells hardened or became larger. In fact, harder and larger nuclei were found in cancer cells (Backman et al., 2000). For modulus jump (Fig. 4.22B), MDA-MB-231 was significantly lower than MCF-7 (or PC3), which meant that the core of MDA-MB-231 was softer than MCF-7 (or PC3), because the cell body size and nucleus of these three types of cells were similar. Previous studies have found that more aggressive cancer cells (such as MDA-MB-231) that undergo epithelial–mesenchymal transition (EMT) usually contain softer nuclei (Cicchillitti et al., 2017). Therefore, the final modulus E_f and the modulus transition D_E can provide insightful information about the physical deformation (hardening or larger) of the nucleus.

4.5.2 Probing migration property of cancer cells under periodic mechanical confinement

Cell migration is a complex cellular process that plays an important role in many physiological events (including cancer progression). Metastatic cells migrate from the primary tumor, pass through the basement membrane, enter the blood and lymph vessels, and finally invade various other tissues to form secondary tumors. Understanding the motility of cancer cells is important for cancer treatment, which requires studying the mechanism of tumor cell migration. In a physically constrained microenvironment, especially under 3D stimulation, the establishment of cell migration assays is essential for studying cancer progression (Paul et al., 2017). Many experimental models have been developed that limit the force to cells in a well-defined microenvironment, such as microfluidic microchannel devices, grooved substrates, and micropatterned ECM wires (Paul et al., 2016). Ma et al. (2018) proposed to use periodic mechanical restriction to compress cancer cells and then probe the migration characteristics of cancer cells.

Ma et al. (2018) developed a microchannel-based cell migration chip to mimic the migration of cancer cells in the microenvironment, and then the migration stability of cancer cells was measured. By adding many vertical contractions along the path of movement on the chip, cancer cells were stimulated by periodic mechanical restrictions as they passed through the chip, similar to the way cancer cells migrate through narrow channels in the internal environment. Fig. 4.23 illustrates a microchannel chip designed to compress cells using microstructures as they pass through the channel. Fig. 4.23A shows a schematic of the designed microchannel chip consisting of an array of microchannels, and each channel is equipped with five constriction structures. Fig. 4.23B shows 36 microchannels on the chip (length of 2000 μm), which is between a cell docking well and a cell collecting well. Both wells have an area of 28.5 mm^2 for cell growth. Each microchannel has a rectangular cross-section with a width of 20 μm and height of 15 μm to allow the cells to pass through. The vertical structure (length of 10 μm and height of 5 μm) reduces the height of the microchannel to 10 μm. The size of the cross-sectional area is 200 μm^2. Adherent MHCC-97L cancer cells and

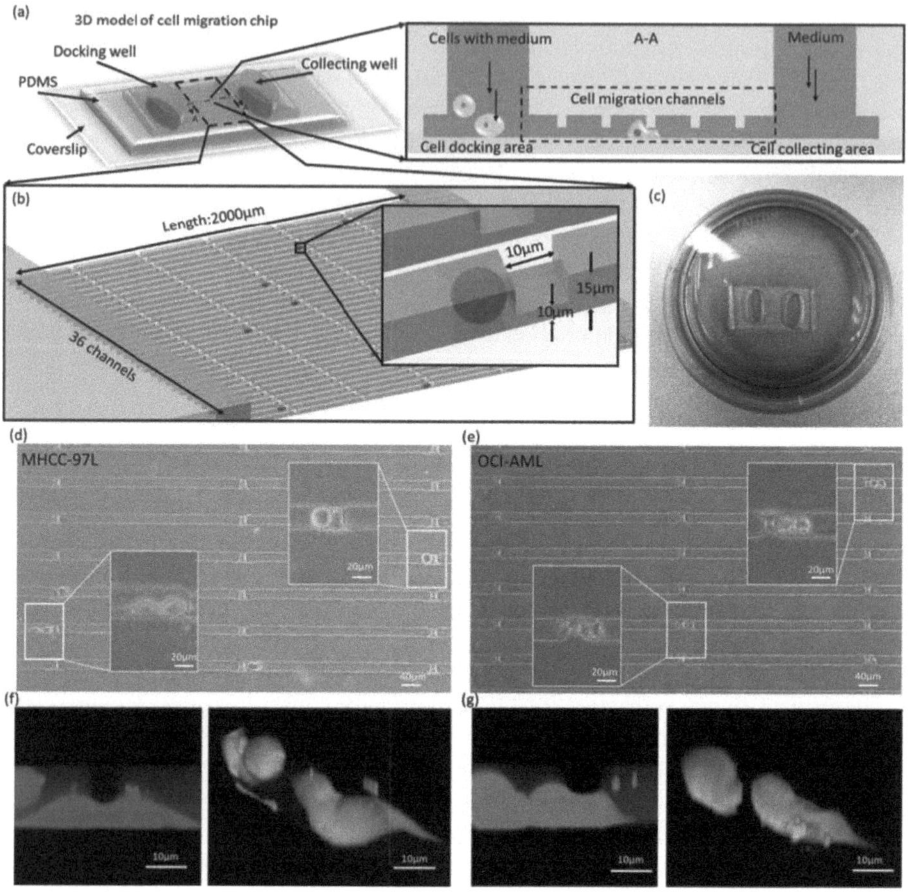

Figure 4.23 On-chip cell migration in confined microchannels (Ma et al. 2018). (A) Chip design. (B) Microchannels on the chip. (C) An image of the chip inside a 35 mm Petri dish. (D) On-chip migration of adherent MHCC-97L cells. (E) On-chip migration of suspended OCI-AML cells. (F) Confocal images of MHCC-97L cells under the vertical constriction structure. (G) Confocal images of OCI-AML cells under the vertical constriction structure.

suspended OCI-AML cells were seeded and cultivated in this designed chip under normal cell culture conditions. The developed chip for the cell migration assays is shown in Fig. 4.23C. Fig. 4.24D illustrates the spreading behavior of the MHCC-97L cells on the flat surface in the cell docking area and when the cells spontaneously migrated into the microchannels. Fig. 4.23E illustrates the spreading behavior of the OCI-AML cells. The cells were compressed when they passed through the chip channels with vertical constriction structures, and such compression was periodic when a number of constriction structures existed. The confined space on the chip can induce cell protrusion and blebbing. Figs. 4.23F and G show 3D reconstructions of the Z-series confocal scanning of cells when passing through the microconstriction structure.

The migration distance was measured based on cell forward traveling displacement for every 48 h starting from day 1. Figs. 4.24A–D (left) show sequential images of persistent cancer cell migration in the confined microchannels for over 9 days. During this time period, the cells entering the 5-constriction chip experienced confinement stimulation once, while the cells entering the 10-constriction chip were stimulated twice. Cell migration distances of five sample cells are illustrated in Figs. 4.24A–D (right). The cell migration speed and 9-day cell migration distances are shown in Figs. 4.24E and F. It was observed that the suspended OCI-AML cells had a faster migration speed and longer migration distance in the microchannels than the adherent MHCC-97 cells. Both types of cells showed a faster migration speed and longer migration distance in the 10-constriction microchannels than in the 5-constriction chip. It

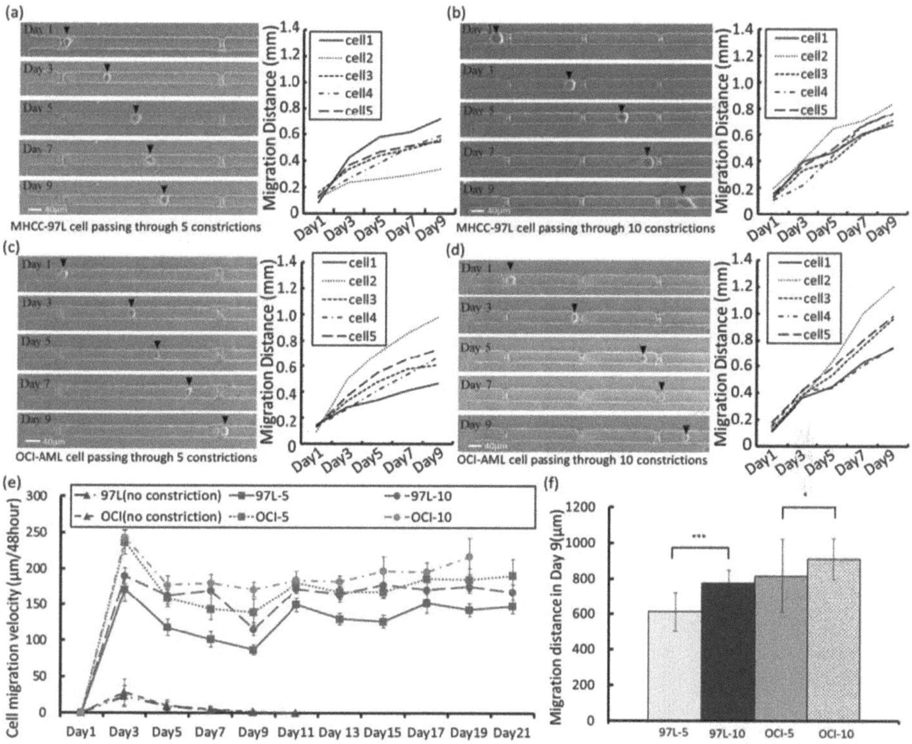

Figure 4.24 Persistent migration of cancer cells under mechanical confinement stimulations (Ma et al., 2018). (A) Displacement of MHCC-97L cells and five sample migration distances for 9 days in the 5-constriction chip. (B) Displacement of MHCC-97L cells and five sample migration distances for 9 days in the 10-constriction chip. (C) Displacement of OCI-AML cells and five sample migration distances for 9 days in the 5-constriction chip. (D) Displacement of OCI-AML cells and five sample migration distances for 9 days in the 10-constriction chip. (E) Average migration velocities in the microchannel chip without constriction and the microchannel chips with 5 and 10 constrictions. (F) Histogram of cell migration distances for 9 days in constriction chips (*$P \leq .05$, **$P \leq .01$, and ***$P \leq .001$).

was also observed that in the 5- and 10-constriction chips, both types of cells had a higher migration speed for the first 2 days and decelerated and accelerated periodically in the remaining days; while the cells migrating in the chip without construction stopped migration after day 9. It could be thus hypothesized that the cell accelerated under the vertical confinement in the microchannel and decelerated without the stimulation. The cells passing through the 10-constriction chip accelerated around day 5, whereas the cells passing through the 5-constriction chip maintained the decreasing trend of velocity. Given that the cancer cells reached the second chokepoint structure in the 10-constriction chip around day 5, the increased migration speed was possibly due to the further vertical confinement stimulation induced by the structure. The above results indicated that the cancer cells migrate faster and longer through vertical constriction in microchannels to produce periodic mechanical confinement on cells. Repeated stimulations on cells would increase cancer cell migration ability.

The mechanical property of the cancer cells was further characterized after they migrated through the designed microchannel chip. After incubation for about 21 days, the cells in the collecting and docking wells were retrieved and expanded for cell deformability tests. The optical stretching method as introduced previously was employed to measure the deformability of the suspended OCI-AML cells. Each cell was stretched by two optical traps, with a stretching force ranging from 7 to 43 pN. Fig. 4.25A shows the cell deformation results under different stretching forces. The Young's modulus was calculated based on the stretching force that induced the largest deformation of cells, as shown in Fig. 4.25D. OCI-AML cells collected from the cell docking well (control group) possessed an average stiffness of 396.9 $\pm$ 74.5 Pa (mean $\pm$ S.D., N = 30). OCI-AML cells migrating through the 5- and 10-constriction microchannel chips were soft, which had an average stiffness of 187.5 $\pm$ 56.7 and 170.5 $\pm$ 31.9 Pa (mean $\pm$ S.D., N = 30), respectively. Cells migrating through the 10-constriction microchannel were softer than those migrating through the 5-constriction microchannels. The optical stretching tests revealed that the cancer cells possessed decreased stiffness after migrating through the confined microchannels. Notably, cancer cells migrating through the 10-constriction microchannel chip were softer than those migrating through the 5-constriction chip.

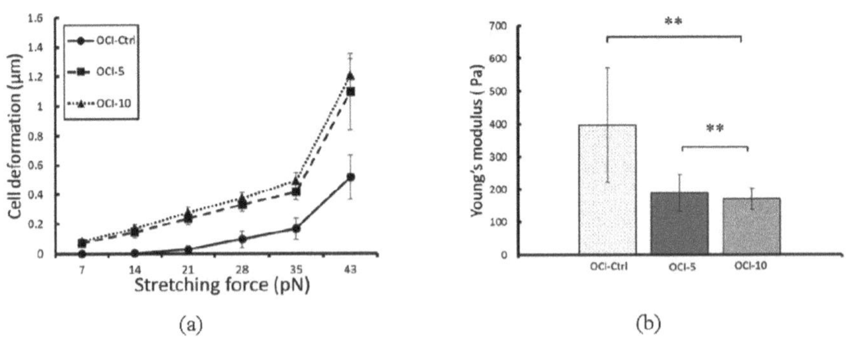

Figure 4.25 Results of cell stiffness characterization (Ma et al. 2018). (A) Force–deformation relationship of OCI-AML cells under optical stretching. (B) Young's modulus of nonmigrating and migrating OCI-AML cells (*$P \leq .05$, **$P \leq .01$, and ***$P \leq .001$).

This result suggested that the enhancement of cells through periodic mechanical confinement stimulations could affect the cell stiffness. The reduced cell stiffness may further facilitate cancer cells to change cell shape and move through the much confined space (Liu et al., 2012). Some soft cancer cells have extremely high tumorigenic ability (Samuel et al., 2011). These findings indicated that periodic mechanical stimulation may contribute to tumor progression.

4.6 Magnet-based cell deformation for intracellular delivery

Finally, a unique method of using magnetic force to induce cell deformation to achieve intracellular delivery is introduced. Living cells can be deformed to generate transient disruption in cell membranes, which allows the surrounding macromolecules to passively diffuse into cytoplasm. However, their inherent limitations are the potential membrane damage and poor throughput. With the advancements of nanotechnology and microfluidics, the penetration of cell membranes through an array of nanowires or nanoneedles achieves delivery of various biomolecules with high throughput. However, these techniques lack the ability to selectively deliver materials into targeted cells in situ. Microinjection and optical transfection can achieve highly selective delivery but at the cost of low throughput. To address these problems, a magnetic force-driven approach can be used to achieve vector-free and selective in situ intracellular delivery. Specifically, millimeter-sized iron rods or spheres driven by magnetic force are used to deform target cells, which in turn generates instantaneous disruption in the cell membrane and enables the foreign materials to enter cytosols (Wang et al., 2018).

Fig. 4.26A shows a schematic of the magnetic force-driven intracellular delivery method. An iron sphere/rod is actuated by a ramped magnetic field generated by a customized micromanipulator-controlled magnet with a sharp pole tip. The actuated sphere/rod exerts forces onto the underlying cells for material delivery that can be modulated by adjusting the distance between the sphere/rod and the magnet. Fig. 4.26B shows the experimental system for the magnetic force-driven intracellular delivery. The setup includes a robotic micromanipulation system with three degrees of freedom (3D), which consists of a motorized *XY* stage and a *Z*-axis linear table. The magnet with a sharp pole tip fixed on the motorized *XY* stage is used to generate an effective magnetic field. A Petri dish with cells is placed on the *Z*-axis table. Cells are loaded by actuating an iron sphere or rod via the magnetic force, which is modulated by controlling the distance between the magnet tip and the sphere/rod. The position of the micromanipulator is robustly controlled by a motion control unit. A CCD camera and a 3× objective mounted at the two ends of an observation tube are used for monitoring the delivery process. Note that the motions are synchronized so that the trajectory of the sphere/rod can be controlled by the magnet. For a sphere, a portion of cells underneath experience the force, thereby making it suitable for selective delivery, including cell pattern formation. For a rod, a large number of cells experience the force, which can achieve efficient delivery.

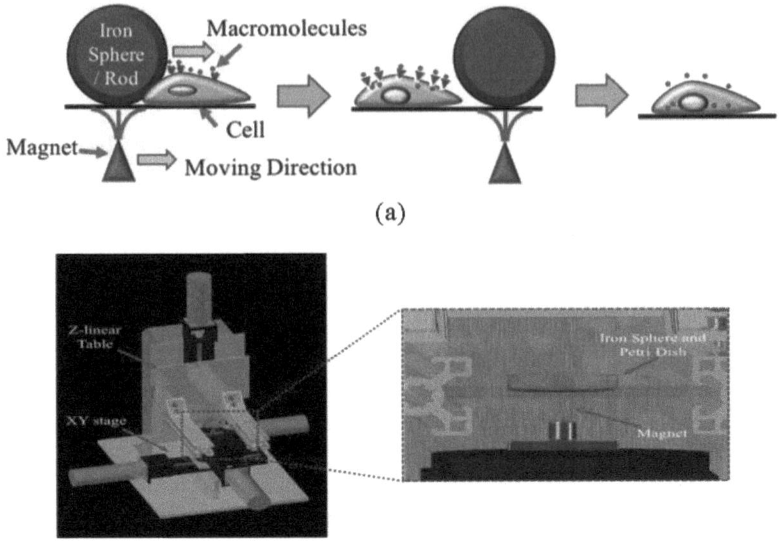

(b)

Figure 4.26 Magnetic force-driven intracellular delivery method. (A) Schematic. (B) Magnetic force injection system.

Wang et al. (2018) reported that FITC-dextran was successfully delivered to human hepatocellular carcinoma (HCC) cells HepG2 on the trajectory of the driving sphere/rod (Fig. 4.27A). When the magnetic force was increased from 0 to 1.9 mN for the sphere and from 0 to 12.5 mN for the rod, the delivery efficiency was increased from 0% to 74% and from 2% to 77%, respectively (Fig. 4.27B), showing that the intracellular delivery depended on the magnitude of magnetic force. This may be due to the fact that larger forces caused higher levels of membrane disruption that could enhance material delivery. In addition, the delivery efficiency was related to molecule concentration under a given force (Fig. 4.27C), which might be due to the molecules at higher concentrations having more chance of passing across the disrupted membranes. The contact area between the sphere/rod and cells could be estimated as the area of cells expressing the fluorescence of delivered materials ($\sim$0.05 mm^2 for the sphere with 1 mm diameter). Therefore, the contact stress was calculated to be 40 kPa for a sphere (1.9 mN), which was at the similar level of 15 kPa solid stress in tissues but much higher than the hemodynamic shear stress in vasculature (within 3 Pa). Note that the duration of force application in this approach was short, at a few milliseconds. Fig. 4.27B also shows the influence of exerted forces on cell functions, including viability, proliferation, and stem cell properties. For both spheres and rods, high magnetic forces (1.9 mN for spheres and 12.5 mN for rods) led to $\sim$90% cell viability with no significant effects on the proliferation of primary human MSCs. Physical forces have the potential to elicit stem cell differentiation.

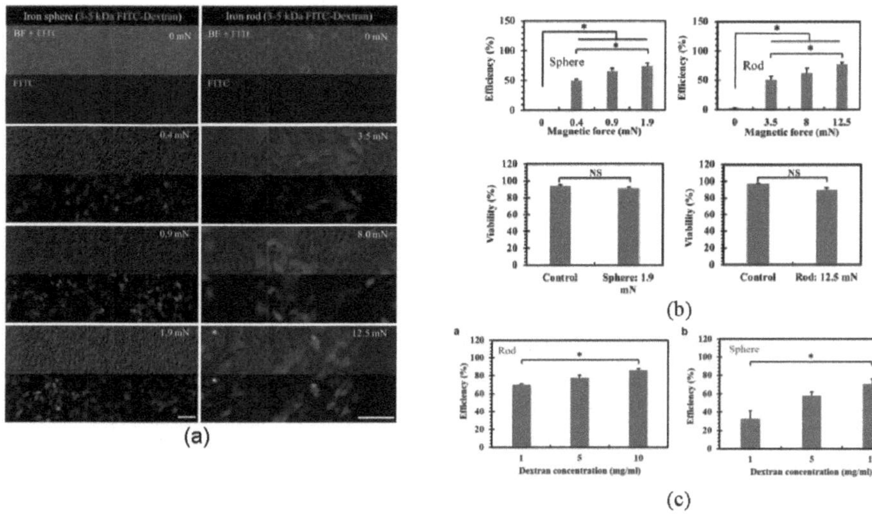

Figure 4.27 Magnetic intracellular delivery results (Wang et al., 2018). (A) The delivery of FITC-dextran into cells using iron sphere (left) or rod (right) depends on force magnitude. Scale bar: 100 μm. Various magnetic forces were used to actuate the sphere or rod, which deformed living cells in the presence of 3–5 kDa FITC-dextran, which was removed after 5 min. The fluorescence images were taken at 24 h after force application. BF: bright field. (B) Quantification of the delivery efficiency and cell viability for both the sphere (left) and rod (right). For the sphere, the FITC-positive and PI-negative cells were counted from the fluorescence images. The efficiency and viability were calculated as the ratio of FITC-positive cells and PI-negative cells over the total cell number, respectively. For the rod, flow cytometry assay was used to quantify the percentage of FITC-positive cells and PI-negative cells. Mean - ± s.e.m. (n = 3). *$P < .05$. NS: no significant difference. (C) The delivery efficiency in relation to molecule concentration. For the rod, under 12.5 mN magnetic force. For the sphere, under 1.9 mN magnetic force.

To test that the proposed magnet-based cell deformation approach can be generally used for intracellular delivery, a series of material delivery experiments were conducted in multiple mammalian cells, including HCC cells HepG2 and MHCC97-L, human dermal fibroblasts, neonatal (HDFn), human cervical cancer cells HeLa, preosteoblast MC3T3 E1, and primary human MSCs. Fig. 4.28 shows that macromolecules were successfully delivered into all cells with high efficiency and viability, suggesting that a magnetic force-driven approach can be applicable across cell types. Further tests were performed to examine whether the method can deliver various types of materials into cells. Fig. 4.29 shows that FITC-dextran with both low (3–5 kDa) and high (2000 kDa) molecular weights can be successfully delivered into HepG2 cells and primary MSCs that are usually difficult to be transfected (Fig. 4.29A and B; top left). The delivery efficiency was lower for large molecules (80% vs. 74% in HepG2; 94% vs. 81% in MSCs) (Fig. 4.29C), probably due to the increasing molecule size, which confirmed that the size-dependent delivery may be mediated by transient membrane disruption. Fluorescence-labeled bovine albumin (FITC-albumin, ~66 kDa) was

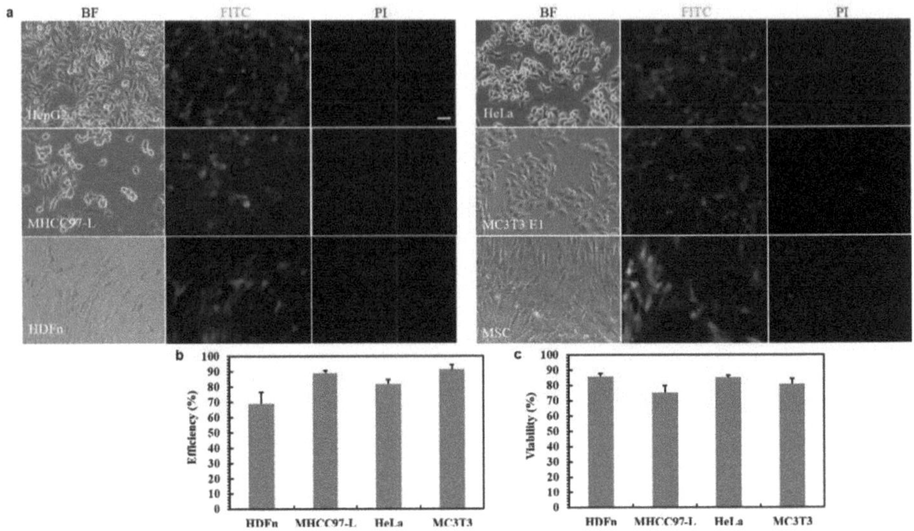

Figure 4.28 Exogenous materials were successfully delivered into various mammalian cells with high efficiency and viability (Wang et al., 2018). Various mammalian cells, including HepG2, MHCC97-L, human dermal fibroblasts, neonatal (HDFn), HeLa, preosteoblast MC3T3 E1, and primary human MSCs, were loaded by the rod under 12.5 mN magnetic forces in the presence of 1 mg/mL FITC-dextran. After 24 h, the treated cells were incubated with 500 nM PI for 15 min before the fluorescence images were taken (A). The delivery efficiency (B) and cell viability (C) were quantified. Scale bar: 50 μm.

also delivered with efficiencies of 66% and 80% for HepG2 and MSCs, respectively (Fig. 4.29A and B; bottom left; Fig. 4.29C). Further, large polystyrene beads (200 nm in diameter) can also be delivered (Fig. 4.29A and B; top right), where 3D reconstruction of the Z-series scanning showed that the delivered beads were inside the cells. In addition, the fluorescence-labeled secondary antibody (donkey anti-goat IgG-CFL 647) was successfully delivered (Fig. 4.29A and B; bottom right), demonstrating that this approach can be used for live cell immunostaining. Moreover, efficient delivery of various materials into mammalian cells did not compromise cell viability (Fig. 4.29D). All these findings demonstrated that the magnetic force-driven method is able to deliver various macromolecules into different types of mammalian cells.

To demonstrate that the delivered materials can be functional in regulating cellular functions, a case study in which siRNAs were delivered to inhibit cancer cell proliferation and migration was reported by Wang et al. (2018). In this study, siRNAs were delivered as an example to target CXCR4, the receptor of cytokine CXCL12, which is overexpressed in various cancer types and crucial in cancer cell proliferation, migration, and metastasis. The data showed that the liposome-based transfection inhibited CXCR4 expression by 32% when the liposome–siRNA mixture was incubated with cells for 2 h (Fig. 4.30A). If the incubation time was 5 min or cells were loaded without

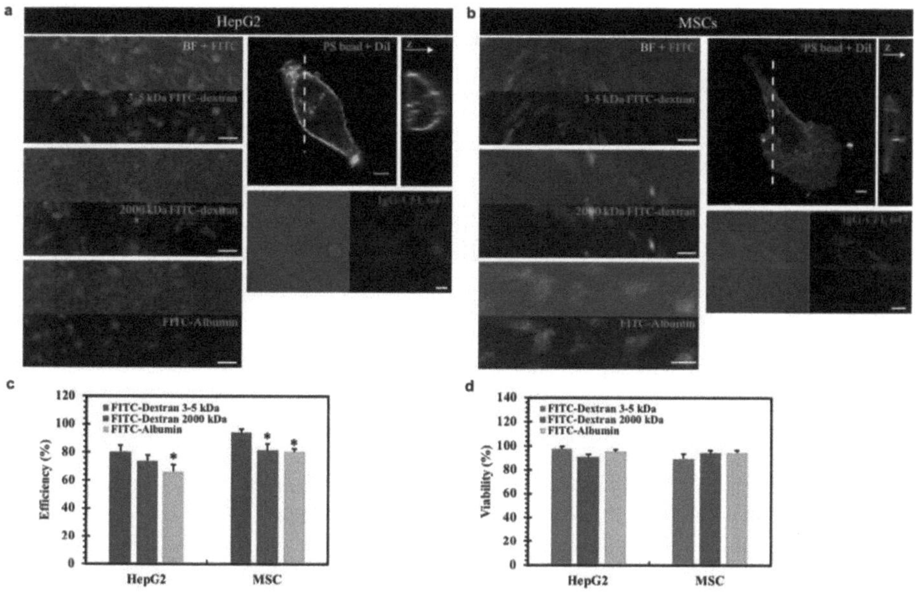

Figure 4.29 Various materials were delivered into mammalian cells across cell types (Wang et al., 2018). A wide range of molecules with sizes from a few nanometers to hundreds of nanometers can be delivered into HepG2 cells (A) and primary MSCs (B) with high efficiency and viability. Cells were deformed with the rod in the presence of 3–5 or 2000 kDa FITC-dextran, FITC-albumin (scale bars: 100 μm), polystyrene (PS) beads (200 nm in diameter; scale bar: 10 μm), and antibody IgG-CFL 647 (scale bar: 20 μm), respectively. Fluorescence images were taken after 24 h. Quantification of the delivery efficiency (C) and cell viability (D). All the cells in (A) and (B) were stained with PI and then used to quantify the efficiency and viability. For cells with PS beads, the Y-Z cross-section images were reconstructed from Z-series fluorescent images of the cell. The sectioning plane is indicated by the dashed line. Cell membrane was counterstained with DiI. $^*P < .05$, representing a significant difference between "FITC-Dextran 3–5 kDa" and other groups.

liposome, no knockdown effects were detected. In contrast, the intracellular delivery approach rapidly delivered the siRNA mixture into cells within 5 min, leading to the knockdown of CXCR4 expression by 75% (Fig. 4.30A), which was much more efficient than the liposome-based transfection. Whether the delivered siRNAs influenced cellular functions, including migration and proliferation, was further tested. The wound-healing assay showed that the delivered CXCR4 siRNA significantly suppressed wound closure (Fig. 4.30B), suggesting that silencing CXCR4 effectively inhibited cell migration, which was consistent with the findings that CXCL12/CXCR4 signaling enhanced the migration and invasion of cancer cells (Singh et al., 2014). The inhibitory effects on cell migration may be mediated by suppressing the downstreams of CXCR4, including β-catenin and vimentin (Fig. 4.30D). The MTT data showed that silencing CXCR4 significantly inhibited cell proliferation (Fig. 4.30C), which was probably due to the downregulation of its downstream

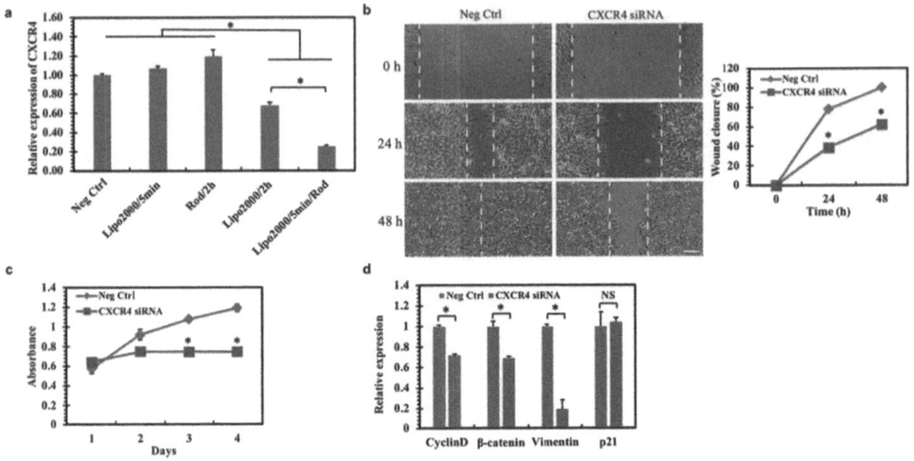

Figure 4.30 Delivered CXCR4 siRNA inhibited gene expression and cancer cell proliferation and migration (Wang et al., 2018). (A) The delivered CXCR4 siRNA effectively silenced gene expression. HepG2 cells were incubated with a mixture of lipofectamine 2000 and negative control siRNA (Neg Ctr) for 2 h, or of lipofectamine 2000 and CXCR4 siRNA for 2 h (Lipo2000/2 h) or 5 min (Lipo2000/5 min) without force application, or of CXCR4 siRNA for 2 h with force application by the rod but no lipofectamine 2000 (Rod/2 h), or of lipofectamine 2000 and CXCR4 siRNA for 5 min with force application by the rod (Lipo2000/5 min/Rod). The expression of CXCR4 was quantified by quantitative RT-PCR after 48 h. (B) Delivered CXCR4 siRNA inhibited cancer cell migration. Left: representative wound-healing figures; right: quantification of wound closure at the indicated times. (C) Delivered CXCR4 siRNA inhibited cancer cell proliferation. The CXCR4 knockdown cells in (B) were cultured in Petri dishes and used for proliferation analysis by MTT assay at days 1, 2, 3, and 4, respectively. (D) Silencing CXCR4 inhibited the expressions of β-catenin, vimentin, and cyclin D, but not p21.

effectors cyclin D and β-catenin (Fig. 4.30D). Note that silencing CXCR4 had no significant effects on p21 expression (Fig. 4.30D). These data suggested that the materials were functional after intracellular delivery.

In summary, the magnetic force-driven and vector-free method utilizes an actuated iron sphere or rod to deform living cells and deliver the surrounding macromolecules into targeted cells, thereby achieving in situ selective intracellular delivery. A wide range of materials from a few nanometers to hundreds of nanometers, including macromolecules, proteins, siRNAs, antibodies, and nanoparticles, have been successfully delivered into various types of mammalian cells with high efficiency while maintaining high viability. Compared to the other transfection methods, this unique approach can efficiently and rapidly deliver various types of materials into those hard-to-transfect cells, such as primary MSCs, and greatly enhance the transfection efficiency. Further, when used for siRNA delivery, the delivered CXCR4 siRNAs silence gene expression, which is much more efficient than the traditional liposome-based method. In addition, CXCR4 siRNAs effectively suppress cell migration and proliferation by inhibiting its downstream genes and signaling, suggesting that the materials are functional inside cells after delivery. The advantage of this method lies in the unique ability to selectively deliver exogenous materials into spatially targeted living cells in situ with relatively high throughput.

4.7 Conclusions

Cell deformation is an important cell manipulation method that can help characterize the biophysical characteristics of cells or achieve intracellular transmission. This chapter introduces the integration of robotics and various micromanipulation tools, including optical tweezers, DEP, microfluidic channels, and magnetic devices, to stretch or compress single cells to characterize cell characteristics or achieve in situ intracellular delivery. Five methods are introduced in this chapter. First, cell stretching with robotically controlled optical tweezers is introduced, which includes optical stretching model and stretching force measurement. Two case studies of stretching hematopoietic cells to understand the property difference under normal and leukemic conditions, and stretching human embryonic stem cells in cardiac differentiation to probe the mechanobiological properties are reported. Second, an actin cytoskeleton model under optical stretching is developed to provide insights into the interrelation between the cell mechanical behavior and alterations in the cell functions. Third, DEP stretching of individual cells is introduced. This method combines microfluidic chip technology, and can provide a larger stretching force in comparison to optical stretching. Fourth, the method of compressing cells through mechanical confinement is further introduced. Compared to the optical and DEP stretching methods, mechanical confinement can cause large cell deformation and thus identify cell biomechanical properties at different levels. A case study of probing migration property of cancer cells under periodic mechanical confinement is also introduced. Finally, a unique method of using magnetic force to deform cells to achieve intracellular delivery is introduced. This method can be used to deliver various types of materials into those hard-to-transfect cells efficiendmntly and rapidly. All the above methods, as well as their experimental tests and case studies, have proved that the cell stretching and compression effects achieved by various robot-assisted operating tools can play important roles in regulating and characterizing cell functions.

References

Antkowiak, M., Torres-Mapa, M.L., Stevenson, D.J., Dholakia, K., Gunn-Moore, F.J., 2013. Femtosecond optical transfection of individual mammalian cells. Nat. Protoc. 8, 1216–1233.

Ashkin, A., Dziedzic, J.M., Bjorkholm, J.E., Chu, S., 1986. Observation of a single-beam gradient force optical trap for dielectric particles. Opt. Lett. 11, 288–290.

Backman, V., Wallace, M.B., Perelman, L., Arendt, J., Gurjar, R., Müller, M., Zhang, Q., Zonios, G., Kline, E., McGillican, T., 2000. Detection of preinvasive cancer cells. Nature 406, 35.

Bai, G., Li, Y., Chu, H.K., Wang, K., Tan, Q., Xiong, J., Sun, D., 2017. Characterization of biomechanical properties of cells through dielectrophoresis-based cell stretching and actin cytoskeleton modeling. Biomed. Eng. Online 16 (41).

Bao, G., Suresh, S., 2003. Cell and molecular mechanics of biological materials. Nat. Mater. 2, 715–725.

Bausch, A.R., Kroy, K., 2006. A bottom-up approach to cell mechanics. Nat. Phys. 2, 231–238.

Beadle, C., Assanah, M.C., Monzo, P., Vallee, R., Rosenfeld, S.S., Canoll, P., 2008. The role of myosin II in glioma invasion of the brain. Mol. Biol. Cell 19, 3357–3368.

Bernick, K.B., Prevost, T.P., Suresh, S., Socrate, S., 2011. Biomechanics of single cortical neurons. Acta Biomater. 7, 1210–1219.

Bonnet, D., Dick, J.E., 1997. Human acute myeloid leukemia is organized as a hierarchy that originates from a primitive hematopoietic cell. Nat. Med. 3, 730–737.

Chang, Y.R., Hsu, L., Chi, S., 2005. Optical trapping of a spherically symmetric Rayleigh sphere: a model for optical tweezers upon cells. Opt. Commun. 246, 97–105.

Chen, J., Abdelgawad, M., Yu, L., Shakiba, N., Chien, W., Lu, Z., Geddie, W.R., Jewett, M.A.S., Sun, Y., 2011. Electrodeformation for single cell mechanical characterization. J. Micromech. Microeng. 21, 054012.

Chen, J., Li, J., Sun, Y., 2012. Microfluidic approaches for cancer cell detection, characterization, and separation. Lab Chip 12, 1753–1767.

Chen, N., Chen, C., Chen, M., Jang, L., Wang, M., 2014. Single-cell trapping and impedance measurement utilizing dielectrophoresis in a parallel-plate microfluidic device. Sensor. Actuator. B Chem. 190, 570–577.

Cheung, A.M.S., Chow, H.C.H., Liang, R., Leung, A.Y.H., 2008. A comparative study of bone marrow and peripheral blood CD34+ myeloblasts in acute myeloid leukaemia. Br. J. Haematol. 144, 484–491.

Chow, Y.T., Chen, S., Wang, R., Liu, C.C., Kong, C.W., Li, R.A., Cheng, S.H., Sun, D., 2016. Single cell transfection through precise microinjection with quantitatively controlled injection volumes. Sci. Rep. 6, 24127.

Chowdhury, F., Na, S., Li, D., Poh, Y.C., Tanaka, T.S., Wang, F., Wang, N., 2010. Material properties of the cell dictate stress-induced spreading and differentiation in embryonic stem cells. Nat. Mater. 9, 82–88.

Cicchillitti, L., Corrado, G., Carosi, M., Dabrowska, M.E., Loria, R., Falcioni, R., Cutillo, G., Piaggio, G., Vizza, E., 2017. Prognostic role of NF-YA splicing isoforms and Lamin A status in low grade endometrial cancer. Oncotarget 8, 7935.

Cross, S.E., Jin, Y.S., Rao, J., Gimzewski, J.K., 2007. Nanomechanical analysis of cells from cancer patients. Nat. Nanotechnol. 2, 780–783.

Darling, E.M., Topel, M., Zauscher, S., Vail, T.P., Guilak, F., 2008. Viscoelastic properties of human mesenchymally-derived stem cells and primary osteoblasts, chondrocytes, and adipocytes. J. Biomech. 41, 454–464.

Ding, X., Stewart, M., Sharei, A., Weaver, J.C., Langer, R.S., Jensen, K.F., 2017. High-throughput nuclear delivery and rapid expression of DNA via mechanical and electrical cell-membrane disruption. Nat. Biomed. Eng. 1, 39.

Doh, I., Lee, W.C., Cho, Y., Pisano, A.P., Kuypers, F.A., 2012. Deformation measurement of individual cells in large populations using a single-cell microchamber array chip. Appl. Phys. Lett. 100, 173702.

Du, E., Dao, M., Suresh, S., 2014. Quantitative biomechanics of healthy and diseased human red blood cells using dielectrophoresis in a microfluidic system. Extreme Mech. Lett. 1, 35–41.

Efremov, Y.M., Bagrov, D.V., Kirpichnikov, M.P., Shaitan, K.V., 2015. Application of the Johnson–Kendall–Roberts model in AFM-based mechanical measurements on cells and gel. Colloids Surf. B 134, 131–139.

Ehler, E., Perriard, J.C., 2000. Cardiomyocyte cytoskeleton and myofibrillogenesis in healthy and diseased heart. Heart Fail. Rev. 5, 259–269.

Engelhardt, H., Gaub, H., Sackmann, E., 1984. Viscoelastic properties of erythrocyte membranes in high-frequency electric fields. Nature 307 (5949), 378–381.

Engler, A.J., Sen, S., Sweeney, H.L., Discher, D.E., 2006. Matrix elasticity directs stem cell lineage specification. Cell 126, 677–689.

Evans, E.A., Skalak, R., 1980. Mechanics and Thermodynamics of Biomembranes. CRC, Boca Raton, FL.

Fortier, H., Variola, F., Wang, C., Zou, S., 2016. AFM force indentation analysis on leukemia cells. Anal. Methods 8, 4421–4431.

Gavara, N., Chadwick, R.S., 2012. Determination of the elastic moduli of thin samples and adherent cells using conical atomic force microscope tips. Nat. Nanotechnol. 7, 733–736.

Gardel, M.L., Shin, J.H., MacKintosh, F.C., Mahadevan, L., Matsudaira, L.P., Weitz, D.A., 2004. Elastic behavior of cross-linked and bundled actin networks. Science 304 (5675), 1301–1305.

Gauthier, R.C., 1997. Theoretical investigation of the optical trapping force and torque on cylindrical micro-objects. J. Opt. Soc. Am. B 14, 3323–3333.

Guido, I., Jaeger, M.S., Duschl, C., 2011. Dielectrophoretic stretching of cells allows for characterization of their mechanical properties. Eur. Biophys. J. 40, 281–288.

Grover, S.C., Skirtach, A.G., Gauthier, R.C., Grover, C.P., 2001. Automated single-cell sorting system based on optical trapping. J. Biomed. Opt. 6, 14–22.

Han, S., Nakamura, C., Obataya, I., Nakamura, N., Miyake, J., 2005. Gene expression using an ultrathin needle enabling accurate displacement and low invasiveness. Biochem. Biophys. Res. Commun. 332, 633–639.

Hochmuth, R.M., 2000. Micropipette aspiration of living cells. J. Biomech. 33, 15–22.

Hou, H.W., Li, Q.S., Lee, G.Y.H., Kumar, A.P., Ong, C.N., Lim, C.T., 2009. Deformability study of breast cancer cells using microfluidics. Biomed. Microdevices 11, 557–564.

Hu, S., Sun, D., 2011. Automatic transportation of biological cells with a robot-tweezer manipulation system. Int. J. Rob. Res. 30 (14), 1681–1694.

Hu, S., Wang, R., Tsang, C.M., Tsao, S.W., Sun, D., Lam, R.H.W., 2018. Revealing elasticity of largely deformed cells flowing along confining microchannels. RSC Adv. 8 (2), 1030–1038.

Hu, Z., Wang, J., Liang, J., 2005. Experimental measurement and analysis of the optical trapping force acting on a yeast cell with a lensed optical fiber probe. Opt Laser. Technol. 39, 475–480.

Jones, T.B., 1995. Electromechanics of Particles. Cambridge University Press, Cambridge (Chapter 2).

Khan, M., Soni, H., Sood, A.K., 2009. Optical tweezer for probing erythrocyte membrance deformability. Appl. Phys. Lett. 95, 233703.

Keyhani, K., Guzmán, H.R., Parsons, A., Lewis, T.N., Prausnitz, M.R., 2001. Intracellular drug delivery using low-frequency ultrasound: quantification of molecular uptake and cell viability. Pharm. Res. 18, 1514–1520.

Lam, W.A., Rosenbluth, M.J., Fletcher, D.A., 2008. Chemotherapy exposure increases leukemia cell stiffness. Blood 109 (8), 3505–3508.

Lam, W.A., Fletcher, D.A., 2011. Cellular Mechanics of Acute Leukemia and Chemotherapy *Cellular and Biomolecular Mechanics and Mechanobiology*, Studies in Mechanobiology, Tissue Engineering and Biomaterials, vol. 4. Springer, Berlin, Heidelberg, pp. 523–558.

Laurent, V.M., Henon, S., Planus, E., Fodil, R., Balland, M., Isabey, D., Gallet, F., 2002. Assessment of mechanical properties of adherent living cells by bead micromanipulation:

comparison of magnetic twisting cytometry vs optical tweezers. J. Biomech. Eng. 124, 408–421.

Lautenschlager, F., Paschke, S., Schinkinger, S., Bruel, A., Beil, M., Guck, J., 2009. The regulatory role of cell mechanics for migration of differentiating myeloid cells. Proc. Natl. Acad. Sci. U.S.A. 106, 15696–15701.

Leung, S.L., Lu, Y., Bluestein, D., Slepian, M.,J., 2016. Dielectrophoresis-mediated electrodeformation as a means of determining individual platelet stiffness. Ann. Biomed. Eng. 44 (4), 903–913.

Levinson, I.J., 1970. Mechanics of Materials. Prentice-Hall, Englewood Cliffs, NJ.

Lim, C.T., Dao, M., Suresh, S., Sow, C., Chew, K., 2004. Large deformation of living cells using laser traps. Acta Mater. 52, 1837–1845.

Liu, J., Tan, Y., Zhang, H., Zhang, Y., Xu, P., Chen, J., Poh, Y.C., Tang, K., Wang, N., Huang, B., 2012. Soft fibrin gels promote selection and growth of tumorigenic cells. Nat. Mater. 11 (8), 734.

MacQueen, L.A., Buschmann, M.D., Wertheimer, M.R., 2010. Mechanical properties of mammalian cells in suspension measured by electro-deformation. J. Micromech. Microeng. 20, 065007.

Mathur, A.B., Collinsworth, A.M., Reichert, W.M., Kraus, W.E., Truskey, G.A., 2001. Endothelial, cardiac muscle and skeletal muscle exhibit different viscous and elastic properties as determined by atomic force microscopy. J. Biomech. 34, 1545–1553.

Martin, M., Mueller, K., Wottawah, F., Schinkinger, S., Lincoln, B., Romeyke, M., Kas, J.A., 2006. Feeling with light for cancer. Proc. SPIE 6080, 60800P.

McCain, M.L., Parker, K.K., 2011. Mechanotransduction: the role of mechanical stress, myocyte shape, and cytoskeletal architecture on cardiac function. Pflug. Arch. Eur. J. Phy. 462, 89–104.

Ma, D., Wang, R., Chen, S., Luo, T., Chow, Y.T., Sun, D., 2018. Microfluidic platform for probing cancer cells migration property under periodic mechanical confinement. Biomicrofluidics 12 (2), 024118.

Mijailovich, S.M., Kojic, M., Zivkovic, M., Fabry, B., Fredberg, J.J., 2002. A finite element model of cell deformation during magnetic bead twisting. J. Appl. Physiol. 93, 1429–1436.

Nawaz, S., Sanchez, P., Bodensiek, K., Li, S., Simons, M., abd Schaap, I.A.T., 2012. Cell viscoelasticity measured with AFM and optical trapping at sub-micrometer deformations. PLoS One 7 (9), 1–9 e45297.

Neuman, K.C., Block, S.M., 2004. Optical trapping. Rev. Sci. Instrum. 75, 2787–2809.

Niederman, R., Amrein, P.C., Hartwig, J., 1983. Three-dimensional structure of actin filaments and of an actin gel made with actin-binding protein. J. Cell Biology 96, 1400–1413.

Nikolaev, N.I., Muller, T., Williams, D.J., Liu, Y., 2014. Changes in the stiffness of human mesenchymal stem cells with the progress of cell death as measured by atomic force microscopy. J. Biomech. 47, 625–630.

Nishimura, S., Nagai, S., Katoh, M., Yamashita, H., Saeki, Y., Okada, J., Hisada, T., Nagai, R., Sugiura, S., 2006. Microtubules modulate the stiffness of cardiomyocytes against shear stress. Circ. Res. 98, 81–87.

Oertel, H., 2004. Prandtl's essentials of fluid mechanics. Appl. Math. Sci. 158, 118–125, 2004.

Paul, C.D., Hung, W.C., Wirtz, D., Konstantopoulos, K., 2016. Engineered models of confined cell migration. Annu. Rev. Biomed. Eng. 18, 159.

Paul, C.D., Mistriotis, P., Konstantopoulos, K., 2017. Cancer cell motility: lessons from migration in confined spaces. Nat. Rev. Cancer 17 (2), 131.

Pathak, A., Kumar, S., 2012. Independent regulation of tumor cell migration by matrix stiffness and confinement. Proc. Natl. Acad. Sci. U.S.A. 109 (26), 10334.

Pohl, H.A., 1951. The motion and precipitation of suspensoids in divergent electric fields. J. Appl. Phys. 22, 869–871.
Palmer, J.S., Boyce, M.C., 2008. Constitutive modeling of the stress-strain behavior of F-actin filament networks. Acta Biometer. 4, 597–612.
Pravincumar, P., Bader, D.L., Knight, M.M., 2012. Viscoelastic cell mechanics and actin remodelling are dependent on the rate of applied pressure. PLoS One 7 (9), 1–10 e43937.
Rosales, C., Lim, K.M., 2005. Numerical comparison between Maxwell stress method and equivalent multipole approach for calculation of the dielectrophoretic force in single-cell traps. Electrophoresis 26 (11), 2057–2065.
Rosenbluth, M.J., Lam, W.A., Fletcher, D.A., 2006. Force microscopy of nonadherent cells: a comparison of leukemia cell deformability. Biophys. J. 90, 2994–3003.
Samuel, M.S., Lopez, J.I., McGhee, E.J., Croft, D.R., Strachan, D., Timpson, P., Munro, J., Schroder, E., Zhou, J., Brunton, J.V.G., Barker, N., Clevers, H., Sansom, O.J., Anderson, K.I., Weaver, V.M., Olson, M.F., 2011. Actomyosin-mediated cellular tension drives increased tissue stiffness and β-catenin activation to induce epidermal hyperplasia and tumor growth. Cancer Cell 19 (6), 776.
Shalek, A.K., Robinson, J.T., Karp, S., Lee, J.S., Ahn, D.R., Yoon, M.H., Sutton, A., Jorgolli, M., Gertner, R.S., Guiral, T.S., MacBeath, G., Yang, E.G., Park, H., 2010. Vertical silicon nanowires as a universal platform for delivering biomolecules into living cells. Proc. Natl. Acad. Sci. U.S.A. 107, 1870–1875.
Simmons, R.M., Finer, J.T., Chu, S., Spudich, J.A., 1996. Quantitative measurements of force and displacement using an optical trap. Biophys. J. 70, 1813–1822.
Singh, S., Singh, U.P., Grizzle, W.E., Lillard, J.W., 2014. CXCL12–CXCR4 interactions modulate prostate cancer cell migration, metalloproteinase expression and invasion. Lab. Invest. 84, 1666–1676.
Snir, M., Kehat, I., Gepstein, A., Coleman, R., Itskovitz-Eldor, J., Livne, E., Gepstein, L., 2003. Assessment of the ultrastructural and proliferative properties of human embryonic stem cell-derived cardiomyocytes. American J. Physiology—Heart and Circulatory Physiology 285, H2355–H2363.
Suresh, S., Spatz, J., Mills, J.P., Micoulet, A., Dao, M., Lim, C.T., Beil, M., Seufferlein, T., 2005. Connections between single-cell biomechanics and human disease states: gastrointestinal cancer and malaria. Acta Biomater. 1, 15–30.
Swaminathan, V., Mythreye, K., O'Brien, E.T., Berchuck, A., Blobe, G.C., Superfine, R., 2011. Mechanical stiffness grades metastatic potential in patient tumor cells and in cancer cell lines. Cancer Res. 71, 5075–5080.
Tan, Y., Sun, D., Wang, J., Huang, W., 2010. Mechanical characterization of human red blood cells under different osmotic conditions by robotic manipulation with optical tweezers. IEEE Trans. Biomed. Eng. 57 (7), 1816–1825.
Tan, Y., Fung, T.K., Wan, H., Wang, K., Leung, A.Y.H., Sun, D., 2011. Biophysical characterization of hematopoietic cells from normal and leukemic sources with distinct primitiveness. Appl. Phys. Lett. 99 (8), 083702.
Tan, Y., Kong, C.W., Chen, S., Cheng, S.H., Li, R.A., Sun, D., 2012. Probing the mechanobiological properties of human embryonic stem cells in cardiac differentiation by optical tweezers. J. Biomech. 45 (1), 123–128.
Tatara, T., 1991. On compression of rubber elastic sphere over a large range of displacements—part 1: theoretical study. J. Eng. Mater. Technol. 113, 285–291.
Titushkin, I., Cho, M., 2009. Regulation of cell cytoskeleton and membrane mechanics by electric field: role of linker proteins. Biophys. J. 96, 717–728.

Treiser, M.D., Yang, E.H., Gordonov, S., Cohen, D.M., Androulakis, I.P., Kohn, J., Chen, C.S., Moghe, P.V., 2010. Cytoskeleton-based forecasting of stem cell lineage fates. Proc. Natl. Acad. Sci. U.S.A. 107, 610–615.

Turdi, S., Guo, R., Huff, A.F., Wolf, E.M., Culver, B., Ren, J., 2009. Cardiomyocyte contractile dysfunction in the APPswe/PS1dE9 mouse model of Alzheimer's disease. PLoS One 4, e6033.

Ujihara, Y., Nakamura, M., Miyazaki, H., Wada, S., 2010. Proposed spring network cell model based on a minimum energy concept. Ann. Biomed. Eng. 38, 1530–1538.

Urbano, R.L., Clyne, A.M., 2016. An inverted dielectrophoretic device for analysis of attached single cell mechanics. Lab Chip 16 (3), 561–573.

Wang, R., Chow, Y.T., Chen, S., Ma, D., Luo, T., Tan, Y., Sun, D., 2018. Magnetic force-driven in situ selective intracellular delivery. Sci. Rep. 8, 14205.

Wang, K., Cheng, J., Cheng, S.H., Sun, D., 2013. Probing cell biophysical behavior based on actin cytoskeleton modeling and stretching manipulation with optical tweezers. Appl. Phys. Lett. 99, 083702.

Wang, K., Sun, D., 2012. Influence of semiflexible structural features of actin cytoskeleton on cell stiffness based on actin microstructural modelling. J. Biomech. 45 (11), 1900–1908.

Wang, X., Wang, X.B., Gascoyne, P.R.C., 1997. General expressions for dielectrophoretic force and electrorotational torque derived using the Maxwell stress tensor method. J. Electrost. 39, 277–295.

Wang, Y., Yang, Y., Yan, L., Kwok, S.Y., Li, W., Wang, Z., Zhu, X., Zhu, G., Zhang, W., Chen, X., Shi, P., 2014. Poking cells for efficient vector-free intracellular delivery. Nat. Commun. 5, 4295–4298.

Warnat, S., King, H., Forbrigger, C., Hubbard, T., 2015. PolyMUMPs MEMS device to measure mechanical stiffness of single cells in aqueous media. J. Micromech. Microeng. 25, 025011.

Wigge, C., Hinssen, H., Reiss, G., Herth, S., 2010. Positioning and stretching of actin filaments by electric fields. Appl. Phys. Lett. 96, 243703.

Wilson, A., Trumpp, A., 2006. Bone-marrow haematopoietic-stem-cell niches. Nat. Rev. Immunol. 6, 93–106.

Wozniak, M.J., Kawazoe, N., Tateishi, T., Chen, G., 2010. Change of the mechanical properties of chondrocytes during expansion culture. Soft Matter 6, 2462–2469.

Wu, Y., Sun, D., Huang, W., 2011. Mechanical force characterization in manipulating live cells with optical tweezers. J. Biomech. 44, 741–746.

Xie, X., Xu, A.M., Leal-Ortiz, S., Cao, Y., Garner, C.C., Melosh, N.A., 2013. Nanostraw–electroporation system for highly efficient intracellular delivery and transfection. ACS Nano 7, 4351–4358.

Yan, S.H., Yao, B.L., 2007. Transverse trapping forces of focused Gaussian beam on ellipsoidal particles. J. Opt. Soc. Am. B 24, 1596–1602.

Yourek, G., Hussain, M.A., Mao, J.J., 2007. Cytoskeletal changes of mesenchymal stem cells during differentiation. Am. Soc. Artif. Intern. Organs J. 53 (2), 219–228.

Zhang, X., Chu, H.K., Zhang, Y., Bai, G., Wang, K., Tan, Q., Xiong, J., Sun, D., 2015. Rapid characterization of the biomechanical properties of drug-treated cells in a microfluidic device. J. Micromech. Microeng. 25, 105004.

Zhang, Y., Nguyen, J., Wei, Y., Sun, Y., 2013. Recent advances in microfluidic techniques for single cell biophysical characterization. Lab Chip 13, 2464–2483.

Cell transport with optical tweezers

5

5.1 Introduction

In biomedical research, such as drug discovery, cell–cell interactions, and tissue engineering, accurate positioning of biological cells has become increasingly important. The huge demand for accuracy and productivity of cell processing highlights the need for automated cell transportation with integrated robotics and microprocessing technology. Optical tweezers use highly focused low-power laser beams that are used to trap and manipulate micron/nano-scale particles, and can be regarded as special robotic "end-effectors" that manipulate biological objects in a noninvasive manner.

Traditionally, many optical tweezers systems use a mouse or vertical joystick to control the optical trap. Although manual operation is robust, it cannot be effectively used in applications that require repetitive and precise manipulations of a large number of cells or coordinated operations of multiple optical traps (Chapin et al., 2006). The open-loop control strategy has been used to automatically control the optical trap (Grover et al., 2001; Tanaka et al., 2008; Arai et al., 2009). Compared with open-loop control, closed-loop control exhibits much improved performance in accuracy, throughput, and robustness, which is crucial in many biological operations. In addition, automatic computer control allows multiple traps to be manipulated at the same time. This will not only increase productivity, but also coordinate multiple traps to achieve more complex manipulation tasks that cannot be achieved with a single optical trap. Some closed-loop control methods for optical trapping have been reported, such as by Ranaweera and Bamieh (2005), Wulff et al. (2007), Wallin et al. (2008), Huang et al. (2009), and Pacoret et al. (2009). All these studies aimed to increase the stiffness of the optical trap and reduce the fluctuation of the trapped particles.

Hu and Sun (2011) proposed incorporating robotics into optical tweezers manipulation to automatically transport biological cells. They built a robotic manipulation system equipped with optical tweezers, and analyzed the dynamics of trapped cells in motion. A single-cell closed-loop control algorithm was developed to transport cells individually, and then a synchronous control method was further developed to solve the multicell transport problem. Chen and Sun (2012) studied the use of robot-controlled holographic optical tweezers (HOT) to automatically move groups of particles into an array. Based on the physical dynamics of trapping, they developed a potential field-based controller to drive each pair of particles to a specified array while preventing collisions between particles. The advantage of the proposed controller is that it can drive two sets of particles into a common array in pairs and control the mutual distance between the pairs of particles. Cheah et al. (2015)

Robotic Cell Manipulation. https://doi.org/10.1016/B978-0-323-85259-3.00017-9

proposed a closed-loop setpoint control algorithm using optical tweezers and showed that a simple control law is effective for closed-loop manipulation, taking into account the dynamic interaction between the laser beam and the cell. Chen et al. (2016) also studied the use of saturation-controlled optical tweezers to automatically transport multiple cells in a crowded microenvironment. To properly plan the motion, Wu et al. (2013) used an improved A* algorithm to plan the path in the process of automated cell transportation. Ju et al. (2014) used a rapid exploration random tree (RRT) algorithm to calculate the collision-free path in the path planner for cell transportation. Banerjee et al. (2010) also developed a random path planning method to automatically transfer particles with optical tweezers.

When trapping a cell with optical tweezers, the cell must be located in the optical trap. If there is no effective control technology that can automatically control the movement of the cells, and at the same time always position the cells in the optical trap, the trapped cells can easily escape, resulting in failure of the manipulation task. Therefore, there is an urgent need for a unified controller to be developed that can simultaneously control cell trapping and cell movement while being robust to environmental interference. For this reason, Li et al. (2015) developed a unified controller that can manipulate cell positioning and cell trapping at the same time. Li et al. (2018) further proposed a method for high-speed manipulation of single suspended cells using robot-assisted optical tweezers. Based on the aim of confining the trapped cells to the high-speed transfer area, a switching geometric model for automatic cell trapping, maintenance of optical trapping, and obstacle avoidance was developed, which helped to achieve high-speed cell transportation. Using the switching geometry model, a controller for high-speed cell transportation was proposed to efficiently transfer target cells to the destination.

Most research into automated cell transport is oriented to single tasks, while many practical applications usually require a series of operational tasks with multiple processing steps. In order to solve this problem, Yang et al. (2017) proposed an automatic cell transportation method that accomplished multiple steps. In their research, they developed a control scheme based on a robotic optical tweezers manipulation system, which controlled the grouped cells to move to different task areas in sequence and without interference. A potential field-based controller was designed to implement multistep process control. In this method, the concepts of contractive coalition and switching region were incorporated into the tweezers—cell coalition. The controller showed the advantages of simultaneously controlling the position of optical tweezers, trapping multiple cells, and avoiding collisions in a unified manner. Yang et al. (2020) further proposed a virtual-based controller for automatic cell transportation with a variable field of view in a dynamic environment. This research aimed to solve the problem of unknown obstacles being suspended outside the field of view that may cling to the target cells, resulting in failure of the cell transport task.

In the following sections, a variety of cell transport control methods using robotically controlled optical tweezers are introduced, including single-cell and multicell transport, group cell pairing, motion planning, high-speed motion control, and cell transfer for multiprocessing task automation.

5.2 Basic theory and methods

Using the force exerted by a strongly focused beam, optical tweezers can act as a special robot end-effector to trap and move objects ranging from tens of nanometers to tens of microns. By integrating robotics technology into optical tweezers, automatic transportation of biological cells can be realized. Hu and Sun (2011) developed a robot-tweezers manipulation system to automatically transport single cells based on the analysis of cell dynamics under the optical trap and the single-cell closed-loop control algorithm. The robot-tweezer system uses a spatial light modulator (SLM) to divide a single collimated laser beam into several separate beams, and each beam can be placed at any position within the focal length of the objective lens. It is assumed that the actual position of the trap after calibration is exactly the same as the desired position.

5.2.1 Dynamics analysis

Optically trapped cells are subjected to five forces: optical force, gravity, buoyancy, viscous drag force, and Langevin force (Banerjee et al., 2010). For convenience, the optical force is divided into the force along the z axis (optical power in the z-axis direction) and the force along the x−y plane (optical trapping force). For stable optical tweezers, the force on the z axis (including the optical force on the z axis, buoyancy, and gravity) is balanced. When considering the movement of the trapped cell in the x−y plane, the force on the z axis does not contribute to the lateral movement, so it can be ignored (Huang et al., 2009). In the process of cell transportation, the Brownian motion caused by the Langevin force is relatively small (Arai et al., 2004), so the Langewin force can also be ignored. Similar analysis can be found in other works of Tan et al. (2008) and Wu et al. (2011). Therefore, the forces that control the motion of the trapped cells include the trapping force from the optical trap and the viscous drag force from the liquid, as shown in Fig. 5.1A.

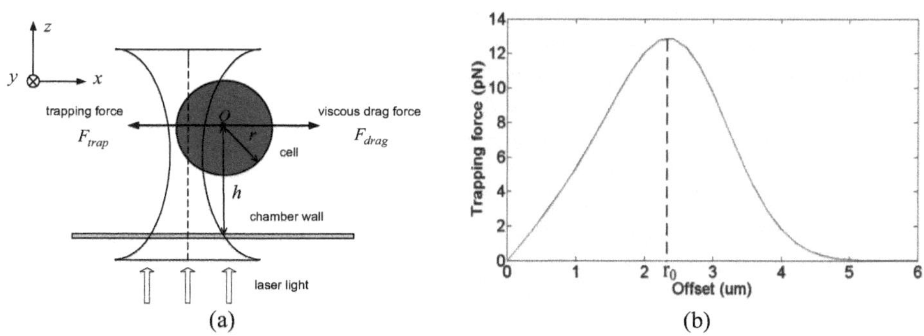

Figure 5.1 Cell trapping diagram (Hu and Sun, 2011). (A) Schematic of a cell in an optical trap. (B) Example of a yeast cell: lateral trapping force versus lateral offset.

The dynamics equation of the motion of the cell in the lateral plane is

$$m\ddot{q} = F_{\text{trap}} - F_{\text{drag}}, \tag{5.1}$$

where m is the cell mass, $q \in R^{2\times 1}$ is the position of the cell in x-y plane, F_{trap} is the optical trapping force, and F_{drag} is the viscous drag force.

It is well known that in the low Reynolds (Re) number environment, the influence of inertia force $m\ddot{q}$ is negligible (Arai et al., 2004; Wu et al., 2011). Considering the small diameter (r_c) and moving speed (v) of cells (for example, most human cells have a diameter less than 20 μm and a moving speed less than 20 μm/ s), the Re number, denoted as Re=$\rho v r_c/\eta$ (where ρ is the density of the suspending medium, and η is the viscosity of the medium) is far less than one. As a result, the inertia force m can be ignored, and Eq. (5.1) can be simplified to

$$0 = F_{\text{trap}} - F_{\text{drag}}. \tag{5.2}$$

The trapping force of the laser beam applied to the cell is generally defined as follows (Svoboda and Block, 1994):

$$F_{\text{trap}} = \frac{Q n_m P}{v_{\text{light}}}, \tag{5.3}$$

where Q is the dimensionless efficiency factor, which depends on the numerical aperture of the objective, laser wavelength, light polarization state, laser mode structure, relative refractive index, and particle geometry (Svoboda and Block, 1994), n_m is the index of refraction of the suspending medium, P is the incident laser power, and v_{light} is the speed of light.

Since the diameter of the cell is usually much larger than the wavelength of the trapping laser (1064 nm), for example, the diameters of the sampled yeast cells and Jurkat T cells are about 5-6 μm and greater than 10 μm, respectively, so the ray optical model can be used to calculate the trapping force. Using the method of Gauthier and Wallace (1995), the force can be calculated numerically, which is a function of the offset between the trap focus and the cell center. Considering a yeast cell with a radius of 3 μm, the trapping force can be obtained as shown in Fig. 5.1B, where r_0 is the critical deviation (or offset) and a further increase in this derivation will lead to a decrease in the trapping force. The parameters in the calculation are as follows:

$$n_m = 1.33, \quad n_o = 1.54, \quad \lambda = 1064\ \text{nm}, \quad W_o = 1.5\ \mu\text{m}, \quad z = 0, \quad r_c = 3\ \mu\text{m}$$

where n_o is the refractive index of the cell, λ is the wavelength of the laser beam, W_o is the radius of the beam waist, r_c is the radius of the cell, and z is the distance from the cell to the minimum beam waist (Gauthier and Wallace, 1995). It can be seen from Fig. 5.1B that when the cell is completely in the center of the trap focus, the trapping force is zero because all the force components are in equilibrium at this position. As the offset between the cell center and the trap center increases, the trapping force increases in an approximately linear relationship until the offset is greater than r_0. When the offset exceeds r_0, the trapping force will decrease as the offset increases, and when the cell is completely outside the trap, the trapping force will become zero. Therefore, it is desirable to limit cell displacement to the range of r_0 in cell transport.

The trapping force can be described as:

$$F_{\text{trap}} = k(l - q), \; \|l - q\| \le r_0, \tag{5.4}$$

where k is the stiffness of the optical trap, $l \in R^{2\times1}$ is the position of the optical trap, and $\|l - q\|$ denotes the deviation (or offset) of the cell from the center of the trap.

The drag force applied to the cell in movement can be calculated by Stokes' law as follows (Svoboda and Block, 1994):

$$F_{\text{drag}} = \beta \dot{q}, \tag{5.5}$$

where β is the drag coefficient expressed as:

$$\beta = \frac{6\pi\eta r_c}{1 - \frac{9}{16}(r_c/h) + \frac{1}{8}(r_c/h)^3 - \frac{45}{256}(r_c/h)^4 - \frac{1}{16}(r_c/h)^5}$$

in which h is the distance from the bottom surface of the chamber to the cell center.

Substituting Eqs. (5.4) and (5.5) into Eq. (5.2) yields the dynamics equation of the motion of the cell in optical trap, expressed as

$$0 = k(l - q) - \beta \dot{q}, \; \|l - q\| \le r_0. \tag{5.6}$$

Eq. (5.6) is rewritten as

$$\frac{\beta}{k}\dot{q} = l - q, \; \|l - q\| \le r_0. \tag{5.7}$$

It can be seen from Eq. (5.7) that the dynamics of the trapped cell is a first-order system subject to the constraint of $\|l - q\| \le r_0$.

5.2.2 Single-cell transport control

Based on the dynamics in Eq. (5.7), the controller for single-cell transportation can be designed as follows (Hu and Sun, 2011):

$$l - q = \begin{cases} c, & \|l - q\| \le r_0 \\ \dfrac{l - q}{\|l - q\|} r_0, & \|l - q\| > r_0 \end{cases}, \tag{5.8}$$

where c is a closed-loop controller. Based on Eq. (5.7), c can be designed as a feedforward plus proportional and integral (PI)-type feedback control in the following format:

$$c = \frac{\beta}{k}\dot{q}^d + K_p e + K_i \int_0^t e d\zeta, \tag{5.9}$$

where K_p and K_i are positive-feedback control gains, ζ is a time variable from 0 to t, and e is the position error between the desired cell position q^d and the actual cell position q, expressed by

$$e = q^d - q. \tag{5.10}$$

Substituting Eqs. (5.8) and (5.9) into Eq. (5.7) yields the following closed-loop dynamics equation when $\|l - q\| \le r_0$,

$$\frac{\beta}{k}\dot{e} + K_p e + K_i \int_0^t e d\zeta = 0. \tag{5.11}$$

Eq. (5.11) implies that the position error $e \to 0$ as time $t \to \infty$ because all β, k, K_p, and K_i are positive.

Using the controller Eqs. (5.8) and (5.9), the cell can move along the desired trajectory as long as the conditions $\|l - q\| \le r_0$ are met. When $\|l - q\| > r_0$, a saturated input based on r_0 can be assigned to the trap position controller, which exerts a maximum trap force to the cell to pull the cell back into the trap. Such a saturation control design ensures that the deviation between the cell and the trip is within the range $[-r_0, r_0]$, so that the cell will not escape from the trap.

5.2.3 Multicell transport control

The single-cell transport controller can be further expanded to transport multiple cells simultaneously. Suppose that multiple traps are used to transport a total of n cells with internal connections. During transportation, the original patterns of the cells must be maintained to avoid destroying the internal connections of the cells. Expanding Eq. (5.7), the dynamics of the ith trapped cell is expressed as

$$\frac{\beta_i}{k_i}\dot{q}_i = l_i - q_i, \ \|l_i - q_i\| \le r_0, \ i = 1, 2, \cdots, n, \tag{5.12}$$

where q_i, β_i, and k_i are the position coordinate, drag coefficient, and stiffness of the ith cell, respectively, and l_i is the position of the ith trap.

The multiagent synchronous control method (Sun, 2010) can be used to solve this multicell transportation control problem. The synchronization control problem can be expressed as guiding and positioning multiple cells along the boundary of a two-dimensional compact set. To this end, a time-varying desired shape denoted by $S(\chi, t)$ is introduced, where χ denotes a 2D position vector and t denotes the time (Sun, 2010). The boundary of $S(\chi, t)$ is parameterized by a two-dimensional planar curve, denoted by $\partial S(\chi, t) = 0$. Assign the target position q_i^d to the ith cell, and q_i^d must be located on the curve such that $\partial S(q_i^d, t) = 0$. The position error of the ith cell is defined as

$$e_i = q_i^d - q_i. \tag{5.13}$$

The control objective is converging each cell to its desired position q_i^d such that $e_i \rightarrow 0$ as time $t \rightarrow \infty$, and meanwhile, maintaining the cell on the desired curve such that $\partial S(q_i, t) = 0$. The former is called the first task, which aims to achieve the transportation control goal of each individual cell. The latter is called the second task, which represents the synchronization control effort in coordinating multicell transportation to maintain the original multicell pattern. Both tasks 1 and 2 are required to be accomplished simultaneously, with a single controller. To ensure that the distances among the cells remain constant, a synchronization control goal is defined as follows

$$e_1 = e_2 = \cdots = e_n. \tag{5.14}$$

Further, divide the goal of Eq. (5.14) into n subgoals of $e_i = e_{i+1}$. Note that when $i = n, n+1$ is denoted as 1. Then the position synchronization errors can be defined as a subset of all possible pairs of two neighboring cells in the following way

$$\varepsilon_1 = e_1 - e_2, \quad \varepsilon_2 = e_2 - e_3, \quad \cdots, \quad \varepsilon_n = e_n - e_1, \tag{5.15}$$

where ε_i denotes the synchronization error of the ith cell. Obviously, if the synchronization error $\varepsilon_i = 0$ for all $i = 1, \ldots n$, the synchronization goal (Eq. 5.14) is achieved automatically.

Finally, the closed-loop controller used to control multicell transportation is designed as follows. The controller is based on the single-cell control architecture (Eq. 5.8), where c, l, and q are replaced by c_i, l_i, and q_i, expressed as

$$\begin{aligned} c_i = {} & \frac{\beta_i}{k_i}\dot{q}_i^d + K_p e_i + K_i \int_0^t e_i d\zeta + K_\varepsilon(\varepsilon_i - \varepsilon_{i-1}) + K_b \int_0^t (\varepsilon_i - \varepsilon_{i-1}) d\zeta \\ & + K_c\left(\dot{\varepsilon}_i - \dot{\varepsilon}_{i-1}\right), \end{aligned} \tag{5.16}$$

where K_p, K_i, K_ε, K_b, and K_c are positive-feedback control gains.

Substituting Eq. (5.16) into the cell dynamics Eq. (5.12), the closed-loop equations can be obtained as follows:

$$\frac{\beta_i}{k_i}\dot{e}_i + K_p e_i + K_i \int_0^t e_i d\zeta + K_e(\varepsilon_i - \varepsilon_{i-1}) + K_b \int_0^t (\varepsilon_i - \varepsilon_{i-1}) d\zeta \\ + K_c\left(\dot{\varepsilon}_i - \dot{\varepsilon}_{i-1}\right) = 0. \tag{5.17}$$

To prove the stability of the controlled system under the controller (Eq. 5.16), the following Lyapunov function candidate can be chosen

$$V = \sum_{i=1}^{n} \frac{1}{2} e_i^T \frac{\beta_i}{k_i} e_i + \sum_{i=1}^{n} \frac{1}{2} \varepsilon_i^T K_c \varepsilon_i + \sum_{i=1}^{n} \frac{1}{2}\left(\int_0^t e_i d\zeta\right)^T K_i \left(\int_0^t e_i d\zeta\right) \\ + \sum_{i=1}^{n} \frac{1}{2}\left(\int_0^t \varepsilon_i d\zeta\right)^T K_b \left(\int_0^t \varepsilon_i d\zeta\right) \tag{5.18}$$

Then the Lyapunov direct approach can show that the position tracking and synchronization errors converge to zero asymptotically, namely, $e_i \rightarrow 0$ and $\varepsilon_i \rightarrow 0$ as time $t \rightarrow \infty$, under the condition of $\|l - q\| \leq r_0$. The details of the proof can be found in Hu and Sun (2011).

5.2.4 Experiments

Experiments were conducted by Hu and Sun (2011) to demonstrate the effectiveness of the cell transport control with optical tweezers. Two types of cells, yeast cells and Jurkat T cells, were used in the experiments. To verify the validity of the dynamic Eq. (5.7) and choose appropriate control parameters, the parameters β and k should be identified first.

It can be seen from Eq. (5.7) that, during the cell transportation process, the value of $(l - q)/\dot{q}$ should remain constant because both β and k are constant. To verify this, in the experiment, the viscous drag force method (Brouhard et al., 2003) was used to measure the value of $(l - q)/\dot{q}$ at different speeds. First, the cell was fixed using optical trap in the suspension medium. At this time, the position of the trap coincided with the position of the cell, denoted as l. Second, the computer-controlled motorized stage moved periodically at a known rate, which created a flow rate in the suspension medium that represented the relative velocity between the trapped cell and the medium, denoted by $\dot{q}$. Due to the drag force of the medium, the cell deviated from the center of the trap under the action of the optical trapping force F_{trap} and the drag force F_{drag}, and reached equilibrium at the new position q. Then, the cell position was retrieved through image-processing technology, and the deviation $l - q$ was obtained. Finally, β/k was calculated according to Eq. (5.7). Fig. 5.2 shows the calibration results of

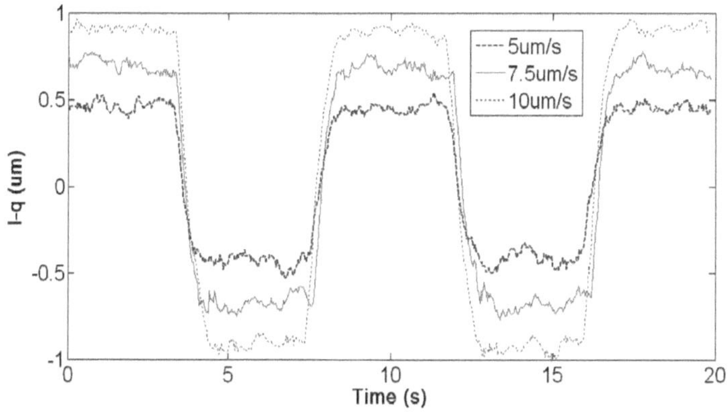

Figure 5.2 Deviations of the cell from the trap center at various cell speeds (Hu and Sun, 2011).

yeast cells at different speeds when the laser power was 0.2 W. The calculation results are given in Table 5.1. It can be seen that all the values of β/k were around 0.09 s, implying that although the speed was different, $(l-q)/\dot{q}$ remained almost unchanged. Therefore, the validity of the dynamic Eq. (5.7) was verified. The Jurkat T cells were further tested with a laser power of 0.4 W, and the results showed that the value of β/ k for Jurkat T cells remained at around 0.27 s.

Using the single cell control method (Eq. 5.8), the yeast cell was then transported along the following circular trajectory:

$$q^d = q^0 + \begin{pmatrix} 20\cos(0.25t) \\ 20\sin(0.25t) \end{pmatrix} \mu\text{m}$$

where q^0 was the center of the circular trajectory. The control gains were $K_p = \text{diag}\{0.4, 0.4\}$ and $K_i = \text{diag}\{0.2, 0.2\}$, which were determined based on the trial-and-error method. Fig. 5.3 shows the position-tracking errors of the cell with good position accuracy.

Then, the experiment of moving multiple Jurkat T-cell cells was performed to demonstrate the effectiveness of the multicell control method. The Jurkat T cell is a cell line derived from human T-cell leukemia. It is used to study acute T-cell leukemia, T-cell signal transduction, and the expression of various chemokine receptors that are susceptible to virus entry. Flexible trapping and manipulation of single or multiple T cells is the key to understanding the behavior of the immune system and other

Table 5.1 Value of β/k of the yeast cell (Hu and Sun, 2011).

Velocity (μm/s)	±5	±7.5	±10
β/ k (s)	0.09	0.1	0.09

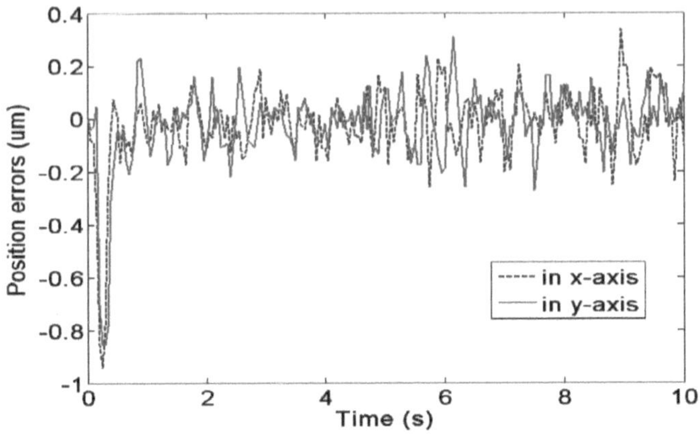

Figure 5.3 Position errors of single-cell transportation (Hu and Sun, 2011).

systems (Harris and McConnell, 2008). For example, CD^{4+} T cells have been placed near Jurkat T cells to study the cell–cell interaction between them (McNerneyet al.,2010). Fig. 5.4 shows that, under appropriate conditions, intercellular channels can be formed between T cells, such as stable adhesion and tunneling nanotubes (TNTs). In order to study the mechanism of molecular transfer and the physiological significance of channels without losing heterogeneity, multiple cells with internal channel connections must be separated from the surrounding background population and transported to the designated target area for further analysis. During the movement, the passage between the cells must be protected in an appropriate manner.

In the experiment, two Jurkat T cells (as shown in Fig. 5.4) were transported along the following circular trajectory while maintaining the distance between them.

$$q_i^d = q_i^0 + \begin{pmatrix} 20\cos(0.15t) \\ 20\sin(0.15t) \end{pmatrix} \mu\text{m}.$$

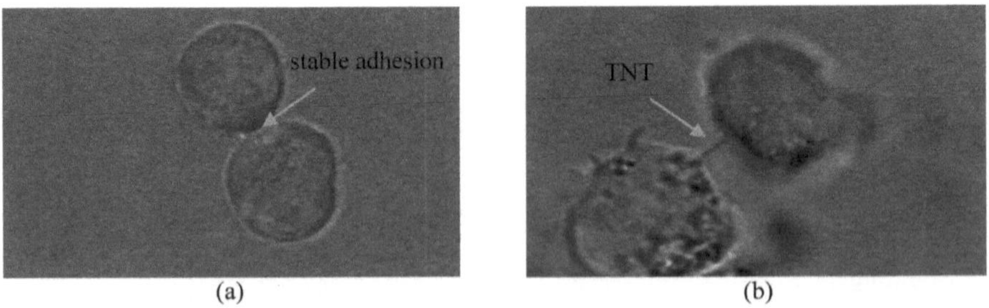

Figure 5.4 Jurkat T cells connected with channels (Hu and Sun, 2011). (A) Jurkat T cells with stable adhesion. (B) Jurkat T cells with TNTs.

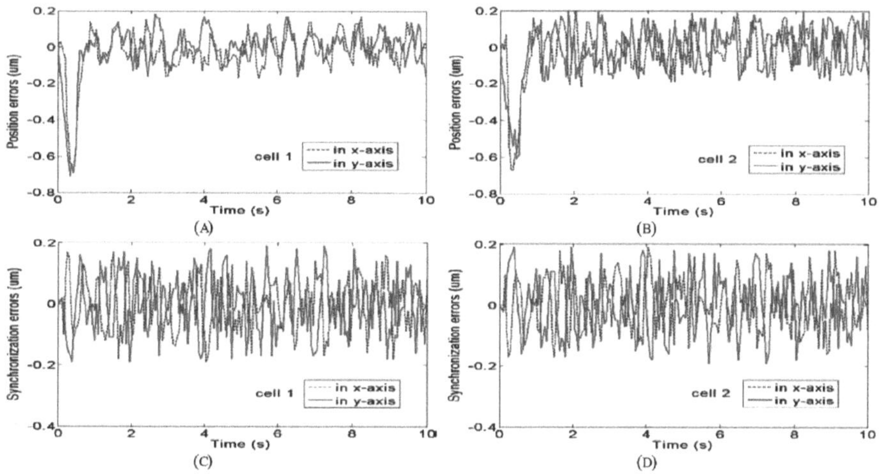

Figure 5.5 Synchronization control results of Jurkat T cells (Hu and Sun, 2011). (A) Position error e_1. (B) Position errors e_2. (C) Synchronization errors ε_1. (D) Synchronization errors ε_2.

where q_i^0 was the center of the circular trajectory of the ith cell. The synchronous controller (Eq. 5.16) was used. The control parameters were set as $K_p = \text{diag}\{0.5, 0.5\}$, $K_i = \text{diag}\{0.2, 0.2\}$, $K_\varepsilon = \text{diag}\{0.08, 0.08\}$, $K_b = \text{diag}\{0.03, 0.03\}$, and $K_c = \text{diag}\{0.02, 0.02\}$. Fig. 5.5 illustrates the position and synchronization errors of the two cells on the x and y axes under the proposed synchronization control. It can be seen that the proposed control method showed good performance in controlling cell position and synchronization errors. The maximum synchronization error was less than 0.2 μm.

5.3 Motion and path planning for automatic cell transportation

5.3.1 Motion planning

In automatic cell transportation, the appropriate design of cell motion is important because it not only determines motion efficiency, but also affects optical trapping performance and laser power requirements. Failure to deal with these factors may lead to undesirable consequences, such as cell escape from the laser trap, laser-induced optical cell damage, and low overall cell-processing throughput efficiency (Hu et al., 2005). Wu et al. (2013) reported the synergy of dynamic analysis and motion planning of cell transportation with optical tweezers. The details of this study are introduced below.

5.3.1.1 Dynamic analysis of cell trapping

As shown in Eq. (5.1), the trapped cell receives the trapping force from the optical trap F_{trap} and the viscous drag force from the liquid during the motion F_{drag}. Define $x = \|l - q\|$ as the distance (or offset) between the center of mass of the cell and the focus of the laser. The cell dynamics equation in Eq. (5.1) can be modified as follows

$$m\ddot{q} = F_{\text{trap}}(x) - F_{\text{drag}}\left(\dot{q}\right), \tag{5.19}$$

where the trapping force $F_{\text{trap}}(x)$ is proportional to the offset x within a certain range, which can be expressed as

$$F_{\text{trap}}(x) = \begin{cases} k_1 x, & 0 < x < r_0 \\ -k_2 x + \text{cont}, & x > r_0 \end{cases}, \tag{5.19}$$

where k_1 and k_2 are the trapping stiffness when the offset is less or greater than the critical displacement r_0, respectively, and cont is a constant.

When the displacement x is within the range of r_0, the trapping force increases with the increase of x, and becomes zero when the cell is completely outside the trap. Several methods for calibrating the trapping stiffness k_1 and k_2 have been reported in the literature, among which the viscous drag method has been widely used. According to Wu et al. (2013), the characterization strategy consists of the following three steps.

In the first step, the numerical solution of x is obtained by solving the cell dynamics (Eq. 5.19). As mentioned in Section 5.2, the influence of inertial force $m\ddot{q}$ is negligible in an environment with low Re number, so it can be ignored. By implementing the so-called "cell-falling" experiment (Wu et al., 2011), it is obtained that $\dot{q} = \dot{x}$. Then, Eq. (5.19) can be simplified to

$$F_{\text{trap}}(x) = F_{\text{drag}}\left(\dot{x}\right). \tag{5.20}$$

Substituting Eqs. (5.19) and (5.5) into Eq. (5.20) and solving the resultant equation yield

$$x = \begin{cases} r_0 \cdot e^{-(k_1/\beta)t}, & 0 < x < r_0 \\ 2r - r_0 \cdot e^{(k_2/\beta)t}, & x > r_0 \end{cases}. \tag{5.21}$$

The second step is to carry out the "cell-falling" experiment. First, a laser is used to trap the cell. Then, the power of the laser is turned off and the cell is moved away from the focus of the laser. When the laser power is turned on again, the cell will fall into the focus of the laser due to the capturing force. During this movement, the trapping force and the viscous drag force are simultaneously exerted on the cell. Using image-processing technology, the cell position can be measured.

In the third step, the actual cell trajectory during the "cell-falling" experiment is fitted according to the numerical solution x, and the stiffness k_1 and k_2 can be determined based on the solution.

Wu et al. (2013) conducted the "cell-falling" experiment on yeast cells, as shown in Fig. 5.6A. The parameters for yeast cell were chosen as $r_c = 2.5\ \mu\text{m}$, $h = 5\ \mu\text{m}$, $\eta = 10^{-3}\ \text{Pa}\cdot\text{s}$, $\beta = 0.08\ \text{pNs}/\mu\text{m}$. In the experiment, the resolution of the CCD camera was set to 688 × 280 pixels, the conversion factor was 0.17 μm/pixel, and the magnification was 40 times. Fig. 5.6B shows the cell displacement x measured in the falling experiment at 10 mW laser power. After repeated experiments, the least square method can be used to obtain the average fitting result as shown below.

$$x = \begin{cases} 2.5e^{-3.94(t-t_0)}, & 0 < x < 2.3\ \mu\text{m} \\ 5 - 2.5e^{3.90(t-t_0)}, & 2.3 < x < 5\ \mu\text{m} \end{cases}, \tag{5.22}$$

where t_0 was the time when $x = r_0 = 2.3\ \mu\text{m}$ during the falling process. The upper and lower bounds of offset x were 2.3 and 5 μm, respectively, which were determined using ray-optic model simulation (Gauthier and Wallace, 1995). Based on Eqs. (5.19) and (5.22), the trapping force of the yeast cell can be calibrated as

$$F_{\text{trap}}(x) = \begin{cases} 0.31x, & 0 < x < 2.3 \\ -0.26x + 1.3, & 2.3 < x < 5 \end{cases}. \tag{5.23}$$

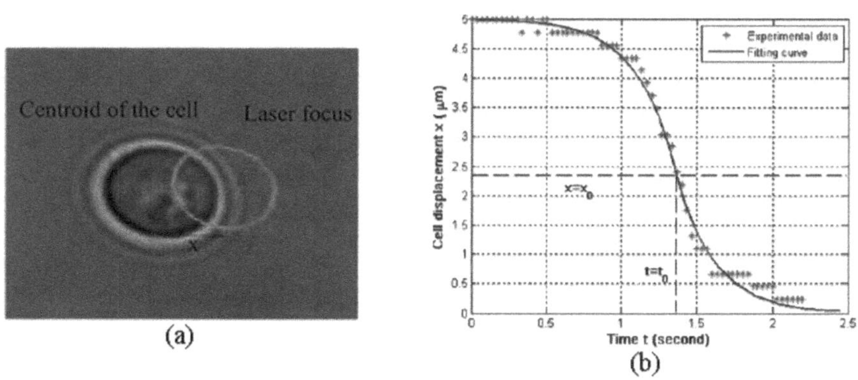

Figure 5.6 Cell-falling example (Wu et al., 2013). (A) Cell-falling experiment on a yeast cell. (B) Measurement of cell offset and curve-fitting result with 10-mW laser power.

Through a series of cell-falling experiments, the trapping stiffness k_1 and k_2 can be finally calibrated according to the laser power P, expressed as

$$k = \begin{cases} 0.03P, & 0 < x < 2.3 \\ -0.02P, & 2.3 < x < 5 \end{cases}. \tag{5.24}$$

5.3.1.2 *Design of movement velocity*

In most optical tweezers systems, after calibration, the optical trap can be accurately generated to make it perfectly coincide with the desired position. Therefore, many efforts have been focused only on designing an appropriate optical trap moving speed to achieve the optimal setting. The design of the moving speed should strike a balance between process efficiency and trapping quality. Rapid cell movement can increase efficiency, but it also creates a risk that cells may escape from the trap. Therefore, the method is to analyze the maximum cell movement speed at which the motorized stage can move cells in a constant motion. When the cell moves at a constant speed (achieved by moving the motorized stage), the cell displacement can be calculated as

$$x = \frac{\beta}{k_1}\dot{q}, \ \|x\| \leq r_0. \tag{5.25}$$

As all forces in constant motion are in equilibrium, $\dot{x} = 0$, and the cell movement velocity $\dot{q}$ is the same as the stage movement velocity v_s. Therefore, the maximum moving velocity of the motorized stage can be determined based on Eq. (5.25).

Note that the properties of the liquid medium and the optical trap may change during cell movement, which will cause the parameters β and k_1 in Eq. (5.25) to change. Eq. (5.5) shows that the drag coefficient β depends on the separation depth h and the viscosity coefficient η. As the cell moves, the liquid medium may vaporize, and the size of the chamber along the moving path may not be fixed, resulting in a change in h. The coefficient η can have different values in different positions of the medium. As a result, the drag coefficient β changes during cell transport. On the other hand, the trapping stiffness k_1 is also affected by many factors, such as changes in the shape and intensity of the laser beam due to unstable laser resources, the laser beam attitude, and the cover glass on the chamber. In addition, some disturbances such as stage mechanical vibration and Brownian motion of the cell will also affect the movement of the cell. Therefore, determination of the cell movement speed should not be based solely on Eq. (5.25).

According to Eq. (5.25), the PI feedback scheme can be used to adjust the cell movement speed online. The PI scheme feeds back the actual cell displacement relative to the laser focus, and uses the error between the actual displacement and the allowable displacement to generate the speed of the stage v_s. Based on image processing, the centroid extraction algorithm can be used to obtain the actual cell displacement x. To avoid overshooting, the allowable displacement denoted by x^d can be set to a value less than r_0. From Eq. (5.25), a higher value of x^d allows faster cell movement speed.

From Eqs. (5.19)–(5.21), the following dynamic equation of the trapped cell within the range of r_0 can be obtained:

$$k_1 x - \beta\left(v_s - \dot{x}\right) = 0. \tag{5.26}$$

Using Laplace transform to yield:

$$X(s) = \frac{\beta}{\beta s + k_1} V_s(s) = G(s)V_s(s), \tag{5.27}$$

where $G(s)$ is the transform function between movement velocity and cell displacement, which can be used to determine control gains k_p and k_i of the PI scheme.

Wu et al. (2013) conducted an experimental test of moving yeast cells at a speed determined by the PI scheme. Before testing, the calibration parameter β and k_1 were used to simulate the motion response, which helped to determine the PI control gain k_p and k_i. During the test, the PI scheme was used to determine the actual movement speed online. The following parameters were used: $x^d = 2\ \mu\text{m}$, $P = 10$ mW, $s = 80\ \mu\text{m}$, $\beta = 0.08\ \text{pN} \times \text{s}/\mu\text{m}$, $k_1 = 0.30\ \text{pN}/\mu\text{m}$, $k_p = 1$, and $k_i = 0.8$. The allowable displacement x^d was set to 2 μm, which was less than the critical value $r_0 = 2.3\ \mu\text{m}$. Fig. 5.7A and B show the moving speed and cell displacement, respectively. When the cell moved at the design speed (Fig. 5.7A), the displacement followed x^d (Fig. 5.7B). This indicated that the cell can move at a relatively high speed if the moving speed is correctly designed using the suggested PI scheme.

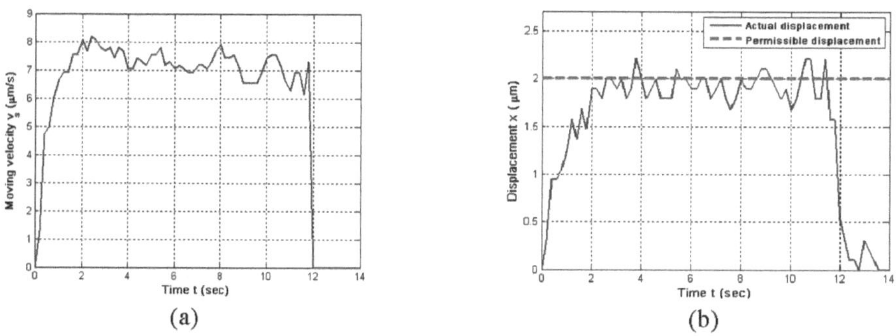

Figure 5.7 Movement velocity test (Wu et al., 2013). (A) Movement velocity determined by the PI scheme. (B) Cell displacement.

5.3.2 Path planning

During cell transportation from the origin to the destination, other cells may block the path. When a laser beam generates force around its focal point, it must maintain a certain distance from other cells. Therefore, proper path planning is required. Two path planning methods are introduced here.

5.3.2.1 A* algorithm-based path planner

The A* algorithm is one of the most classic heuristic path-planning algorithms, which finds the path between the starting point and the ending point at the lowest possible cost (ChongSeet and Lin, 2004). Considering that the optical trap will change the direction of cell movement at the waypoint, the cell may have a large displacement to the laser focus at the waypoint, which may cause the cell to easily escape from the optical trap. Therefore, it is necessary to smooth (or simplify) the path by reducing the number of waypoints. In the dynamic environment, the A* algorithm can help generate an optimal path at the low cost.

The A* algorithm can be modified to plan the path for cell transportation. The entire moving area of the cell is represented by a grid diagram, as shown in Fig. 5.8. When a cell is trapped by a laser, the trapped cell must keep a safe distance from its neighboring cells to avoid the laser's influence on other cells. The safety distance depends on the power of the laser and the characteristics of the trapped cell. Without loss of generality, the safety distance can be set to

$$\frac{\sqrt{2}}{2}d > 2r_c, \tag{5.28}$$

where r_c, as defined earlier, denotes the radius of the cell, and d denotes the minimum grid size of square of the laser beam.

The A* algorithm can be modified by adding an additional item, denoted by $\eta(i,j)$, to the movement cost $F(i,j)$ to penalize the nodes whose movement direction changes. The cost estimation algorithm is expressed as

$$F(i,j) = G(i,j) + H(i,j) + \eta(i,j), \tag{5.29}$$

where $F(i,j)$ denotes the total movement cost at the given node (i,j), $G(i,j)$ denotes the movement cost from the starting point to the node (i,j), and $H(i,j)$ denotes the estimated movement cost from the given node (i,j) to the final destination. If there is a waypoint between node (i,j) and the next position, then $\eta(i,j)$ is a positive number; otherwise, it is zero. The value of $\eta(i,j)$ is determined by the balance between smoothness and movement cost.

Fig. 5.8 illustrates the different paths generated by the A* algorithm with different values of η, where the movement cost of each single grid in the x or y direction was set to 9, and the grid size was set to 15. Fig. 5.8A shows the original image with the starting position and destination. Using the standard A* algorithm, five waypoints were

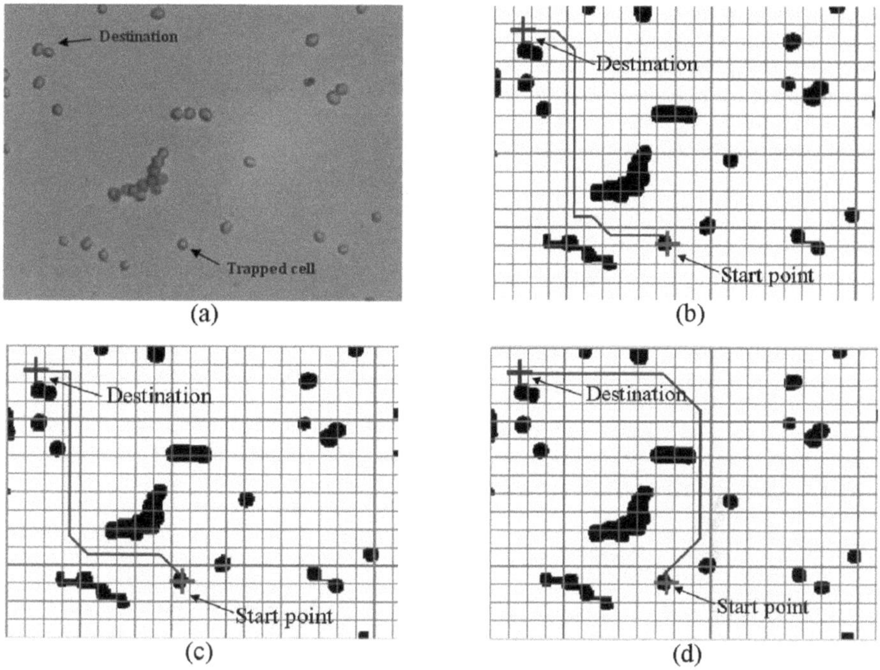

Figure 5.8 Path generation with standard and modified A* algorithms in a binary image (Wu et al., 2013). (A) Original image. (B) The path generated by standard A* algorithm with $\eta = 0$ (five waypoints). (C) The path generated by modified A* algorithm with $\eta = 10$ (four waypoints). (D) The path generated by modified A* algorithm with $\eta = 1000$ (three waypoints). The cross-points denote the starting position and destination.

generated along the path, as shown in Fig. 5.8B. When using the modified A* algorithm by adding the additional cost $\eta = 10$, the number of waypoints was reduced to four, as shown in Fig. 5.8C, and the path became smoother. If η was further increased to 1000, only three waypoints were generated, as shown in Fig. 5.8D, and the movement cost increased significantly. After conducting a series of tests on yeast cells, it was found that choosing a value of η between 5 and 25 could ideally balance the path smoothness and movement cost in the experiment.

Fig. 5.9 illustrates the transportation of a yeast cell along the generated path given in Fig. 5.8C. The moving direction was along the x or y axis, or at an angle of 45 degrees. The cell always moved in a straight line. The PI scheme was used to adjust the movement speed online to ensure that the cell moved at the maximum possible speed. Due to the dynamic change of the liquid environment, certain background cells might change their positions and block the cell movement path. In the experiment, this problem was solved through software design. That is, after the trapped cell reaches a specific position, the next grid is checked at to whether it is occupied. If the next grid is occupied, it is marked as "1" in the grid diagram and the path is replanned. If the next grid is not occupied, it is marked as the default "0" in the map, and the cell continues to move along the designed path.

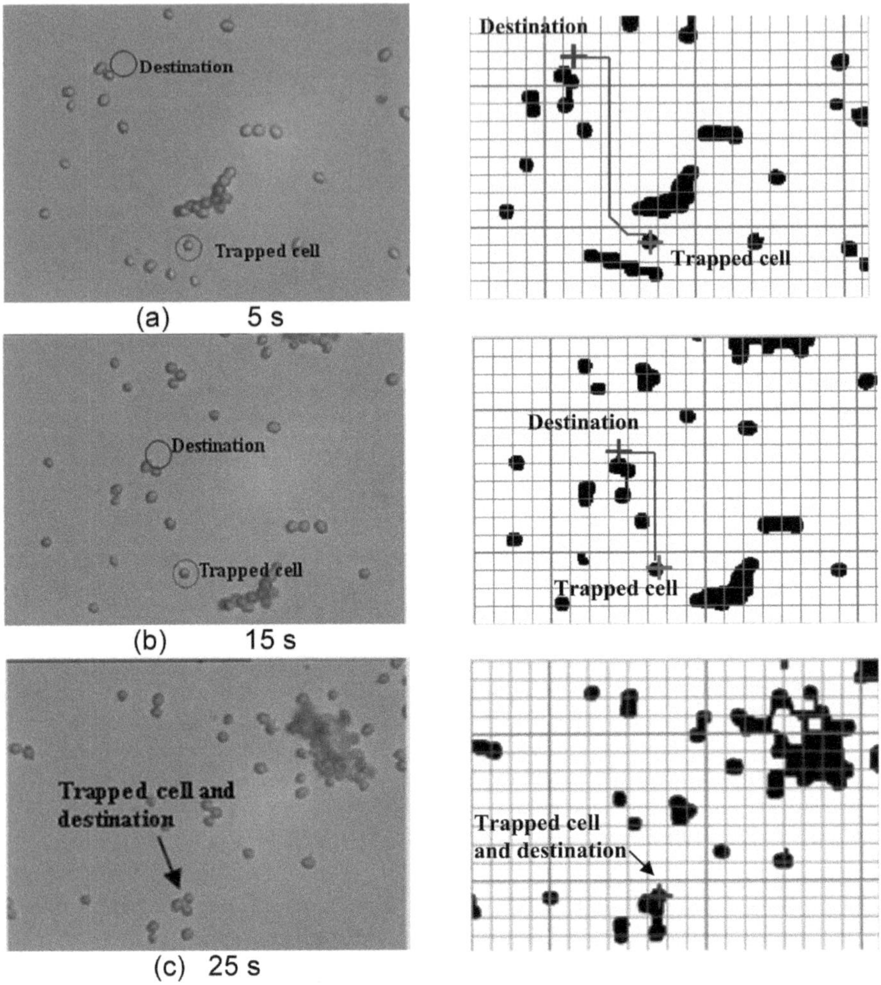

Figure 5.9 Cell transport path (Wu et al., 2013). (A) and (B) Original images. (C) Corresponding binary images.

5.3.2.2 RRT-based path planner

A path can also be generated by using an RRT-based path planner, which has two steps based on the binary map of the liquid level captured image. The main idea of these two steps is as follows.

The first step is generating an initial collision-free geometric path by expanding a random tree containing a series of vertices. As shown in Fig. 5.10A, the random tree is initialized from its starting state q_{init}, which is inserted as the first vertex. A control law is used to limit the motion of the cell, denoted as $q_{\gamma+1} = f\left(q_{\gamma}, u_{\gamma}\right)$, $q_{\gamma} \in C$, $u_{\gamma} \in U$, where γ is the index of each vertex, C represents the configuration space, and U

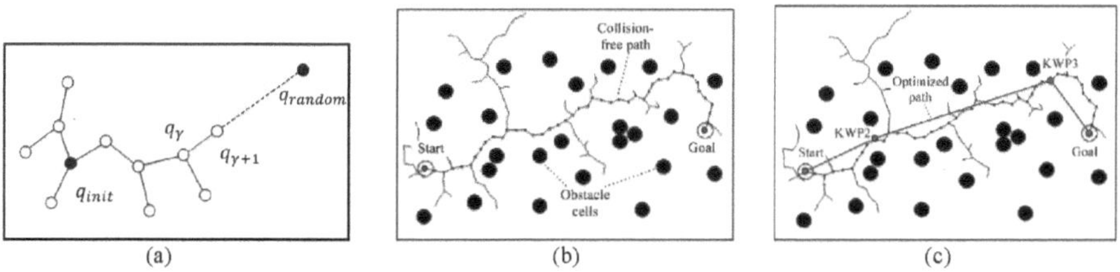

Figure 5.10 RRT path generation (Ju et al., 2014). (A) Growth of RRT. (B) Waypoints of the collision-free path. (C) The generated KWP path.

represents the length space on C. A point q_{random} on C is randomly selected, and the nearest neighbor q_k is found in the tree with the shortest distance to q_{random}. Then select a control law u_γ to expand the tree from q_γ to q_{random}. A new vertex is formed to represent a new state $q_{\gamma+1} = f\left(q_\gamma, u_\gamma\right)$, thereby specifying a new edge between q_γ and $q_{\gamma+1}$. Only when the edge has no collision on C, can the vertex $q_{\gamma+1}$ be regarded as a product of q_γ in the tree. To access the target location, the vertex q_{random} can be selected using the following steps during path planning. First, select the target position q_{goal} with probability P_b, and select the random point with probability $(1 - P_b)$ in C. Second, repeat the process until the target q_{goal} is inserted into the tree and the initial collision-free path is generated. Fig. 5.10B shows the simulation result of the collision-free path generated based on the RRT algorithm. The result shows that the initial collision-free path can be generated by expanding the random exploration tree from the starting position to the target position.

The second step is optimizing the initial path through key waypoint (KWP) decisions. Generating too many waypoints during the first step will result in a reduction in natural movement during cell transportation in a tortuous path and lower efficiency. Therefore, this step aims to use the KWP determination method to smooth the jagged path. This can be done by selecting the appropriate KWP to guide the path and discarding unnecessary waypoints. The path generated in the first step is defined as $\{c_1, \ c_2, \ ..., \ c_\gamma, \ ...\}$, where c_γ is the position of the waypoint and γ is the position index. The start position and the target position are designated as the initial KWP and the last KWP, respectively. Only when the straight line between $c^{\text{pre}}_{\gamma,kwp}$ and $c_{\gamma+1}$ intersects obstacles, c_γ is designated as a KWP, where $c^{\text{pre}}_{\gamma,kwp}$ represents the previous KWP of c_γ. The graphical representation of the KWP decision in Fig. 5.10C shows that the generated path can be further optimized using the KWP determination method, which has fewer waypoints and improved efficiency.

It should be noted that the path planning introduced above is ideally used for liquid solutions with small Brownian motion of cells or particles. If the target cell is small or the solution temperature is high enough, the Brownian motion of the cell may be strong enough to significantly affect cell transport. To solve this problem, Ju et al. (2014) proposed a dynamic path planner that considered the Brownian motion of cells.

5.4 Unified motion control design

When trapping a cell with optical tweezers, the cell must be located in the optical trap. To prevent the trapped cell from escaping easily and thus ensure the success of the cell transport task, an effective controller must be designed to always position the cell in the optical trap during the automatic control of cell transport. Li et al. (2015) proposed a so-called unified controller that can simultaneously control cell trapping and cell movement, and is robust to environmental disturbances. Using this method, a geometric model was first established to confine the cell to the local region around the optical trap. On this basis, the connection between the cell and the optical trap was formed by using the concept of cell—tweezers (C—T) coalition. Then, based on the defined potential field function, a robust controller was designed to drive the C—T coalition to a desired state while avoiding collisions with other obstacles in the environment. The details of the study are introduced below.

5.4.1 Model

In the low Re number environment, the influence of inertial force can be ignored. Eq. (5.7) gives the dynamic model of the trapped cell. Fig. 5.11 shows the cell in the optical trap. The target cell is represented by a solid sphere, and the optical trap is represented by a dashed sphere. The optical tweezers trap the cell only when the cell centroid is located in the trapping area. In other words, the center of the laser beam must be controlled to keep it "connected" with the trapped cell during the manipulation, so that the cell is always located in the trapping area. Here, the cell-tweezer connection is defined as the C—T coalition, which is similar to multirobot connection control (Li et al., 2013).

Introduce a constraint function for maintaining the C—T coalition as follows:

$$G_{C-T} = \frac{1}{2}\left(r_0^2 - \|l - q\|^2\right). \tag{5.30}$$

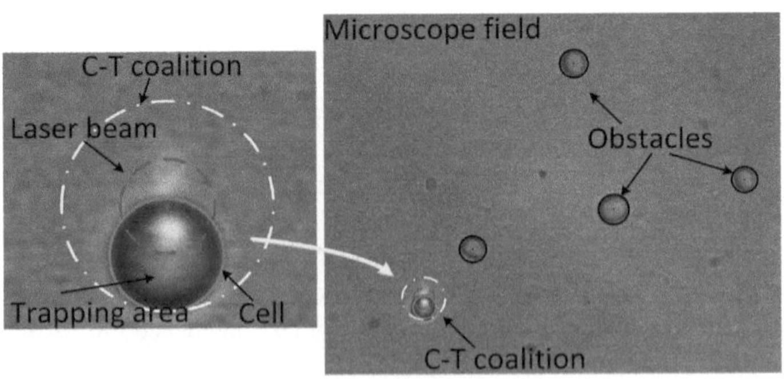

Figure 5.11 Illustration of C—T coalition (Li et al., 2015).

It is worth noting that $G_{C-T} > 0$ indicates that the cell is located in the optical trap and that the C−T coalition is maintained. Using the constraint function (Eq. 5.30), the C−T coalition can be regarded as a virtual sphere defined as follows:

Definition 5.1 (C−T coalition) C−T coalition is defined as a virtual sphere centered at l with a radius of R_{C-T}, which satisfies the C−T coalition constraint $G_{C-T} > 0$.

Notably, R_{C-T} should be set large enough so that the defined C−T coalition can cover the cell and laser beam. Then consider how the C−T coalition avoids other conflicts during manipulation. Without loss of generality, all other particles can be expressed as a spherical obstacle centered at q_ς with a radius of R_ς, where a total of m other particles exist and the index $\varsigma \in \{1, \cdots, m\}$. Introduce a constraint function for obstacle avoidance as

$$G_O = \prod_{\varsigma=1}^{m} \left(\frac{1}{2} \left(\|l - q_\varsigma\|^2 - (R_{C-T} + R_\varsigma)^2 \right) \right) = \prod_{\varsigma=1}^{m} \alpha_\varsigma. \tag{5.31}$$

If $G_O > 0$, there is no collision between C−T coalition and other particles.

By combining the constraint functions for C−T coalition and obstacle avoidance, a new workspace called *free coalition manipulation space* is defined as follows:

Definition 5.2 (free coalition manipulation space)

$$F = \{ l | G = G_{C-T} G_O > 0 \}. \tag{5.32}$$

In space F, the cell is located in the optical trap to maintain the C−T coalition and is collision-free.

Denote $u = \dot{l} \in \Re^2$ as the velocity of the optical trap, which is also regarded as a control input. Then, the following coalition manipulation problem can be formulated.

Consider the cell manipulation system with dynamic (Eq. 5.7). *Under the initial configuration of* $G(0) > 0$, *determine the control input u applied to the optical tweezers to drive the target cell to a desired position while maintaining* $G(\mathrm{t}) > 0$, $\forall t > 0$.

5.4.2 Control

Define a bounded potential field function as follows:

$$\phi = \frac{\gamma}{(\gamma^\delta + G)^{\frac{1}{\delta}}}, \tag{5.33}$$

where δ is a positive parameter, $\gamma = \frac{1}{2} e_{C-T}^T e_{C-T}$ is a criterion function, $e_{C-T} = l - q^d$ denotes the position error of the C−T coalition, and q^d denotes the desired position of the cell. The control input, which is the velocity of the optical trap, is designed as the negative gradient of the potential function ϕ expressed by

$$u = -k_{\text{cont}}\frac{\partial \phi}{\partial l}, \tag{5.34}$$

where k_{cont} is a positive control gain.

Theorem 5.1. Consider a cell manipulation system equipped with optical tweezers, which is subject to dynamics (Eq. 5.7). Under the initial configuration of $G(0) > 0$, the control law Eq. (5.34) gives rise to: (1) $G(t) > 0, \forall t > 0$; (2) the trapped cell is confined within the optical trap; (3) the C−T coalition is collision-free.

Proof: Denote $\partial f = \{l | G_{C-T} = 0 \cup G_O = 0\}$ as the boundary of the free coalition manipulation space F and $\nabla_l G$ as the gradient of G. Thus, the vector $\nabla_l G$ is normal to ∂f and toward the internal of F ($G > 0$) over the boundary ∂f. The velocity of the C−T coalition u can be simplified over the boundary ∂f as follows:

$$u = k_{\text{cont}}\frac{\nabla_l G}{\delta \gamma^{\delta}}. \tag{5.35}$$

Taking the inner product of vectors u and $\nabla_l G$ over the boundary ∂f yields

$$u\nabla_l G = k_{\text{cont}}\frac{(\nabla_l G)^T}{\delta \gamma^{\delta}}\nabla_l G = \frac{k}{\delta \gamma^{\delta}}\|\nabla_l G\|^2. \tag{5.36}$$

The following will show that the cell can always stay in the free joint coalition manipulation space F as given in Eq. (5.32). It is worth noting that, in the initial configuration, the centroid of the C−T coalition is located inside F. If the constraint (Eq. 5.32) is broken and the center of the C−T coalition is located on the boundary ∂f, one of the following two cases will hold.

Case 1: The target cell almost escapes from the optical trap, and the center of the C−T coalition is located on the boundary ∂f formed by $G_{C-T} = 0$.

Case 2: The C−T coalition collides with the ςth obstacle, and the center of the C−T coalition is located on the boundary ∂f formed by $\alpha_\varsigma = 0$.

In Case 1, there exist $G_{C-T} = 0$ and $q - l = r_0$ such that

$$\|\nabla_l G\| = \left\| G_O(q-l) + \sum_{\varsigma=1}^{m} G_{C-T}\overline{\alpha}_\varsigma(l - q_\varsigma) \right\| = G_O r_0, \tag{5.37}$$

where $\overline{\alpha}_\varsigma = \prod_{\tau \neq \varsigma} \alpha_\tau$, and $\tau \in \{1, \cdots, m\}$. Substituting Eq. (5.37) into Eq. (5.36) yields

$$u\nabla_l G = \frac{k_{\text{cont}}}{\delta \gamma^{\delta}}(G_O r_0)^2 > 0. \tag{5.38}$$

The inequality (Eq. 5.38) indicates that when the target cell is located on the boundary ∂f formed by $G_{C-T} = 0$, the velocity of the optical tweezers is consistent with the vector $\nabla_l G$, and the optical trap converges into the space F. Therefore, $G_{C-T} = 0$ will never happen, and thus the boundary formed by $G_{C-T} = 0$ will not be reached.

In Case 2, a similar result to that of Case 1 can be obtained as follows:

$$u\nabla_l G > \frac{k_{\text{cont}}\left(G_{C-T}\overline{\alpha}_{\varsigma}(R_{C-T} + R_{\varsigma})\right)^2}{\delta\gamma^{\delta}} > 0. \tag{5.39}$$

Similarly, the inequality (Eq. 5.39) indicates that when the C−T coalition almost hits the ςth obstacle, the velocity of the optical tweezers will converge to $G > 0$ for avoiding collision. Therefore, $\alpha_{\varsigma} = 0, \forall \varsigma \in \{1, \cdots, m\}$ will never happen, and the boundary of the free manipulation space formed by $\alpha_{\varsigma} = 0, \forall \varsigma \in \{1, \cdots, m\}$ will not be reached.

Finally, it is concluded that the boundary of the free manipulation space ∂f cannot be reached under the controller (Eq. 5.34), so that $G(t) > 0, \forall t \geq 0$. The optical tweezers can adjust its motion adaptively so that the target cell is confined in the optical trap while avoiding collisions with other obstacles during manipulation.

Theorem 5.2. The parameter δ has a positive lower bound $\widehat{\delta}$ so that the desired cell position q^d is the only critical point for the C−T coalition in the free coalition manipulation space F.

Proof: The destination q^d is clearly a nondegenerated minimum of ϕ, and the proof of this part is omitted here. The following description will discuss how δ is chosen such that q^d is the only critical point of ϕ.

The simplified estimation of ϕ, expressed as $\widehat{\phi} = \gamma^{\delta}/G$, will be used here to analyze the polar property of ϕ (Li et al., 2013). Denote l' (which is not equal to q^d) as a critical point of $\widehat{\phi}$. Taking the gradient of $\widehat{\phi}$ at l' yields

$$\gamma\nabla_{l'}G = \delta G\nabla_{l'}\gamma. \tag{5.40}$$

Taking the norm of both sides of Eq. (5.40) and expanding, the term $\nabla_{l'}G$ yields:

$$\delta \leq \frac{\gamma}{\|\nabla_{l'}\gamma\|}\left(\frac{r_0}{G_{C-T}} + \sum_{\varsigma=1}^{m}\frac{\|l - q_{\varsigma}\|}{\alpha_{\varsigma}}\right) = \frac{e_{C-T}}{2}\left(\frac{r_0}{G_{C-T}} + \sum_{\varsigma=1}^{m}\frac{\|l - q_{\varsigma}\|}{\alpha_{\varsigma}}\right) \underline{\underline{\Delta}} \widehat{\delta}. \tag{5.41}$$

If inequality (Eq. 5.41) does not hold, l' is not the critical point of $\widehat{\phi}$. Therefore, if $\delta \geq \widehat{\delta}$, there is no other critical point, and q^d is the only critical point of ϕ. In practical application, one can choose the lower bound for δ.

Theorem 5.3. Consider an optical tweezers cell manipulation system with initial configuration of $G(0) > 0$. Controller (Eq. 5.34) gives rise to: (1) the dynamic system (Eq. 5.7) is global asymptotically stable; (2) $e_{C-T} \rightarrow 0$ is asymptotically expressed as $t \rightarrow \infty$; and (3) $e \rightarrow 0$ as $t \rightarrow \infty$, where $e = q - q^d$ denotes the position error of the target cell.

Proof: Define $V = \phi$ as the Lyapunov function candidate. Differentiating V with respect to time yields

$$\dot{V} = \frac{\partial \phi}{\partial l}\frac{\partial l}{\partial t} + \frac{\partial \phi}{\partial q}\frac{\partial q}{\partial t} = -k\frac{\partial \phi}{\partial l}\frac{\partial \phi}{\partial l} - \frac{\gamma G_O(l-q)}{\delta(\gamma^\delta + G)^{\frac{1}{\delta}+1}}\frac{k(l-q)}{\beta}$$
$$= -k\left(\frac{\partial \phi}{\partial l}\right)^2 - \frac{k\gamma G_O}{\beta\delta(\gamma^\delta + G)^{\frac{1}{\delta}+1}}(l-q)^2 \leq 0. \tag{5.42}$$

Therefore, system (Eq. 5.7) is global asymptotically stable under controller (Eq. 5.34). From Theorem 5.2, it is known that $\dot{V} = 0$ holds only at equilibrium q^d. Therefore, the C–T coalition converges to the destination q^d asymptotically, and $e_{C-T} \rightarrow 0$ as $t \rightarrow \infty$.

Considering the Lyapunov function candidate $V' = \frac{l-q^2}{2}$, taking the time derivation of V' yields

$$\dot{V}' = (q-l)\dot{q} = -\frac{k}{\beta}(q-l)^2 \leq 0. \tag{5.43}$$

$V' = 0$ holds at $q = l = q^d$. Therefore, $e \rightarrow 0$ as $t \rightarrow \infty$, and q converges to q^d asymptotically.

In the presence of disturbances, the trapped cell can easily escape from the optical trap during manipulation, resulting in unexpected behavior. To overcome the interference, the continuous function Δu within a finite time can be used as an additional control item of the velocity control input (Eq. 5.34), expressed as

$$u_r = u + \Delta u = -k\frac{\partial \phi}{\partial l} + \Delta u(t) \tag{5.44}$$

Li et al. (2015) has proved that the controller (Eq. 5.44) is robust under the initial configuration of $G(0) > 0$.

5.4.3 Experiments

The above control development has been verified in experiments using a robot-controlled optical tweezers manipulation system to transport yeast cells (Li et al., 2015). After calibration with a digital power and energy meter, 5 mW laser power on the trapped cells was considered safe when handling living cells. A CCD camera was used to obtain an image of the working space with 640×480 pixels at a magnification of 60, and each pixel was calibrated to 0.1025 μm. In the experiment, the safety offset r_0 was set to 30 pixels (3.073 μm), and the sampling time was about 50 ms. When the position error was within 10 pixels (1.025 μm), the experiment was stopped.

As in many other works, the cells were modeled as spheres. In this experiment, cells with irregular shapes and cell clumps were represented by virtual spherical obstacles. Image-processing technology was used to process obstacle recognition in three steps. First, the original image acquired from the CCD was converted into a grayscale image, and a threshold algorithm was used to separate the cells from the background. Second, the contour of the cell was detected from the binary image. Third, the minimum circumscribed circle of the outline of each cell was determined, and the minimum circumscribed circles that acted as virtual sphere obstacles were used to represent the actual cells.

Fig. 5.12 illustrates the manipulation process in the experiments. The optical tweezers were represented by small circles, and other cells and particles, enclosed by large circles, were regarded as obstacles in the working space. The target position was indicated by a cross, and the trajectory of the transferred cell was indicated by a dotted line. Fig. 5.12A shows the initial configuration, while Fig. 5.12B and C show the manipulation process at different times. Fig. 5.12D shows that the cell reached the target position successfully. The control performance of the proposed controller is shown in Fig. 5.13. Fig. 5.13A shows that the position error of the target cell converged to the termination condition, which meant that the cell transportation task was successfully completed. Fig. 5.13B shows the time course of the offset $\|l-q\|$

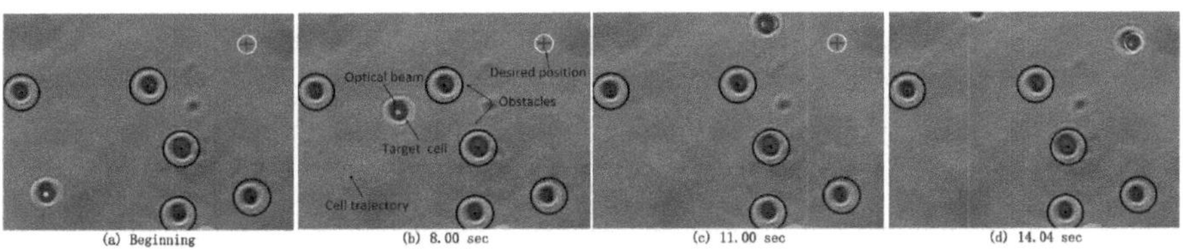

Figure 5.12 Coalition manipulation of yeast cells (Li et al., 2015).

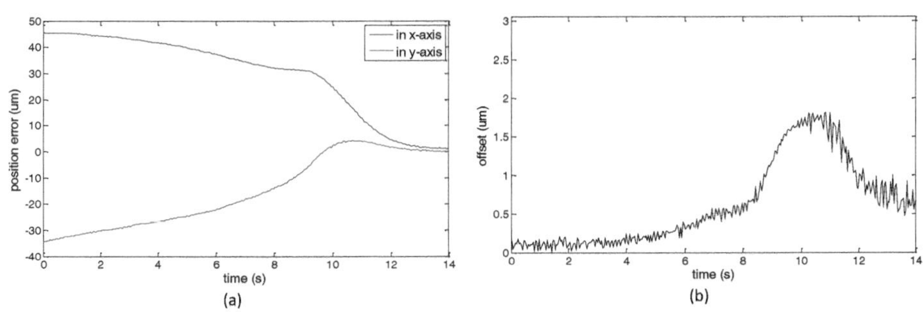

Figure 5.13 Control performance (Li et al., 2015). (A) Manipulation performance. (B) Offset during manipulation.

during manipulation. The offset was well limited within the safety offset $r_0 = 3.075\ \mu m$, indicating that the C–T coalition remained unchanged. A total of 15 sets of cell samples were prepared, and more than 120 experiments were performed using the proposed control method. In all experiments, the target cells were successfully transferred to the destination without escaping from the optical trap.

5.5 Multiple cell transportation for cell pairing

In many bioengineering applications, cells need to be paired to observe cell–cell interaction phenomena, such as cell fusion. Cell pairing can help in studying the attack of cancer cells and natural killer cells, the contact of cells with DNA, the reaction of cancer cells to B cells, and the response of cells to drugs. Some cells need to be transported to a designated conventional buffer for further manipulation, such as batch fertilization of egg cells (Kuncova and Kallio, 2004), drug discovery (Walther and Stein, 2000), DNA microencapsulation (Alexakis et al., 1995), and cell separation (Wang et al., 2011). Buffers are usually constructed as tiny arrays of containers in which cells can be manipulated precisely. In these bioengineering tasks, high-precision and high-productivity cell transportation and pairing are required.

In practical applications, cells are always randomly distributed in the workspace. The cell-pairing task is difficult and can lead to negative results (for example, two or more cells collide and mix together). In addition, the random distribution of cells makes bulk transportation inconvenient, especially when it is necessary to transport the cells in pairs into a regular array buffer. In order to overcome the shortcomings of low efficiency and low accuracy of existing transportation and pairing methods, it is necessary to develop an automatic method to effectively pair and move batch cells into a regular array. Chen and Sun (2012) reported an automatic control method that used a robot-tweezer manipulation system to move cell populations into the array. This section introduces this method.

5.5.1 Model

Extending Eqs. (5.1), (5.4), and (5.5), the dynamic model of the ith cell can be expressed as

$$m_i\ddot{q}_i = F_{\text{trap}} - F_{\text{drag}} = k_i(l_i - q_i) - \beta_i\dot{q}_i \tag{5.45}$$

Consider $2n$ cells whose positions are represented by $q_{2n} = \{q_1, \cdots, q_{2n}\}$. These cells belong to two groups, and each group contains n cells. Determine the control input $L_{2n} = \{l_1, \cdots l_{2n}\}$ to drive the cells to the desired array without collisions, while forming cell–cell pairs during the array process. In each pair, the two cells are from two different groups, and the distance between them is well controlled.

The bottleneck assignment method (Burkard et al., 2009) can be used to allocate two sets of cells to a common array. Any two cells from different groups but assigned to a common destination are treated as a pair. Based on the assignment result, the desired configuration of all $2n$ cells is expressed as $q_{2n}^d = \{q_1^d, \cdots, q_{2n}^d\}$, where $q_i^d \in R^2$ denotes the destination of the ith cell, which is fixed during the manipulation. Given that cell i and κ are both assigned to a common destination, where $i = 1, \cdots, 2n$, $\kappa = 1, \cdots, 2n$, and $i \neq \kappa$, there is $q_i^d = q_\kappa^d$.

All $2n$ cells must move toward the destination while avoiding collisions. The cells in the optical traps cannot be close to each other, otherwise, the cell may be dragged into the force area of another cell. To prevent collisions, the minimum distance between any two cells must be defined. This minimum distance is called the safe distance, denoted by d, and is restricted by the following constraint function

$$g_{ij}\left(\Delta q_{ij}\right) = \left\|\Delta q_{ij}\right\|^2 - d^2 \geq 0 \tag{5.46}$$

where $\left\|\Delta q_{ij}\right\| = \left\|q_i - q_j\right\|$ is the Euclidean distance between cells i and j.

The artificial potential field method (Cheah et al., 2009) can be used to achieve collision avoidance. A local potential function is defined as follows.

Definition 5.3 (local potential function) Define the potential function Q_{ij} as a nonnegative function of the distance $\left\|\Delta q_{ij}\right\|$ between cell i and j, which satisfies three conditions:

1. $Q_{ij}\left(\Delta q_{ij}\right) \rightarrow \infty$, as $\left\|\Delta q_{ij}\right\| \rightarrow 0$;
2. $Q_{ij}\left(\Delta q_{ij}\right) = 0$, when $\left\|\Delta q_{ij}\right\| \geq d$;
3. $Q_{ij}\left(\Delta q_{ij}\right)$ is smooth when $\left\|\Delta q_{ij}\right\| > 0$.

Under condition (1), the two cells will not overlap. Under condition (2), the repulsive force is activated only when the cell distance is less than the safety distance d. Condition (3) is necessary for the controller design (which is discussed later).

Consider the following potential function candidate:

$$Q_{ij}\left(\Delta q_{ij}\right) = \left(\max\left(0, g_{ij}\right)\right)^2 \left(1 + k_l / \left\|\Delta q_{ij}\right\|\right)^2 \tag{5.47}$$

where k_l is a positive constant, and the function $\max\left(0, g_{ij}\right)$ returns the larger of 0 and g_{ij}. Obviously, the function (Eq. 5.47) satisfies conditions (1) and (2) in the definition of local potential function (5.3).

Differentiating Eq. (5.47) with respect to Δq_{ij} yields

$$\begin{aligned} \frac{\partial Q_{ij}}{\partial \Delta q_{ij}} &= -\max\left(0, g_{ij}\right)\left(1 + k_l / \left\|\Delta q_{ij}\right\|\right) \\ &\quad \left(2\left(1 + k_l / \left\|\Delta q_{ij}\right\|\right) + \max\left(0, g_{ij}\right)\left(k_l / \left\|\Delta q_{ij}\right\|^3\right)\right)\Delta q_{ij} \end{aligned} \tag{5.48}$$

Because $\partial Q_{ij} / \partial \Delta q_{ij} = 0$ when $\left\| \Delta q_{ij} \right\| = d$, the function (Eq. 5.47) is smooth when $\left\| \Delta q_{ij} \right\| > 0$. Therefore, the function (Eq. 5.47) is a local potential function and will be used in the following analysis.

Based on Eq. (5.47), the objective function for collision avoidance is given as

$$Q = \frac{1}{2} k_c \sum_{i=1}^{2n} \frac{1}{2} \sum_{j \in N_i} Q_{ij}\left(\Delta q_{ij}\right) = \frac{1}{2} k_c \sum_{i=1}^{2n} \frac{1}{2} \sum_{j \in N_i} \left(\max\left(0, g_{ij}\right)\right)^2 \left(1 + k_l / \left\| \Delta q_{ij} \right\|\right)^2 \tag{5.49}$$

where k_c is a positive constant and N_i is a set of neighbors around the cell i. To determine whether a cell is concentrated in neighbors, an artificial interaction range $r_N > d$ can be introduced. Any cell whose distance to cell i is shorter than r_N is defined as a neighbor of cell i. Note that the function $Q_{ij}\left(\Delta q_{ij}\right)$ is activated only when the distance between cell i and its neighboring cell is less than d. Otherwise, $Q_{ij}\left(\Delta q_{ij}\right) = 0$.

5.5.2 Controller design

The control design aims to drive the pair of cells into the required array while controlling the distance between the two cells in each pair. In order to achieve this goal, the concept of a free region B_i corresponding to each cell is introduced. The free region is a circular area with a radius R and q_i^d $(i = 1, \cdots 2n)$ as the center, as shown in Fig. 5.14. Note that when the two cells i and κ are assigned to the same target location, their free regions are the same (i.e., $B_i = B_\kappa$). After cell i enters the interior B_i, it is only affected by repulsive force. The distance $\|\Delta q_{i\kappa}\|$ can be adjusted by changing the size of the free region. Without loss of generality, the objective of distance control can be determined as follows:

$$\|\Delta q_1\| = \|\Delta q_2\| = \cdots = \|\Delta q_{2n}\| \tag{5.50}$$

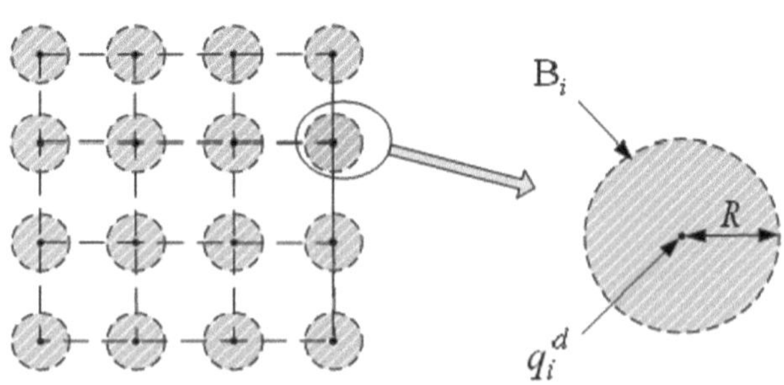

Figure 5.14 Definition of free regions (Chen and Sun, 2012).

$$\|\Delta q_{i\kappa}\| = d_{i\kappa}^{d} \tag{5.51}$$

where $\Delta q_i = q_i - q_i^d$ denotes the position error of the ith cell, and $d_{i\kappa}^d$ denotes the desired distance between cells i and κ, which can be the same for all pairs.

Based on the above analysis, the control objective of the array manipulation can be expressed as:

$$E = \sum_{i=1}^{2n}\left\{\frac{1}{2}k_q\left(\max\left(0, \|\Delta q_i\|^2 - R^2\right)\right)^2 + \frac{1}{2}k_p\dot{q}_i^T\dot{q}_i\right\} + Q \rightarrow 0, \text{ as } t \rightarrow \infty \tag{5.52}$$

According to Eq. (5.52), all cells are driven to their desired free regions in the desired array when E converges to zero. A feedback controller to achieve this goal is given by

$$u_i = -k_q \tanh\left(\max\left(0, \ \|\Delta q_i\|^2 - R^2\right)\right)\Delta q_i - k_p\dot{q}_i - k_c\Delta\xi_i + q_i \tag{5.53}$$

where k_q and k_p are positive control gains. Here, $\Delta\xi_i$ is the combined repulsive forces from all neighboring particles, which are calculated by

$$\begin{aligned}\Delta\xi_i &= \frac{1}{2}\sum_{j\in N_i}\left(\partial Q_{ij}/\partial\Delta q_{ij}\right)\\ &= -\sum_{j\in N_i}\max\left(0, g_{ij}\right)\left(1 + k_l/\left\|\Delta q_{ij}\right\|\right)\left(2\left(1 + k_l/\left\|\Delta q_{ij}\right\|\right)\right.\\ &\quad\left. + \max\left(0, g_{ij}\right)\left(k_l/\left\|\Delta q_{ij}\right\|^3\right)\right)\Delta q_{ij}\\ &= -\sum_{j\in N_i}A_{ij}\Delta q_{ij}\end{aligned} \tag{5.54}$$

where

$$\begin{aligned}A_{ij} &= \max\left(0, g_{ij}\right)\\ &\quad\left(1 + k_l / \left\|\Delta q_{ij}\right\|\right)\left(2\left(1 + k_l / \left\|\Delta q_{ij}\right\|\right) + \max\left(0, g_{ij}\right)\left(k_l / \left\|\Delta q_{ij}\right\|^3\right)\right)\end{aligned} \tag{5.55}$$

Note that the first term in Eq. (5.53) denotes the attractive force that drives cell i to its free region, which equals zero when cell i enters into the region. The second term is the damping term. The third term is used to handle the repulsive force caused by the neighboring cells.

Substituting Eq. (5.53) into the dynamic Eq. (5.45) yields the following closed-loop dynamic equation:

$$\ddot{q}_i = -\frac{a_i}{m_i}k_q \tanh\left(\max\left(0,\ \|\Delta q_i\|^2 - R^2\right)\right)\Delta q_i - \left(\frac{a_i}{m_i}k_p + \frac{b_i}{m_i}\right)\dot{q}_i - \frac{a_i}{m_i}k_c\Delta\xi_i \tag{5.56}$$

Theorem 5.4. Consider two groups of cells with dynamics described by Eq. (5.45), where each group contains n cells. Given the grid size of the desired array as $d_g \geq 2d$ and the size of free regions as $R \leq d/2$, the control law (Eq. 5.53) gives rise to:

1. Each pair of particles moves into a circular region with radius not less than R.
2. $\|\Delta q_i\| = \|\Delta q_\kappa\| = \|\Delta q_{i\kappa}\|/2$.
3. The cell velocity $\dot{q}_i \rightarrow 0$ for all $i = 1, \cdots, 2n$ as time $t \rightarrow \infty$.

The proof can be seen by referring to Chen and Sun (2012). Theorem 5.4 shows that when $R < d/2$, the value of $\|\Delta q_{i\kappa}\|$ cannot be easily calculated due to the existence of both repulsive and attractive forces. Therefore, the only solution to satisfy Eqs. (5.50) and (5.51) is $R = d/2$ (see Fig. 5.15), in which the distance $\|\Delta q_{i\kappa}\| = 2R = d$.

Note that the controller (Eq. 5.53) can be slightly modified as follows to control a group of cells into the array:

$$u_i = -k_q \tan h\left(\|\Delta q_i\|^2\right)\Delta q_i - k_p\dot{q}_i - k_c\Delta\xi_i + q_i \tag{5.57}$$

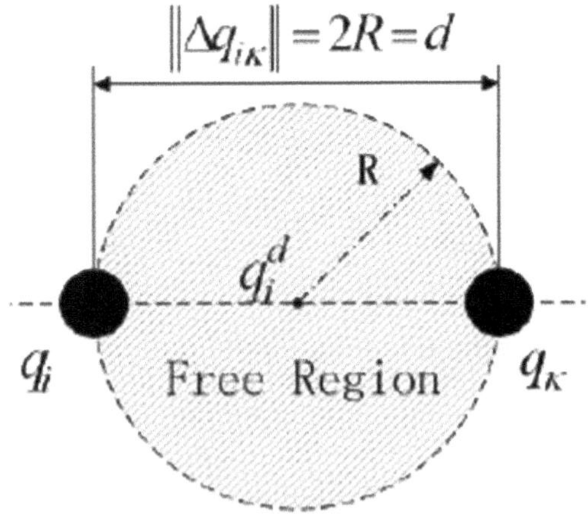

Figure 5.15 Desired spatial relationship between the pair of cells i and κ (Chen and Sun, 2012).

With Eq. (5.57), cells are directly driven to their destinations without free regions, namely $R = 0$. The controller (Eq. 5.57) can be further simplified as

$$u_i = -k_q\Delta q_i - k_p\dot{q}_i - k_c\Delta\xi_i + q_i \tag{5.58}$$

The controllers Eqs. (5.57) and (5.58) represent special forms of the controller (Eq. 5.53) used to control a single group of cells into the array.

Theorem 5.5. Consider a group of n cells with the dynamics of Eq. (5.45). The control law (Eq. 5.58) gives rise to $\Delta q_i \rightarrow 0$ $\Delta\xi_i \rightarrow 0$, and $\dot{q}_i \rightarrow 0$ for all $i = 1, \cdots, n$, as $t \rightarrow \infty$, provided that the grid size of the desired array $d_g \geq 2d$.

The proof of Theorem 5.5 is similar to that of Theorem 5.4, which can be referred to in Chen and Sun (2012).

In a similar manner to Eq. (5.53), the control objective of the array manipulation under controller (Eq. 5.58) can be expressed as:

$$E = \sum_{i=1}^{n}\left\{\frac{1}{2}k_q\Delta q_i^T\Delta q_i + \frac{1}{2}k_p\dot{q}_i^T\dot{q}_i\right\} + \frac{1}{2}k_c\sum_{i=1}^{n}\frac{1}{2}\sum_{j\in N_i}Q_{ij}\left(\Delta q_{ij}\right) \rightarrow 0, \text{ as } t \rightarrow \infty \tag{5.59}$$

5.5.3 Experimental study

To verify the proposed controller Eqs. (5.53) and (5.58), experiments were conducted on two sets of cells and particles. These were silica beads with a size of $r_b = 2$ μm and yeast cells with an average size of $r_c = 5$ μm. The particles were dissolved in an aqueous solution. The laser power on each trapped particle/cell was set to 5 mW, which was shown to be safe for cell operation (Banerjee et al., 2010). As shown in Fig. 5.1B, the safety distance d between two adjacent particles/cells should be at least greater than $2r_0$ to prevent the effect of optical traps from interacting with each other. According to the calibration results in Hu and Sun (2011), r_0 was set to 2.5 μm. The physical size of each pixel used in the experiment was approximately $\sigma = 0.12$ μm; therefore, r_0 is approximately $r_0/\sigma \approx 20$ pixels. The safety distance d was set to 50 pixels. When using controllers Eqs. (5.53) and (5.58), the saturation control was used based on $r_0/\sigma \approx 20$. This degree of saturation ensured that the cells would not escape from the trap. It is worth noting that the number of particles/cells that the optical tweezers system can handle simultaneously is subject to constraints of the size of workspace, the size of each particle/cell, and the power used to manipulate the particles/cells. Because it is sometimes difficult to move particles/cells of larger size or weight in a single optical trap, multiple optical traps are needed (Koss et al., 2011). In this experimental study, a single light trap (5 mW) can process one bead or yeast cell, and the entire system can effectively manipulate dozens of particles/cells in parallel.

In the first experiment, the controller Eq. (5.53) was used to pair and move two groups of particles and cells into a common array without collisions. One group contained 10 beads and the other contained 10 yeast cells. The system parameters and

Table 5.2 System parameters and control gains (Chen and Sun, 2012).

r_c	d_g	r_b	k_l	k_q	k_c	k_p
60 (pixels)	100 (pixels)	25 (pixels)	0.01	1.5	0.001	0.1

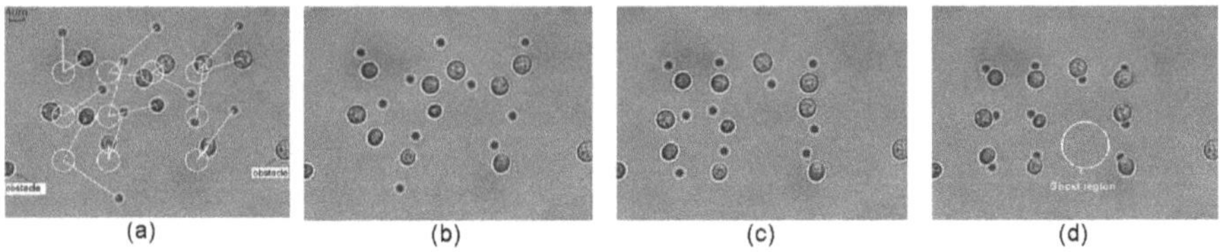

Figure 5.16 Snapshots of the arraying experiment of two groups of particles and cells (Chen and Sun, 2012): (A) 0 s; (B) 1 s; (C) 3.5 s; (D) 4.5 s.

control gain were as seen in Table 5.2. The sampling time was set to 80 ms. The bottleneck assignment algorithm (Burkardet al.,2009) was used to assign targets to particles and cells. Fig. 5.16 illustrates the position of all particles and cells at different times under the controller Eq. (5.53). As shown by the circles and lines in Fig. 5.16A, 10 beads and 10 yeast cells were assigned to their destinations. Two obstacles were detected and then fixed in place by the optical trap. Fig. 5.16 shows that the particles and cells gradually moved into the free area of the desired array within 3.5 s, and all the interdistances between the pairs of particles and cells were the same. As shown in Fig. 5.16D, each pair of beads is allowed to make physical contact with yeast cells to simulate the interaction process of many biomedical applications (such as cell fusion). The "ghost region" shown in Fig. 5.16D was due to the scattering effect of the laser beam, which existed in a fixed position in the field of view. The "ghost region" here is defined as an area with obstacles, and the controller should prevent particles and cells from entering this area. Fig. 5.17 illustrates the position error of

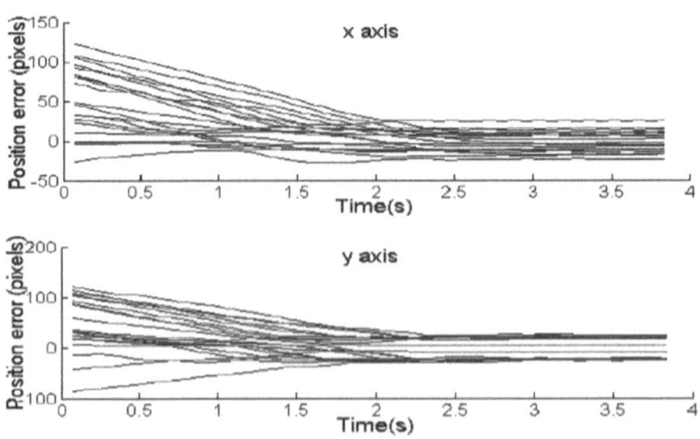

Figure 5.17 Position errors of 20 particles and cells in the x (upper) and y (bottom) axes (Chen and Sun, 2012).

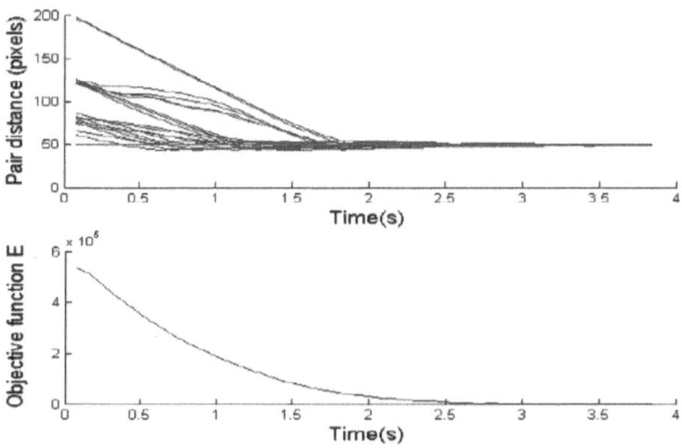

Figure 5.18 Time response of the interdistances between pair members (upper), and time response of the objective function E (bottom) (Chen and Sun, 2012).

particles and cells in the x and y directions. Because the control law Eq. (5.53) aimed to drive each pair of particles and cells into its corresponding free zone, the position error converged to a steady-state value instead of zero. Finally, as shown in Fig. 5.18, all the distances $||\Delta q_{i\kappa}||$ between the paired particles and cells converged to the required free region diameter, that was $d = 50$ pixels. The objective function E defined in Eq. (5.52) gradually converged to zero.

In the second experiment, the controller Eq. (5.58) was used to move a group of yeast cells to the desired array. The same parameters and control gain as in the first experiment were used. Fig. 5.19 illustrates the positions of 20 yeast cells used in the experiment at different times under the controller Eq. (5.58). It was found that all cells moved quickly into the desired array. In 0.5 s, the saddle was detected and the destinations of the two participating cells were exchanged. Fig. 5.20 illustrates the position error. Fig. 5.21 illustrates the objective function defined in Eq. (5.52). It can be seen that all position errors and objective functions converged to zero successfully. Note that some position errors in Fig. 5.21 varied greatly. This is because a saddle point or near-saddle point was detected in the process and the cells were triggered to exchange their destinations.

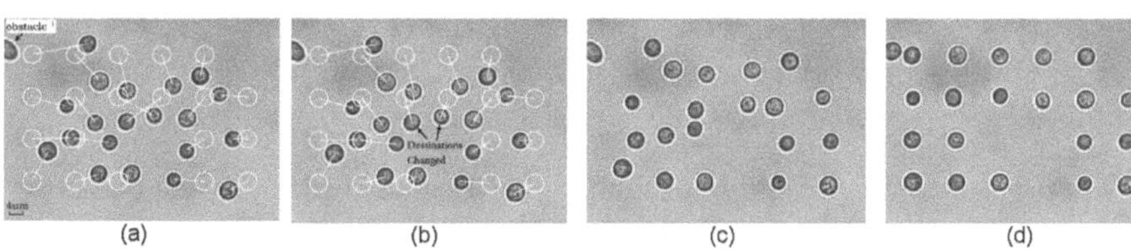

Figure 5.19 Snapshots of the arraying experiment of a group of yeast cells (Chen and Sun, 2012): (A) 0 s; (B) 0.5 s; (C) 1.5 s; (D) 2.5 s.

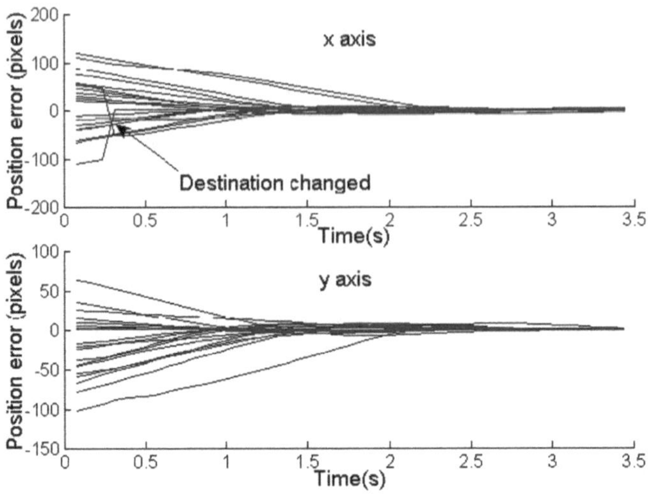

Figure 5.20 Position errors of 20 yeast cells in x (upper) and y (bottom) axis (Chen and Sun, 2012).

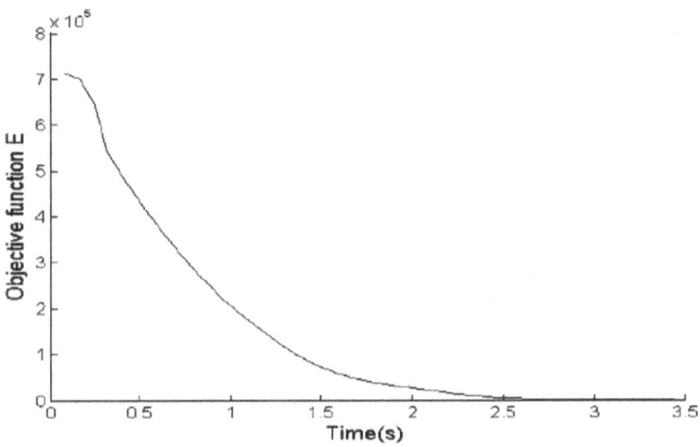

Figure 5.21 Time response of the objective function E (Chen and Sun, 2012).

5.6 Cell transportation for multiprocessing automation tasks

Most reported research on automated cell transportation is single-task oriented. The results of these studies can hardly meet the growing demand for emerging cell therapy procedures, which usually require a series of manipulation tasks with multiple processing steps. Fig. 5.22 illustrates an example of intracellular organelle extraction, which requires several processing steps. First, the target cells are transported into task region 1 for reorientation. Second, the cells are transported to task region 2 for organelle extraction. Then, the cells are transported to another work area for subsequent steps

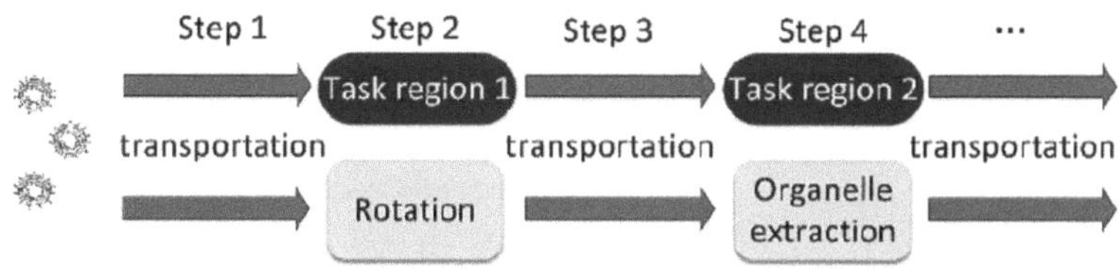

Figure 5.22 Multiple steps of a complete cell therapeutic operation (Yang et al., 2017).

such as cell fusion and injection. In addition to automating the single task in each step, the automation network is also required that links all processing steps through the automatic transportation of grouping cells. Therefore, in order to achieve automated cell therapy operations, it is necessary to develop a control strategy that connects all sequential steps to accomplish a complete therapeutic operation.

Yang et al. (2017) reported an automated cell transportation method that used a robot-assisted optical tweezers manipulation system to complete the multistep process in cell therapy. In this study, the grouped cells were manipulated to continuously enter different task regions without interference. A potential field-based controller was designed to implement multistep process control. In this method, the concepts of contractive coalition and switching region were incorporated into the tweezers–cell coalition. The advantage of this controller is that it can simultaneously control the position of optical tweezers, trap multiple cells, and avoid collisions in a unified manner. This section introduces this method.

5.6.1 Modeling

Fig. 5.23 illustrates the expected manipulation using the holographic optical tweezers (HOT) system. At the beginning, the contour detection algorithm is used to detect all positions of cells and other biological particles through an image-processing program (Castleman, 1996). First, optical tweezers are used to label and trap the target cells. Then, the sensor module of the HOT system starts to track the cells and provide visual feedback of the cell position. Under the guidance of the proposed control strategy, the cells are automatically transferred to the first task region to complete the first task. After that, the cells are transported to the second task in the second task region, and so on. Collisions between cells and obstacles are avoided during operation. Fig. 5.24 shows the flow chart of the subsequent cell manipulation process.

5.6.1.1 Effective trapping

The dynamics of the ith cell trapped by the ith optical tweezers has been given in Eq. (5.45). In the low Re number environment, it can be further simplified as

$$\dot{q}_i = \frac{k_i}{\beta_i}(l_i - q_i). \tag{5.60}$$

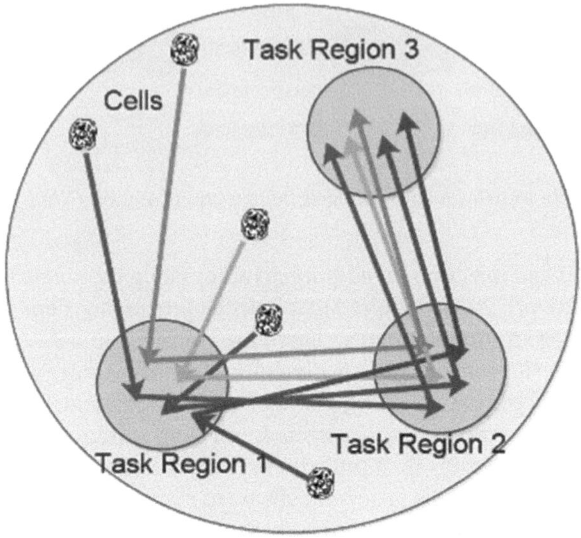

Figure 5.23 Automated sequential transportation of multiple cells to different task regions sequentially (Yang et al., 2017).

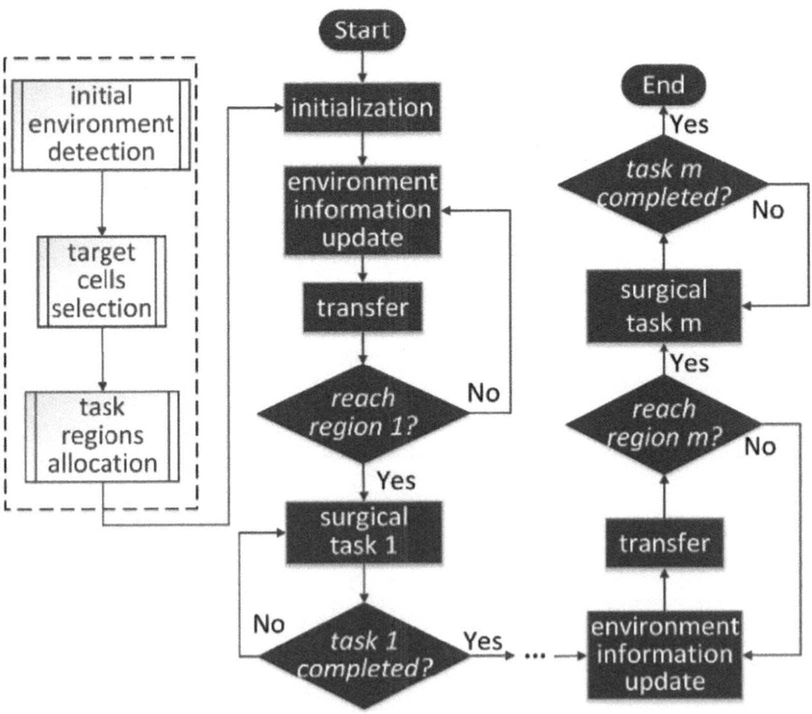

Figure 5.24 Flowchart of transporting cells to multiple task regions (Yang et al., 2017).

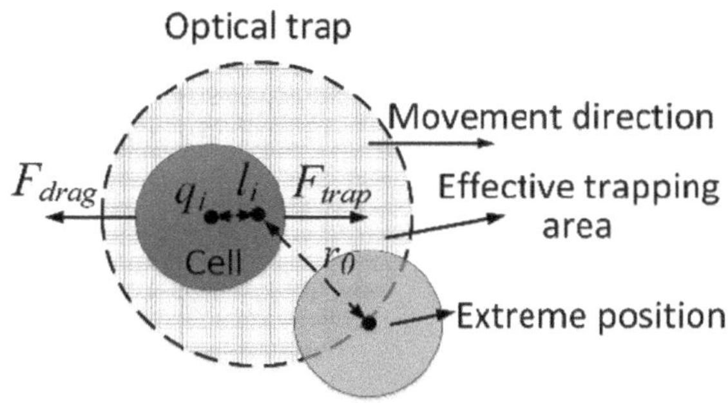

Figure 5.25 Schematic of an optically manipulated cell (Yang et al., 2017).

When the offset between the cell and the optical trap is greater than the threshold r_0, the cell escapes from the optical trap. Therefore, the cell must be confined within the effective trapping area. In other words, it should be ensured that $l_i - q_i < r_0$ during manipulation. Fig. 5.25 illustrates a schematic diagram of optical manipulation of cells.

Define the trapping area of the ith cell as follows:

$$C_i = \left\{ q_i | r_0^2 - \|l_i - q_i\|^2 > 0 \right\}. \tag{5.61}$$

If $q_i \varepsilon C_i$, then the cell is located inside the effective trapping area.

Denote n cells by the position $q_n = \{q_1, \cdots, q_i, \cdots, q_n\}$ and radius $r_n = \{r_1, \cdots, r_i, \cdots r_n\}$. Suppose that n optical traps, denoted by the position $L_n = \{l_1, \cdots, l_i, \cdots, l_n\}$, are applied to the cells. Therefore, the above dynamics indicate that only when the center of mass of the ith cell is located inside the trapping area C_i can the robot-tweezers system effectively manipulate the ith cell. Yang et al. (2017) defined this tweezers−cell spatial relationship as the T−C alliance, similarly to Li et al. (2015).

A constraint function is then introduced to maintain the ith T−C coalition as follows:

$$G_i^{T-C} = \frac{1}{2}\left(r_0^2 - \|l_i - q_i\|^2\right). \tag{5.62}$$

The T−C coalition can be modeled as a virtual circle defined as follows:

Definition 5.4 (T−C coalition): T−C coalition is defined as a virtual circle centered at q_i with a radius of r_i^{T-C}, which satisfies the T−C coalition constraint $G_i^{T-C} > 0$.

5.6.1.2 Cell transfer

At the beginning of the operation, the target cells may be located far away from the work area and need to be transferred to the first task region. Without loss of generality, all the m different task regions are denoted as circular regions, centered at $t_j \in \Re^2$ with a radius $tr_j, j\varepsilon\{1, \cdots, m\}$. A binary factor denoted by Flag_j is used to denote the status of the jth task. That is, $\mathrm{Flag}_1 = 1$ means that task 1 is ongoing; $\mathrm{Flag}_1 = 0$ and $\mathrm{Flag}_2 = 1$ mean that task 1 is completed and task 2 is ongoing.

Introduce contractive coalition as follows, which is defined as a potential field-based constraint function:

$$G_i^c = \sum_j^m \frac{1}{2}\left(cr_i^{j2} - \|l_i - t_j\|^2\right) \cdot \mathrm{Flag}_j = \sum_j^m G_i^j \cdot \mathrm{Flag}_j, \tag{5.63}$$

where $cr_i^j = q_i - t_j + \rho$, and ρ is a buffer distance that is greater than r_0 (i.e., $\rho > r_0$). $G_i^c > 0$ indicates that the cell is located in the contractive coalition. The boundary of the coalition is set to be always close to the cell. This condition means that the cells are driven away from the boundary and move toward the center of the contractive coalition. The center of the contractive coalition is set to be the same as the center of the task region. In the case that the cell is always in the contractive coalition, the cell is pushed to the task region through the contractive coalition boundary. The coalition boundary coincides with the task region boundary, which means that the cell has been transferred to the task region. Therefore, the contractive coalition is considered to be a virtual circle with a variable radius as defined below.

Definition 5.5 (contractive coalition): Contractive coalition is defined as a virtual circle centered at t_j with a variable radius of cr_i^j, which satisfies the contractive coalition constraint $G_i^c > 0$.

Fig. 5.26 illustrates the concept of the proposed contractive coalition.

5.6.1.3 Task switching

After the current task is completed, the control algorithm switches to the next task. This switching process requires a continuous and smooth contractive coalition G_i^c.

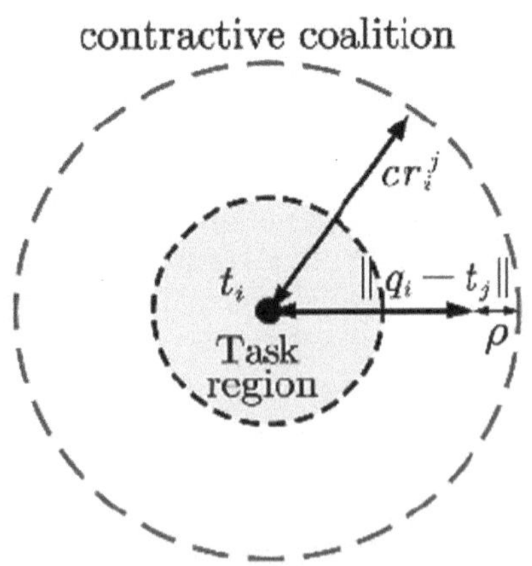

Figure 5.26 Illustration of contractive coalition (Yang et al., 2017).

For this purpose, a switching region S_i^j is introduced here. The region is defined as a circle centered at $q_i(t_j)$ with a radius rs, where $q_i(t_j)$ denotes the cell position at the time when the jth task is completed. A smooth switching process is ensured by updating the status factor Flag_j as follows when the cell is located in the switching region:

$$\text{Flag}_j = \begin{cases} \sin^2\left(\dfrac{\pi\|\boldsymbol{q}_i - \boldsymbol{q}_i(t_{j-1})\|}{2rs}\right), & q_i \in S_i^{j-1},\ \text{Flag}_{j-1} < 1 \\ 1, & q_i \notin S_i^{j-1},\ \text{Flag}_{j+1} = 0 \\ 1 - \sin^2\left(\dfrac{\pi\|\boldsymbol{q}_i - \boldsymbol{q}_i(t_j)\|}{2rs}\right), & q_i \in S_i^j,\ \text{Flag}_{j+1} > 0. \end{cases} \tag{5.64}$$

Note that the first term Flag_1 can be neglected when the first task is performed. The selection of sine function makes G_i^c continuous and smooth. The switching regions are shown in Fig. 5.27A, and the value of Flag_j is illustrated in Fig. 5.27B.

Definition 5.6 (switching region): Switching region is defined as a virtual circle centered at $q_i(t_j)$ with a variable radius of rs for smooth transfer among different tasks.

5.6.1.4 Obstacle avoidance

The proposed controller should be equipped with a collision avoidance function to ensure that no target cells will collide with other particles or cells. There may be

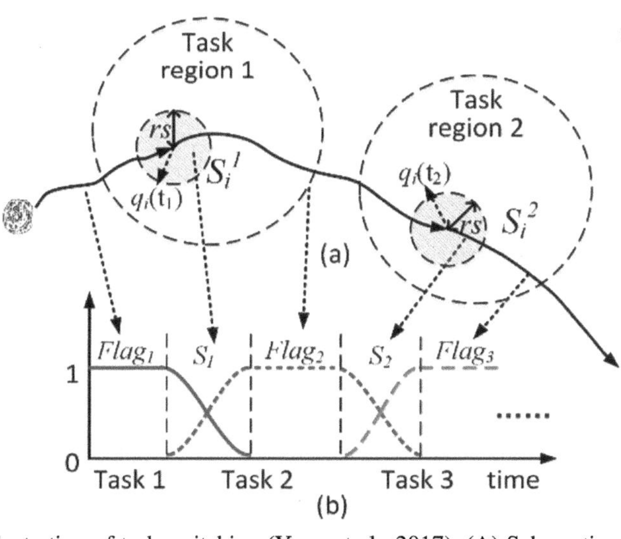

Figure 5.27 Illustration of task switching (Yang et al., 2017). (A) Schematic of switching region. (B) Illustration of Flag_j variation.

two obstacles in the workspace, namely, immovable particles attached to the substrate and floating particles. After identifying them, the cells can be controlled to simply stay away from the immovable particles. Floating particles can be marked and then trapped with optical tweezers to move to a predefined storage area. Compared with the current target cell, other moving target cells are also regarded as movable obstacles.

All the obstacles in the workspace are denoted as circular obstacles centered at $O_k(t)$ with a radius of ro_k, where $k \in \{1, \cdots, p\}$ and p is the total number of obstacles. All the other targeted cells are also regarded as obstacles with respect to the ith targeted cell. Therefore, the number of obstacles with respect to the ith cell is $p + n - 1$ for n targeted cells in the workspace. All obstacles with respect to the ith cell are denoted as circles centered at $O_k(t)$ with a radius of ro_k for $k \in \{1, \cdots, p, \cdots p + n - 1\}$, where $O_{p+a}(t) = q_b(t)$ and $ro_{p+a} = r_b$, $a \in \{1, \cdots, n-1\}$, and $b \in \{1, \cdots, n\}(b \neq i)$. Hence, a constraint function is introduced below to guarantee that no collision occurs during cell transportation:

$$G_i^o = \prod_k \frac{1}{2}\left(\|l_i - O_k\|^2 - (r_0 + r_i + ro_k)^2\right) = \prod_k \alpha_k. \tag{5.65}$$

If $G_i^o > 0$, there is no collision between the target cell and the other particles or cells.

5.6.1.5 Free manipulation space

Free manipulation space is a workspace that integrates all constraint functions of T−C coalitions, contractive coalition, and obstacle avoidance. The free manipulation space for the ith cell is defined as follows.

Definition 5.7 (free manipulation space)

$$F_i = \{l_i | G_i(l_i(t)) = G_i^{T-C} G_i^c G_i^o > 0\}. \tag{5.66}$$

The cells in the free manipulation space are located within the effective trapping area of optical tweezers and the contractive coalition region. All cells are collision-free.

5.6.2 Controller design

The velocity of the ith optical trap applied on the ith cell is denoted as $u_i = \dot{l}_i \in \Re^2$, which is defined as the control input to the ith optical tweezer manipulator. The center of the final task region is set as the goal point, denoted as $g \in \Re^2$. The problem of automatic cell transportation for multiple cell surgery tasks is formulated as follows:

Consider n cells in multiple cell surgery tasks with dynamic (Eq. 5.61). *Under the initial configuration of* $G_i(l_i(0)) > 0$, *the control input* $u = \{u_1, \cdots, u_i, \cdots u_n\}$ *is determined for optical tweezers manipulators that can sequentially drive the cells to the task regions centered at* $t = \{t_1, \cdots, t_j, \cdots t_m\}$ *and finally reach the goal region centered at* g *while maintaining* $G_i(l_i(t)) > 0$, $\forall t > 0$.

A bounded potential field function $\phi \in [0, 1]$ is designed as follows:

$$\phi_i = \frac{\gamma_i(l_i)}{\left(\gamma_i^\delta(l_i) + G_i(l_i)\right)^{\frac{1}{\delta}}}, \tag{5.67}$$

where δ is a positive parameter, $\gamma_i(l_i) = \frac{1}{2}e_{gi}^T e_{gi}$ is a criterion function to denote the position error of the ith T−C coalition to the final goal g, and $e_{gi} = l_i - g$. Then, the control input is designed as the negative gradient of the potential field function ϕ_i, expressed as follows:

$$u_i = -k_i \frac{\partial \phi_i}{\partial l_i}, \tag{5.68}$$

where k_i is the positive control gain.

Yang et al. (2017) has proved that under the initial configuration of $G_i(l_i(0)) > 0$, the control law Eq. (5.68) gives rise to the following: (1) $G_i(l_i(0)) > 0, \ \forall t > 0$; (2) the trapped cell is always located within the effective trapping area and the contractive coalition boundary; and (3) the cells are collision-free. Further, the parameter δ has a positive lower bound $\widehat{\delta}$, such that the desired position g is the only critical point in the free manipulation space F_i.

5.6.3 Experiments

Experiments were conducted to transport a group of yeast cells to different task areas in sequence while avoiding collisions with immovable or floating obstacles. The diameters of yeast cells ranges from 4 to 6 μm. Images of the manipulation process were acquired through a CCD camera under 60× magnification with a resolution of 0.1075 μm/pixel. The parameters were set as follows: the critical offset was $r_0 = 10$ pixel ≈ 1.0 μm, which was used for maintaining the cell in the effective trapping area (Wu et al., 2011); the buffer distance was $\rho = 5$ pixel ≈ 0.54 μm, which was used to push cells forward; the radius of the switching region was $rs = 5$ pixel ≈ 0.54 μm, and the radius of the task region was 80 pixel = 8.6 μm, both for effective task switching. The target cells were scattered in the liquid environment, and the other particles were marked as obstacles.

In the first experiment, the immovable obstacles attached to the substrate were considered. Table 5.3 lists the initial configuration of yeast cells, obstacles, and task areas. The operation process is shown in Fig. 5.28. The optical tweezers trapped the target cell, which was represented by a solid circle. The task region was marked as a solid black circle, and obstacles were represented by green discs. As seen in Fig. 5.28A, the target cells were initially located far from the task region 1. The cells were driven to approach task region 1 under the proposed controller, as seen in Fig. 5.28B and C. Then, the cells were driven to task region 2 when the first task was completed, as seen in Fig. 5.28D and E. Finally, all target cells were transported to task region 3 successfully, as seen in Fig. 5.28F.

Table 5.3 Initial configurations of the yeast cells, obstacles, and task regions (Yang et al., 2017).

Position (μm)		$q_i(0)$	O_k	t_j
Index	1	(9.8, 14.6)	(36.2, 17.2)	(12.9, 37.6)
	2	(44.8, 30.7)	(34.8, 39.0)	(53.8, 40.9)
	3	(49.0, 46.5)	(59.4, 24.8)	(55.7, 9.0)
	4	(28.0, 47.3)	(17.0, 7.0)	

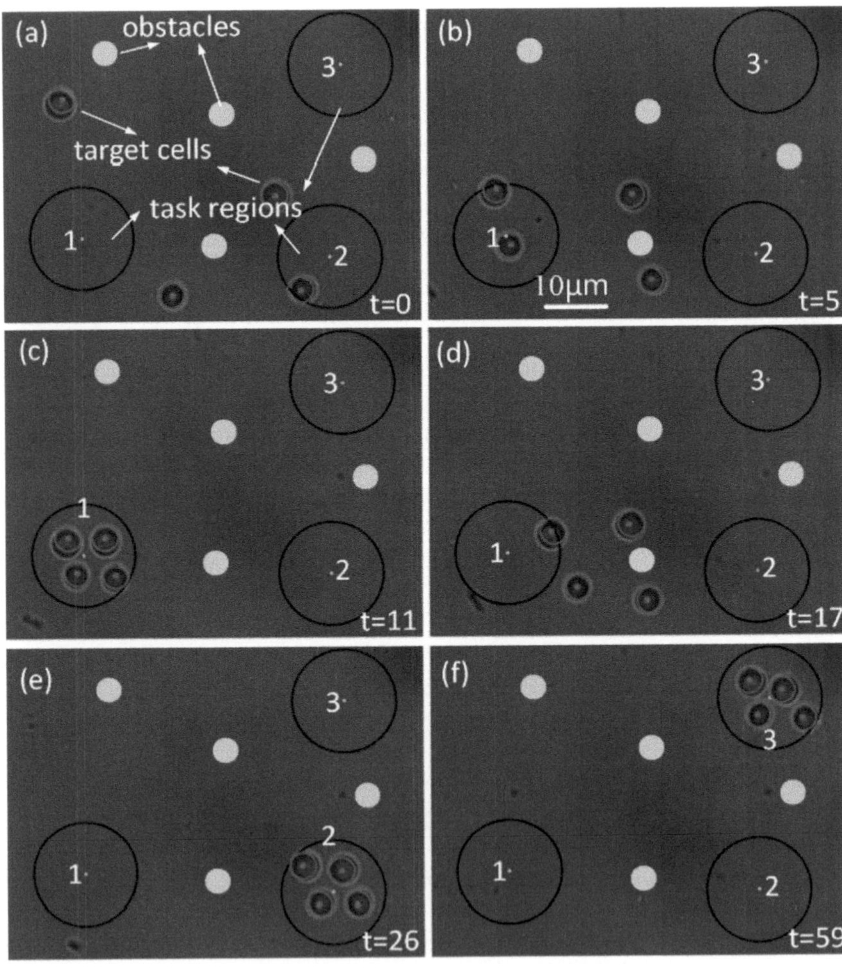

Figure 5.28 Experimental process of transporting cells into different task regions with fixed obstacles (Yang et al., 2017). (A) Initial positions. (B, C) The cells arrived in the first task region successively. (D, E) The cells arrived in the second task region after the first task was completed. (F) All cells arrived in the final task region.

Fig. 5.29 illustrates the experimental control performance. Fig. 5.29A–C show the time response of the distance $q_i - t_j$ between the target cell and the center of the three task regions. The radius of the task region tr_j was equally set to 8 μm so that all target cells arrived in the assigned task regions sequentially. After all the cells reached each task area, they stopped for 5 s to perform the task, which was marked accordingly in the figures. Fig. 5.29D illustrates the offset $l_i - q_i$ during the cell transfer process, indicating that the optical tweezers effectively trapped all cells. These experimental results demonstrated that the proposed control approach can successfully achieve all the control objectives.

In the second experiment, floating particles were introduced as movable obstacles. These floating particles were moved to the obstacle storage area and fixed in the area by optical tweezers. The same steps as in the first experiment were then implemented. The initial configurations of the experiment are listed in Table 5.4, where t_o represents the center of the obstacle storage area.

The experimental process is shown in Fig. 5.30. The target cells trapped by optical tweezers were represented by solid circles, and obstacles were represented by blue disks. The task area and obstacle storage area were marked as solid black and orange

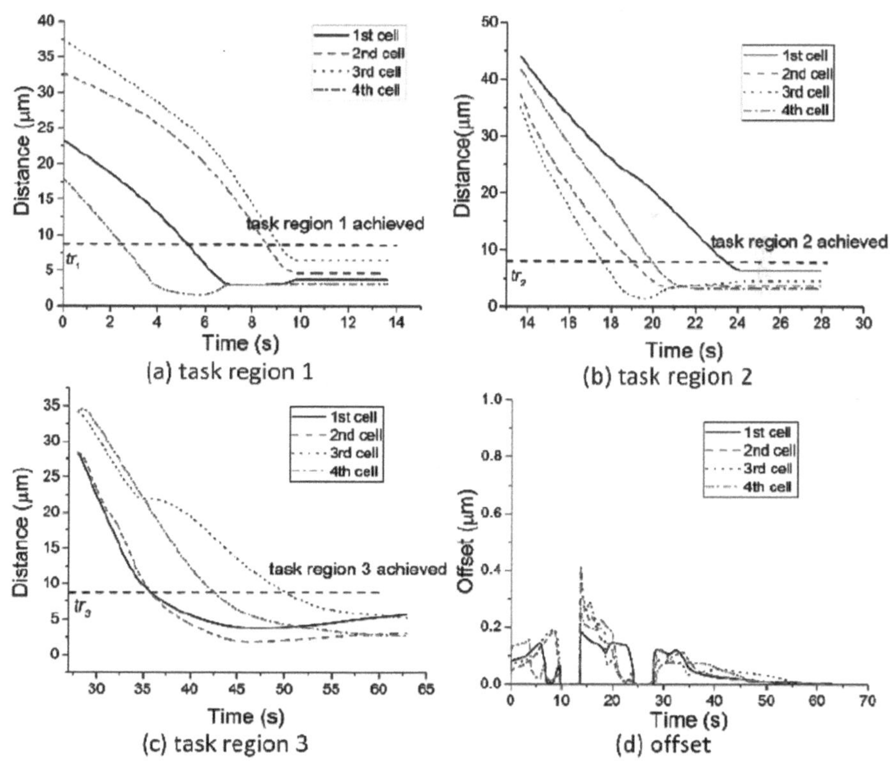

Figure 5.29 Experimental control performance (Yang et al., 2017). (A–C) Position distance between the cells and the three task points. (D) Offset between the traps and cells.

Table 5.4 Initial configurations of the experiment with movable obstacles (Yang et al., 2017).

Position (μm)		$q_i(0)$	$O_k(0)$	t_j	t_o
Index	1	(9.7, 17.7)	(11.0, 36.7)	(12.9, 40.9)	(12.9, 10.8)
	2	(33.5, 43.1)	(22.1, 30.3)	(53.8, 40.9)	
	3	(36.7, 43.1)	(15.2, 22.7)	(53.9, 12.9)	
	4	(21.0, 14.6)	(34.4, 18.8)		
	5		(36.3, 8.4)		

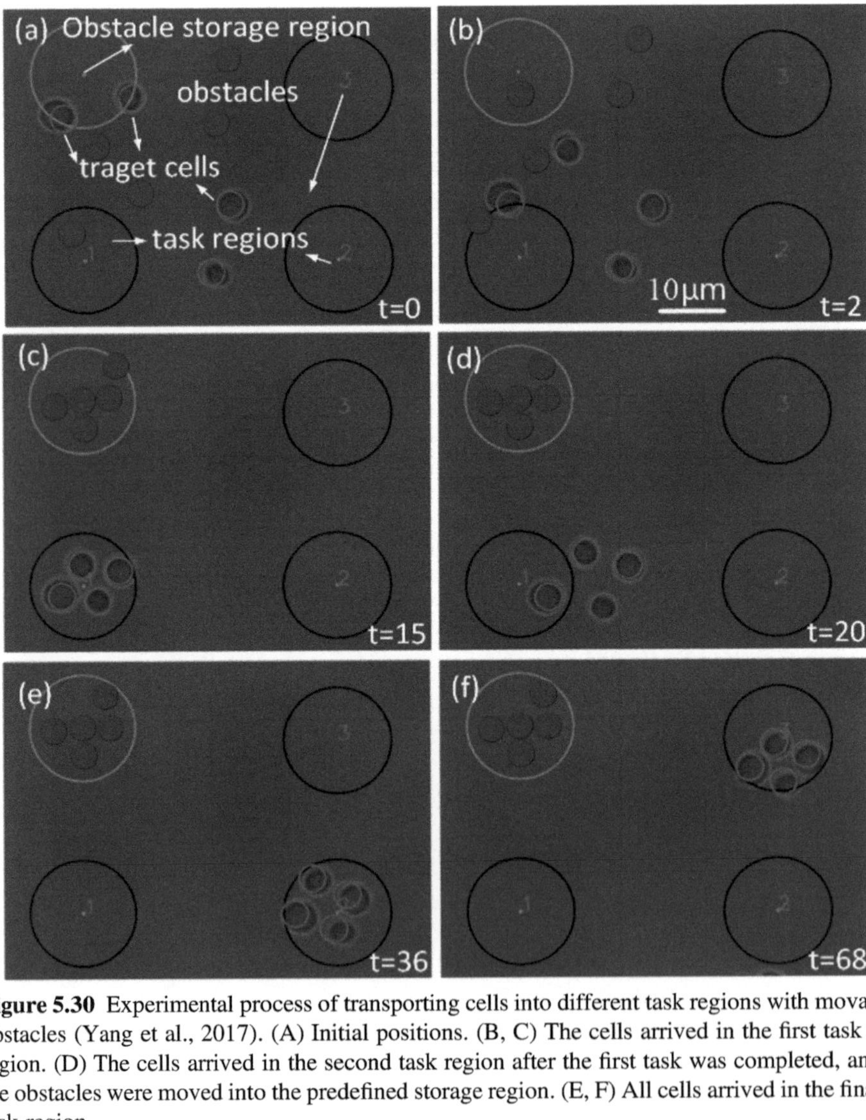

Figure 5.30 Experimental process of transporting cells into different task regions with movable obstacles (Yang et al., 2017). (A) Initial positions. (B, C) The cells arrived in the first task region. (D) The cells arrived in the second task region after the first task was completed, and the obstacles were moved into the predefined storage region. (E, F) All cells arrived in the final task region.

circles. The cells were driven to different task regions in turn, and obstacles were simultaneously transferred to the storage area. Finally, all target cells were successfully transported to task region 3, and obstacles were stored in the obstacle area. Fig. 5.31 illustrates the control performance. As shown in Figs. 5.31A–D, the cells were successfully transported to the three task regions, and the cells were effectively trapped

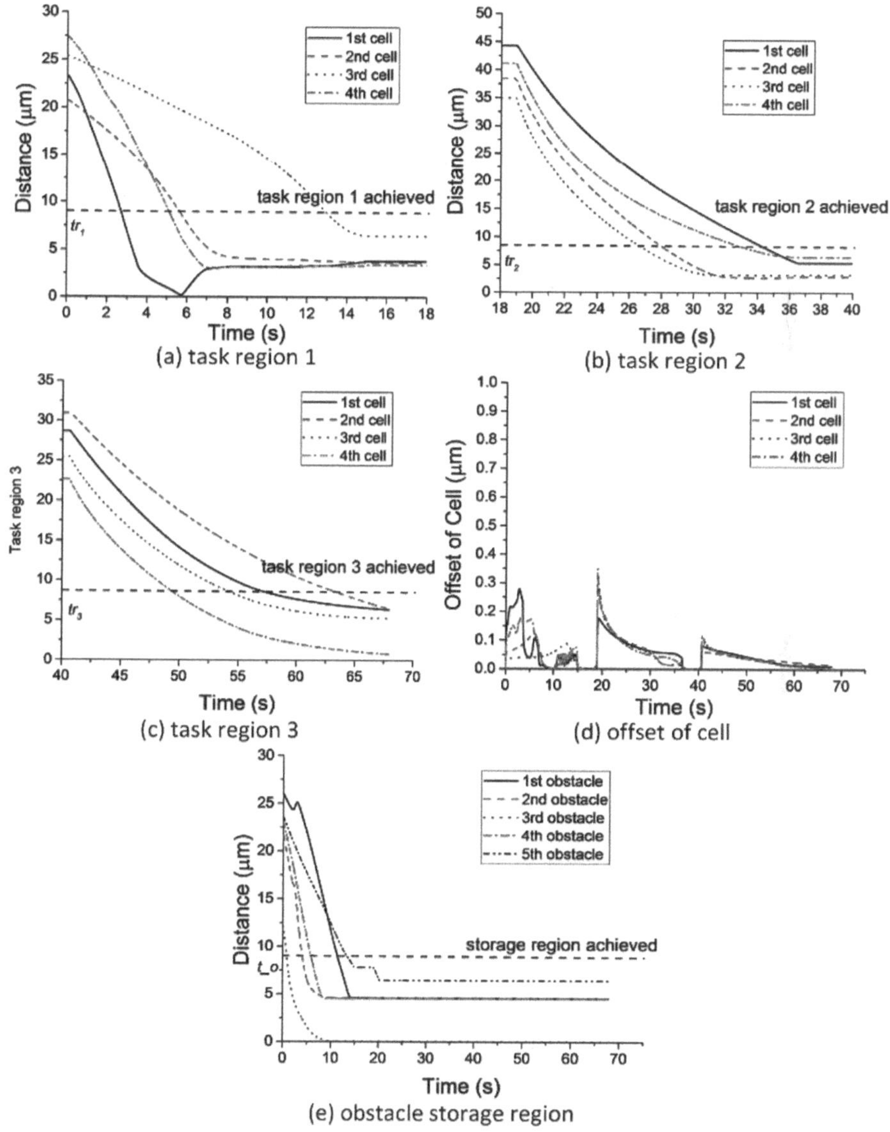

Figure 5.31 Experimental control performance (Yang et al., 2017). (A–C) Position/distance between the cells and the three task points. (D) Offset between the traps and cells. (E) Distances between the obstacles and the storage region center.

during the transport process. Fig. 5.31E shows the distance between the obstacle and the center of the obstacle storage area, indicating that all the obstacles were moved into the storage area and were kept in this area during the entire operation.

5.7 Conclusions

Automating cell transport with optical tweezers requires sophisticated dynamic analysis, motion planning, and motion controller design. This chapter introduces a variety of methods to automatically transport single or multiple cells by integrating robotics technology into optical tweezers manipulation. Five topics are introduced.

First, the basic theory and method of automatic cell transportation using the robotic optical tweezers system are reported. Analysis of the dynamics of the trapped cells shows that deviation of the trapped cells must be in the optical trap to prevent the cells from escaping the optical trap during transportation. A feedback controller is introduced that can control single and multiple cells in automatic transportation without knowing the precise values of the trapping stiffness and drag coefficient.

Second, the motion and path planning of automatic cell transportation are introduced. The optimal motion parameters are determined by calibrating the trapping force on living cells, and the PI scheme is used to adjust the motion speed online so that the cells can move efficiently while maintaining their positions within the optical trap. To plan the path in automatic cell transportation, a modified A* algorithm and RRT-based path planner are introduced.

Third, a unified feedback controller to effectively manipulate cells in cell transportation is presented. The controller can transfer the target cell to the destination while always placing it in the optical trap and avoiding collisions with other particles in the environment. The design of the controller is based on the use of a geometric C−T coalition model, which aims to confine the cell to the optical trap while considering obstacle avoidance. Compared with other cell transport control methods, the unified controller can simultaneously control cell positioning, cell trapping, and obstacle avoidance without the need for an additional trajectory planner.

Fourth, a control method that can move a group of cells or particles into an array is introduced. This method can drive different groups of cells or particles into a common array for pairing. Based on the physical dynamics of trapping, a potential field-based controller is presented to drive each pair of cells to a specified array while preventing collisions between them. The advantage of this controller is that it can drive the two sets of cells or particles into a common array of correct pairs, and control the distance between the pairs.

Finally, an automated cell transportation control method for the multistep process in cell therapy is introduced. The presented controller can sequentially transfer a group of cells to a series of task regions, while keeping the cells in an effective trapping area and avoiding conflicts. A geometric model is designed to formulate the controller by using tweezers−cell coalition, contractive coalition, and switching region. The controller can simultaneously control cell positions, cell trapping, and collision avoidance in a coordinated manner, and continuously transfer cells to different task regions without interference.

This chapter has clearly demonstrated that robotic optical tweezers technology can achieve automated cell transport successfully. The precise positioning of cells through efficient and automated cell transport can support many biomedical applications, such as drug discovery, cell–cell interactions, and tissue engineering.

References

Alexakis, T., Boadi, D.K., Quong, D., Groboillot, A., O'Neill, I., Poncelet, D., Neufeld, R.J., 1995. Microencapsulation of DNA within alginate microspheres and crosslinked chitosan membranes for in vivo application. Appl. Biochem. Biotechnol. 50, 93–106.

Arai, F., Yoshikaw, K., Sakami, T., Fukuda, T., 2004. Synchronized laser micromanipulation of multiple targets along each trajectory by single laser. Appl. Phys. Lett. 85, 4301–4303.

Arai, F., Onda, K., Iitsuka, R., Maruyama, H., 2009. Multi-beam Laser Micromanipulation of Microtool by Integrated Optical Tweezers. IEEE Int Conf Robotics and Automation, Kobe, Japan, pp. 12–17.

Banerjee, A.G., Pomerance, A., Losert, W., Gupta, S.K., 2010. Developing a stochastic dynamic programming framework for optical tweezer based automated particle transport operations. IEEE Trans. Automat. Sci. Eng. 7, 218–227.

Brouhard, G.J., Schek, H.T., Hunt, A.J., 2003. Advanced optical tweezers for the study of cellular and molecular biomechanics. IEEE Trans. Biomed. Eng. 50, 121–125.

Burkard, R., Dell'Amico, M., Martello, S., 2009. Assignment Problems. SIAM, Philadelphia, PA.

Castleman, K.R., 1996. Digital Image Processing. Prentice-Hall, Englewood Cliffs, NJ, USA.

Chapin, S.C., Germain, V., Dufresue, E.R., 2006. Automated trapping, assembly, and sorting with holographic optical tweezers. Opt. Expr. 14, 13095–13100.

Cheah, C.C., Hou, S.P., Slotine, J.J.E., 2009. Region-based shape control for a swarm of robots. Automatica 45, 2406–2411.

Cheah, C.C., Li, X., Yan, X., Sun, D., 2015. Simple PD control scheme for robotic manipulation of biological cell. IEEE Trans. Automat. Control 60 (5), 1427–1432.

Chen, H., Sun, D., 2012. Moving groups of microparticles into array with a robot-tweezers manipulation system. IEEE Trans. Robot. 28 (5), 1069–1080.

Chen, H., Wang, C., Li, X., Sun, D., 2016. Transportation of multiple biological cells through saturation-controlled optical tweezers in crowded microenvironments. IEEE/ASME Trans. Mechatron. 21 (2), 888–899.

ChongSeet, B., Lin, G., 2004. A-STAR: a mobile ad hoc routing strategy for metropolis vehicular communications. Networking 3042, 989–999.

Gauthier, R.C., Wallace, S., 1995. Optical levitation of spheres: analytical development and numerical computations of the force equations. J. Opt. Soc. Am. B 12, 1680–1685.

Grover, S.C., Skirtzch, A.G., Gauthier, R.C., Grover, C.P., 2001. Automated single-cell sorting system based on optical trapping. J. Biomed. Opt. 6, 14–22.

Harris, J., McConnell, G., 2008. Optical trapping and manipulation of live T cells with a low numerical aperture lens. Opt. Expr. 16, 14036–14043.

Hu, S., Sun, D., 2011. Automatic transportation of biological cells with a robot-tweezer manipulation system. Int. J. Robot. Res. 30 (14), 1681–1694.

Hu, Z., Wang, J., Liang, J., 2005. Experimental measurement and analysis of the optical trapping force acting on a yeast cell with a lensed optical fiber probe. Opt. Laser Tech. 39 (3), 475–480.

Huang, Y., Zhang, Z., Menq, C.H., 2009. Minimum-variance Brownian motion control of an optically trapped probe. Appl. Opt. 48, 5871–5880.

Ju, T., Liu, S., Yang, J., Sun, D., 2014. Rapidly exploring random tree algorithm-based path planning for robot-aided optical manipulation of biological cells. IEEE Trans. Automat. Sci. Eng. 11 (3), 649–657.

Koss, B., Chowdhury, S., Aabo, T., Gupta, S.K., Losert, W., 2011. Indirect optical gripping with triplet traps. J. Opt. Soc. Am. B 28, 982–985.

Kuncova, J., Kallio, P., 2004. Challenges in capillary pressure microinjection. In: Proc. 26th Annu. IEEE Int. Conf. Eng. Med. Biol. Soc, pp. 4998–5001.

Li, X., Sun, D., Yang, J., 2013. Bounded controller for multirobot navigation while maintaining network connectivity in the presence of obstacles. Automatica 49 (1), 285–292.

Li, X., Yang, H., Wang, J., Sun, D., 2015. Design of a robust unified controller for cell manipulation with a robot-aided optical tweezers system. Automatica 51 (5), 279–286.

Li, X., Yang, H., Huang, H., Sun, D., 2018. A switching controller for high speed cell transportation by using a robot-aided optical tweezers system. Automatica 89, 308–315.

McNerney, G.P., Hübner, W., Chen, B.K., Huser, T., 2010. Manipulating CD4+ T cells by optical tweezers for the initiation of cell-cell transfer of HIV-1. J. Biophoton. 3, 216–223.

Pacoret, C., Bowman, R., Gibson, G., Haliyo, S., Carberry, D., Bergander, A., et al., 2009. Touching the microworld with force-feedback optical tweezers. Opt. Expr. 17, 10259–10264.

Ranaweera, A., Bamieh, B., 2005. Modeling, identification, and control of a spherical particle trapped in an optical tweezer. Int. J. Robust Nonlin. Control 15, 747–768.

Sun, D., 2010. Synchronization and Control of Multiagent System. Taylor & Francis Group, LLC, London.

Svoboda, K., Block, S.M., 1994. Biological applications of optical forces. Annu. Rev. Biophys. Biomol. Struct. 23, 247–332.

Tan, Y., Sun, D., Huang, W., Cheng, S.H., 2008. Mechanical modeling of biological cells in microinjection. IEEE Trans. NanoBiosci. 7, 257–266.

Tanaka, Y., Kawada, H., Hirano, K., Ishikawa, M., Kitajima, H., 2008. Automated manipulation of non-spherical microobjects using optical tweezers combined with image processing techniques. Opt. Expr. 16, 15115–15122.

Wallin, A.E., Ojala, H., Hæggström, E., Tuma, R., 2008. Stiffer optical tweezers through real-time feedback control. Appl. Phys. Lett. 92, 224104.

Walther, W., Stein, U., 2000. Viral vectors for gene transfer: a review of their use in the treatment of human diseases. Drugs 60, 249–271.

Wang, X., Chen, S., Kong, M., Wang, Z., Costa, K., Li, R.A., Sun, D., 2011. Enhanced cell sorting and manipulation with combined optical tweezer and microfluidic chip technologies. Lab Chip 11 (21), 3656–3662.

Wu, Y., Sun, D., Huang, W., 2011. Mechanical force characterization in manipulating live cells with optical tweezers. J. Biomech. 44, 741–746.

Wu, Y., Sun, D., Huang, W., Xi, N., 2013. Dynamics analysis and motion planning for automated cell transportation with optical tweezers. IEEE/ASME Trans. Mechatron. 18 (2), 706–713.

Wulff, K.D., Cole, D.G., Clark, R.L., 2007. Servo control of a optical trap. Appl. Opt. 46, 4923–4931.

Yang, H., Li, X., Liu, Y.H., Sun, D., 2017. Automated transportation of biological cells for multiple processing steps in cell surgery. IEEE Trans. Automat. Sci. Eng. 14 (4), 1712–1721.

Yang, H., Li, X., Li, X., Sun, L., Sun, D., 2020. A virtual assisted controller for biological cell transportation in a dynamic environment with variable field of view. IEEE/ASME Trans. Mechatron. 25 (3), 1255–1265.

Cell rotation

6

6.1 Introduction

In many cell therapy applications, cells must be oriented properly so that micromanipulation tools can access target components with minimal damage to cells. These applications include cell injection (Huang et al., 2009; Xie et al., 2010), in vitro fertilization (IVF) (Lin et al., 2007), preimplantation genetic diagnosis (PGD) (Braude et al., 2002), intracytoplasmic sperm injection (ICSI) (Yoshida and Perry, 2007), and organelle extraction analysis and diagnosis (Shelby et al., 2005; Ando et al., 2008). These procedures require noninvasive rotation of cells in three-dimensional (3D) space to orient target cell structures or components for various micromanipulation tasks. In the microelectromechanical system field, micromotors and microfans also rotate for microfluidic applications, such as mixing processes, used to drive and manufacture micromachines (Kim and Breuer, 2007; Luo et al., 2000). Cells usually have a structural orientation (polarity) that determines cell physiology and function (Reffay et al., 2011; Lee and Vasioukhin, 2008), in terms of membrane potential or membrane protein distribution. Therefore, in experimental biological procedures, the ability to orient cells under microscopy is important for studying their physiological functions. In addition, rotation manipulation is also important for studying the behavior of twisted macromolecules, biological enzyme motors, and the operating mechanism of bacterial flagella (Min et al., 2009). Therefore, the orientation control of cells has become a basic and important cell micromanipulation technique required in many cell therapy applications.

As explained in detail in earlier chapters, optical tweezers are a scientific instrument that uses a low-power laser beam to apply trapping force and torque to microscopic particles (Ashkin et al., 1987). The use of optical tweezers to control cell orientation has been reported in the literature. The oscillating linear optical trap was used to rotate rod-shaped bacterial cells (Carmon and Feingold, 2011). The fast oscillating trap was generated by a galvanometer. By changing the oscillation amplitude, the cell can rotate about 90 degree relative to the optical axis. Linearly polarized optical tweezers were used to orient flat particles (Galajda and Ormos, 2003), in which the rotating torque came from the anisotropic scattering of laser light by particles. As reported by Bingelyte et al. (2003), the 3D rotation of microscopic particles can be controlled via a spatial light modulator to create a pair of optical traps to fix different parts of the cell, and then rotate the trapped cell around three coordinate axes. Other methods of controlling cell orientation using optical tweezers were also proposed, including by Tanaka et al. (2008), Habaza et al. (2015), and Cao et al. (2017).

In addition to optical tweezers, other methods to achieve cell rotation control include microneedles (Zhuang et al., 2018), dielectrophoresis (Jiang and Mills, 2015), electromagnetic field drive methods (Kilinc and Lee, 2014), rotating stage

Robotic Cell Manipulation. https://doi.org/10.1016/B978-0-323-85259-3.00003-9

(Liu et al., 2011), hydrodynamic methods (Leung et al., 2012), and acoustic waves (Ahmed et al., 2016). The microneedling method can cause mechanical damage to cells due to direct contact. Dielectrophoresis and electromagnetic orientation can only achieve a single degree of freedom (DOF) through a rotating platform, and the cell orientation is limited by the distribution of electric and magnetic fields. Hydrodynamic and acoustic wave methods can achieve multi-DOF cell rotation control, but the manipulation procedures are complicated and it is difficult to achieve active control of cells. Table 6.1 provides a summary of existing cell rotation control methods. Given that high-precision, high-complexity, and high-flexibility cell manipulations are becoming a trend, it is of great significance to develop an autonomous system that can perform multi-DOF cell rotation control. Here, rotation in the optical plane of the microscope refers to in-plane rotation. In contrast, out-of-plane rotation refers to rotation around an axis out of the optical plane of the microscope.

Xie et al. (2016) reported the use of robotically controlled holographic optical tweezers (HOT) to automatically rotate in-plane suspended cells. A general dynamic model of motion was established, which took cell rotation into account. The T matrix method was used to characterize the relationship between the torque applied to the cell and the trapping coordinates within the cell (Nieminen et al., 2011). A vision-based controller was developed to rotate the cell in-plane. Xie et al. (2019) further studied the dynamic model of out-of-plane rotation of suspended cells using optical tweezers. Compared with the in-plane cell rotation control, the out-of-plane cell rotation control faces greater challenges when identifying and tracking the rotation angle of the cell under 2D microscopy. An image-processing algorithm was designed to determine the out-of-plane orientation angle of the cell. Based on the simplified dynamic equation

Table 6.1 Cell orientation control methods (Xie et al., 2019).

Tools	Mechanisms (principle)	Discriminating parameters	Disadvantages
Optical tweezers	Altering its trapping force and torque	Particle size and refractive index	Optical damage to laser-sensitive cells
Mechanical tools	Mechanical contact	Cell size and deformability	Mechanical damage
Electric tools	DEP force	Size and electric properties	Constrained by the electric field distribution
Magnetic tools	Magnetic gradient field	Magnetic properties of cells	Constrained by the magnetic field distribution
Hydrodynamic tools	Hydrodynamic inertial force	Cell size	Failure to have active control on cells
Acoustic waves	Axial acoustic forces	Size, density, and compressibility	Failure to have active control on cells

used to model the out-of-plane cell orientation, a visual-based robust controller was designed to perform closed-loop control of cell out-of-plane rotation. The remainder of this chapter introduces in-plane and out-of-plane cell rotation control and its applications.

6.2 Automated in-plane rotation of cells using a robot tweezers manipulation system

6.2.1 Dynamic model of single-cell rotation

The HOT cell manipulation system has been introduced in earlier chapters. The system includes three modules, namely, execution, sensory, and control modules. The execution module includes an x−y positioning platform with a resolution of 10 nm in both x and y directions, a z-axis motion stage used to adjust the height of objective lens, and an in-house assembled 3-DOF micromanipulator. The execution module includes a micropipette installed on the 3-DOF micromanipulator for cell micromanipulation and organelle extraction, a manually controlled microinjector connected to the micropipette, and the HOT device. The sensory module includes a microscope and a CCD camera mounted on the z axis. The control module consists of two motion controllers for the x−y positioning platform and the z-axis motion stage, an assembled 3-DOF micromanipulator, a liquid crystal spatial light modulator (SLM) for HOT equipment, and a host computer. All mechanical parts are supported on the antivibration table.

Two optical tweezers are used to rotate a single suspended cell to the desired direction under closed-loop control. Assuming that the cell will not be significantly deformed when subjected to the optical trapping force during rotation, the cell can be modeled as a 3D rigid body. The following describes the dynamic model of suspension cells.

6.2.1.1 A general dynamic model

When the cell of interest is selected, the sensor module of the HOT system starts tracking the cell and provides visual feedback of the position and speed of the cell to the SLM control module. Once the cell is positioned in the center of the field of view, the cell rotation control starts to process based on the visual feedback of the cell. The state variables of the trapped cell used for rotation are the rotation angle and angular velocity, which are obtained using the optical flow method (Barron et al., 1994), as shown in Fig. 6.1. During in-plane rotation, the 2D motion field and feature points of the cell are extracted by optical flow. Using the optical flow method, corner detection is performed on the previous image frame $i-1$ to calculate the feature points to be tracked. A motion field vector is formed according to the positions of these feature points in the current frame (denoted as i), and then the rotation direction (counterclockwise or clockwise) and the rotation angle θ_z around the z axis are extracted. The position vectors of the feature points relative to o, denoted by

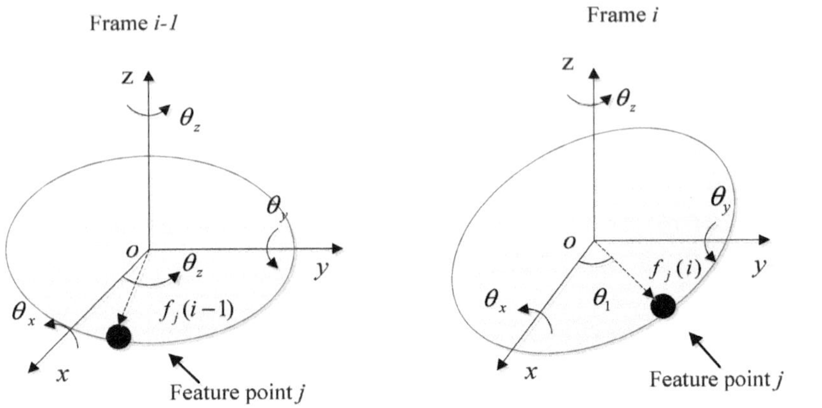

Figure 6.1 Detection of cell rotation angle along the z axis with optical flow method (Xie et al., 2016).

$f_j(i-1)$ and $f_j(i)$ in Fig. 6.1, are calculated by subtracting the coordinate o from the coordinates of each feature point in the $i-1$st frame and the ith frame, respectively, where j denotes the number of feature points. The rotation angle θ_z can then be calculated by averaging the dot product of $f_j(i-1)$ and $f_j(i)$ pair as follows:

$$\theta_z = \frac{1}{N}\sum_{j=1}^{N} \arccos \frac{f_j(i-1) \cdot f_j(i)}{\left\| f_j(i-1) \right\| \left\| f_j(i) \right\|} \tag{6.1}$$

Note that a positive result in Eq. (6.1) indicates that the trapped cell rotates in a counter-clockwise direction, and a negative result indicates rotation in a clockwise direction.

As shown in Fig. 6.2, two coordinate frames are defined to describe the motion equation of suspended cells. The first coordinate frame is fixed in space, denoted as the inertial frame $O-XYZ$. The second coordinate frame is attached to the center of mass o of the cell, which is the body frame $o\text{-}xyz$ with the three rotation angles θ_x, θ_y, and θ_z, as shown in Fig. 6.2. After using one optical trap to translate the suspended cell to the center of the field of view, two optical traps are then used to rotate the cell.

The external force and torque produced by the optical trap on any point P on the cell are expressed as F_P and M_P, respectively, and both vectors are expressed with respect to the body frame. The angular velocity of the cell relative to the inertial frame is expressed as $\omega(t)$. As shown in Fig. 6.2, the position of the center of mass of the cell (represented by o) relative to the inertial frame is presented by the vector $q(t)$, and the position vector from point o to the optical trap P relative to the inertial frame

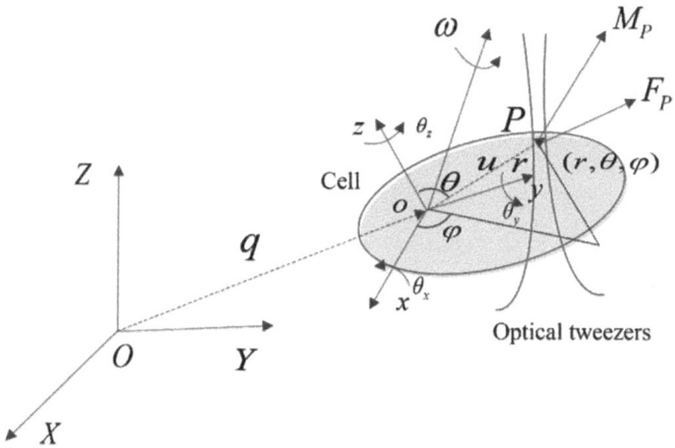

Figure 6.2 Schematic of the cell rotation with a single optical tweezers. $O - XYZ$ is the inertial frame, *o-xyz* is the body frame, and (r, θ, ϕ) denotes the spherical coordinates of optical trap *P* with respect to the body frame (Xie et al., 2016).

is denoted by $u(t)$. The position of the optical trap *P* can also be described as (r, θ, ϕ) in spherical coordinates relative to the body frame, as shown in Fig. 6.2, where r is the radial coordinate of the optical trap P, θ is the polar angle, and ϕ is the azimuth angle.

To establish the dynamic equation of motion of the cell, the force F_P and torque M_P at point *P* must be expressed relative to the inertial frame. The transforming force and torque at the center of mass of the cell are expressed as:

$$F_{CM} = R(t)F_P, \tag{6.2}$$

$$M_{CM} = R(t)M_P + u(t) \times F_{CM}, \tag{6.3}$$

where F_{CM} and F_{CM} are the transforming force and torque relative to the inertial frame, and $R(t)$ is the 3×3 rotation matrix between the two coordinate frames.

Considering the linear and rotational viscous resistance in the dynamic equation, the force and torque on the trapped cell are expressed as:

$$F_{CM} = R(t)F_P + F_d, \tag{6.4}$$

$$M_{CM} = R(t)M_P + u(t) \times F_{CM} + R(t)M_r, \tag{6.5}$$

$$F_d = -d_l\dot{q}(t), \tag{6.6}$$

$$M_r = -d_r\omega(t), \tag{6.7}$$

where F_d and M_r are the linear translational drag force and rotational viscous drag torque, respectively, $\omega(t)$ is the angular velocity of the rotated cell, and d_l and d_r are the linear and rotational viscous coefficients, respectively.

The dynamic model of the cell trapped by single optical trap takes the following form:

$$\ddot{q}(t) = \frac{F_{CM}}{m}, \tag{6.8}$$

$$\dot{\omega}(t) = I^{-1}(t)(M_{CM} - \omega(t) \times (I(t)\omega(t))), \tag{6.9}$$

where $q \in R^{1\times 2}$ is the position coordinate of the center o of the cell, m is the mass of the cell, and $I(t)$ is the 3×3 matrix of the inertial mass moment of the cell body relative to the center of mass of the inertial frame. The relationship between the inertial mass moment in the body frame and that in the inertial frame is as follows:

$$I(t) = R(t) I_{\text{body}} R(t)^T, \tag{6.10}$$

where I_{body} is a constant matrix of the inertial mass moment relative to the body frame at its center of mass, which can be calculated based on the given material and geometry of the cell.

6.2.1.2 A simplified dynamic model

Fig. 6.3 illustrates the control problem of using an optical trap to translate a cell in the x−y plane, and then using two optical traps to rotate the cell around the z axis. These two optical traps move along a circular trajectory on the x−y plane and act as dipoles to control cell rotation.

Using the T-matrix method (Nieminen et al., 2007) to model the optical tweezers, a sine function can be used to express the relationship between the applied torques M_x, M_y and the polar angle θ (with a fixed radial coordinate r and azimuth angle ϕ). The relationship between the applied torque M_z and θ is a cosine function, where r and ϕ are fixed. Here M_x, M_y, and M_z represent the torques around the x, y, and z axes, respectively. In addition, the relationship between the applied torques M_x, M_y and the azimuth angle ϕ with fixed radial coordinates r and polar angle θ are cosine and sine functions, respectively. The torque M_z has nothing to do with ϕ, where r and θ are fixed. Note that the period of $T = 2\pi$ is used by all sine and cosine functions.

According to the above analysis, when the dual optical tweezers are applied to the cell rotation control in a symmetrical position around the cell centroid in the x−y plane, the components of the force acting on the x and y axes and the component of the torque acting around the x and y axes are canceled out. The force component in the z axis is balanced by buoyancy and gravity (Hu and Sun, 2011). Therefore, only the net torque acting around the z axis acts on the suspended cell, and the trapped

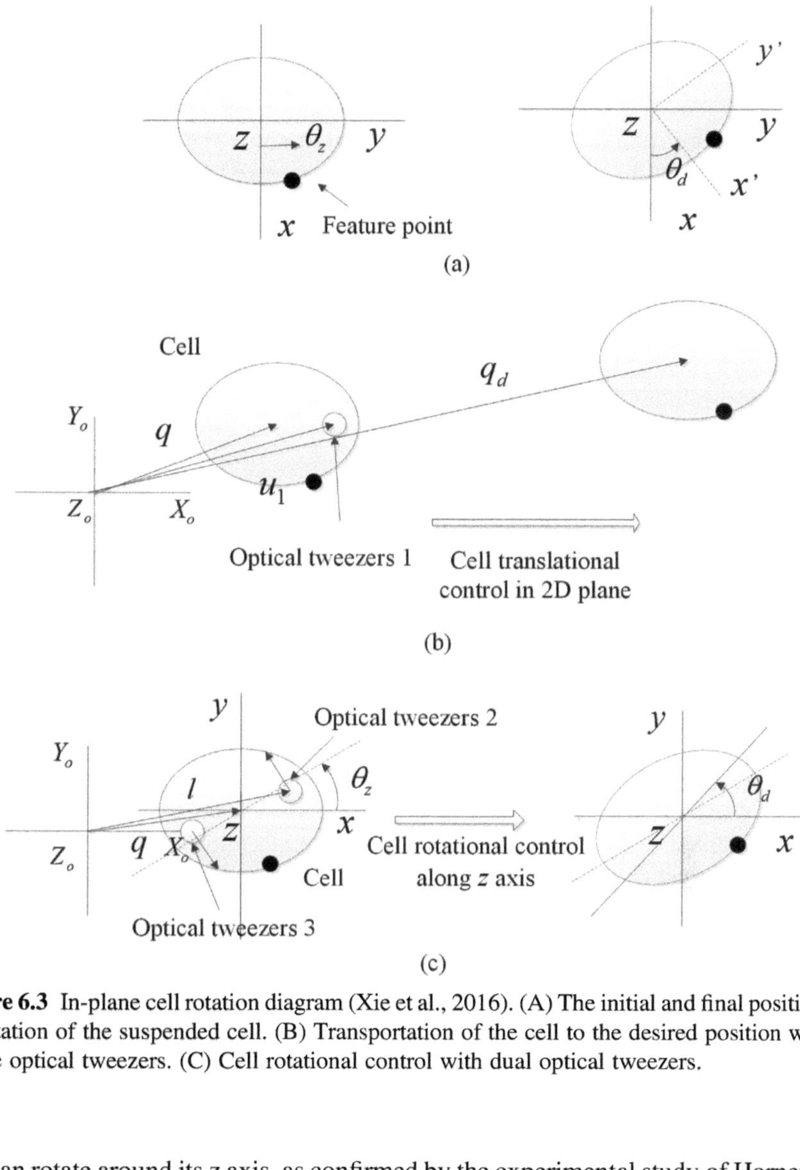

Figure 6.3 In-plane cell rotation diagram (Xie et al., 2016). (A) The initial and final position and orientation of the suspended cell. (B) Transportation of the cell to the desired position with a single optical tweezers. (C) Cell rotational control with dual optical tweezers.

cell can rotate around its z axis, as confirmed by the experimental study of Horner et al. (2010). The simplified dynamic model of the cell is expressed as follows:

$$m\ddot{q}(t) = R(t)F_P + F_d,$$

$$I(t)\ddot{\theta}_z = M_{CM} - \omega(t) \times (I(t)\omega(t)), \tag{6.11}$$

where θ_z denotes the angle of rotation of the trapped cell around the z axis.

Three remarks in this regard are given here.

Remark 1. Using a contour detection algorithm and feature extraction algorithm, the centroid o of the cell and its position coordinate can be extracted. Once the position coordinate of point o is obtained, the offset between the cell and the optical trap can be calculated according to the proposed control algorithm. The trapping point of the optical tweezers can then be determined.

Remark 2. The power provided by the optical trap to the cell is low. In the research of Banerjee et al. (2011), the process of cell rotation lasted a few seconds only, and the laser power of each optical trap was set to 1.81 mW, which was proven to be safe and effective for stable manipulation of a single cell. Therefore, the effect of thermal damage on living cells is limited. Directing the laser scissors at a certain point on the embryo zona around the cell that is not in contact with the nuclear material will provide maximum protection to the nucleus from potential laser thermal damage. The damage to cells caused by laser application must be carefully controlled, as discussed in detail by Yu et al. (2009).

Remark 3. When the dual optical tweezers are applied to a symmetrical position around the center of mass of the cell in the x−y plane, the method can also be extended to rotate the trapped cells along the y axis. The force and torque analysis is similar to analysis of the rotating the cell along the z axis, and so it is omitted here. As a result, 2-DOF rotation control of the cell can be achieved using dual optical tweezers.

It is worth noting that the cell translation and rotation controls are regarded as two separate issues, and these two tasks should be performed in a sequential manner. First, in the process of cell translation control, the cell is manipulated by a single tweezers, called tweezers 1, and the orientation of the trapped cell is not considered at this moment, as shown in Fig. 6.3B. When the cell of interest is translated to the desired position, Tweezer 1 is closed, and then two new optical tweezers (called tweezers 2 and 3) are applied to the cell and move along a circular trajectory to rotate the cell to the desired orientation, as is shown in Fig. 6.3C. The dual optical tweezers can prevent cell translation during cell rotation. Here, $I(t)$ can be approximately treated as a constant, and the dynamic model (6.11) can be further simplified as follows:

$$m\ddot{q} = F_{\text{trap}} - F_{\text{drag}} = K_t(u_1 - q) - d_l\dot{q}, \tag{6.12}$$

$$I\ddot{\theta}_z = M_{CM} = M_z - d_r\dot{\theta}_z, \tag{6.13}$$

where K_t is the trapping stiffness of the optical tweezers, u_1 is the position coordinate of optical tweezers 1, d_l and d_r are linear and rotational viscous coefficients, respectively, and M_z is the moment about the z axis from the optical tweezers 2 and 3.

For the fixed value of θ, the relationship between M_z and the optical trap spherical coordinates in the cell can be described by the following function:

$$M_z = B(r, \theta, \phi)K_r r, \tag{6.14}$$

where $B(r, \theta, \phi)$ represents the nonlinear fitting function between the torque and the optical trapping spherical coordinates, K_r is torsional stiffness of the dual optical tweezers, which depends on incident laser power and optical frequency, and r is the radial coordinate of optical tweezers.

By using the T-matrix method to model the optical tweezers and the multivariate data fitting method, the nonlinear fitting function (6.14) can be linearized near equilibrium, as shown here:

$$M_z = K_r r. \tag{6.15}$$

Eq. (6.15) indicates that for a fixed value of θ, the torque applied from the dual optical traps around the z axis has nothing to do with ϕ, and depends only on r. Considering the control problem of rotating the cell around the z axis in the x−y plane, the following equation holds:

$$r = \|l - q\|, \tag{6.16}$$

where l is the position coordinate of optical tweezers 2, as shown in Fig. 6.3C, and $\|\cdot\|$ denotes the Euclidean distance.

Similar to the linear motion equation of optical tweezers acting on suspended cells, the rotational motion equation is modeled as

$$I\ddot{\theta}_z = M_z - d_r\dot{\theta}_z = K_r r - d_r\dot{\theta}_z, \tag{6.17}$$

where d_r is the rotational viscous drag coefficient, and θ_z is the angular position of the cell, which represents the rotation angle of the cell.

Finally, the dynamic Eqs. (6.12) and (6.13) can be rewritten as:

$$m\ddot{q} = K_t(u_1 - q) - d_l\dot{q}, \tag{6.18}$$

$$I\ddot{\theta}_z = K_r r - d_r\dot{\theta}_z. \tag{6.19}$$

6.2.2 Controller design for automated cell transportation and rotation

Based on the cell dynamic model in Eqs. (6.18) and (6.19), the cell translational and rotational control problem is formulated as follows:

Consider the suspended cell of interest with the position coordinate denoted by q. Determine the control input u_1 for optical tweezers 1 to transport the cell to the desired position q^d. Once the cell arrives in the desired position, determine the control input r for optical tweezers 2 to rotate the cell around the z axis to the desired angle θ_z^d in a counterclockwise direction. During the cell rotational control process, the position of the trapped cell is fixed at q^d.

The problem described above can be divided into two subproblems. The first subproblem is the linear translation control, which is designed to transport the trapped cell to the desired position q^d. The controller is represented as:

$$u_1 = q + k_1 e + k_2 \dot{e}, \tag{6.20}$$

where u_1 is the position coordinate of optical trap 1, $e = q^d - q$ is the position error, and k_1 and k_2 are control gains.

The second subproblem is the nonlinear rotation control after the cell is translated to the desired position. As mentioned earlier, two optical traps are used to provide rotational torque. The rotation controller is proposed as follows:

$$r = k_3 \theta_e - k_4 \dot{\theta}_z, \tag{6.21}$$

where $\theta_e = \theta_z^d - \theta_z$ is the angular error when rotating around the z axis, and k_3 and k_4 are control gains.

Theorem 6.1. Consider a suspended cell with dynamic equation given by Eqs. (6.18) and (6.19). The controllers Eqs. (6.20) and (6.21) give rise to the convergence of $e \to 0$ and $\theta_e \to 0$ as $t \to \infty$.

Proof:

Substituting Eq. (6.20) into Eq. (6.19) yields:

$$m\ddot{q} = K_t\left(k_1 e + k_2 \dot{e}\right) - d_l \dot{q}. \tag{6.22}$$

Considering that q^d is a constant, $\dot{q}^d = \ddot{q}^d = 0$, and therefore, $\dot{e} = -\dot{q}$ and $\ddot{e} = -\ddot{q}$. Then, Eq. (6.22) can be rewritten as:

$$m\ddot{e} + (K_t k_2 + d_l)\dot{e} + K_t k_1 e = 0. \tag{6.23}$$

Eq. (6.23) implies that $e \to 0$ as $t \to \infty$. By appropriately choosing the control gains k_1 and k_2, the roots of Eq. (6.23) are strictly negative.

Substituting Eq. (6.21) into Eq. (6.19) yields:

$$I\ddot{\theta}_z = K_r\left(k_3 \theta_e - k_4 \dot{\theta}_z\right) - d_r \dot{\theta}_z. \tag{6.24}$$

Considering that θ_d is a constant, Eq. (6.23) can be rewritten as:

$$I\ddot{\theta}_e + (d_r + K_r k_4)\dot{\theta}_e + K_r k_3 \theta_e = 0. \tag{6.25}$$

Eq. (6.25) implies that $\theta_e \to 0$ as $t \to \infty$. By appropriately choosing the gains k_3 and k_4, the roots of Eq. (6.25) are strictly negative. Hence, the proof of *Theorem 6.1* is completed.

According to the above stability analysis and the derivation of Eqs. (6.23) and (6.25), both the position error and the angle error are affected by the second-order dynamics. Since the cell inertia is negligible in the low Reynolds (Re) number environment, first-order exponential decay is expected for both translational and rotational motions under the proposed control design.

6.2.3 Experiments

Experiments were performed to demonstrate the effectiveness of the proposed control method. In the experiment, yeast cells with buds (called feature points) were used, which can estimate the position and angle of the cells in the plane. The laser power of each optical trap was set to 1.81 mW, which was proven to be safe and effective for stable manipulation of a single cell (Banerjee et al., 2011). A CCD camera (640 × 480 pixels) was used to capture images of yeast cells under a 60X microscope. Referring to the previous calibration results (Chowdhury et al., 2014), the conversion coefficient from CCD image pixels to metric units was 0.12 μm/pixel. The trap stiffness of each trap was calibrated to 0.12 pN/(μm mW), the torsional stiffness of the two optical tweezers was calculated to be 0.6 pN/mW, and the linear and rotational viscosity coefficients were 0.08 pN s/μm and 0.5 pN μm s/rad, respectively. The control gain was set to $k_1 = 5$, $k_2 = 5$, $k_3 = 10$, and $k_4 = 10$. The sampling and update rate of the control system was set to 125 Hz, which corresponded to an 8 ms update time.

The yeast cells with feature points were selected for translation control. Fig. 6.4 illustrates the image of the cell translation process, where the desired position was set to $q^d = [370, 490]^T$ pixel. After the yeast cell was transported to the desired position by optical tweezers 1 under the controller (Eq. 6.20), the tweezers 1 were turned off, and the two new optical tweezers were turned on to rotate the cell around the z axis. Fig. 6.5 illustrates a series of images of cells in this process. The desired rotation angle was set to $\theta_z^d = 360$ degree. Fig. 6.5A shows alignment of the two new optical traps with the cell. Figs. 6.5B–D show that under the action of the controller (Eq. 6.21), the trapped cells were gradually rotated along the z axis to the desired direction. Fig. 6.6 shows the time response of angular error during cell rotation. Although the cell rotation dynamics is first-order, the response is actually approximately linear.

6.3 Automated out-of-plane rotation of cells using a robot tweezers manipulation system

The previous section introduced cell in-plane rotation control. Many practical applications require more out-of-plane rotation of cells, which represents a significant increase in single-cell manipulation capabilities. Automated out-of-plane cell orientation will

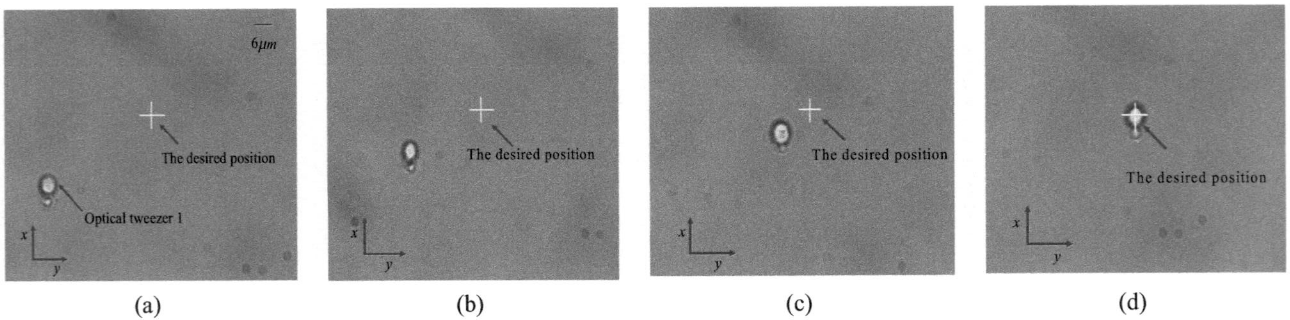

Figure 6.4 Experimental results of translating a single yeast cell with optical tweezers (Xie et al., 2016). The vertical cross represents the desired position of the translated cell. (A) A yeast cell with feature points was detected and trapped by a single optical tweezer 1. (B) Position of the cell after 1 s. (C) Position of the cell after 2.5 s. (D) Final desired position of the trapped cell.

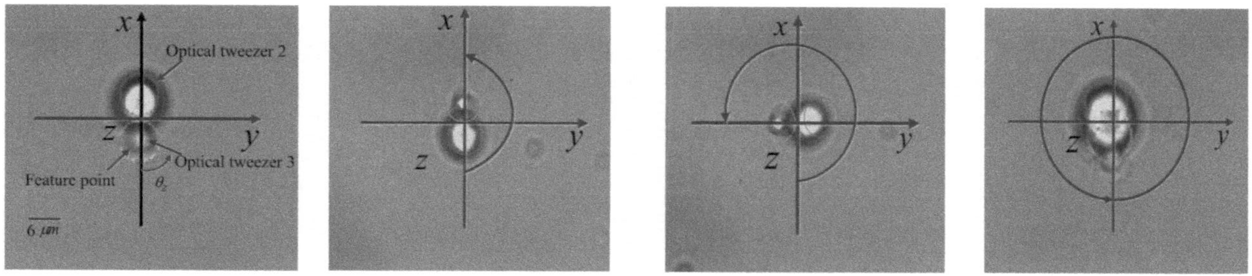

(a) (b) (c) (d)

Figure 6.5 Experiment of rotating a single yeast cell with two optical tweezers (Xie et al., 2016). The semicircular arcs with arrows indicate the positive direction of rotation. (A) The yeast cell of interest is trapped by two optical tweezers at the desired position, and the rotation angle $\theta_z = 0$. (B) Orientation of the cell after rotating the angle of $\theta_z = \pi$. (C) Orientation of the cell after rotating the angle of $\theta_z = 1.5\pi$. (D) The final orientation of the cell after rotating the angle of $\theta_z = 2\pi$.

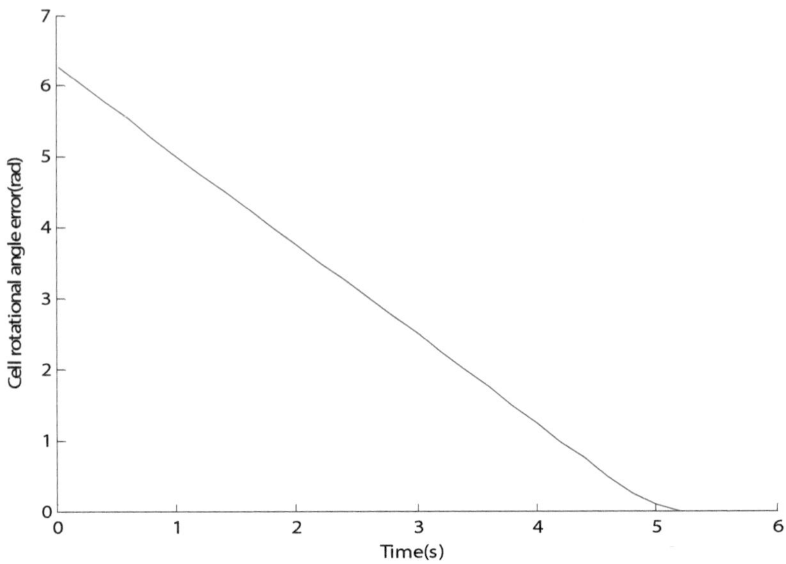

Figure 6.6 Time response of angle errors during the process of cell rotation (Xie et al., 2016).

improve cell-processing capabilities and complexity, and meet the growing requirements of multi-DOF cell orientation control in many cell therapy applications. Xie et al. (2019) reported the use of a robotic optical tweezers manipulation system to achieve automatic out-of-plane orientation control of cells. They demonstrated that multiple optical tweezers can perform stable multi-DOF cell rotation control, in which torsional stiffness can be used to characterize the mechanical properties of the optical tweezers, and the cell out-of-image plane rotation angle can be estimated based on 2D image slices obtained from optical microscopy. The following introduces an integrated framework that combines cell rotation control and cell-oriented enucleation operations, showing the necessity and importance of cell rotation control in many cell surgery operations.

6.3.1 Model

In many cell manipulation tasks, such as cell enucleation, the cells of interest should be oriented in the proper direction so that the organelles can be imaged by microscopy. Reorientation of cells allows access via micromanipulation tools and also avoids damage to other components of cells. Once the cell is correctly oriented, cell surgery can be performed. Fig. 6.7 illustrates a flowchart of a cell manipulation example, including cell orientation control and cell enucleation. To rotate the cell successfully, the sensory module of the robotic optical tweezers system tracks the target cell and provides visual feedback of the cell orientation to the control module. SLM then activates the HOT device according to the control algorithm to update the position of the optical trap. The vision-processing algorithm is developed to estimate the out-of-plane orientation

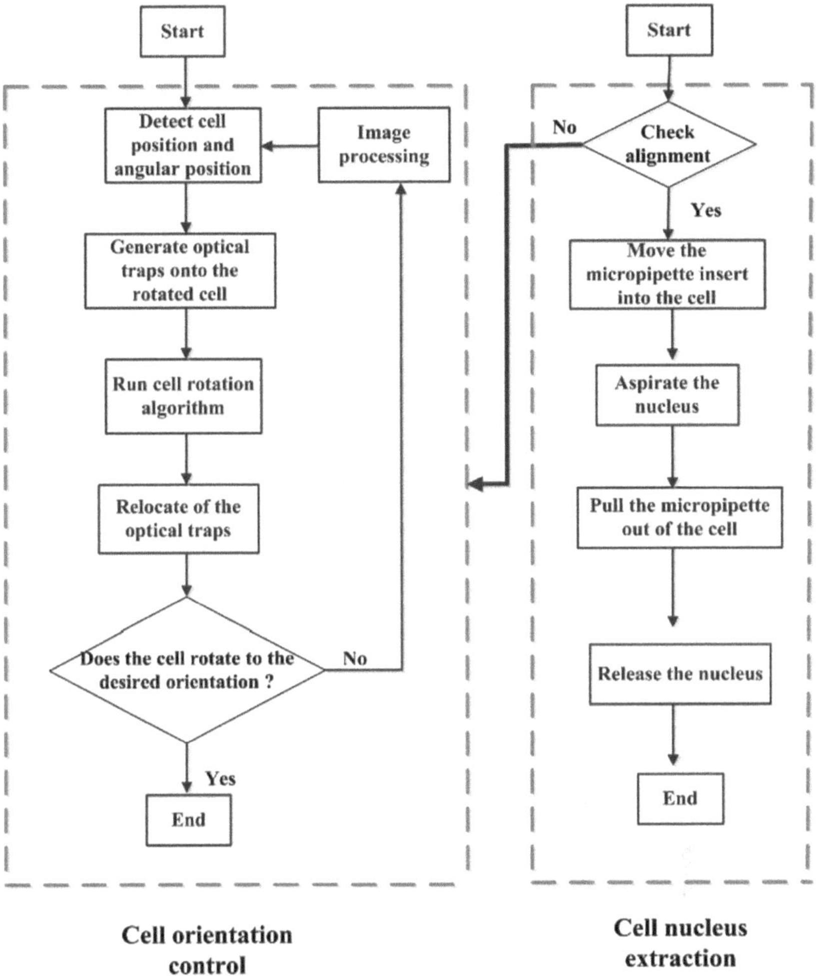

Figure 6.7 Flowchart of cell out-of-plane rotational control and cell enucleation (Xie et al., 2019).

angle of the cell. The state variables required for cell orientation control include rotation angle and corresponding angular velocity. After rotating the cell to the proper direction, cell enucleation can be performed. Only when the nucleus is aligned with the tip of the pipette can the cell be properly denucleated. Subsequent procedures include inserting the micropipette into the cell, aspirating the nucleus, removing the micropipette from the cell, and releasing the nucleus extracted from the micropipette. Stained nuclei can be identified by fluorescence microscopy.

To design an automated framework for the cell out-of-plane rotation control, a dynamic model of suspended cells under the action of optical tweezers is developed first. Similar to the method of simulating in-plane rotation of cells (Xie et al. 2016), the suspended cells rotating out of plane are assumed to be rigid bodies in 3D space. This assumption is based on the fact that the cell of interest will not be significantly deformed during the rotation under the action of the applied optical traps.

Fig. 6.8 schematically shows the optical trapping force and torque applied to the cell. As detailed in the previous section, two coordinate frames are defined to model the dynamic equation of the trapped cell. As shown in Fig. 6.8, the inertial coordinate frame *O-XYZ* is defined and fixed in inertial space, and the body coordinate frame *o-xyz* whose origin is at the center of mass *o* of the cell is introduced. The trapping force and torque applied to the suspended cells in the body coordinate frame are denoted as F and T, respectively. The position coordinates of the cell and the optical trap and the angular velocity of the cell are represented by q, u, and $\omega(t)$, respectively, which are all described relative to the inertial coordinate system. Relative to the spherical coordinates, the position coordinates of the applied optical trap can also be described as shown in Fig. 6.8.

Based on the general dynamic equation of planner motion of the trapped cell in Eqs. (6.2)–(6.10), the general dynamic equation of out-of-plane rotation can be described as

$$\ddot{\theta}(t) = I^{-1}(t)\left(T_{CM} - \dot{\theta}(t) \times \left(I(t)\dot{\theta}(t)\right)\right), \tag{6.26}$$

$$T_{CM} = R(t)T + u(t) \times F_{CM} + R(t)T_r, \tag{6.27}$$

where $\theta = [\theta_x \quad \theta_y \quad \theta_z]^T$ is the angle that the cell rotates out of the image plane, T_{CM} represents the torque relative to the inertial frame, T is torque acting about the x-y plane

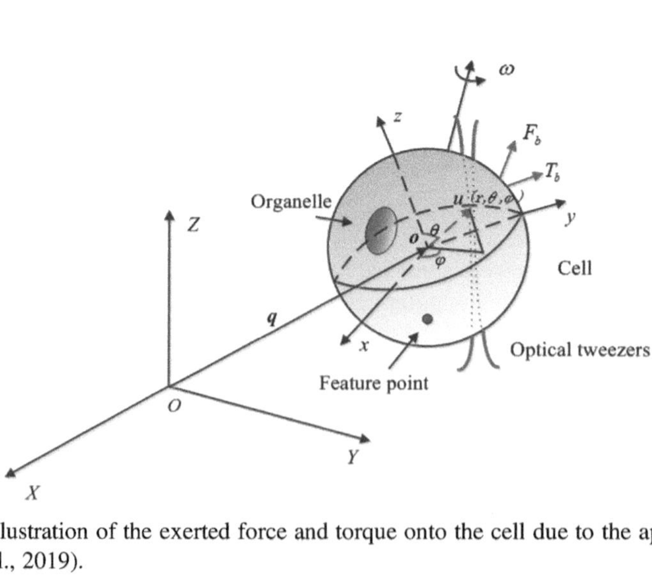

Figure 6.8 Illustration of the exerted force and torque onto the cell due to the applied optical trap (Xie et al., 2019).

from the two optical traps, $R(t) \in R^{3\times3}$ is the rotation matrix between the two coordinate frames, T_r denotes the rotational viscous drag torque, and $\dot{\theta}(t) = \omega(t)$. Note that the suspended cell buoyancy forces are ignored.

The optical trapping force and torque that allow cells to be manipulated and rotated originate from the laser tweezers transferring the linear and angular momentum of light to the particles, which causes the particle momentum to change due to light scattering. Therefore, the calculation of optical trapping force and torque can be regarded as the calculation of light scattering (Nieminen et al., 2007). As mentioned in the previous section, the T-matrix method provides a mechanism to model light scattering. After laser scattering is calculated once, it can be used repeatedly to calculate the trapping force and torque (Nieminen et al., 2007). Based on the optical tweezers computational toolbox developed in MATLAB, the relationship between the applied force F $[F_x\ F_y\ F_z]^T$, torque $T\ [T_x\ T_y\ T_z]^T$, and the spherical coordinates (r, θ, ϕ) of the optical trap within the cell have been calibrated in the previous section (Xie et al., 2016).

Here, two optical traps are used to rotate the cell out of the image plane. Two optical traps that are originally located in the x-y plane of the cell and symmetrical about the center o of the cell are applied to rotate the suspended cell by changing the Z-axis coordinate of the two optical traps, where x and y coordinates the cell are fixed, as shown in Fig. 6.9. When two optical traps are applied at a symmetrical position outside the x-y plane around the cell center o, the optical trapping force and torque are cancelled out. Therefore, by changing the Z-axis coordinates of the two optical traps in opposite directions simultaneously while fixing the x- and y-axis coordinates of the cell, a rotational torque is generated along the x-y plane, so the cell can rotate out of the image plane about the x-y plane. Fig. 6.9 shows a schematic diagram of the cell out-of-plane rotation. The rotation axis in the x-y plane is perpendicular to the line where the optical trap plane intersects the x-y plane, as shown in Fig. 6.9C. The dynamic equation of cell out-of-plane rotation can be expressed as follows:

$$I\ddot{\theta} = T - d_r\dot{\theta}. \tag{6.28}$$

where d_r has been early defined as rotational viscous coefficient.

The applied torque T can be derived from the two optical traps as follows. Suppose that the position coordinates of the two optical tweezers (denoted as OT_1 and OT_2) are $[x_1, y_1, z_1]^T$ and $[-x_1, -y_1, -z_1]^T$, respectively. The position coordinate of OT_1 can also be expressed as (r_1, θ_1, ϕ_1) with respect to the spherical coordinate. When the two optical traps move synchronously along the z axis to the new position $[x_1, y_1, z_1 + \Delta Z]^T$ and $[-x_1, -y_1, -(z_1 + \Delta Z)]^T$, respectively, the torque applied from the optical trap can be calculated as follows

$$\|T\| = 2\|\Delta Z \times F_{\text{trap}}\| = 2\|\Delta Z\|\|F_{\text{trap}}\|\sin\theta_1 = 2\|\Delta Z\|kr_1\sin\theta_1 = 2k\rho\|\Delta Z\|. \tag{6.29}$$

where $\|\cdot\|$ denotes the Euclidean norm of a vector, k is the trapping stiffness, and $\rho = \sqrt{x_1^2 + y_1^2}$ is fixed.

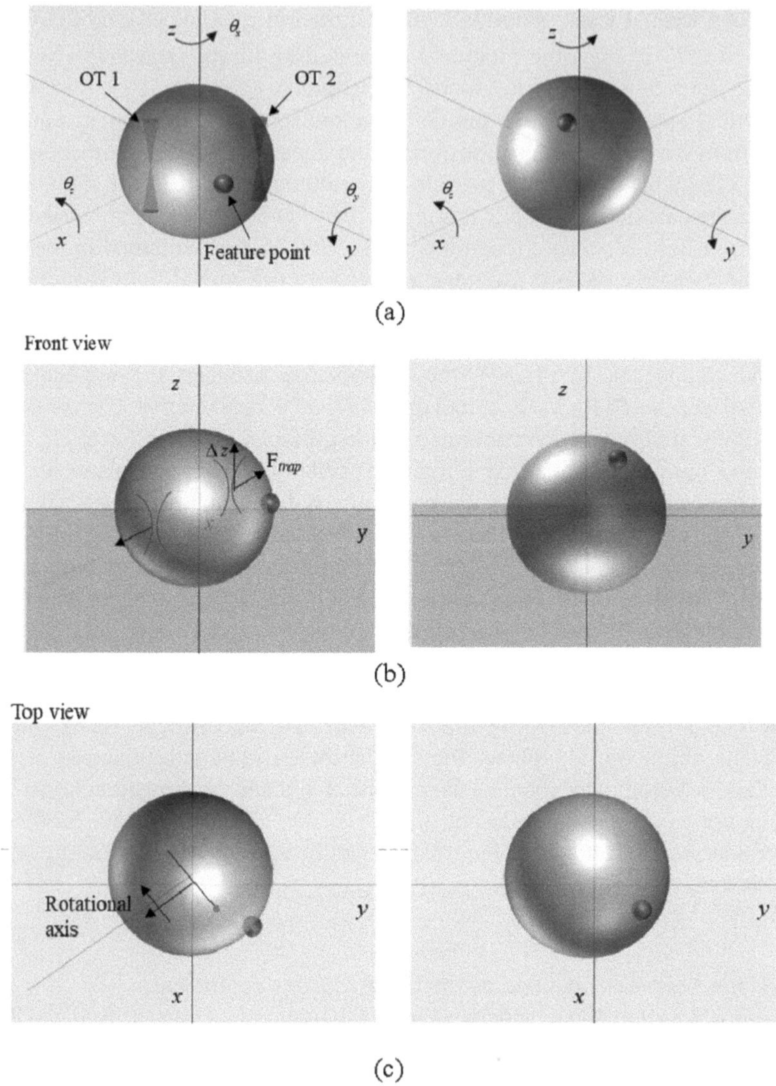

Figure 6.9 Schematic diagram of cell out-of-plane rotation under the action of two optical traps. (A) The cell can be rotated out of the image plane by adjusting the relative vertical height of the two optical traps in the z-axis direction. (B) The front view of cell rotation, and the cell arrives at a new orientation after the cell rotating an angle θ_1. (C) The top view of cell rotation.

Torsional stiffness can be used to describe the mechanical properties of optical tweezers during the rotation of cells, expressed as

$$T = K_r \tau, \tag{6.30}$$

where K_r is defined as the torsional stiffness about the x−y plane of the dual optical traps, and $\tau = 2||\Delta Z||$ is the relative vertical height of the two optical traps along the z axis and is regarded as the control input. Note that K_r can be determined through calibration, as reported by Wu et al. (2011).

Therefore, the dynamic model Eq. (6.28) can be rewritten as

$$I\ddot{\theta} + d_r\dot{\theta} = K\tau, \tag{6.31}$$

and the dynamic model of cell out-of-plane rotation (6.31) can be written as

$$I\ddot{\theta} + d_r\dot{\theta} = Y\left(\dot{\theta}, \ddot{\theta}\right)\delta, \tag{6.32}$$

where $Y\left(\dot{\theta}, \ddot{\theta}\right) \in \Re^{2\times n_1}$ is a dynamic parameter regressor matrix, $\delta = [\delta_1, ...\delta_{n_1}]^T$ denotes a set of physical parameters, and n_I represents the number of unknown physical parameters.

6.3.2 Cell out-of-plane rotational control

To develop a feedback controller for cell out-of-plane rotation control, the orientation angle of the cell must be obtained using a vision extraction algorithm. In this section, an image-processing algorithm is presented to calculate the orientation angle of suspended cells outside the x−y plane, and a robust feedback controller is then introduced to stabilize the cell rotation control system.

6.3.2.1 Image-processing algorithm

To obtain the orientation angle of the target cell, a geometric model can be used to estimate the orientation of the cell outside the image plane based on 2D image slices obtained from the optical microscope. Fig. 6.10 shows the method of using the position coordinates of the feature points on the x−y plane to estimate the position coordinates along the z axis. Consider biological cells as a sphere with a radius of r_c, which can be obtained from a 2D microscopy image. The position coordinate of the feature point on the z axis is derived as:

$$z = \sqrt{R^2 - (x^2 + y^2)}. \tag{6.33}$$

When the cell rotates outside the x−y plane, the feature point captured by microscopy in the 2D slice moves from point P_1 to point P_2 in a different optical focal plane,

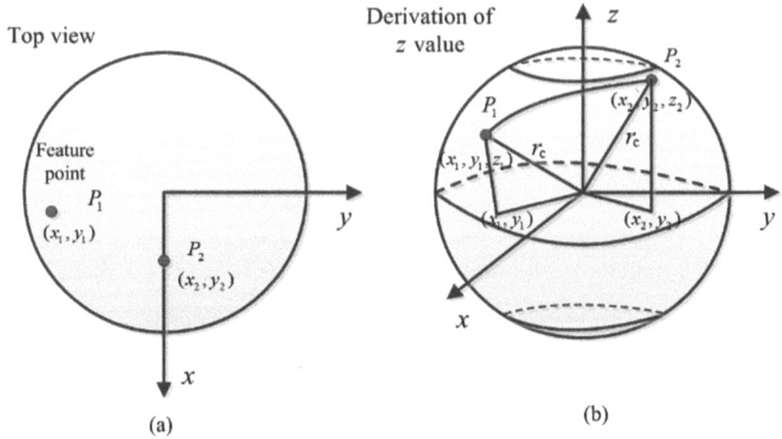

Figure 6.10 Geometrical model to estimate cell orientation angle by tracking the position coordinates of the feature point within the cell (Xie et al., 2019). (A) Two-dimensional image acquired from CCD camera; (B) derivation of the z-coordinate value of the feature point.

as shown in Fig. 6.10A. The rotation angle θ can be calculated by using the position coordinates of P_1 (x_1, y_1, z_1) and P_2 (x_2, y_2, z_2), expressed as

$$\theta = \frac{\pi}{180} \arccos\left(\frac{P_1 \cdot P_2}{|P_1||P_2|}\right). \tag{6.34}$$

The angular velocity of the cell is $\omega = \theta r_c / t_s$, where t_s is the sampling interval.

Fig. 6.11 shows the procedure of image processing for detecting cell centroid and its characteristic points from images taken by fluorescence microscopy. Fig. 6.11A shows the original image. It is converted into a binary image, as shown in Fig. 6.11B. Then morphological closing operation is performed to remove small particles and noise in the binary image, as shown in Fig. 6.11C, which is followed by a morphological filling operation to identify the feature points marked with dark speckles, as shown in Fig. 6.11D. The contour detection algorithm is further applied to obtain the contours of the pixels and feature points, where circular curves are used to fit the contours of the pixels and feature points respectively. As shown in Fig. 6.11E, the geometric centers of the fitted circles are regarded as the centers of the cell and the feature point, denoted as o, and o_n, respectively.

The imaging accuracy is affected by the recognition of feature points with a low-contrast brightfield microscope and the deletion of those irrelevant points retaining the features of interest. The binary image of the original image can be obtained based on the accurate threshold of the feature points, and the threshold can be obtained using the calibrated pixel values of the feature points. The matching template can also be used to obtain the desired feature points. Using the above method, the accuracy of the imaging system can reach 0.05 *rad* in cell orientation control (Xie et al., 2019).

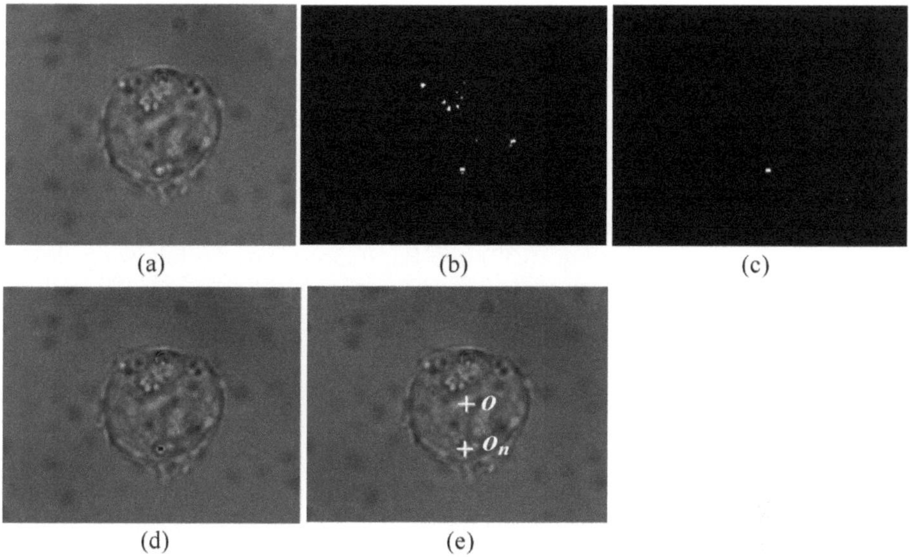

Figure 6.11 Visual extraction of feature point (Xie et al., 2019). (A) Original image. (B) Binary image. (C) Morphological close operation to remove noise and small particles. (D) Morphology filling operation. (E) Detected cell center and its feature point center.

6.3.2.2 Controller design

Introduce a sliding mode variable S_θ as follows:

$$S_\theta = \dot{\theta} - \dot{\theta}_r = \dot{\theta} - \left(\dot{\theta}^d - \Lambda\widetilde{\theta}\right) = \dot{\widetilde{\theta}} + \Lambda\widetilde{\theta}, \tag{6.35}$$

where θ^d denotes the desired rotation angle, $\widetilde{\theta} = \theta - \theta^d$ is the angular error, $\dot{\theta}_r = \dot{\theta}^d - \Lambda\widetilde{\theta}$ is a reference vector, and Λ is a positive constant.

Utilizing the sliding variable S_θ, the dynamics Eq. (6.31) can be rewritten as:

$$I\dot{S}_\theta + d_r S_\theta = K\tau - I\ddot{\theta}_r - d_r\dot{\theta}_r = K\tau - Y\left(\dot{\theta}_r, \ddot{\theta}_r\right)\delta. \tag{6.36}$$

An adaptive controller is then designed as:

$$\tau = K^{-1}\left(Y\left(\dot{\theta}_r, \ddot{\theta}_r\right)\widehat{\delta} - K_d S_\theta\right), \tag{6.37}$$

where $\widehat{\delta}$ is the estimated value of the parameter δ, and K_d is a positive control gain. The estimated parameter $\widehat{\delta}$ is updated by the following update law:

$$\dot{\widehat{\delta}} = -\Gamma Y^T\left(\dot{\theta}_r, \ddot{\theta}_r\right)S_\theta, \tag{6.38}$$

where Γ is a positive definite gain matrix.

Substituting the controller Eq. (6.37) into Eq. (6.36) yields the following closed-loop dynamics:

$$I\dot{S}_\theta + (d_r + K_D)S_\theta + Y\left(\dot{\theta}_r, \ddot{\theta}_r\right)\widetilde{\delta} = 0, \tag{6.39}$$

where $\widetilde{\delta} = \delta - \widehat{\delta}$ is the estimated error of the parameter δ.

Using the controller Eq. (6.37) and Eqs. (6.29) and (6.30), the z-axis coordinate value of OT_1 at the fixed point (x_1, y_1), denoted as z_1, can be calculated. Based on the fact that the two optical traps are symmetrical about the cell center o, the position coordinate of OT2 can be further calculated as $[-x_1, -y_1, -z_1]^T$.

To prove the stability of the closed-loop system Eq. (6.39), define a Lyapunov-like function candidate as:

$$V = \frac{1}{2}S_\theta^T I S_\theta + \frac{1}{2}\widetilde{\delta}^T \Gamma^{-1}\widetilde{\delta}. \tag{6.40}$$

Differentiating V with respect to time yields:

$$\dot{V} = S_\theta^T I \dot{S}_\theta + \widetilde{\delta}^T \Gamma^{-1}\dot{\widetilde{\delta}}. \tag{6.41}$$

Considering $\dot{\widetilde{\delta}} = -\dot{\widehat{\delta}}$ and further combining with Eq. (6.38), Eq. (6.41) can be rewritten as follows:

$$\begin{aligned}\dot{V} &= -S_\theta^T(d_r + K_D)S_\theta - S_\theta^T Y\left(\dot{\theta}_r, \ddot{\theta}_r\right)\widetilde{\delta} + \widetilde{\delta}^T Y^T\left(\dot{\theta}_r, \ddot{\theta}_r\right)S_\theta \\ &= -\,S_\theta^T(d_r + K_D)S_\theta \leq 0.\end{aligned} \tag{6.42}$$

Therefore, both S_θ and $\widetilde{\delta}$ are bounded. According to Eq. (6.35), the angular error $\widetilde{\theta}$ can be regarded as the output of a first-order linear system with a transfer function $1/(S + \Lambda)$ and input S_θ, so $\widetilde{\theta}$ is also bounded. The boundedness of S_θ and $\widetilde{\theta}$ guarantees the boundedness of $\dot{\widetilde{\theta}}$ according to Eq. (6.35). In practical applications, the term

$Y(\dot{\theta}_r, \ddot{\theta}_r)\widetilde{\delta}$ in Eq. (6.39) is bounded and therefore $\dot{S}_\theta$ is also bounded. As a result, S_θ is uniformly continuous. Finally, according to Barbalat's lemma, $S_\theta \to 0$ and $\widetilde{\theta} \to 0$ as time $t \to \infty$.

6.3.3 Experiments

Experiments were performed to demonstrate the effectiveness of the cell out-of-plane rotation control method. Human acute promyelocytic leukemia cells (NB4) with an average radius of 10 μm were selected in experiments. The laser power of each optical trap was set to 1.5 mW. The size of each pixel on the CCD camera was 0.12 μm under 60× magnification. The resolution of the CCD camera was 640 × 480 pixels. Based on the previous calibration results of Wu et al. (2011), the torsional stiffness was set to $K = 1.08 \times 10^{-6} N$ in experiments. The initial system parameter was set to $\delta_0 = \left[2 \times 10^{-22} \quad 3 \times 10^{-15}\right]^T$, the parameter of the update law was $\Gamma = \text{diag}\{10, 10\}$, and the control gains were chosen as $K_d = 10$ and $\Lambda = 10$. The sampling time of the control system was $T = 10$ ms. Note that the control gains were selected using the trial-and-error method under two principles. The first principle was that the weight of the differential item in Eqs. (6.37) and (6.35) should not be too large. This is because a larger differential term will cause a larger overshoot, leading to instability of the closed-loop system (Eq. 6.39). The second principle was that the control gains were chosen to obtain a proper convergence speed of cell rotation.

In the first experiment, two optical traps were used to rotate the cell clockwise out of the plane. Using the image-processing scheme to track the orientation angle of the cell, the feature point in the cell can be identified. The two optical traps were initially applied symmetrically on the x−y plane of the cell. By adjusting the z-axis coordinate of the two optical traps in two directions, the cell was rotated out of plane. The desired rotation angle was set to $\theta_d = 30$ degree. Fig. 6.12 shows the orientation of the cell at different times under the action of the controller (Eq. 6.37) and the adaptation law (Eq. 6.38). As shown in Fig. 6.12A, two optical traps represented by OT1 and OT2 were applied on the NB4 cell. Fig. 6.12B−C show that by changing the relative vertical height of the two optical traps, the cell was gradually rotated out of the image plane. Since the feature point that was initially not in the image plane was gradually rotated into the image plane as the rotation progressed, it can be seen more clearly. Fig. 6.13 illustrates the angular error response, showing that the cell was rotated out of plane successfully to its desired direction.

In the second experiment, a polystyrene bead coated with streptavidin was attached to NB4 cells so that the rotation effect could be seen more clearly. The attached bead was regarded as a feature point for calculating the angular position of the rotating cell. Two optical traps were used to rotate the cell out of plane in a counterclockwise direction. The desired rotation angle was set to $\theta^d = -30$ degree. Figs. 6.14 and 6.15, respectively, show the image and the rotation angle error of the cell rotation. At the start, part of the attached bead was shown in the image plane, as seen in

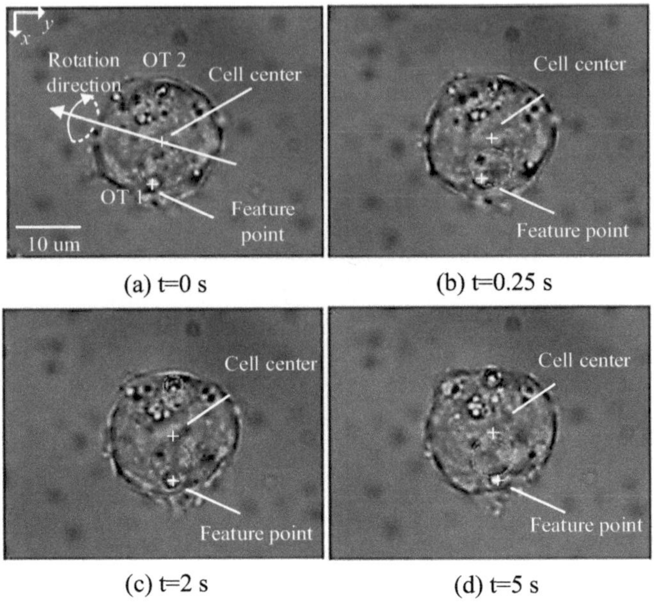

Figure 6.12 Results of the first experiment. The cell is rotated out of the image plane in a clockwise direction utilizing two controlled optical traps (Xie et al., 2019). (A) Initial orientation of the NB4 cell $\theta_d = 0$ degree. (B) New cell orientation after rotating $\theta_d = 10$ degrees. (C) Cell orientation at $\theta_d = 25$ degrees. (D) Final cell orientation at $\theta_d = 30$ degrees.

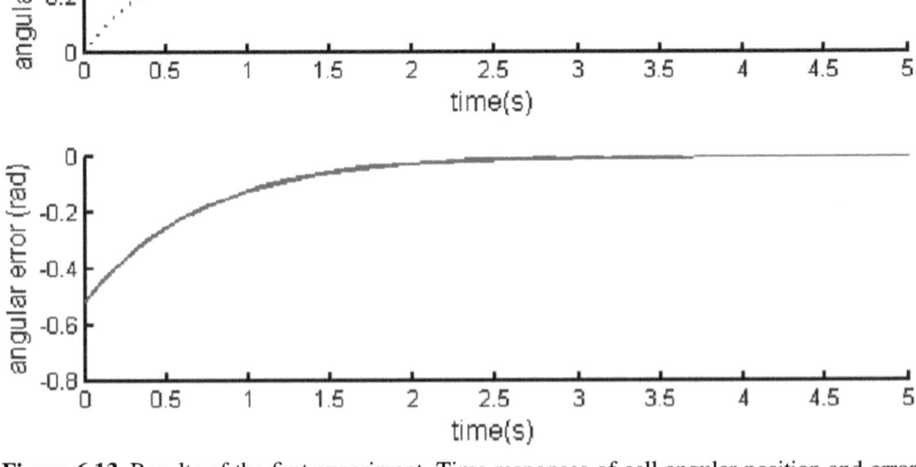

Figure 6.13 Results of the first experiment. Time responses of cell angular position and error (Xie et al., 2019).

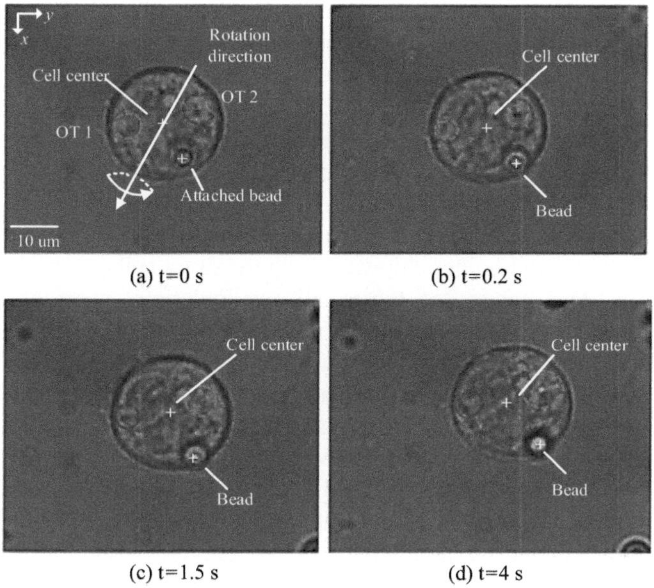

Figure 6.14 Results of the second experiment. The cell was rotated out of image plane in a counterclockwise direction (Xie et al., 2019). (A) Initial orientation of the NB4 cell $\theta^d = -30$ degrees. (B) New cell orientation after rotating $\theta^d = -25$ degrees. (C) Cell orientation at $\theta^d = -5$ degrees. (D) Final cell orientation at $\theta^d = 0$ degree.

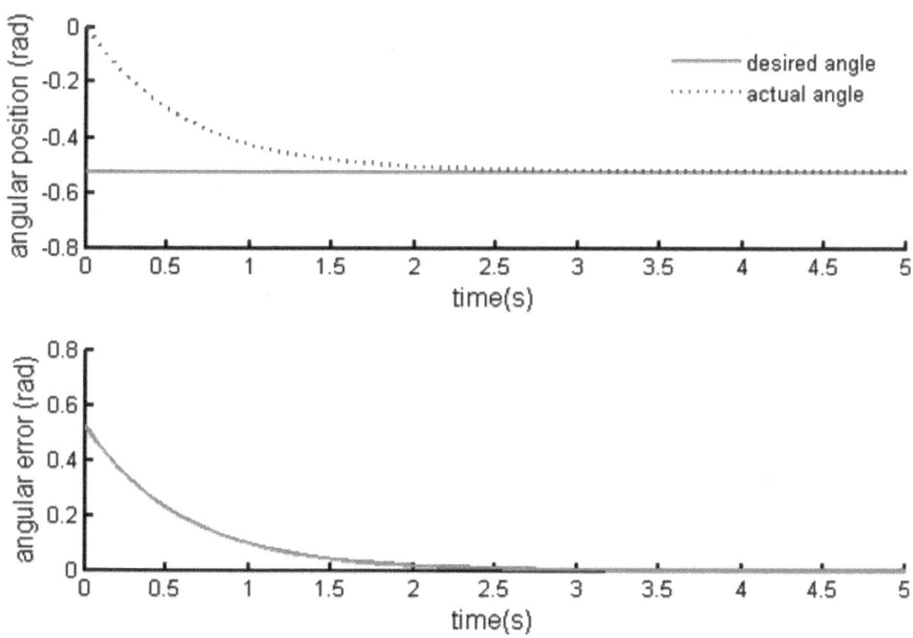

Figure 6.15 Results of the second experiment: time responses of cell angular position and error, respectively, when the cell was rotated out of the image plane in a counterclockwise direction (Xie et al., 2019).

Fig. 6.14A. Under the action of the controller (Eq. 6.37), the bead gradually rotated into the image plane and can be seen more clearly, as shown in Fig. 6.14B–D. Fig. 6.15 illustrates the convergence of the angular error to zero.

In the third experiment, a case study of cell nucleus extraction was performed after cell rotation. The cell must be rotated to the preferred direction before extracting the nucleus. As mentioned earlier, once the cell nucleus is in the image plane, close to and aligned with the pipette tip, the cell is considered to be in the ideal orientation, as this can avoid damage to irrelevant components and is easy to penetrate and aspirate. The microfluidic cell holder chip was designed to fix cells when performing nuclear extraction. The images of these cell manipulations were observed under fluorescence microscopy, as shown in Fig. 6.16. Fig. 6.16A shows the initial orientation of the cell, indicating that the stained nucleus of the cell was not in the image plane or aligned with the sharp tip of the micropipette. Then, the cell was rotated into the image plane and moved out of the image plane in turn, so that the nucleus was located in the image plane and aligned with the tip of the micropipette, as shown in Fig. 6.16B. After that, the reoriented cell was translated to the channel of the microfluidic chip using two optical traps operating in the translation mode, and the cell was well trapped in the microfluidic channel by applying negative pressure using a syringe pump. Fig. 6.16C illustrates the process of trapping the cell in the channel and penetrating

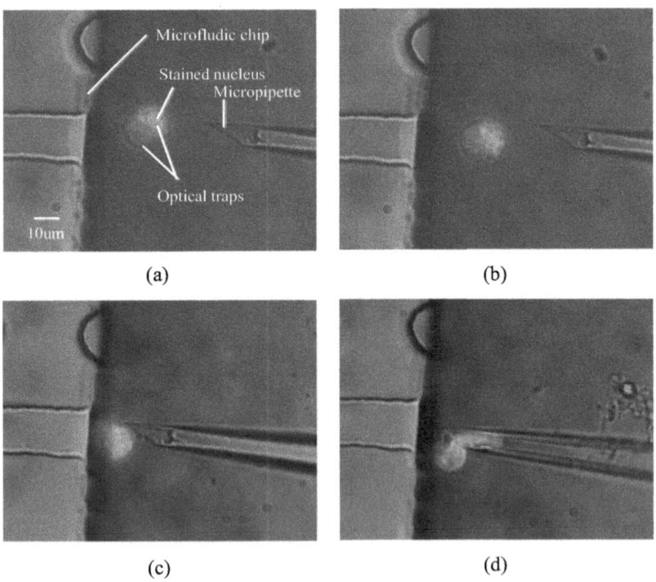

Figure 6.16 Results of the third experiment. Snapshots of cell rotation and nucleus extraction observed under fluorescence microscopy (Xie et al., 2019). (A) Initial position and orientation of the cell of interest. (B) New orientation of the cell after in-plane and out-of-plane rotation controls. (C) Translating the cell to the microfluidic cell holder channel, and then penetrating the micropipette into the cell. (D) Aspirating the nuclear into the pipette using microinjector.

the cell with the micropipette. Fig. 6.16D shows aspirating part of the cell nuclei into the micropipette using a microinjector. By rotating the microinjector clockwise, the aspirated nucleus can be released.

6.4 Conclusions

This chapter introduces the control of cell rotation using robotic optical tweezers-based manipulation. First, the dynamics and control of in-plane cell rotation around an axis are presented. After establishing the general dynamic equation of suspended cells in rotation, the controller is developed to realize the one-DOF in-plane rotation control of the suspended cell. The position control of the cells is also considered for cell translation before rotation. Second, an automated control scheme for out-of-plane cell rotation is introduced. After establishing a dynamic model of the cell in out-of-plane rotation and developing an image-processing algorithm to estimate the orientation of the cell out of the image plane, a vision-based adaptive controller is introduced to achieve closed-loop rotation control. Experiments are performed to illustrate the performance of in-plane and out-of-plane cell rotation control methods. Cell rotation control represents the advancement of single-cell manipulation and has the potential to contribute to many cell-oriented therapeutic applications, such as nuclear biopsy and transplantation, cloning technology, and PGD.

References

Ahmed, D., Ozcelik, A., Bojanala, N., Nama, N., Upadhyay, A., Chen, Y., Hanna-Rose, W., Huang, T.J., 2016. Rotational manipulation of single cells and organisms using acoustic waves. Nat. Commun. 7, 11085.

Ando, J., Bautista, G., Smith, N., Fujita, K., Daria, V.R., 2008. Optical trapping and surgery of living yeast cells using a single laser. Rev. Sci. Instrum. 79, 103705.

Ashkin, A., Dziedzic, J.M., Yamane, T., 1987. Optical trapping and manipulation of single cells using infrared laser beams. Nature 330, 769−771.

Banerjee, A.G., Chowdhury, S., Losert, W., Gupta, S.K., 2011. Survey on indirect optical manipulation of cells, nucleic acids, and motor proteins. J. Biomed. Opt. 16 (5), 051302.

Barron, J.L., Fleet, D.J., Beauchemin, S.S., 1994. Performance of optical flow techniques. Int. J. Comput. Vis. 12, 43−77.

Bingelyte, V., Leach, J., Courtial, J., Padgett, M.J., 2003. Optically controlled three-dimensional rotation of microscopic objects. Appl. Phys. Lett. 82, 829−831.

Braude, P., Pickering, S., Flinter, F., Ogilvie, C.M., 2002. Preimplantation genetic diagnosis. Nat. Rev. Genet. 3, 941−955.

Cao, B., Kelbauskas, L., Chan, S., Shetty, R.M., Smith, D., Meldrum, D., 2017. Rotation of single live mammalian cells using dynamic holographic optical tweezers. Opt. Laser. Eng. 92, 70−75.

Carmon, G., Feingold, M., 2011. Rotation of single bacterial cells relative to the optical axis using optical tweezers. Opt. Lett. 36, 40−42.

Chowdhury, S., Thakur, A., Svec, P., Wang, C., Losert, W., Gupta, S.K., 2014. Automated manipulation of biological cells using gripper formations controlled by optical tweezers. IEEE Trans. Autom. Sci. Eng. 11 (2), 338–347.

Galajda, P., Ormos, P., 2003. Orientation of flat particles in optical tweezers by linearly polarized light. Opt. Expr. 11, 446–451.

Habaza, M., Gilboa, B., Roichman, Y., Shaked, N.T., 2015. Tomographic phase microscopy with 180 rotation of live cells in suspension by holographic optical tweezers. Opt. Lett. 40, 1881–1884.

Horner, F., Woerdemann, M., Muller, S., Maier, B., Denz, C., 2010. Full 3D translational and rotational optical control of multiple rod-shaped bacteria. J. Biophot. 3, 468–475.

Hu, S., Sun, D., 2011. Automatic transportation of biological cells with robot-tweezers manipulation system. Int. J. Robot. Res. 30 (14), 1681–1694.

Huang, H., Sun, D., Mills, J.K., Cheng, S.H., 2009. Robotics cell injection system with position and force control: towards automatic batch biomanipulation. IEEE Trans. Robot. 25 (3), 727–737.

Jiang, C., Mills, J.K., 2015. Planar cell orientation control system using a rotating electric field. IEEE/ASME Trans. Mech. 20, 2350–2358.

Kilinc, D., Lee, G.U., 2014. Advances in magnetic tweezers for single molecule and cell biophysics. Integr. Biol. 6, 27–34.

Kim, M.J., Breuer, K.S., 2007. Controlled mixing in microfluidic systems using bacterial chemotaxis. Anal. Chem. 79 (3), 955–959.

Lee, M., Vasioukhin, V., 2008. Cell polarity and cancer-cell and tissue polarity as a non-canonical tumor suppressor. J. Cell Sci. 121, 1141–1150.

Leung, C., Lu, Z., Zhang, X.P., Sun, Y., 2012. Three-dimensional rotation of mouse embryos. IEEE Trans. Biomed. Eng. 59 (4), 1049–1056.

Lin, G., Quyang, Q., Zhou, X., Gu, Y., Yuan, D., Li, W., Liu, G., Liu, T., Lu, G., 2007. A highly homozygous and parthenogenetic human embryonic stem cell line derived from a one-pronuclear oocyte following in vitro fertilization procedure. Cell Res. 17, 999–1007.

Liu, X., Lu, Z., Sun, Y., 2011. Orientation control of biological cells under inverted microscopy. IEEE/ASME Trans. Mech. 16, 918–924.

Luo, Z.P., Sun, Y.L., An, K.N., 2000. An optical spin micrometer. Appl. Phys. Lett. 76, 1779–1781.

Min, T.L., Maers, P.J., Chubiz, L.M., Rao, C.V., Golding, I., Chemla, Y.R., 2009. High-resolution, long-term characterization of bacterial motility using optical tweezers. Nat. Methods 6, 831–835.

Nieminen, T.A., Loke, V.L.Y., Stilgoe, A.B., Knoner, G., Branczyk, A.M., Heckenbera, N.R., Rubinsztein-Dunlop, H., 2007. Optical tweezers computational toolbox. J. Opt. Pure Appl. Opt. 9, 196–203.

Nieminen, T.A., Loke, V.L.Y., Stilgoe, A.B., Heckenbera, N.R., Rubinsztein-Dunlop, H., 2011. T-matrix method for modelling optical tweezers. J. Mod. Opt. 58, 528–544.

Reffay, M., Petitiean, L., Coscoy, S., Grasland, E., Amblard, F., Buguin, A., Silberzan, P., 2011. Orientation and polarity in collectively migrating cell structures: statics and dynamics. Biophys. J. 100, 2566–2575.

Shelby, J.P., Edgar, J.S., Chiu, D.T., 2005. Monitoring cell survival after extraction of a single subcellular organelle using optical trapping and pulsed-nitrogen laser ablation. Photochem. Photobiol. 81, 994–1001.

Tanaka, Y., Kawada, H., Hirano, K., Ishikawa, M., Kitajima, H., 2008. Automated manipulation of non-spherical micro-objects using optical tweezers combined with image processing techniques. Opt. Expr. 16, 15115–15122.

Wu, Y., Sun, D., Huang, W., 2011. Mechanical force characterization in manipulating live cells with optical tweezers. J. Biomech. 44, 741–746.

Xie, Y., Sun, D., Liu, C., Tse, H.Y., Cheng, S.H., 2010. A force control approach to a robot-assisted cell microinjection system. Int. J. Robot. Res. 29 (9), 1222–1232.

Xie, M., Mills, J.K., Wang, Y., Mahmoodi, M., Sun, D., 2016. Automated translational and rotational control of biological cells with a robot-aided optical tweezers manipulation System. IEEE Trans. Autom. Sci. Eng. 13 (2), 543–551.

Xie, M., Shakoor, A., Shen, Y., Mills, J.K., Sun, D., 2019. Out-of-plane rotation control of biological cells with a robot-tweezers manipulation system for orientation-based cell surgery. IEEE Trans. Biomed. Eng. 66 (1), 199–207.

Yoshida, N., Perry, A.C., 2007. Piezo-actuated mouse intracytoplasmic sperm injection (ICSI). Nat. Protoc. 2, 296–304.

Yu, L., Mohanty, S., Liu, G., Genc, S., Kim, M., Chen, Z., Berns, M., 2009. Quantitative phase evaluation of dynamic changes on the cell membrane during laser microsurgery. Proc. SPIE 7182.

Zhuang, S., Lin, W., Zhong, J., Zhang, G., Li, L., Qiu, J., Gao, H., 2018. Visual servoed three-dimensional rotation control in zebrafish larva heart microinjection system. IEEE Trans. Biomed. Eng. 65 (1), 64–73.

Three-dimensional image reconstruction and intracellular surgery

7

7.1 Introduction

In recent years, intracellular surgery, such as cell injection (Chow et al., 2016), intracellular component extraction (Shakoor et al., 2019), and preimplantation genetic diagnosis (Braude et al., 2002), has aroused great interest. Obtaining the positions of cells and micromanipulators in 3D mode is critical to the success of these operations. A template-matching algorithm (Sun and Nelson, 2002) and an entropy calculation algorithm (Zhang et al., 2009) were proposed to adjust the height of the pipette used for cell injection. In the application of polystyrene beads (Xie et al., 2019), cells were rotated around the focal plane to achieve enucleation. Obtaining the precise location of small organelles (such as mitochondria) within a cell is a large challenge. Traditionally, manual control of the extraction of organelles and determination of the extraction location empirically were performed, which requires a great deal of aspiration pressure and multiple extraction attempts, resulting in cell disruption (Actis et al., 2013). To improve the success rate and reduce the operation damage through intracellular surgery, three-dimensional (3D) information of intracellular organelles is required, which can be obtained via image reconstruction methods.

3D image reconstruction methods are based on optical sectioning technologies, such as medical computer tomography (CT), magnetic resonance imaging (MRI), confocal fluorescence microscopy (CFM), and wide-field fluorescence microscopy (WFFM). CT and MRI are widely used to visualize tissues, organs, and other large-scale specimens (Chan et al., 2008), and CFM can eliminate out-of-focus blurs. However, CFM suffers from limitations, such as high cost of purchase and operations, slow scanning speed, and high-intensity light, which may lead to short fluorescence lifetime and photon toxicity in living cells (Shaw, 2006). WFFM can be easily integrated with robot-assisted manipulations at a relatively low cost. Given that images sampled by WFFM contain out-of-focus blurs and noises, the restoration of original images is required.

Deconvolution methods have been developed in the past few years, such as Janson–Van–Cittert (JVC) constrained deconvolution, Tikhonov–Miller gradient descent, and Richardson–Lucy maximum likelihood deconvolution. These methods ignore the spherical aberration and use a spatially invariant point spread function (PSF), which will cause artifacts during restoration. Several space-varying deconvolution methods have been recently proposed. A linear interpolation method was used to simulate PSF of different depths (Preza and Conchello, 2004). A weight function was introduced to solve the spatial invariance of a given PSF (Hadj and Blanc-Féraud, 2011). A principal component analysis (PCA) method was developed to decompose multiple PSFs into several principal components and corresponding coefficients

Robotic Cell Manipulation. https://doi.org/10.1016/B978-0-323-85259-3.00011-8

(Arigovindan et al., 2010). These methods used a limited number of PSFs to approximate PSFs of other optical depths. The restoration accuracy decreased as the number of PSFs derived from the approximation increased. These methods can reduce the processing time and computational complexity, so they are suitable for thick specimens. In intracellular surgery, however, the size of organelles is usually small (e.g., the size of mitochondria in human cells is about 2 μm only). Moreover, the motion resolution of the objective lens is limited, indicating that the number of PSFs is small. Gao et al. (2019) used microscope lens movement to obtain a series of optical cross-sections along the vertical direction, and implemented deconvolution, segmentation, and reconstruction processes to achieve 3D image reconstruction.

3D image reconstruction technology will enable intracellular surgery that relies on cell 3D information. Intracellular delivery is the process of transporting exogenous elements into cells. This method has been widely used in biomedical applications, such as the delivery of micro/nanorobots to embryos to achieve cell or drug release (Li et al., 2018) and the study of nuclear mechanical polarity (Wang et al., 2019). Some tracking macromolecules are delivered into mammalian cells to study intracellular mechanisms, such as the entry of cytoplasmic molecules into primary cilia (Kee et al., 2012) and the release of spliced mRNA from the nuclear spot domain (Dias et al., 2010). Transferring DNA (Wang et al., 2014) and RNA molecules (Montecalvo et al., 2011) to different cell types for genome-editing cell transfection has also aroused a great deal of interest. The precise delivery of these exogenous materials to certain intracellular components is crucial to the success of these operations. DNA normally performs its function in the nucleus, and delivery of DNA to the cytoplasm will reduce the activity of DNA. This feature indicates that the direct delivery of DNA in the nucleus is highly preferred (Ding et al., 2017). The existing delivery methods are divided into two categories. The first category is the use of vector-based biological/chemical methods, such as vesicles (Montecalvo et al., 2011) and viruses (Anokye-Danso et al., 2012). The second category is the use of a physical destruction method, such as electroporation (Bodles-Brakhop et al., 2009), extrusion via microfluidic chips (Sharei et al., 2013), and magnetic bead force-driving methods (Wang et al., 2018). In these methods, exogenous substances are delivered into the cytoplasm and diffused passively. As a result, only part of the delivered materials can pass through the membranes of intracellular organelles. Micro/nanopipette-based injection has the ability of membrane penetration, accurate dosage, and timing control, and has unique advantages in precise intracellular delivery. Micropipettes were used to implant large embryos (Huang et al., 2009; Xie et al., 2010). In recent years, micropipettes were used to deposit fluorescent molecules into the cytoplasm and nucleus (Shekaramiz et al., 2016; Liu et al., 2015; Guillaume-Gentil et al., 2013). In these works, the injection was implemented on adherent cells with flat morphology and the intracellular organelles were easily positioned (Esmaeilsabzali et al., 2011). Given the greater cortical tension (Cartagena-Rivera et al., 2016) and higher penetration depth (Pan et al., 2020), intracellular delivery of flat attached cells is more difficult than with floating cells. Considering that some cells naturally suspend without attaching to the surface, the suspended cells are close to a spherical shape in culture, and the height of these cells is greater than the height of the attached cells. Therefore, it is difficult for the micropipette to penetrate the cell membrane given incorrect height positioning.

3D cell information is necessary to ensure the success of intracellular delivery tasks. Gao et al. (2020) proposed an accurate and automated intracellular delivery method that implements 3D image reconstruction of cells on a robotic microscopy system. With this method, a series of optical cross-sectional images are sampled and restored to the computer through a moving objective lens, and the region of interest (ROI) containing the target organelles is automatically selected and cropped. The NRMLE deconvolution algorithm can be used to process the cropped images for deblurring and denoising. To reduce the computational complexity, the deconvolution calculation is conducted in the frequency domain. To reconstruct the 3D model of the sample from these segmented images, an adaptive filtering process is implemented before the segmentation process. A robust controller is developed to control the micropipette to the desired position in the cell and deliver foreign materials.

The remainder of this chapter introduces 3D image reconstruction methods, the operation of intracellular delivery based on 3D image reconstruction on robotic cell microscopy systems, and case studies.

7.2 3D image reconstruction

7.2.1 Wide-field fluorescence microscopy 3D reconstruction system

Fig. 7.1 illustrates a robot-assisted wide-field fluorescence microscopy system for 3D reconstruction (Gao et al., 2019). The system has three main modules, namely, imaging, control, and executive. The imaging module contains an inverted wide-field fluorescence microscopy (Nikon, TE2000) with a CCD camera (FOculus, FO124SC). The

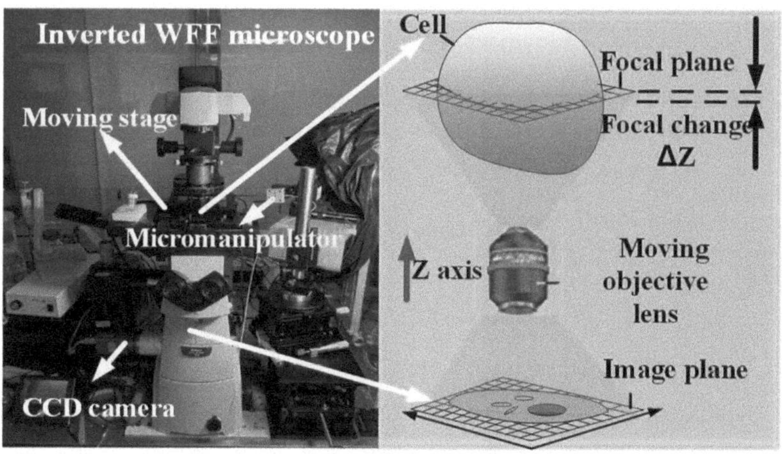

Figure 7.1 Robot-assisted wide-field fluorescence microscopy system for 3D reconstruction (Gao et al., 2019).

control module includes a motorized x−y moving stage, a z-axis movable objective lens, and in-house assembled three degrees-of-freedom (3-DOF) micromanipulator (Sensapex, UMP). The executive module consists of a micropipette (Sutter, B-100-78-15) mounted on the manipulator and a controllable microinjector (MicroData, PM6000) linked to the micropipette for cell surgical operations.

The objective lens moves along the z axis with step size Δz such that the entire specimen can be scanned from the bottom to the top. Optical sections from the CCD camera are restored in the computer. Each optical section combines sharp in-focus features with blurred features from out-of-focus planes and noises, which can be expressed by PSF. The measured optical section is a convolution of PSF functions and the real object, and is given as follows:

$$g(x_i, y_i, z_i) = \sum_{s} \sum_{(x_o, y_o)} h_s(x_i - x_o, y_i - y_o, z_i - z_o) f(x_o, y_o, z_o) \tag{7.1}$$

where (x_i, y_i, z_i) is the selected point on the focal plane of the image space, (x_o, y_o, z_o) represents the selected light source point of the object space, $g(x_i, y_i, z_i)$ denotes the pixel intensity value of the corresponding focal point from the CCD camera, $f(x_o, y_o, z_o)$ indicates the intensity value of the source point, $h_s(x_i - x_o, y_i - y_o, z_i - z_o)$ refers to a PSF describing the projection behavior on point (x_i, y_i, z_i), and subscript s denotes that PSF is calculated on the s plane wherein the source point (x_o, y_o, z_o) lies. Fig. 7.2 illustrates the operation flowchart with 3D reconstruction feedback. Sampled sections are deconvoluted to eliminate most blurs and noises. The processed sections are then segmented to obtain a clear boundary and reconstructed into a 3D model. This model provides straightforward position information for cell surgery and thus improves accuracy and success rate.

7.2.2 Methods

7.2.2.1 Point spread function (PSF)

Several methods have been proposed to estimate intrinsic PSF, and they can be classified into two categories, namely, experimental measurement (Monvel et al., 2003;

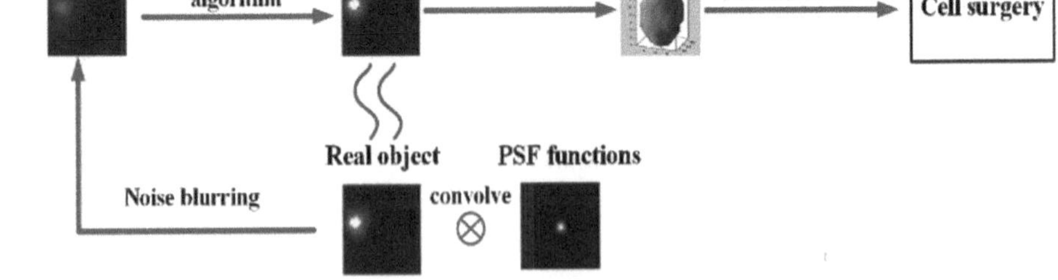

Figure 7.2 Operation with 3D reconstruction feedback (Gao et al., 2019).

Tiedemann et al., 2006) and theoretical calculation (Gibson and Lanni, 1991; Zhang et al., 2007). Experimental methods have difficulty in obtaining PSF with good quality at an arbitrary depth regardless of complicated experimental procedures. Alternatively, a theoretical model can be used to calculate PSF. Gao et al. (2019) used the Gibson–Lanni model to calculate PSF at each sample section. Spherical aberrations show that the trajectory difference between the ideal and actual light rays are caused by the mismatch of refractive indices between the lens immersion medium and specimen and the discrepancy between the ideal and real parameters of the microscopy system. The aberrations can be characterized with the optical path difference (OPD) (Gibson and Lanni, 1991), described as follows:

$$OPD = z_i + t'_{im}\sqrt{n_{im}^2 - (NAp)^2} + z_o\sqrt{n_s^2 - (NAp)^2} - t'_{im}\sqrt{n'^2_{im} - (NAp)^2} + t_c\sqrt{n_c^2 - (NAp)^2} - t'_c\sqrt{n'^2_c - (NAp)^2}, \tag{7.2}$$

On the basis of OPD function, PSF function can be expressed as

$$h_s = \left| A\int_0^1 e^{iOPD} J_0\left(\frac{2\pi}{\lambda}\sqrt{(x_i - x_o)^2 + (y_i - y_o)^2}\, NAp\right) p dp \right|^2, \tag{7.3}$$

where p is the normalized distance between the focal (x_i, y_i, z_i) and light source (x_o, y_o, z_o) points on the x–y plane; NA represents the numerical aperture; n_{im}, n_c, and n_s refer to the refractive indices of the lens immersion medium, coverslip, and specimen, respectively; t_{im}, t_c, and t_s indicate the thickness of the corresponding layers; the superscript $'$ stands for the ideal value of each parameter; λ denotes the emission light wavelength; A is a constant complex amplitude; and J_0 represents the Bessel function of the first type of order zero. Notably, multiple PSFs can be generated at different depth of sampling sections.

In the PSF calculation, the depth interval between optical sections, d_z, is not equal to the size of lens movement Δz due to the geometric distortion that arises from the difference among the refractive indices of layers through which the focal light passes (Snyder et al., 1993). This interval can be expressed as

$$d_z = \frac{\tan\left(\arcsin\dfrac{NA}{n_{im}}\right)}{\tan\left(\arcsin\dfrac{NA}{n_s}\right)}\Delta z. \tag{7.4}$$

7.2.2.2 Maximum likelihood estimation deconvolution

This algorithm incorporates multiple PSFs at each sampling depth into the Richardson–Lucy method. It is assumed that each focal point $g(x_i, y_i, z_i)$ of the image space is statistically independent from the others. Based on the Poisson distribution with a mean value of $\widehat{g}(x_i, y_i, z_i)$ (Sibarita, 2005), the following equation holds

$$P(g(x_i, y_i, z_i)|\widehat{g}(x_i, y_i, z_i)) = \frac{\widehat{g}(x_i, y_i, z_i)^{g(x_i,y_i,z_i)} e^{-\widehat{g}(x_i,y_i,z_i)}}{g(x_i, y_i, z_i)!}. \tag{7.5}$$

The log-likelihood function of the entire image space is as follows:

$$\begin{aligned} L = & -\prod_{(x_i,y_i,z_i)} \ln[P(g(x_i, y_i, z_i)|\widehat{g}(x_i, y_i, z_i))] \\ & -\sum_{(x_i,y_i,z_i)} [\widehat{g}(x_i, y_i, z_i) - g(x_i, y_i, z_i)\ln(\widehat{g}(x_i, y_i, z_i)) + \ln(g(x_i, y_i, z_i)!)] \end{aligned} \tag{7.6}$$

$$\widehat{g}(x_i, y_i, z_i) = \sum_{z_o} \sum_{(x_o,y_o)} h_s(x_i - x_o, y_i - y_o, z_i - z_o)\widehat{f}(x_o, y_o, z_o). \tag{7.7}$$

Let the derivative of the likelihood with respect to the estimation value $\widehat{f}(x_o, y_o, z_o)$ be zero. Given $g(x_i, y_i, z_i)$, the equations with an interactive form are expressed as

$$\widehat{f}^{k+1}(x_o, y_o, z_o) = \frac{\widehat{f}^{k}(x_o, y_o, z_o)}{H(x_o, y_o, z_o)} \sum_{(x_o,y_o,z_o)} h_s(x_i - x_o, y_i - y_o, z_i - z_o) \frac{g(x_i, y_i, z_i)}{\widehat{g}^{k}(x_i, y_i, z_i)}, \tag{7.8}$$

$$\widehat{g}^{k}(x_i, y_i, z_i) = \sum_{z_o} \sum_{(x_o,y_o)} h_s(x_i - x_o, y_i - y_o, z_i - z_o)\widehat{f}^{k}(x_o, y_o, z_o), \tag{7.9}$$

$$H(x_o, y_o, z_o) = \sum_{s} \sum_{(x_i,y_i,z_i)} h_s(x_i - x_o, y_i - y_o, z_i - z_o), \tag{7.10}$$

where $\widehat{f}^{k+1}(x_o, y_o, z_o)$ is the estimation of the real object at the (k+1)th interaction, $\widehat{g}^{k}(x_i, y_i, z_i)$ denotes the sample mean of the Poisson distribution at the (k+1)th interaction, and $H(x_o, y_o, z_o)$ represents an energy conservation constant.

7.2.2.3 Noise regulation

The measured optical sections are corrupted by various noises. The proposed maximum likelihood estimation deconvolution algorithm amplifies these noises and thus generates artifacts during interactions (Markham and Conchello, 1997). Adding a regulation term to the log-likelihood function is a practically used method to attenuate this problem. The regularized log-likelihood function ϕ can be defined as

$$\phi = L_R - \alpha R\left(\widehat{f}_R(x_o, y_o, z_o)\right), \tag{7.11}$$

where $R(\bullet)$ denotes the regulation function, α is the regulation factor, and $\widehat{f}_R(x_o, y_o, z_o)$ refers to the noise-regulated estimation. Notably, regularized log-likelihood function uses $\widehat{f}_R(x_o, y_o, z_o)$ and $\widehat{f}(x_o, y_o, z_o)$ to replace $\widehat{g}(x_i, y_i, z_i)$ and $g(x_i, y_i, z_i)$, respectively. Hence, this function is different from Eq. (7.5). Here, the regulation function is defined in the form of Conchello's intensity function proposed by Conchello and McNally (1996). This function can achieve better resolution than other regulation functions, such as Good's roughness (Goodd and Gaskins, 1971) and total regulation (Dey et al., 2006). $R(\bullet)$ is defined as

$$R\left(\widehat{f}(x_o, y_o, z_o)\right) = \sum_{(x_o, y_o, z_o)} \left[\widehat{f}_R(x_o, y_o, z_o)\right]^2. \tag{7.12}$$

Substituting Eq. (7.12) into Eq. (7.11) yields

$$L_R = -\sum_{(x_o, y_o, z_o)} \left[\widehat{f}_R(x_o, y_o, z_o) - \widehat{f}(x_o, y_o, z_o)\ln\left(\widehat{f}_R(x_o, y_o, z_o)\right.\right.$$
$$\left.\left. \times\right) + \ln\left(\widehat{f}(x_o, y_o, z_o)!\right)\right] - \alpha\left[\widehat{f}_R(x_o, y_o, z_o)\right]^2. \tag{7.13}$$

Let the derivative of ϕ with respect to the noise-regulated estimation $\widehat{f}_R(x_o, y_o, z_o)$ be zero. Then,

$$2\alpha\left[\widehat{f}_R(x_o, y_o, z_o)\right]^2 + \widehat{f}_R(x_o, y_o, z_o) - \widehat{f}(x_o, y_o, z_o) = 0. \tag{7.14}$$

The solution to Eq. (7.14) is as follows:

$$\widehat{f}_R(x_o, y_o, z_o) = \frac{-1 + \sqrt{1 - 8\alpha\widehat{f}(x_o, y_o, z_o)}}{4\alpha}. \tag{7.15}$$

Substituting $\widehat{f}^k(x_o, y_o, z_o)$ into Eq. (7.8) with the noise-regulated estimation $\widehat{f}^k_R(x_o, y_o, z_o)$, the following estimation value $\widehat{f}^{k+1}(x_o, y_o, z_o)$ can be obtained

$$\widehat{f}^{k+1}(x_o, y_o, z_o) = Fourier^{-1}\left[\eta\widehat{F}^k(w_{xo}, w_{yo}, w_{zo}) \sum_k H_k(w_{xo}, w_{yo}, w_{zo}) \frac{G(w_{xo}, w_{yo}, w_{zo})}{\widehat{G}^n(w_{xo}, w_{yo}, w_{zo})}\right], \tag{7.16}$$

$$\widehat{g}^k(x_i, y_i, z_i) = Fourier^{-1}\left[\sum_k H_k(w_{xo}, w_{yo}, w_{zo})\widehat{F}^k(w_{xo}, w_{yo}, w_{zo})\right], \tag{7.17}$$

where $Fourier^{-1}()$ is the inverse Fourier transform function, $\widehat{g}^k(x_i, y_i, z_i)$ is the $(n+1)$ th update of the measured point $g(x_i, y_i, z_i)$, and η represents an energy conservation constant. The complete interactive process will be calculated in the frequency domain to reduce time consumption. The final estimation $\widehat{f}^{k+1}(x_o, y_o, z_o)$ is transformed back to the time domain with Eq. (7.6). The interactive noise-regulated estimation $\widehat{f_R}^{k+1}(x_o, y_o, z_o)$ is

$$\widehat{f_R}^{k+1}(x_o, y_o, z_o) = \frac{-1 + \sqrt{1 - 8\alpha\widehat{f}^{k+1}(x_o, y_o, z_o)}}{4\alpha}, \tag{7.18}$$

which should be the restoration result with a satisfactory resolution.

Notably, $\widehat{f}_R^{k+1}(x_o, y_o, z_o)$ can be calculated with Eq. (7.15) for the next interaction. After a number of interactions, the blurred optical sections can be restored with a satisfactory resolution.

7.2.2.4 Boundary segmentation and 3D reconstruction

The grayscale values of several object points may exceed their upper limitations or fall behind the correct ones due to the ringing effect (Sage et al., 2017) that produces local over- and undershoots. The fluorescence intensities of intracellular components are assumed to be solid and homogeneous, and the overshoot points are set to 255. However, the remaining boundary renders itself indistinct and unclear, which causes difficulty during 3D model reconstruction. To solve this problem, a localized region-based segmentation algorithm (Lankton and Tannenbaum, 2008) can be used to obtain distinct restoration. The boundary contour is derived on the basis of the energy function and is given as

$$\begin{aligned} E(\Psi(x_o, y_o)) = {} & \\ & \sum_{(x_o, y_o)} \partial I(\Psi(x_o, y_o)) \sum_{(x_a, y_a)} \left[M(x_o, y_o, x_a, y_a)F\left(\widehat{f}_R(x_a, y_a), \Psi(x_a, y_a)\right)\right] \\ & + \lambda \sum_{(x_o, y_o)} \left[\partial I(\Psi(x_o, y_o)) \| \nabla\Psi(x_o, y_o)\| \right], \end{aligned} \tag{7.19}$$

where $I(\Psi)$ represents the interior of contour Ψ, $\partial I(\Psi)$ denotes the derivative of $I(\Psi)$ with respect to Ψ, mask $M(x_o, y_o, x_a, y_a)$ is used to define the narrow gap containing point (x_a, y_a) near contour Ψ, and $F\left(\widehat{f}_R(x_a, y_a), \Psi(x_a, y_a)\right)$ indicates a force function calculated at point (x_a, y_a) with the deconvoluted result $\widehat{f}_R(x_a, y_a)$ and contour function value $\Psi(x_a, y_a)$.

Taking the first variation of Eq. (7.19) with respect to Ψ and calculating the minimum energy, the contour movement is calculated as

$$\frac{\partial \Psi(x_o, y_o)}{\partial n} = \partial I(\Psi(x_o, y_o)) \sum_{(x_a, y_a)} \left[M(x_o, y_o, x_a, y_a) \frac{\partial F\left(\widehat{f}_R(x_a, y_a), \Psi(x_a, y_a)\right)}{\partial \Psi} \right] + \lambda \partial I(\Psi(x_o, y_o)) \nabla \left(\frac{\nabla \Psi(x_o, y_o)}{|\nabla \Psi(x_o, y_o)|} \right), \tag{7.20}$$

where n is the interaction number. After interacting a few times, the optical sections can have a clear boundary, where the grayscale values of the interior part can be set to 255 under the previous assumption. Notably, the produced overshoots in some sample images that originally contain no objects may misguide the segmentation algorithm and produce artificial boundaries. To solve this problem, an adaptive filter process can be used before segmentation. The light intensity distribution of the object along the depth direction is similar to a square wave, in which the boundary points should have the largest difference between their forward and backward derivations. The filter process can obtain the sampling depth of these points, and the segmentation algorithm only processes images within this range (Kaufman and Mueller, 2005).

A 3D model of the specimen can be reconstructed after obtaining a series of possessed sections. Reconstruction methods are classified into two main categories. One is based on surface rendering, such as the classical marching cube algorithm (Lorensen and Cline, 1987), and the other is based on volume rendering (Kaufman and Mueller, 2005). In comparison with surface plotting methods that require an excessive amount of geometric primitives to approximate surfaces and lose considerable information contained within sections, volume rendering is relatively straightforward, free from an intermediate surface extraction step, and capable of reconstructing specimens with good resolution. Therefore, a 3D model of the specimen is reconstructed from these segmented images with the ISOSURFACE function.

7.2.3 Evaluations

The accuracy of the above algorithm was tested through simulations and experimental measurement of fluorescence microspheres. The restoration quality of the simulated object was examined through a comparison with the actual object function, which was exactly known. A fluorescence microsphere with a fixed dimension was used to extract authentic PSFs from the developed microscopy system and verify if the proposed methods can be applied to 3D information feedback of intracellular surgery. Two metrics were used for the performance evaluation. The first was the normalized mean square error (*NMSE*) of the deconvoluted results $\widehat{f}_R(x, y, z)$ in comparison with the real object $f(x, y, z)$, expressed as

$$NMSE = \frac{||\hat{f}_R(x,y,z) - f(x,y,z)||^2}{||f(x,y,z)||^2}. \tag{7.21}$$

The second was the error point ratio (*EPR*), described as

$$EPR = \frac{EPN}{TPN}, \tag{7.22}$$

where *EPN* is the error number of sections after segmentation and reconstruction in comparison with the real object $f(x, y, z)$, and *TPN* stands for the total pixel number in the created 3D space.

7.2.3.1 Simulations

A 3D space with dimensions of 64 × 64 × 64 pixels was generated, which included in the center a sphere with a diameter of 20 pixels. The voxel size of the space was 0.123 μm, and the grayscale value of the voxel containing the sphere was 255. Eq. (7.3) was used to calculate 64 PSFs at each section. The parameters are listed in Table 7.1. The space was blurred with 64 PSFs. The blurred objects were restored in two quantitative cases. One was the noiseless case in which the blurred space was free of noises. The other was the noisy case in which Poisson and Gaussian noises at various levels were added to the blurred result.

First, the noiseless case with a noise regulation factor $\alpha = 0$ was analyzed, and the results were compared with those of the PCA approximating method (Arigovindan et al., 2010). Fig. 7.3A illustrates the *NMSE* values during interactions of the two methods. With the proposed algorithm of Gao et al. (2019), *NMSE* decreased and reached a constant value of 0.0451 after 10,000 interactions. With the PCA method, *NMSE* initially decreased and reached a minimum value of 0.0665, and then increased. Fig. 7.3B shows the process flow of the two methods with the optimal

Table 7.1 Parameters of PSFs (Gao et al., 2019).

Symbol	Name	Value
n_i	Refractive index of the lens immersion medium (oil)	1.515
n_c	Refractive index of the coverslip	1.52
n_s	Refractive index of the specimen	1.33
t_i	Thickness of the lens immersion medium	0.160 μm
t_c	Thickness of the coverslip	0.170 μm
NA	Numerical aperture	1.2
λ	Wavelength	0.590 μm
N	Number of PSFs	64
	Dimension	64 × 64 × 64
	Voxel size	0.123 μm
d_z	Thickness interval	0.123 μm

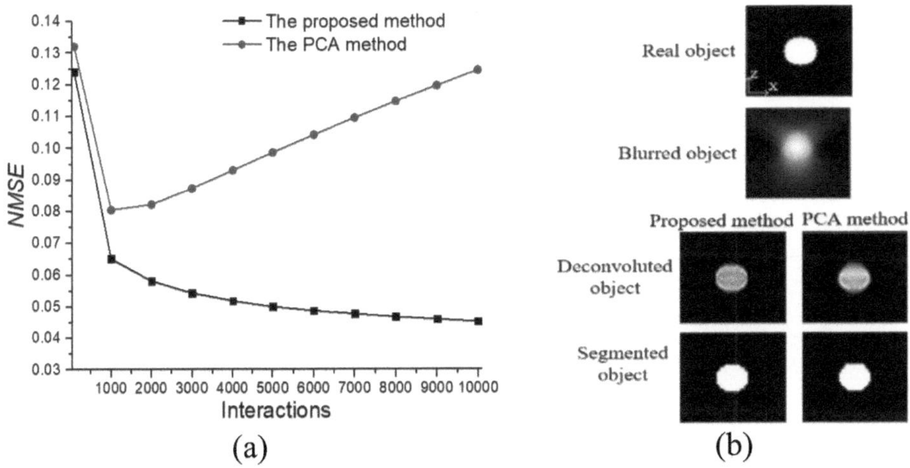

Figure 7.3 Results of the noiseless case (Gao et al., 2019). (A) Relationship between *NMSE* and interactions. (B) Process flow of noiseless data with the two methods, as shown on the x−z plane.

interaction numbers. After segmentation, *EPN* reached 170 and 374 pixels under Gao et al. (2019)'s method and the PCA method, respectively.

Second, the noisy case with different Poisson and Gaussian noises was analyzed. The Poisson noise originates from the Poisson nature of light emission, and the Gaussian noise is derived from the detector readout. Both noises are signal independent and incorporated with the measured sections. In the simulation, the Poisson noise was generated in the same manner as in Conchello and Hansen (1990). Two noise levels with mean photon densities of 4000 and 100 photons/pixel (SNR_1 and SNR_2, respectively) were generated. Two levels of Gaussian noise with a mean value of 0 and standard variations of 0.5 (SNR_3) and 2 (SNR_4) were generated also. The blurred object was corrupted in case SNR_5, which had combined Gaussian noise from case SNR_4 and Poisson noise from case SNR_1. The blurred object was also corrupted in case SNR_6, which had combined Gaussian noise from case SNR_4 and Poisson noise from case SNR_2. The noise-corrupted object was quantified in terms of its signal-to-noise ratio (*SNR*), which was defined as

$$SNR = 10\log 10\frac{\sigma_{noisy}}{\sigma_{noise}}, \tag{7.23}$$

where σ_{noisy} is the standard variation of the noise-adding object and σ_{noise} represents the standard variation of the noise. Fig. 7.4 illustrates the *SNR* of each section in the six cases. Optimal noise regulation factor α was determined by the minimum *NMSE*. Fig. 7.5 displays the relationship between noise regulation factor α and corresponding *NMSE* in the six noise cases. The optimal noise regulation factor α is given in Table 7.2.

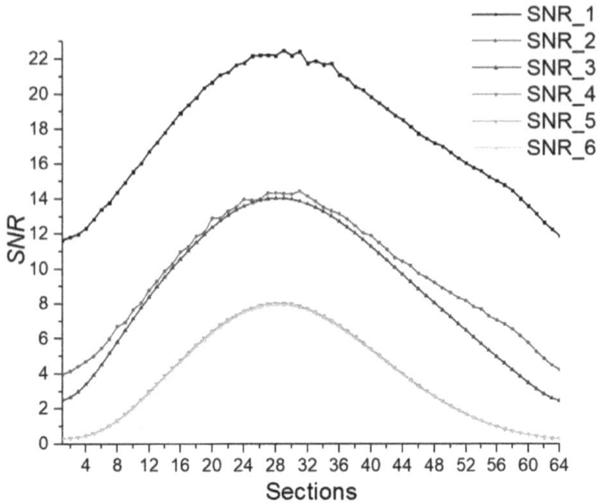

Figure 7.4 SNR of each section in the six noise cases (Gao et al., 2019).

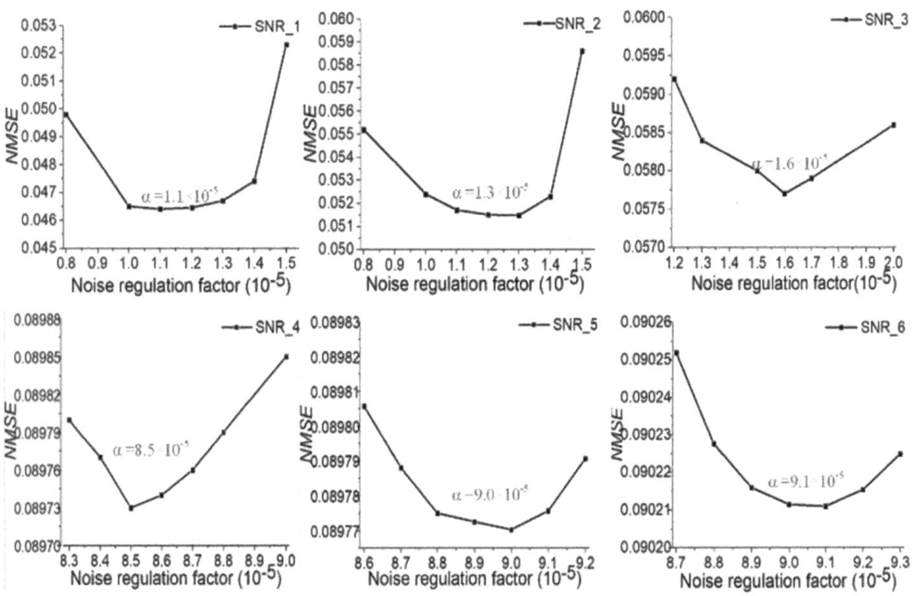

Figure 7.5 Optimal noise regulation factor α in six noise cases (Gao et al., 2019).

Table 7.2 Performance metrics (Gao et al., 2019).

Case	α	*NMSE*	*EPN*	*EPR*
SNR_1	1.1×10^{-5}	0.0464	170	0.0649%
SNR_2	1.3×10^{-5}	0.0515	179	0.0683%
SNR_3	1.6×10^{-5}	0.0577	232	0.0885%
SNR_4	8.5×10^{-5}	0.0897	264	0.1007%
SNR_5	9.0×10^{-5}	0.0898	271	0.1034%
SNR_6	9.1×10^{-5}	0.0902	274	0.1045%

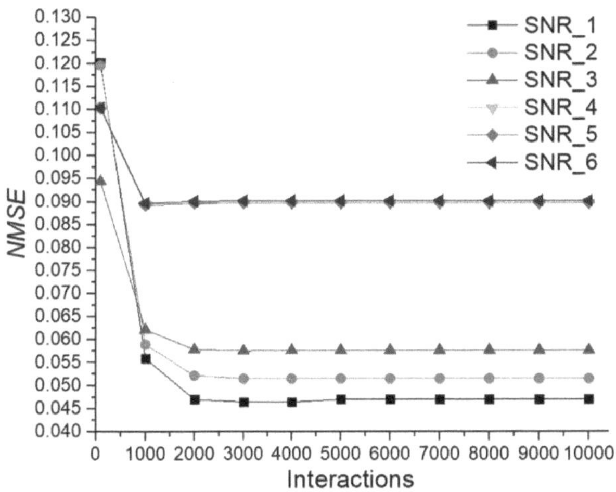

Figure 7.6 Relationship between *NMSE* and interactions with optimal factor α (Gao et al., 2019).

Fig. 7.6 presents the *NMSE* values with different optimal noise regulation factors (α) during the interactions. Similar to the noiseless case, the *NMSE* values decrease as the interactions increase and finally reach a constant level. Deconvoluted results after 10,000 interactions are used in the following segmentation process.

Fig. 7.7 illustrates the processing flow of the six cases, and Fig. 7.8 shows the gray-scale value profiles along the central line on the *XZ* plane in the six cases. After segmentation, the processed objects exhibit a more distinct boundary than the deconvoluted objects, which greatly benefits the 3D reconstruction. Table 7.2

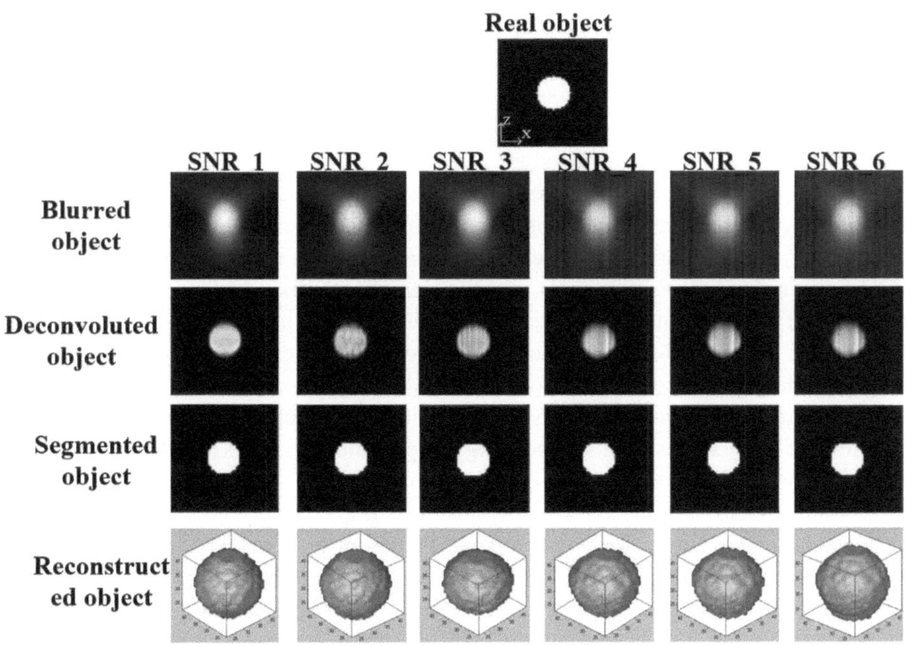

Figure 7.7 Processed flow of the six cases (Gao et al., 2019).

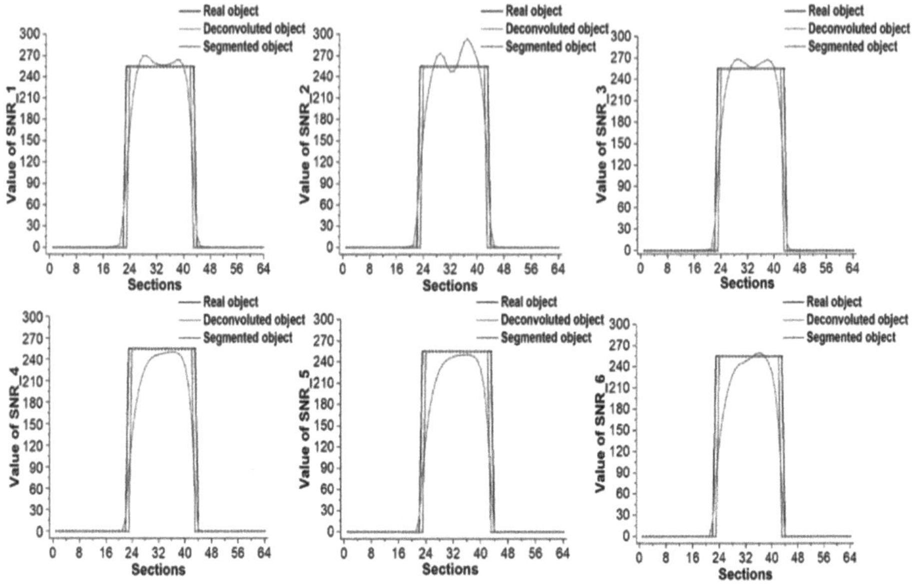

Figure 7.8 Intensity profiles along the central line on the *XZ* plane of the six cases (Gao et al., 2019).

illustrates the evaluation metrics of the six cases. Case SNR_1 has the lowest *NMSE* and *EPR* because it has the highest *SNR*, whereas SNR_6 has the highest *NMSE* and *EPR*. In addition, the maximum *EPN* among the six cases is 274 pixels, whereas the maximum *EPR* is less than 0.105%. These results verify that the proposed method exhibits excellent restoration performance.

7.2.3.2 Experiments

Fluorescent microspheres (TetraSpec, T-14792) with 4 μm diameter were used to test the accuracy of the developed robot-assisted microscopy method. In the experiments, an objective lens with 60× magnification was immersed in water. The resolution of the CCD camera was 640 × 480 pixels, and the size of each pixel on the CCD camera was 0.123 μm. The depth interval of two focal planes was 0.2 μm. The microspheres were mounted on a slide and fixed with optical cement with a refractive index of 1.57. The refractive index of the cover glass was 1.52, and its thickness was 0.17 mm. Filter GFP was selected, and the emission wavelength of the microspheres was set to 515 nm.

A total of 161 sections were scanned. Fig. 7.9 presents the results of the center area with dimensions of 100 × 100 pixels in each section. Fig. 7.9A shows the x−z plane of the tested microsphere, and Fig. 7.9B shows the x−z plane of theoretical blurred sections without adding any noises. In the theoretical calculation, an ellipse with a lateral diameter of 32 pixels and a vertical diameter of 20 pixels was generated on a 100 × 100 × 161 pixel space and centered at point (51, 51, 81). One hundred and sixty-one PSFs with a depth interval of 0.2 μm from the bottom to the top of the ellipse were computed. The

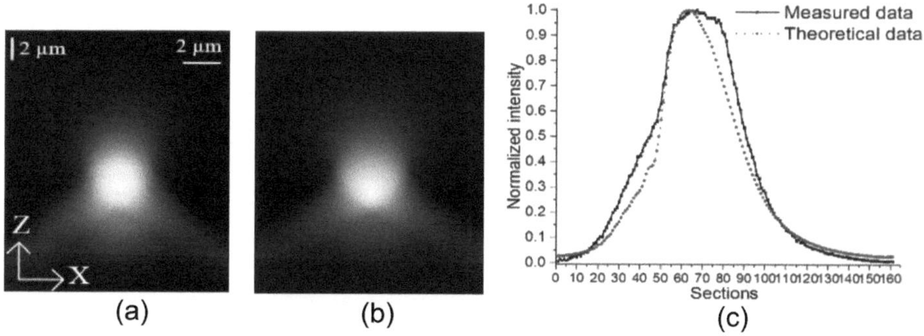

Figure 7.9 Images of the scanned microsphere (Gao et al., 2019). (A) XZ plane of measured sections. (B) XZ plane of theoretical sections. (C) Normalized intensity of the central line in images (A) and (B).

proposed model was used to generate theoretical blurred sections. Fig. 7.9C illustrates the normalized intensity of the central line in the image in Fig. 7.9A and B. The *NMSE* among the 161 theoretical and measured sections was 0.036, indicating that the theoretical calculation was in good agreement with the measured results.

The measured sections were deconvoluted given a noise regulation factor $\alpha = 0.00008$. Fig. 7.10A illustrates the comparison of deconvoluted, segmented, and synthetic objects. Fig. 7.10B presents the central line intensity of the three x−z plane images. The blur details around the microsphere were eliminated after deconvolution. The *NMSE* between the deconvoluted object and synthetic microsphere was 0.247, which was relatively larger than that in the simulation analysis. In addition, most errors were observed in the lateral dimension because the shape of the tested sample was not a perfect sphere with a diameter of 4 μm, and its fluorescence was nonuniform. The *EPR* of the reconstructed microsphere was 0.0975%, as shown in Fig. 7.10A. These results not only demonstrated the accuracy of the proposed method but also calibrated the PSFs of the system, rendering the system capable of providing 3D reconstructed position information for intracellular surgery.

7.3 Robot-assisted intracellular delivery with 3D image reconstruction information

This section presents a precise and automated intracellular delivery approach using a robotic microscopy system. The intracellular transmission is a comprehensive process, where a series of optical section images are sampled and restored in a computer by moving objective, and a region of interest (ROI) containing organelles is automatically selected and cropped. The deconvolution algorithm reported in the previous section can be used here to process these cropped images for deblurring and denoising. Deconvolution calculations are performed in the frequency domain to reduce the computational complexity. Given that the light intensity of intracellular organelles may not be uniform, an adaptive

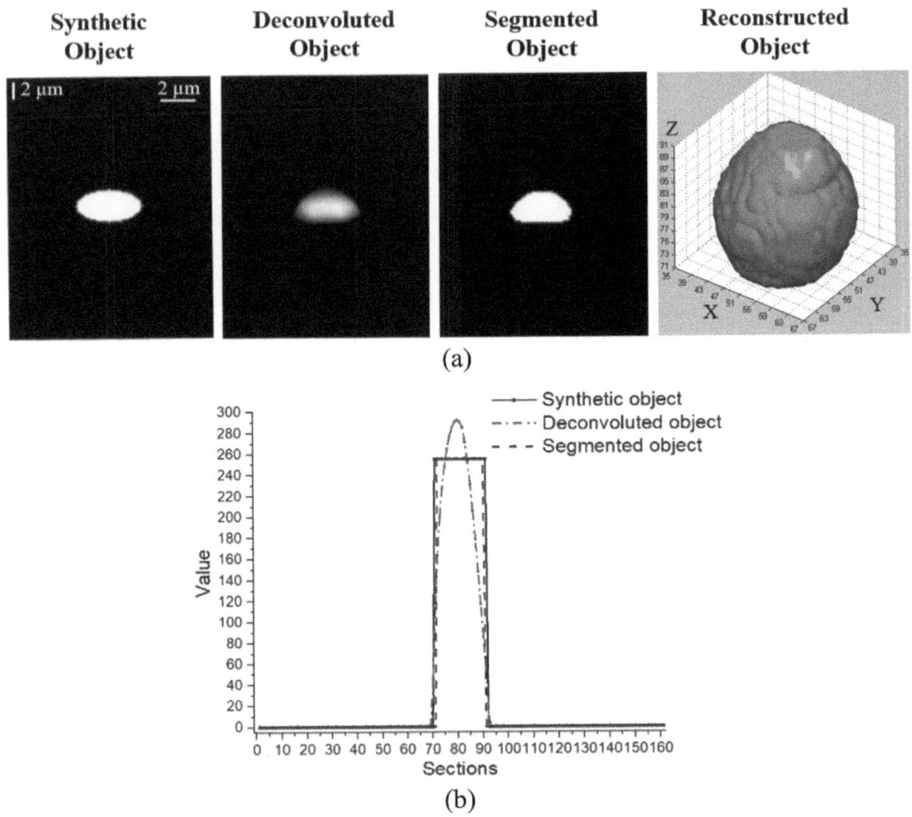

Figure 7.10 Processing results of recorded sections (Gao et al., 2019). (A) x−z plane of synthetic, deconvoluted, segmented objects, and reconstructed 3D model (The resolution in the z-axis is 0.2 μm, and that in the x−y plane is 0.12 μm.) (B) Value of the central line in three images.

filtering process is implemented before the segmentation process to reconstruct a 3D model of the samples from these segmented images. An articulated 3D geometric analysis is developed to provide the optimal operating position. A robust controller is further developed to manipulate the micropipette to this position and deliver foreign material, and the controller can compensate for external disturbances. Experimental results are finally reported to verify the effectiveness of the method.

7.3.1 Intracellular delivery method

Fig. 7.11 shows the procedures of the precise intracellular strategy. First, the relative position of the original focal plane and the micropipette tip is calibrated. The original focal plane can be placed in the bottom surface of the chip channel, so the movable objective lens can scan the entire trapped cell. Second, the system searches the trapped cell in the current image field. After finding the cell, the objective lens moves along the z-axis

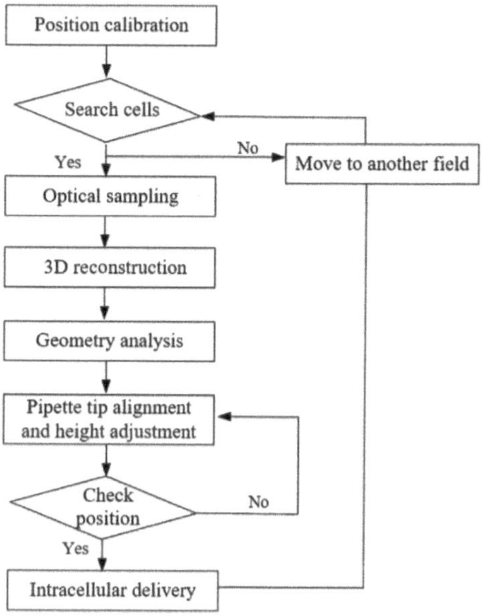

Figure 7.11 Operation procedures of an automated intracellular delivery system (Gao et al., 2020).

with a step size to sample the cell optically. These optical section images are corrupted by out-of-focus blurs and noises owing to the limitation of the WFFM and must be restored by image restoration algorithms. Using the 3D reconstruction algorithm reported in the previous section, the optical sections can be deconvoluted to deblur and denoise, followed by a segmentation process for clear boundaries and reconstruction into a 3D model. The system then performs the geometric analysis of the reconstructed model to determine an optimized operation position depending on the given tasks. The controller adjusts the height of the micropipette and then moves the motorized stage along the y-axis to coincide with the pipette tip with the optimal destination position laterally, as shown in Fig. 7.12. Finally, the stage moves and facilitates the penetration of micropipette in the cell membranes to conduct the intracellular delivery task.

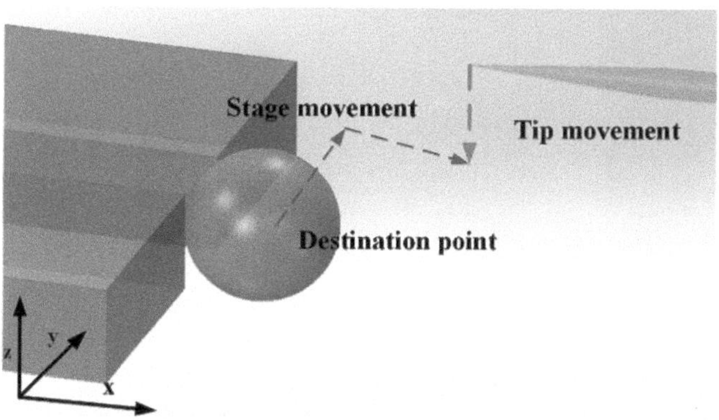

Figure 7.12 Motion strategy of an automated intracellular delivery system (Gao et al., 2020).

7.3.1.1 3D geometry analysis

Once the reconstructed 3D model of the specimen is obtained, a customized geometry analysis is conducted to calculate the optimal operation position to guide the motion of the micropipette. For the intracellular delivery, the operation position is essential because the main challenge of intracellular delivery is to penetrate the cytomembrane and organelle membrane to push out exogenous materials successfully. The plane with the largest section area should be selected. However, such a plane may lie in the height away from its central plane due to the irregularity of the organelles in suspended cells. This feature leads to failure of the penetration due to the tilting movement caused by micropipette thrust force, as shown in Fig. 7.13A. Therefore, a comprehensive volume-based model is required to facilitate successful delivery. In the current research, the plane with the highest section area $P_{\max}$ is searched, and the object boundary is fitted by an ellipse with long axis $a_{\max}$ and short axis $b_{\max}$. Meanwhile, the boundaries of each segmented section are also fitted by ellipses. The entire 3D model can be separated into two parts, namely, the upper part with volume V_u and the lower part with volume V_l, which are calculated as follows:

$$V_u = \sum_{i \geq P_{\max}} V_{ui}, \tag{7.24}$$

$$V_{ui} = \sum_{i \geq P_{\max}} \pi \Delta z \left(\frac{a_{i+1} b_{i+1}}{3} + \frac{a_{i+1} b_i}{6} + \frac{a_i b_{i+1}}{6} + \frac{a_i b_i}{3} \right), \tag{7.25}$$

$$V_l = \sum_{i \leq P_{\max}} V_{ui}, \tag{7.26}$$

$$V_{li} = \sum_{i \leq P_{\max}} \pi \Delta z \left(\frac{a_i b_i}{3} + \frac{a_{i-1} b_i}{6} + \frac{a_i b_{i-1}}{6} + \frac{a_i b_i}{3} \right), \tag{7.27}$$

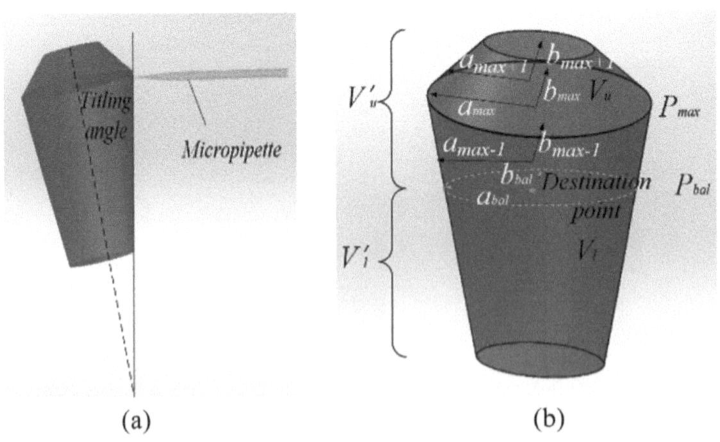

Figure 7.13 Geometric analysis for a reconstructed 3D model (Gao et al., 2020). (A) Optimal delivery point analysis. (B) Titling movement by inappropriate operation height.

where V_{ui} and V_{li} are the volumes between the two image planes, a_i and b_i are long and short axes in each plane, respectively, and Δz is the focal distance between two image planes.

The optimal position for delivery should lie in the plane P_{bal}, resulting in the modified upper volume $V_u' = V_u \pm V_{bal}$, which is equal to the low-volume $V_l' = V_l \pm V_{bal}$. V_{bal} is balance volume and given as

$$V_{bal} = \sum_{\min(P_{bal}, P_{\max}) \le i \le \max(P_{bal}, P_{\max})} V_{bali}. \tag{7.28}$$

P_{bal} can be derived through $V_u' = V_l'$. The destination point should be the center of the ellipse in the balance plane to ensure the successful penetration and delivery, as shown in Fig. 7.13B.

7.3.1.2 Motion control

The moving stage and the micropipette move toward the destination position, as shown in Fig. 7.14A. The micropipette adjusts its height into the balance plane along the z-axis. The moving stage aligns the micropipette tip along the y-axis and then coincides. After that, the controller moves the stage to penetrate the cell membrane and conducts the delivery task. The dynamics of the system can be described using Lagrange's equation of motion as follows:

$$M\ddot{q} + B\dot{q} + G + \tau_d = \tau, \tag{7.29}$$

where M, B, and G represent mass, damping, and gravity matrices of the system, respectively, τ is the input torque vector, τ_d is a disturbance term, and $q = [x_o, y_o, z_o]^T$ is the stage coordinate position vector in object space, which has the following relationship with the image coordinate:

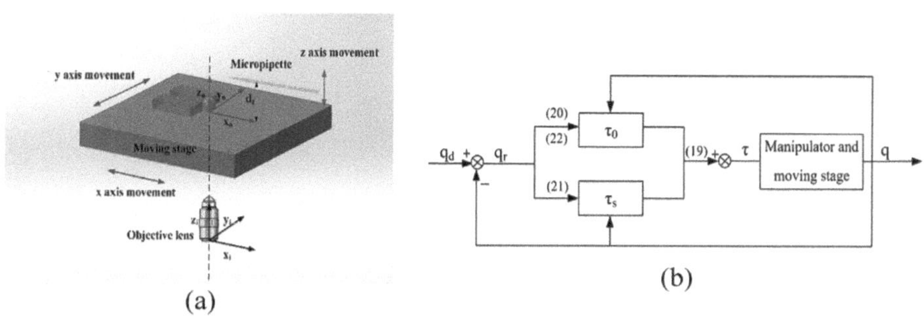

Figure 7.14 Motion control of the system (Gao et al., 2020). (A) Control coordinates of the camera, moving stage, and manipulator. (B) Scheme of the proposed controller.

$$q = \begin{bmatrix} x_o \\ y_o \\ z_0 \end{bmatrix} = T \begin{bmatrix} x_i \\ y_i \\ z_i \end{bmatrix} + \begin{bmatrix} 0 \\ 0 \\ d_z \end{bmatrix}, \tag{7.30}$$

where $[x_i, y_i, z_i]^T$ is the image coordinate position vector, $T = diag[T_x, T_y, T_z]^T$ is the diagonal transformation matrix, and T_x, T_y are constant transformation factors along the x- and y-axes, respectively. $T_z = \frac{\tan\left(\arcsin\frac{NA}{n_{im}}\right)}{\tan\left(\arcsin\frac{NA}{n_s}\right)}$ is the geometric distortion factor along the z-axis that depends on the refractive index of the lens immersion medium and specimen (Snyder et al., 1993), and d_z denotes the relative vertical distance between two coordinate frames.

Model uncertainties of the system and external disturbances (such as vibration) may fail the manipulation process. Therefore, a sliding mode controller is designed to improve the system robustness. Assuming $\widehat{\sigma}$ is a 3D vector containing the unknown elements in the dynamic equation, the estimated dynamics of the system is expressed as follows:

$$\widehat{M}\ddot{q}_r + \widehat{B}\dot{q}_r + \widehat{G} + \tau_d = Y\widehat{\sigma}, \tag{7.31}$$

where $\widehat{M}$, $\widehat{B}$, and $\widehat{G}$ are estimated mass, damping, and gravity matrices, respectively, $\dot{q}_r$ is defined as $\dot{q}_d - \varepsilon q_e$, q_d is the desired position point, ε is a positive constant, and $q_e = q_d - q$ is the position error. Y is a regression matrix and is independent of dynamic parameters. The sliding vector S is defined as $S = \dot{q} - \dot{q}_r$. The robust sliding controller is then designed as

$$\tau = \tau_0 + \tau_s, \tag{7.32}$$

where τ_0 accounts for the model uncertainties and external disturbances, and τ_s regulates the desired trajectory. They are given by

$$\tau_0 = \widehat{M}\ddot{q}_r + \widehat{B}\dot{q}_r + \widehat{G} + \tau_d, \tag{7.33}$$

$$\tau_s = -K\arctan(S), \tag{7.34}$$

$$\dot{\widehat{\sigma}} = -\Gamma Y^T S, \tag{7.36}$$

where $K = diag[K_x, K_y, K_z]$ is a gain matrix, $\arctan(S)$ is the arctangent function for the sliding vector S, and Γ is a constant positive definite matrix. The vector $\dot{q}_r$ is obtained based on q and q_d, which is used to calculate the differential model estimated vector $\dot{\widehat{\sigma}}$, the torque vector τ_s, and the regression matrix Y. After a set of integration processes, the estimator $\widehat{\sigma}$ is updated for vector τ_0. The manipulator and moving stage move under the inputs of τ_0 and τ_s, while the position q is updated for the next movement, as shown in Fig. 7.14B.

The stability of the control system can be analyzed by introducing a Lyapunov function calculated with the estimated error $\widetilde{\sigma}$, described as

$$V = \frac{1}{2}S^T MS + \frac{1}{2}\widetilde{\sigma}^T \Gamma^{-1} \widetilde{\sigma}. \tag{7.36}$$

Differentiating V with respect to time and considering the skew-symmetric property of the Lagrangian formulation (Slotine and Li, 1987) yield the following equation:

$$\begin{aligned} \dot{V} &= -S^T \tau_s - S^T Y \sigma + \sigma^T \Gamma^{-1} \dot{\sigma} \\ &= -\sum_{axis=x,y,z} K_{axis} S_{axis} \arctan(S_{axis}). \end{aligned} \tag{7.37}$$

Given K_x, K_y, and K_z are positive, $K_{axis}S_{axis} \arctan(S_{axis}) \geq 0$ for any S. Therefore, $\dot{V} \leq 0$, and the motion controller Eqs. (7.32–7.35) can drive the micropipette to the destination position without interferences to the model uncertainties and external disturbances.

7.3.2 Experiments

7.3.2.1 3D reconstruction of organelles

To demonstrate the accuracy of the image reconstruction method, a robotic WFFM system was used to generate 3D reconstructed models of intracellular organelles, and the results were then compared with those obtained by the CFM. Biological specimens are largely transparent to visible light. To obtain high-contrast images at different sampling depths, neonatal human dermal fibroblasts (HDFn) were stained with Hoechst (Invitrogen, nucleic acid probes) to prevent genotoxicity by appropriate dye concentration and luminous flux (Purschke et al., 2010; Kakasi et al., 2012). In the tests, cells in movement were solidly trapped in the microfluidic channel during the intermittence between the robotic manipulation system and confocal fluorescence microscopy, as shown in Fig. 7.15A. For a comparison of the reconstruction performance, an assessment metric named discriminated point ratio (DPR) was used, which was defined as

$$DPR = \frac{DPN}{TPN}, \tag{7.38}$$

where DPN is the discriminated number of the reconstructed models of the two microscopes, and TPN represents the total pixel number in the 3D space.

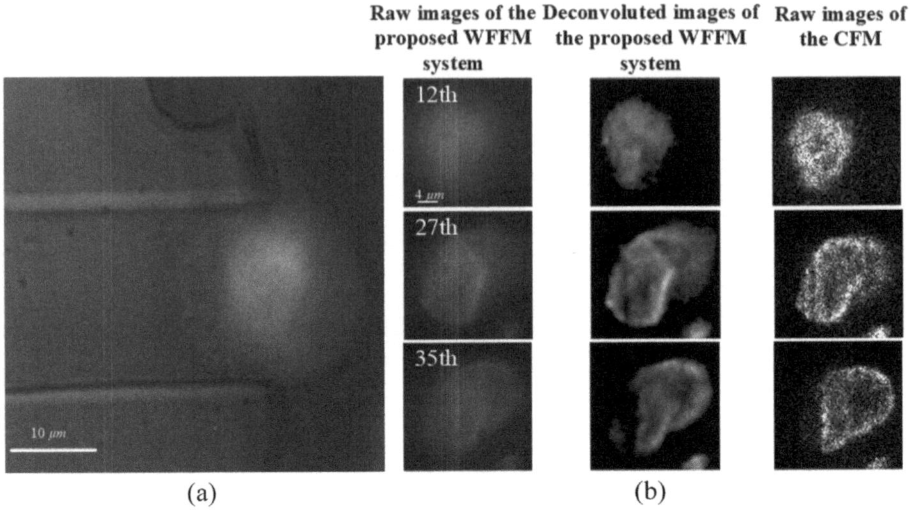

Figure 7.15 Trapped HDFn cell (Gao et al., 2020). (A) HDFn nucleus stained with Hoechst. (B) Comparison of the processed images of WFFM in the proposed system and CFM.

In each observation, 50 images were sampled with a lens step size of 0.4 μm. For WFFM, a water-immersed objective lens with a pixel size of 0.123 μm and 60× magnification, similar to that of confocal measurements, was used. Fig. 7.15B shows the region containing the nucleus of the three sampled images in planes with different optical heights. Compared with images sampled by confocal microscopy, the raw images from WFFM were corrupted by noises and out-of-focus blurs. However, most of these corruptions were eliminated by the proposed deconvolution algorithm, and the processed images matched the confocal results well. Fig. 7.16A shows the y−z section of two measurements. Fig. 7.16C and D present the normalized intensity profiles along two certain characteristic lines of the two y−z section images. These results were in good agreement, reflecting that the processed images also had feature restoration along the height direction. Image series in the proposed WFFM system and CFM were reconstructed into similar 3D models, as shown in Fig. 7.16B. The DPN of the two models was 1.76%. These results demonstrated the accuracy of the proposed reconstruction method and its capability of providing intracellular delivery with 3D information.

7.3.2.2 Intracellular delivery tests

The intracellular delivery tests were performed on HDFn. Cells were cultured in Dulbecco's modified Eagle medium (DMEM) mixed with 10% fetal bovine serum (FBS). Before experiments, cells were stained with Hoechst and Fluo-4 Calcium Imaging (Invitrogen, Cell Viability Probe) with emission wavelengths of 461 and 526 nm, respectively. The cells were then detached enzymatically from the culturing dish and trapped in the microfluidic chip by negative pressure. The chip was bonded to the coverslip with a thickness of 0.17 mm and a refractive index of 1.59 and sterilized

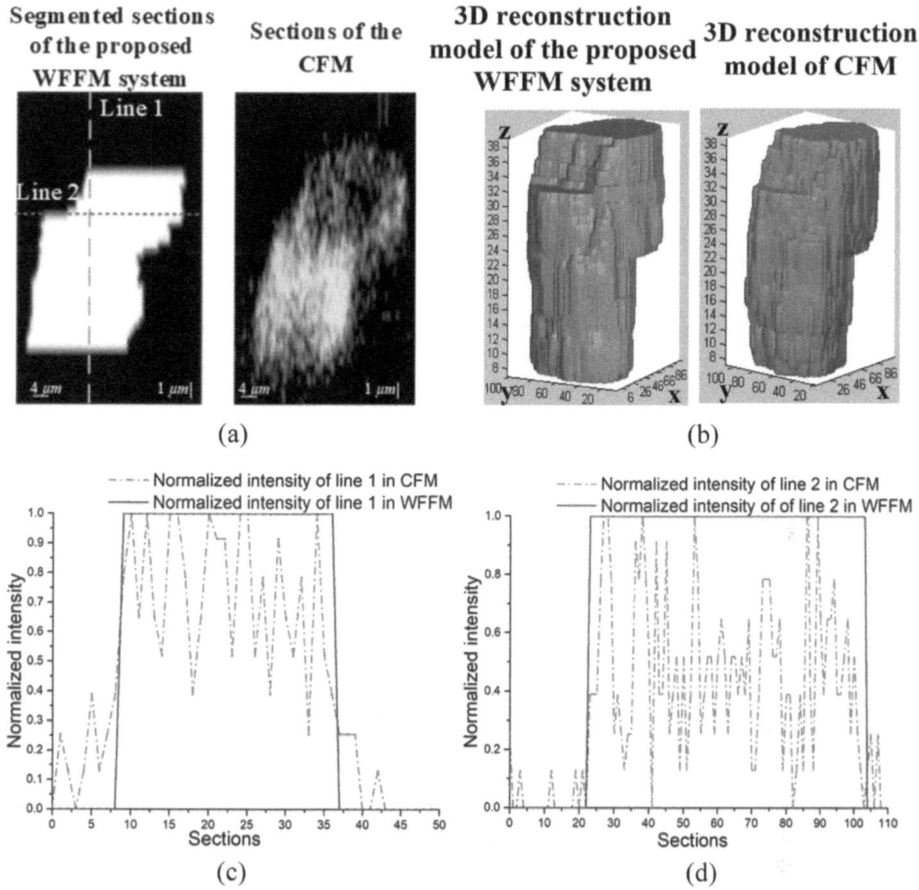

Figure 7.16 Processing images of two microscopes (Gao et al., 2020). (A) y−z sections of image series in the proposed WFFM system and CFM. (B) Reconstructed 3D model of two microscopes. (C) Intensity profile of the selected feature line 1 in y−z section. (D) Intensity profile of the selected feature line 2 in y−z plane.

under UV light for 30 min before cell trapping. The micropipette was loaded with the hydrophilic tracker dextran-tetramethylrhodamine with 1 mg/mL concentration, 580 nm emission wavelength, and 70,000 Da molecular weight to verify the delivery performance. The high molecular weight ensured that the tracker could not pass through the nuclear membrane once it was injected into the cytoplasm.

Note that the microchannel trapping will not produce harmful effects on cell viability for several reasons. First, the microfluidic chip was made of PDMS (polydimethylsiloxane), which was a widely used nontoxic and biocompatible material. Second, once the PDMS material and cells were in contact, they created an adhesive force between them. In the tests, the negative trapping pressure was set at less than 100 Pa, which rarely deformed trapped cells during fixation. Third, most trapping cells attached to the substrate 24 h after the delivery process. Therefore, the harmful effects on the trapping cells in the microfluidic channel can be negligible.

Calibrating the relative position of the micropipette and the focal plane was crucial at the beginning of experiments. The micropipette tip was driven to contact the cover-slip and the focal plane, and the height of the focal plane and the 3D tip position were recorded at the same time. The objective lens was then moved upward with a step size of 0.4 μm. The system used a 60× objective lens immersed with water and a CCD camera with a pixel resolution of 0.123 μm. After each movement, a section image was sampled with a size of 640 × 480 pixels and saved in the system. A total of 50 images were sampled, as shown in Fig. 7.17.

To reduce the complexity, the ROI containing the selected organelle was chosen automatically. The system selected the image with the highest optical density (which was the 18th image) and binarized the image using a threshold. The binarized image was fitted with a bounding box, which recorded the center position and the side length. The ROI area was a square centered on the center of the bounding box, and its side length was longer than the long side of the bounding box, as shown by the ROI box in Fig. 7.17. All sampled images were cropped with the ROI with a size of 170 × 170 pixels and then gray-scaled, as shown in Fig. 7.18A. The NRMLE method

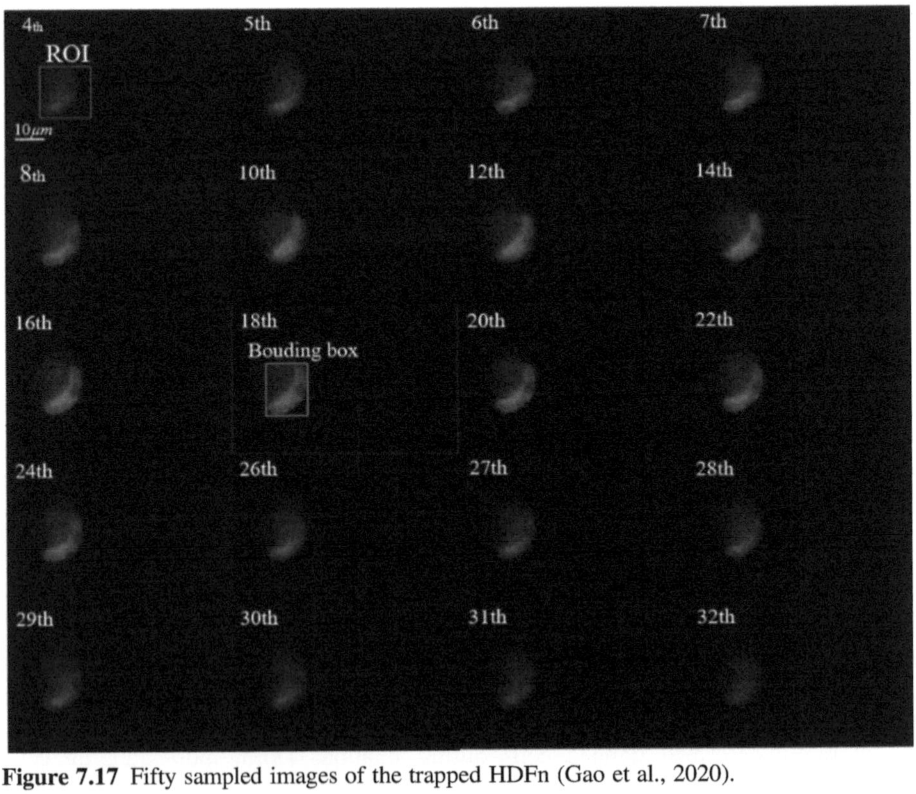

Figure 7.17 Fifty sampled images of the trapped HDFn (Gao et al., 2020).

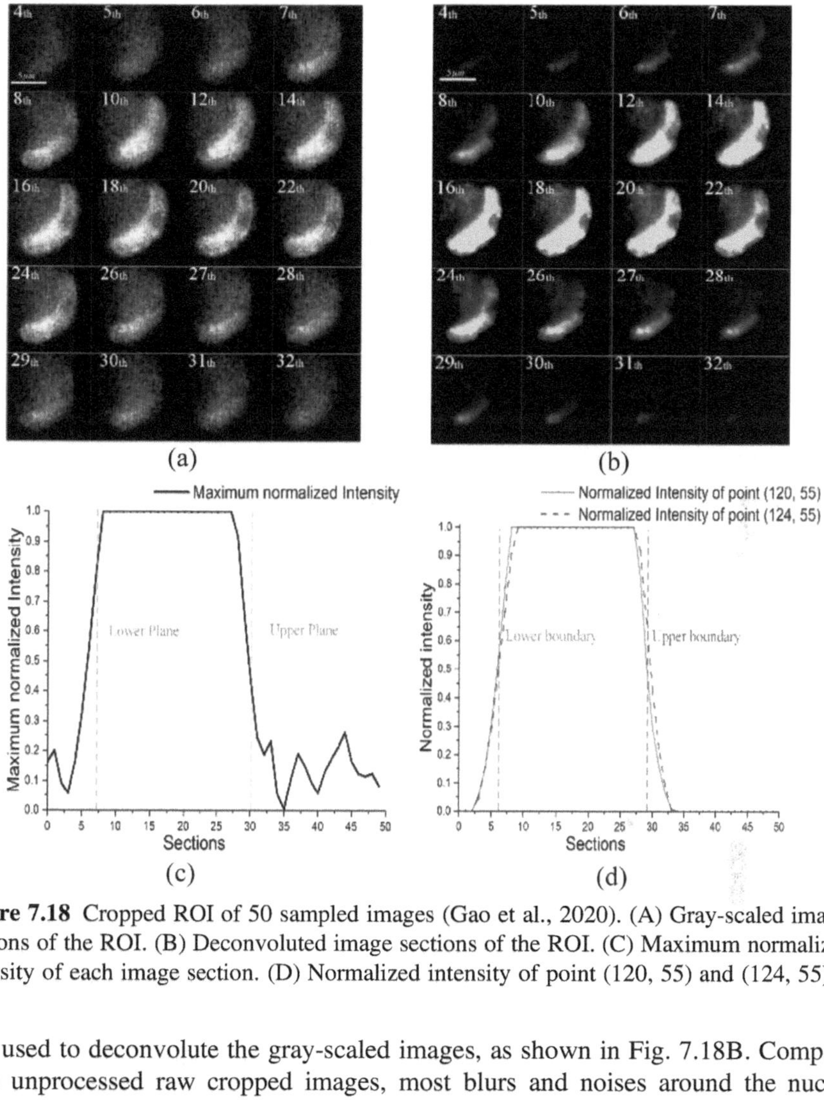

Figure 7.18 Cropped ROI of 50 sampled images (Gao et al., 2020). (A) Gray-scaled image sections of the ROI. (B) Deconvoluted image sections of the ROI. (C) Maximum normalized intensity of each image section. (D) Normalized intensity of point (120, 55) and (124, 55).

was used to deconvolute the gray-scaled images, as shown in Fig. 7.18B. Compared with unprocessed raw cropped images, most blurs and noises around the nucleus were removed. After that, the deconvoluted images were segmented. Before segmentation, the filter process was used to avoid the segmentation of image planes without objects, which included the following steps. First, the maximum grayscale intensity of all section images was scanned and then one lower and one upper plane were selected with the largest maximum intensity difference with neighboring planes as well as their maximum intensity position. In this case, the seventh and the 30th images were the lower and upper planes, respectively, as shown in Fig. 7.18C. Points (120, 55) and (124, 55) were the maximum positions in the two planes. Second, intensity profiles of such two points are analyzed among deconvoluted image sections, as shown in Fig. 7.18D. The sixth image is selected as the lower boundary, which had the largest intensity difference in the point (120, 55) profile. The 29th image was the upper boundary derived from point (124, 55) profile. The section images from the 6th to 29th were segmented, as shown in Fig. 7.19A. A 3D model was generated based on the segmentation results, and the time consumption for the whole image processes was within 20 s. The 18th image was the plane with the largest section area. The upper volume V_u was larger than the lower volume V_l. The balance plane was on the 16th image, in which an ellipse was fitted, as shown in Fig. 7.19B. The center of the fitted ellipse was (87, 86) and selected as the optimal delivery point in this case.

Fig. 7.20 illustrates the delivery process to the nucleus after the optimal delivery position was determined. Fig. 7.20A shows that the micropipette was moved vertically to place its tip on the target plane. The tip with a diameter of less than 1 μm was then moved horizontally to align with the delivery point, as shown in Fig. 7.20B. Fig. 7.20C shows that the micropipette penetrated the cytoplasm and nucleus membrane and reached the delivery point. Meanwhile, a positive pressure of 1 psi was provided to push the interior dextran-tetramethylrhodamine. After that, the micropipette was retrieved to the original position and the cell remained intact, as shown in Fig. 7.20D. Fig. 7.20E shows the delivery result, in which dextran was solely delivered into the nucleus and no residual was observed in the cytoplasm. Notably, the nucleus rarely moved laterally during the delivery process owing to the resistance force from surrounding components.

The designed robust controller was examined during the delivery process. The control gains were selected by using the trial-and-error method based on two principles. First, the diagonal elements in matrix K should not be large, in order to avoid large overshoots. Second, the magnitude of Γ was chosen to obtain a proper converging

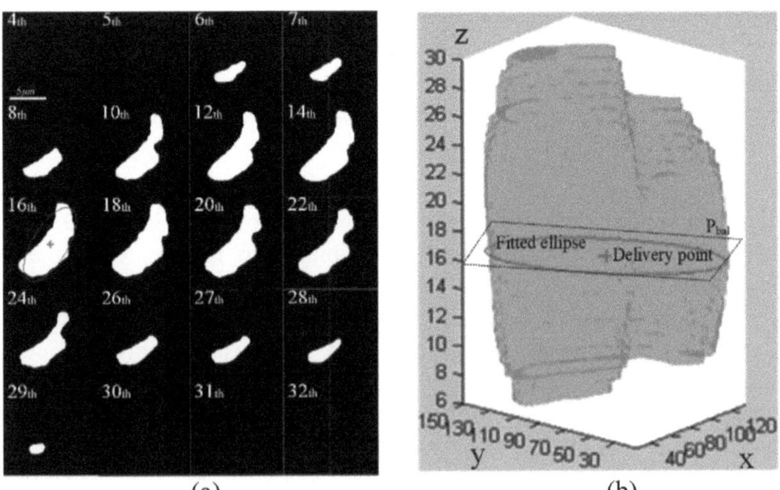

Figure 7.19 Reconstruction processes of the deconvoluted image sections (Gao et al., 2020). (A) Segmentation results of the deconvoluted image sections. (B) Reconstructed 3D model with optimal delivery position from model analysis.

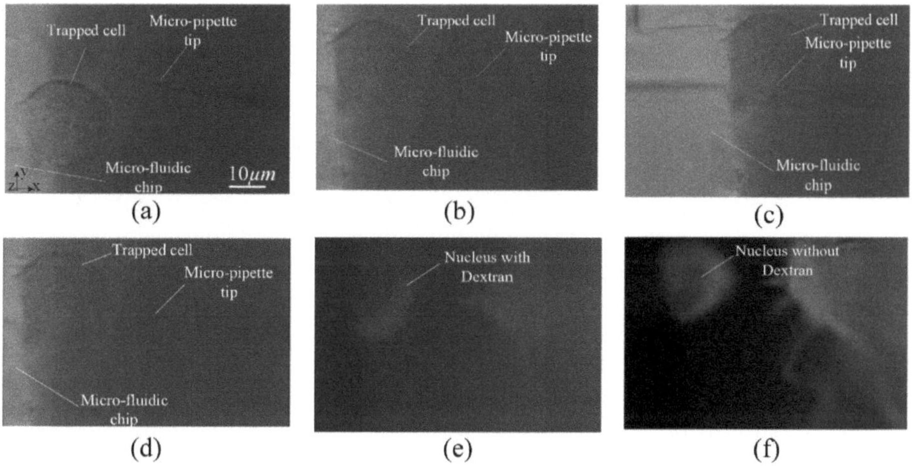

Figure 7.20 Delivery process of the trapped HDFn (Gao et al., 2020). (A) Height adjustment of the pipette tip. (B) Pipette alignment with the delivery position along the y-axis. (C) Penetration movement along the x-axis to conduct the delivery task. (D) Retrieval of the pipette. (E) Successful delivery to the nucleus with 3D information. (F) Delivery to the cytoplasm that frequently occurred with 2D information.

speed. In the experiments, the initial system parameter estimator was set to $\sigma_0 = 0$, the gain $K_{axis} = 1.35$, $\varepsilon = 5$, and the magnitude of matrix $\Gamma = 3.3 \times 10^{-7}$. After unit transformation between pixels and micrometers, the initial micropipette position was (40.86, 22.72, 0) μm while the optimal destination point of the nucleus was (22.11, 38.75, 6.40) μm. The micropipette was adjusted to its height along the z-axis within 1.2 s, with a position error of 0.05 μm, as shown in Fig. 7.21A. The moving stage then moved along the y-axis to align the pipette tip with the destination point laterally. After the tip and destination coincided, the moving stage was driven along the x-axis. Fig. 7.21B illustrates this process, in which the micropipette reached (40.86, 38.66, 6.45) μm and the position error along the y-axis was −0.09 μm. When the hover

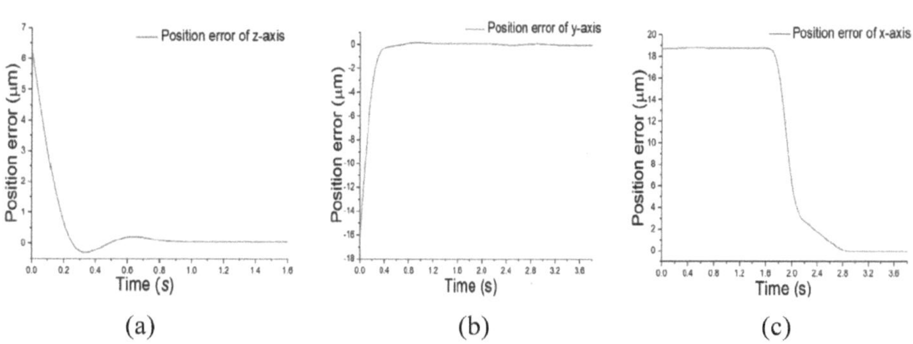

Figure 7.21 Position errors of the controllers during the delivery experiments (Gao et al., 2020). (A) Position error of the z-axis. (B) Position error of the y-axis. (C) Position error of the x-axis.

movement was around the destination point, considerable damage was inflicted on the cell. The moving stage was stopped once the position error was less than 0.1 μm. Finally, the micropipette was moved to (22.06, 38.72, 6.45) μm, with the position errors of −0.05, −0.03, and 0.05 μm along the x-, y-, and z-axes, respectively.

Delivery experiments without the 3D reconstruction information were also conducted for comparison. In the 2D experiment, normal practice was that the micropipette was initially aligned with the trapped cell vertically and then maintained on this initially focused plane for succeeding experiments. The delivery efficiency was summarized in Table 7.3. The positive success rate (PSR) was defined as the ratio between the number of dextran cells delivered into the nucleus and the total number of cells. The negative success rate (NSR) accounted for the case in which the fluorescent medium was delivered into the cytoplasm. The fail rate (FR) indicated the case in which no fluorescence was pushed out and inside the cell. The test results showed that the overall PSR of 3D experiments was 71%, which was much higher than the 48% obtained with 2D experiments. The NSR of 2D experiments accounted for a large proportion of 33% and more than 17% of 3D experiments. Fig. 7.21F shows a case where only the fluorescent medium was injected into the cytoplasm and no fluorescence was observed in the nuclear space. Improper delivery locations in 2D experiments can easily lead to failure of nuclear membrane injection. Moreover, the FR of 3D experiments was 12%, while that of 2D experiments was 19%. Similarly, failure usually occurred when the tip of the pipette was blocked by an intracellular organelle and no internal medium was pushed out. In the 2D experiments, the height of the pipette tip was fixed, which may not be appropriate for most cell membrane penetration attempts, therefore it was easy for the pipette tip to become clogged. Therefore, finding an optimal plane from 3D image reconstruction was important for successful delivery.

Calcium flux is an effective marker of cell viability (Actis et al., 2013), and it drops sharply in severely damaged cells (Shakoor et al., 2019). All cells were stained with Fluo-4 Calcium Imaging before delivery experiments. Fig. 7.22A demonstrates the calcium flux image before and after the delivery process. The intensity of green fluorescence remained approximately stable after delivery experiments, indicating that the damage to the processed cells was negligible. The ability of HDFn to attach after delivery should be further evidence of cell survival (Shakoor et al., 2019). The survival rate was defined as the ratio between the number of cells that can attach and the total number of cells. Fig. 7.22B illustrates the cell status at 24 h incubation after delivery. The survived cells exhibited normal shape and were attached to the coverslip substrate,

Table 7.3 Delivery experimental results (Gao et al., 2020).

Method	Number	PSR (%)	NSR (%)	FR (%)
3D info	100	71	17	12
2D info	100	48	33	19

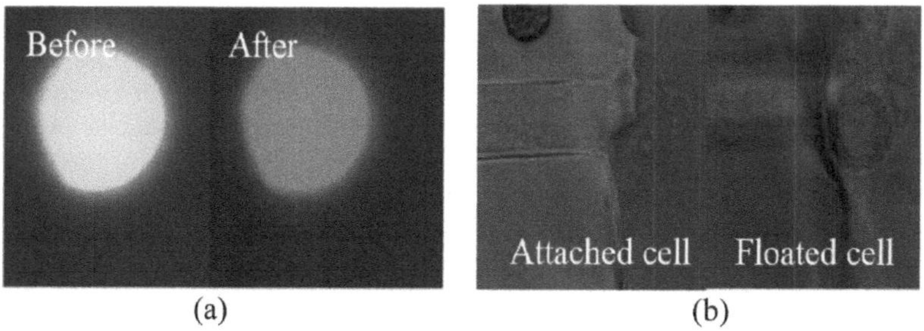

Figure 7.22 Cell validity test after intracellular delivery (Gao et al., 2020). (A) Calcium imaging of the cells before and after the delivery experiment. (B) Cell status at 24 h after experiments.

while damaged cells were detached from the substrate and suspended in the culture medium. The survival rate for HDFn was approximately 85%, indicating the feasibility of the proposed approach.

7.4 Conclusions

This chapter introduced 3D image reconstruction technologies for intracellular surgery using a robot-assisted microscopy system. First, a 3D image reconstruction method was introduced, which utilizes the objective lens movement to sample the targeted cells optically. The sampled optical sections are then deconvoluted by the maximum likelihood estimation-based deconvolution algorithm, which uses multiple PSFs in combination with a noise regulation function. A localized region-based segmentation algorithm is utilized to obtain a clear boundary, and a volume-rendering method is proposed to obtain a 3D reconstruction model of the specimen. Experimental results illustrate the effectiveness of the presented approach by using simulated spheres with various noise levels and measuring fluorescence microspheres with a specific dimension. Second, a precise intracellular delivery method with 3D image reconstruction information is introduced. The 3D model is reconstructed with the segmented sections. The optimal delivery position is derived from the volume-based model in the geometric analysis of the reconstructed model. Based on this position, a robust controller is proposed to drive the moving stage and the micropipette tip to execute the delivery task without the influence of external disturbances. Reconstruction tests on the nucleus of HDFn are conducted, and the results are compared with a confocal microscope to show the improvement of accuracy of the proposed method. Intracellular nucleus delivery experiments are successfully conducted using the proposed system with 3D reconstruction information. The delivery performance exhibits remarkable advantages over existing methods without the use of 3D information. In summary, the 3D image reconstruction method for intracellular surgery has great potential for various biomedical applications requiring precise delivery.

References

Actis, P., Maalouf, M.M., Kim, H.J., Lohith, A., Vilozny, B., Seger, R.A., Pourmand, N., 2013. Compartmental genomics in living cells revealed by single-cell nanobiopsy. ACS Nano 8 (1), 546–553.

Anokye-Danso, F., Trivedi, C.M., Juhr, D., Gupta, M., Cui, Z., Tian, Y., Zhang, Y., Yang, W., Gruber, P.J., Epstein, J.A., Morrisey, E.E., 2012. Highly efficient miRNA-mediated reprogramming of mouse and human somatic cells to pluripotency. Cell Stem Cell 11 (6), 853.

Arigovindan, M., Shaevitz, J., McGowan, J., Sedat, J.W., David, A., Agard, D.A., 2010. A Parallel Product-Convolution approach for representing the depth varying Point Spread Functions in 3D widefield microscopy based on principal component analysis. Opt. Express 18 (7), 6461.

Bodles-Brakhop, A.M., Heller, R., Draghia-Akli, R., 2009. Electroporation for the delivery of DNA-based vaccines and immunotherapeutics: current clinical developments. Mol. Ther. 17 (4), 585–592.

Braude, P., Pickering, S., Flinter, F., Ogilvie, C.M., 2002. Preimplantation genetic diagnosis. Nat. Rev. Genet. 3 (12), 941–953.

Cartagena-Rivera, A.X., Logue, J.S., Waterman, C.M., Chadwick, R.S., 2016. Actomyosin cortical mechanical properties in nonadherent cells determined by atomic force microscopy. Biophys. J. 110 (11), 2528–2539.

Chan, P., Dinniwell, R., Haider, M.A., Cho, Y.B., Jaffray, D., Lockwood, G., Levin, W., Lee, M., Fyles, A., Milosevic, M., 2008. Inter- and Intrafractional tumor and organ movement in patients with Cervical cancer undergoing radiotherapy: a cinematic-MRI point-of-interest study. Int. J. Radiat. Oncol. Biol. Phys. 70 (5), 1507–1515.

Chow, Y.T., Chen, S., Liu, C., Liu, C.C., Li, L., Kong, C.W., Cheng, S.H., Li, R.A., Sun, D., 2016. A high throughput automated microinjection system for human cells with small size. IEEE/ASME Trans. Mechatron. 21 (2), 838–850.

Conchello, J., Hansen, W., 1990. Enhanced 3-D reconstruction from confocal scanning microscope images 1: deterministic and maximum likelihood reconstructions. Appl. Opt. 29 (26), 3795–3804.

Conchello, J., McNally, J.G., 1996. Fast regularization technique for expectation maximization algorithm for optical sectioning microscopy. In: Three-Dimensional Microscopy: Image Acquisition and Processing III.

Dey, N., Blanc-Feraud, L., Zimmer, C., Rous, P., Kam, Z., Olivo-Marin, J.C., Zerubia, J., 2006. Richardson–Lucy algorithm with total variation regularization for 3D confocal microscope deconvolution. Microsc. Res. Tech. 69 (4), 260–266.

Dias, A.P., Dufu, K., Lei, H., Reed, R., 2010. A role for TREX components in the release of spliced mRNA from nuclear speckle domains. Nat. Commun. 1, 97.

Ding, X., Stewart, M.P., Sharei, A., Weaver, J.C., Langer, R.S., Jensen, K.F., 2017. High-throughput nuclear delivery and rapid expression of DNA via mechanical and electrical cell-membrane disruption. Nat Biomed Eng. 1, 39.

Esmaeilsabzali, H., Sakaki, K., Dechev, N., Burke, R.D., Park, E.J., 2011. Machine vision-based localization of nucleic and cytoplasmic injection sites on low-contrast adherent cells. Med. Biol. Eng. Comput. 50 (1), 11–21.

Gao, W., Shakoor, A., Xie, M., Chen, S., Guan, Z., Zhao, L., Jiang, Z., Sun, D., 2020. Precise automated intracellular delivery using a robotic cell microscope system with three-dimensional image reconstruction information. IEEE/ASME Trans. Mechatron. 25 (6), 2870–2881.

Gao, W., Shakoor, A., Zhao, L., Jiang, Z., Sun, D., 2019. 3-D image reconstruction of biological organelles with a robot-aided microscopy system for intracellular surgery. IEEE Robot. Autom Lett. 4 (2), 231–238.

Gibson, S., Lanni, F., 1991. Experimental test of an analytical model of aberration in an oil-immersion objective lens used in three-dimensional light microscopy. J. Opt. Soc. Am. A 8 (10), 1601.

Goodd, I., Gaskins, R.A., 1971. Nonparametric roughness penalties for probability densities. Biometrika 58 (2), 255–277.

Guillaume-Gentil, O., Potthoff, E., Ossola, D., Dörig, P., Zambelli, T., Vorholt, J.A., 2013. Microfluidics: force-controlled fluidic injection into single cell nuclei. Small 9 (11), 1870.

Hadj, S.B., Blanc-Féraud, L., 2011. Restoration method for spatially variant blurred images. INRIA 7654.

Huang, H., Sun, D., Mills, J.K., Cheng, S.H., 2009. Robotics cell injection system with position and force control: towards automatic batch biomanipulation. IEEE Trans. Robot. 25 (3), 727–737.

Kakasi, B., Kováts, N., S. Nagy, S., 2012. Assessment of the genotoxic potential of Hoechst 33342, SYBR-14 and PI using the SOS ChromoTest™. Biotech. Histochem. 87 (5), 372–375.

Kaufman, A., Mueller, K., 2005. Overview of Volume Rendering. Visualization Handbook. Academic Press, New York, USA, pp. 127–174.

Kee, H., Dishinger, J., Blasius, T.L., Liu, C., Margolis, B., Verhey, K., 2012. A size-exclusion permeability barrier and nucleoporins characterize a ciliary pore complex that regulates transport into cilia. Nat. Cell Biol. 14 (4), 431–437.

Lankton, S., Tannenbaum, A., 2008. Localizing region-based active contours. IEEE Trans. Image Process. 17 (11), 2029–2039.

Li, J., Li, X., Luo, T., Wang, R., Liu, C., Chen, S., Li, D., Yue, J., Cheng, S.H., Sun, D., 2018. Development of a magnetic microrobot for carrying and delivering targeted cells. Sci. Robot. 3 (19), eaat8829.

Liu, J., Siragam, V., Gong, Z., Chen, J., Fridman, M.D., Leung, C., Lu, Z., Ru, C., Xie, S., Luo, J., Hamilton, R.M., Sun, Y., 2015. Robotic adherent cell injection for characterizing cell–cell communication. IEEE Trans. Biomed. Eng. 62 (1), 119–125.

Lorensen, W., Cline, H.E., 1987. Marching cubes: a high resolution 3D surface construction algorithm. In: Proc. 14th Annual Conference on Computer Graphics and Interactive Techniques.

Markham, J., Conchello, J.A., 1997. Tradeoffs in regularized maximum-likelihood image restoration. In: Three-Dimensional Microscopy: Image Acquisition and Processing IV.

Montecalvo, A., Larregina, A.T., Shufesky, W.J., Stolz, D.B., Sullivan, M.L.G., Karlsson, J.M., Baty, C.J., Gibson, G.A., Erdos, G., Wang, Z., Milosevic, J., Tkacheva, O.A., Divito, S.J., Jordan, R., Lyons-Weiler, J., Watkins, S.C., Morelli, A.E., 2011. Mechanism of transfer of functional microRNAs between mouse dendritic cells via exosomes. Blood 119 (3), 756–766.

Monvel, J., Scarfone, E., Calvez, S.L., Ulfendahl, M., 2003. Image-adaptive deconvolution for three-dimensional deep biological imaging. Biophys. J. 85 (6), 3991–4001.

Pan, F., Chen, S., Jiao, Y., Guan, Z., Shakoor, A., Sun, D., 2020. Automated high-productivity microinjection system for adherent cells. IEEE Robot. Autom. Lett. 5 (2), 1167–1174.

Preza, C., Conchello, J.A., 2004. Depth-variant maximum-likelihood restoration for three-dimensional fluorescence microscopy. J. Opt. Soc. Am. A 21 (9), 1593.

Purschke, M., Rubio, N., Held, K.D., Redmond, R.W., 2010. Phototoxicity of Hoechst 33342 in time-lapse fluorescence microscopy. Photochem. Photobiol. Sci. 9 (12), 1634.

Sage, D., Donati, L., Soulez, F., Fortun, D., Schmit, G., Seitz, A., Guiet, R., Vonesch, C., Unser, M., 2017. DeconvolutionLab2: an open-source software for deconvolution microscopy. Methods 115, 28–41.

Shakoor, A., Xie, M., Luo, T., Hou, J., Shen, Y., Mills, J.K., Sun, D., 2019. Achieving automated organelle biopsy on small single cells using a cell surgery robotic system. IEEE Trans. Biomed. Eng. 66 (8), 2210–2222.

Sharei, A., Zoldan, J., Adamo, A., Sim, W.Y., Cho, N., Jackson, E., Mao, S., Schneider, S., Han, M.J., Lytton-Jean, A., Basto, P.A., Jhunjhunwala, S., Lee, J., Heller, D.A., Kang, J.W., Hartoularos, G.C., Kim, K.S., Anderson, D.G., Langer, R., Jensen, K.F., 2013. A vector-free microfluidic platform for intracellular delivery. Proc. Natl. Acad. Sci. U. S. A. 110 (6), 2082–2087.

Shaw, P.J., 2006. Comparison of widefield/deconvolution and confocal microscopy for three-dimensional imaging. Handb. Biol. Confocal Microsc. 453–467.

Shekaramiz, E., Varadarajalu, G., Day, P.J., Wickramasinghe, H.K., 2016. Integrated electrowetting nanoinjector for single cell transfection. Sci. Rep. 6, 29051.

Sibarita, J., 2005. Deconvolution microscopy. In: Proc. Microsc. Techn. Berlin, Germany, pp. 201–243.

Slotine, J.J.E., Li, W., 1987. On the adaptive control of robot manipulators. Int. J. Robot Res. 6 (3), 49–59.

Snyder, D.L., Hammoud, A.M., White, R.L., 1993. Image recovery from data acquired with a charge-coupled-device camera. J. Opt. Soc. Am. A 10 (5), 1014.

Sun, Y., Nelson, B.J., 2002. Biological cell injection using an autonomous microrobotics system. Int. J. Robot Res. 21, 861–868.

Tiedemann, M.V., Fridberger, A., Tomo, I., Monvel, J., 2006. Image adaptive point-spread function estimation and deconvolution for in vivo confocal microscopy. Microsc. Res. Tech. 69 (1), 10–20.

Wang, Y., Yang, Y., Yan, L., Kwok, S.Y., Li, W., Wang, Z., Zhu, X., Zhu, G., Zhang, W., Chen, X., Shi, P., 2014. Poking cells for efficient vector-free intracellular delivery. Nat. Commun. 5, 4466.

Wang, R., Chow, Y.T., Chen, S., Ma, D., Luo, T., Tan, Y., Sun, D., 2018. Magnetic force-driven in situ selective intracellular delivery. Sci. Rep. 8, 14205.

Wang, X., Ho, C., Tsatskis, Y., Law, J., Zhang, Z., Zhu, M., Dai, C., Wang, F., Tan, M., Hopyan, S., McNeill, H., Sun, Y., 2019. Intracellular manipulation and measurement with multipole magnetic tweezers. Sci. Robot. 4 (28), eaav6180.

Xie, Y., Sun, D., Liu, C., Tse, H.Y., Cheng, S.H., 2010. A force control approach to a robot-assisted cell microinjection system. Int. J. Robot Res. 29 (9), 1222–1232.

Xie, M., Shakoor, A., Shen, Y., Mills, J.K., Sun, D., 2019. Out-of-plane rotation control of biological cells with a robot-tweezers manipulation system for orientation-based cell surgery. IEEE Trans. Biomed. Eng. 66 (1), 199–207.

Zhang, B., Zerubia, J., Olivo-Marin, J.C., 2007. Gaussian approximations of fluorescence microscope point-spread function models. Appl. Opt. 46 (10), 1819.

Zhang, Y., Tan, K.K., Huang, S., 2009. Vision-servo system for automated cell injection. IEEE Trans. Ind. Electron. 56 (1), 231–238.

Cell sorting and separation

8

8.1 Introduction

In biological research and clinical medicine, sorting specific target cells from heterogeneous mixtures is an important process. Although conventional cell-sorting methods, such as gradient centrifugation, magnetically activated cell sorting, and fluorescence-activated cell sorting, are widely used given their mature engineering development and high-throughput advantages, these methods require the use of a large number of samples. In many applications, target cells such as stem cells or primary cells are rare and difficult to obtain.

Due to the many excellent properties of microfluidics, such as laminar flow, easy integration with mechanical, electrical, and optical systems, and low-cost manufacturing, microfluidics-based methodologies for cell sorting and manipulation have been extensively studied (Dittrich et al., 2006). Using the microfluidic cell sorter, a small number of samples can be processed, and the reagents used in this microenvironment are greatly reduced. In addition, the microfluidic cell sorter uses a closed platform, which can reduce infection of the sorted cells. The microfluidic chip technology allows the application of multiple force fields, which can be combined with the hydrodynamic force in microchannels to realize complex cell manipulations that are difficult to achieve with traditional large-scale cell sorters. Examples include the use of electric mechanisms (Yao et al., 2004), optical mechanisms (MacDonald et al., 2003), magnetic mechanisms (Ramadan et al., 2006), acoustic mechanisms (Petersson et al., 2005), and photoelectric mechanisms (Shah et al., 2009).

Microfluidic flow cytometry has attracted widespread attention for handling a small number of cells (Lenshof and Laurell, 2010). Most importantly, it can be applied to a variety of force fields, such as magnetic fields (Pamme and Manz, 2004), electric fields (Braschler et al., 2008), optical fields (Wang et al., 2011), and acoustic fields (Petersson et al., 2007), to combine the hydrodynamics in microchannels to realize multifunctional cell manipulations. One limitation of microfluidic flow cytometry is the snapshot of instant cell information during the examination, which makes it unsuitable for measuring dynamic cell responses over time. The other limitation of microfluidic flow cytometry is the random distribution of isolated cells in the collection container, which makes it difficult to further perform high-precision manipulations on these cells. Therefore, the cells must be removed from the collection container through a pipette or an output fluid interface, which may cause cell damage or cell loss. There is a need to develop an advanced manipulation tool that can isolate cells of interest from rare cell populations and deposit these separated cells accurately at a predetermined location.

To solve these problems, array-based platforms (such as microwell arrays) can be combined with programmable time-resolved live cell imaging to monitor the cellular

Robotic Cell Manipulation. https://doi.org/10.1016/B978-0-323-85259-3.00009-X

information of hydrodynamically restricted cells with high spatiotemporal resolution (Park et al., 2011; Skelley et al., 2009). Precise and dynamic manipulation of individual cells is a prerequisite for the development of such advanced manipulation tools in combination with the array-based platform. Of particular interest are optical manipulation methods that use scattering or gradient forces from a laser beam to push or trap cells in any preferred medium in a noninvasive manner. Kovac and Voldman (2007) used the scattering force of infrared lasers to make the cells of interest propagate along the light from the microfluidic microwell array to the flow field for collection. Optical tweezers use the gradient force exerted by a focused laser beam to precisely and dynamically manipulate dielectric particles or cells with pico-Newton force, which undoubtedly makes them one of the most attractive and functional tools in a number of biological applications (Tan et al., 2010; Hu and Sun, 2011; Chen and Sun, 2012). Wang et al. (2011) reported on a universal single-cell manipulation tool that integrates optical tweezers and microfluidic chip technologies to handle small-cell population sorting with high accuracy. Based on this work, Wang et al. (2013) further proposed an optical tweezers manipulation technology based on a uniquely designed microwell array to achieve a series of manipulation tasks, including identification, separation, assembly, transportation, and deposition cells of interest. Therefore, this tool is not only an independent cell sorter, but also an integrated cell operating system.

The separation and purification of cells is a necessary pretreatment process in disease diagnosis and treatment. Over the past few decades, various strategies have been adopted, such as DEP field flow separation (DEP-FFF) and 3D lateral DEP (LDEP) to accurately separate biological cells based on size differences (Park et al., 2005; Cheng et al., 2015; Han et al., 2011). In recent years, the DEP method has been used to isolate cells of similar size based on the difference in dielectric properties, such as human mesenchymal stem cells and their differentiated progeny (osteoblasts) (Song et al., 2015). Most reported DEP separators require a sheath flow or well-designed electrodes to actively prefocus the input cell mixtures to the side/center of the microfluidic channel before they enter the DEP separation zone. The use of sheath flow requires a complicated and cumbersome peripheral system for multichannel fluid control, and this requirement hinders integration of the DEP separation system with other microfluidic functions. In addition, the use of sheath buffer dilutes the sample and reduces the actual throughput of the sample processing (Kanai et al., 2004). Most existing electric prefocusing methods use dielectrophoresis or electroosmosis. Dielectrophoresis depends to a large extent on the DEP force of the particles and requires a well-designed electrode structure. Therefore, cell mixtures with large differences in size and dielectric properties are difficult to focus (Jen et al., 2011). Although electroosmosis can focus cells with different sizes and dielectric properties into the flow, the focusing efficiency is low when the flow rate is high (>1 μL/min), so its application in high-throughput sample processing remains limited (Ren et al., 2016). In this regard, passive nonsheathed cell prefocusing can be combined with active DEP separation to separate cells based on size and dielectric properties, with the advantages of simplicity, label free, and high throughput.

In many researches, the combination of passive and active methods can separate cells more efficiently. Porous flow fractionation is combined with dielectrophoresis to separate breast cancer cells from blood samples in a label-free and continuous manner (Sollier et al., 2014). However, this method is still based on the size difference between cancer cells and blood cells. The electrophoresis method is combined with the DEP method to perform size-based cell separation (Yan et al., 2015) and plasma separation (Yan et al., 2014) from diluted whole blood. This combination can control the lateral position of the particles by adjusting the external voltage without redesigning the microfluidic channel, which shows great flexibility. However, cell separation based on this combination still depends on size, and the prefocusing efficiency is highly dependent on the DEP response of the cell sample. By combining deterministic lateral displacement (DLD) and DEP technology, adjustable cell size and polarization rate and high-resolution separation can be achieved (Beech et al., 2009). The design and manufacturing accuracy of DLD chips depend to a large extent on the size distribution of cell samples. Dependence on the size of cells processed limits the flexibility of these methods for different samples.

Luo et al. (2018) proposed a method that combined gravity-sedimentation-based sheathless prefocusing and DEP separation in a simple microfluidic setup for the continuous separation of cells on the basis of size and dielectric property. This approach exhibits two unique advantages. First, from the perspective of sheathless focusing, this method utilizes the gravity sedimentation of cells in a tubing for the sheathless focusing of a cell mixture in a wide range of flow rates. Second, from the perspective of cell separation, this method utilizes an oblique interdigitated electrode array located at the bottom of the microchannel for the generation of a nonuniform electric field and production of a positive DEP force for cell manipulation.

The remainder of this chapter introduces three topics in cell sorting and separation. The first is the universal single-cell manipulation tool that integrates robotically controlled optical tweezers and microfluidic chip technology for handling small cell population sorting with high accuracy (Wang et al., 2011). The second is the automated cell manipulation tool with combined optical tweezers and microwell array, which functions for recognition, isolation, assembly, transportation, and deposition of the interesting cells (Wang et al., 2013). The third is the simplified sheathless cell separation approach that combines gravity-sedimentation-based sheathless prefocusing and DEP separation (Luo et al., 2018). Experiments and case studies are introduced for each part.

8.2 Cell sorting using combined optical tweezers and microfluidic chip technology

This section will introduce an active cell sorter, which consists of a microfluidic chip for cell focusing and optical tweezers for cell manipulation. Using digital image processing that recognizes multiple features such as size and fluorescence, target cells can be detected and identified based on intrinsic or extrinsic features of the cells. In order to successfully isolate target cells without focusing single-cell flow, optical tweezers are used to move these cells for a certain distance from the sample flow to the buffer flow.

These cells are then collected in the collection outlet. Yeast cells and human embryonic stem cells (hESC) are sorted separately to prove the effectiveness of the proposed cell sorter.

8.2.1 Methods

8.2.1.1 Operation principle and system setup

Fig. 8.1 shows a schematic diagram of the cell sorting procedure. The sample stream and the buffer stream are driven into the sorter from the upper and lower inlets, respectively, using the syringe pump. The CCD camera is used to capture the image when the cell passes through the region of interest (ROI). Digital image processing technology is used to detect and identify target cells. After detection and identification, an optical trap is positioned on the target cell and then moves the cell from the sample stream to the buffer stream. Multiple optical traps can also work on multiple cells at the same time. After the target cell reaches the desired destination, the optical trap releases the cell and the cell flows into the outlet for collection in the buffer stream. Other cells or particles flow into the outlet as waste together with the sample stream.

Fig. 8.2 shows the setup of a cell sorter that combines optical tweezers and a microfluidic chip. A holographic optical trapping device is used to engrave a continuous wave (CW) laser beam (V-106C-3000 OEM J series, Spectra Physics) with a wavelength of 1064 nm, and multiple optical traps can be created at the same time. After the laser beam is reflected by the dichroic mirror (DM1), it enters the microscope objective lens (Nikon 60X, numerical aperture = 1.2, water) to produce a three-dimensional optical trap. The microfluidic chip with biological samples is connected to a syringe pump (KDS 200P, KD Scientific) through tubing, and placed on a two-dimensional x−y motorized stage (ProScan, Prior Scientific) with a positioning accuracy of 15 nm. When the halogen lamp is on, the CCD camera can see the bright field of the microfluidic channel. The fluorescent image can be captured by turning on the

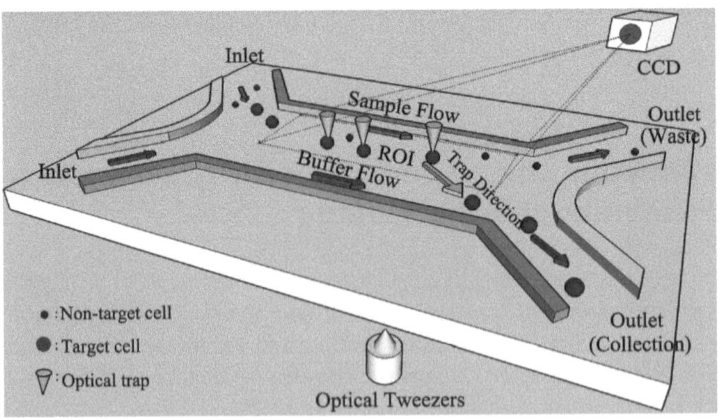

Figure 8.1 Schematic of the cell-sorting procedure (Wang et al., 2011).

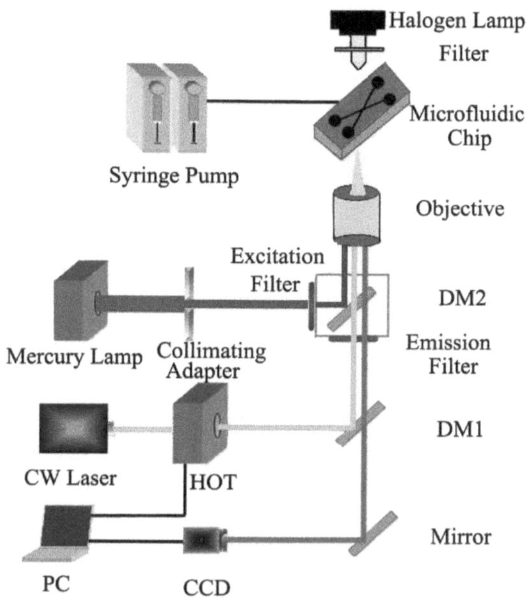

Figure 8.2 Cell sorter setup that combines optical tweezers and a microfluidic chip (Wang et al., 2011).

mercury lamp. The excitation beam of the mercury lamp is filtered by an excitation filter (450–490 nm), reflected by DM2 (500 nm), and then focused on the microfluidic channel by the objective lens. An emission filter (515 nm) is used to collect the fluorescence signal through the objective lens. A CCD camera with high sensitivity is used to capture fluorescence images. The location of target cells can be determined by digital image processing, and they serve as feedback to guide the sorting process. All mechanical parts are supported by the antivibration platform.

Fig. 8.3A illustrates the overall structure and size of an example microfluidic chip. The microfluidic cell sorter consists of four branches with two inlets and two outlets. The sample stream and buffer stream come from reservoirs A and B, respectively. The waste and target particles enter reservoirs C and D, respectively. The widths of the two

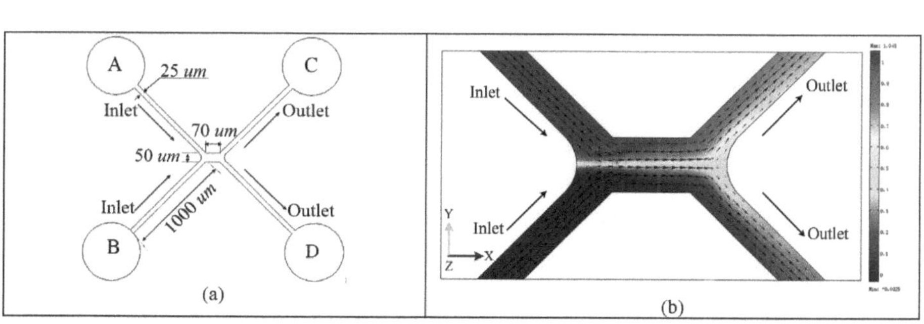

Figure 8.3 Microfluidic chip design (Wang et al., 2011). (A) Structure and dimension of the microfluidic chip. The *arrow* represents the flow direction within the microchannel. (B) Simulation of flow behavior of the designed microfluidic chip.

inlet channels and the two outlet channels are both 25 μm and the length is 1000 μm, and the width of the conjunction channel is 50 μm and the length is 70 μm. The diameter of the four containers is 1 mm. The height of the microchannel is 50 μm. In order to better understand the microenvironment inside the microfluidic chip, the MEMS module with "incompressible Navier–Stokes" and "convection and diffusion" application modes through the Comsol Multiphysics finite element program is used to simulate the flow behavior of fluid in microchannels. Fig. 8.3B shows the simulation results. The slice graph shows the concentration distribution of the flow. The sample flow from the upper inlet channel does not diffuse into the buffer flow from the lower inlet channel. The arrow graph represents the velocity distribution of laminar flow in the microchannel.

8.2.1.2 Target cell recognition with image processing

An image-processing method based on multiple cell characteristics is needed to identify target cells. In the following discussion, two characteristics are considered: cell size and fluorescent markers (such as GFP). The image-processing algorithm is applied to each frame of the CCD camera. Due to the mobility of target cells caused by fluid flow, the time for cell center-based image processing must be short enough that cell location information can be updated in time. Therefore, image processing is ideally suited to a small ROI, which can be done within the time interval (e.g., 33 ms) between consecutive frames. The two image-processing methods are described below.

Size-dependent method: If the size of the target cell is different from other cells, the cell can be detected based on the size difference. Fig. 8.4 illustrates the use of a size-dependent method to detect yeast cells from a mixture of beads and yeast cells. First,

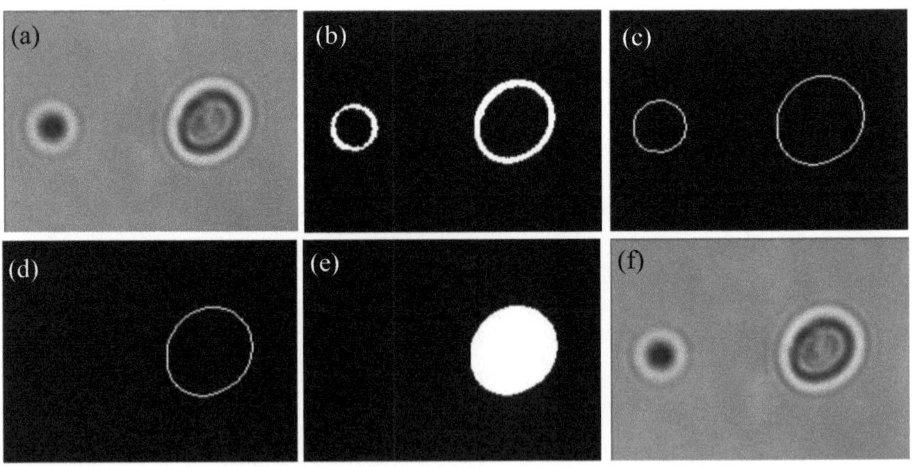

Figure 8.4 Separation of a yeast cell from a mixture of microbead and yeast cell using the size-dependent method (Wang et al., 2011): (A) original RGB image, (B) image after threshold segmentation, (C) contours of the particles, (D) removal of small contour, (E) filling the contour, and (F) center of the yeast cell.

the original color image in the ROI is converted into a grayscale image, and a threshold segmentation algorithm is used to separate the particles from the background. Then the outline of the particle from the binary image is identified. Depending on the size of the contour, the particle with smaller contour than the yeast cell is a microbead. Based on the outline of the target cell, the center of the cell can be calculated by the first-order moment of the filled contours.

Fluorescence-dependent method: When the size difference between the target cell and other particles is not sufficient to identify the target cell in the image processing, extrinsic features such as fluorescent label can be used for identification. Fig. 8.5 shows the result of identifying and locating cells with green fluorescent protein (GFP). The process of this fluorescence-dependent method is described as follows. Assume that the image is composed of low-frequency background, random noise, and fluorescent signals emitted from fluorescent proteins. The first step is to extract data from the green channel of the fluorescence image and correct it using a smoothing filter to increase the signal-to-noise ratio. The second step is to set an appropriate threshold according to the fluorescence intensity. After the image is binarized, the morphological opening operation (erosion and expansion) is used to eliminate the influence of small areas in the binary image.

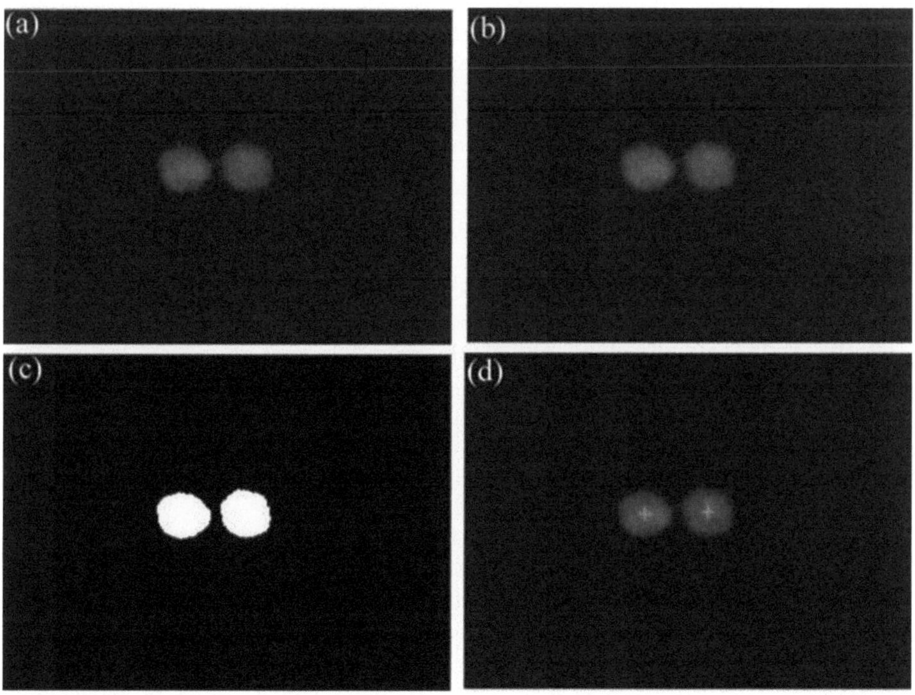

Figure 8.5 Separation of cells with GFP using the fluorescence-dependent method (Wang et al., 2011): (A) original fluorescence image, (B) green value after smoothing filter, (C) threshold and opening operation, and (D) center of the fluorescence cell.

8.2.1.3 Cell transportation by optical tweezers

After identifying the target cells, optical tweezers are used to transport the cells to the desired destination. In order to optimize the motion control of the optical traps in cell transportation, the cell motion dynamics is analyzed here.

When the target cell is trapped and moved by the optical tweezer, both the fluid drag force denoted by F_{drag} and the optical trapping force denoted by F_{trap} act on the cell simultaneously. The dynamics of the cell movement is

$$m\frac{d^2q}{dt^2} = F_{\text{trap}}(q) + F_{\text{drag}}(q), \tag{8.1}$$

where m denotes the mass of the cell, $q = [q_x, q_y]^{\mathrm{T}}$ is the central position of the cell, and t is the time interval determined by the frame rate of the camera. Given the velocity of the flow V_s, according to Stokes' law, the drag force F_{drag} can be expressed by

$$F_{\text{drag}}(q) = 6\pi\eta r_c\left(V_s - \frac{dq}{dt}\right), \tag{8.2}$$

where η is the fluid viscosity coefficient, and r_c is the radius of the cell. When the cell reaches the maximum velocity, its acceleration is zero, implying that the fluid drag force and optical trapping force are in equilibrium. Therefore, Eq. (8.1) can be simplified as follows:

$$\frac{dq}{dt} - V_s = \frac{F_{\text{trap}}(q)}{6\pi\eta r_c}. \tag{8.3}$$

Define the x coordinate direction as being along the direction of flow. The speed of the optical trap in the x direction is the same as the flow velocity. As a result, there is no need to apply a trapping force on the target cell in the flow direction. Due to the laminar nature of microflow, the fluid velocity perpendicular to the flow direction is zero. As a result, Eq. (8.3) is simplified as

$$\frac{dq_y}{dt} = \frac{F_{\text{trap}}\left(q_y\right)}{6\pi\eta r_c}. \tag{8.4}$$

In the y coordinate direction, the optical trap drives the target cell to move as fast as possible. The movement speed is determined to prevent cells from escaping from the optical trap (Wu et al., 2011). In the low range, the trapping force of the optical trap is approximately proportional to the laser power (Wright et al., 1994). When using 100 mW tweezers with a wavelength of 1064 nm, the temperature has been confirmed to increase by 1–2°C (Peterman et al., 2003). To avoid damage to the cell by the laser, the lowest possible laser power should be used.

The increase in the moving speed of the cell leads to an increase in operating efficiency. In order to effectively trap cells with low laser power, the relationship between the maximum cell moving speed and laser power should be calibrated. The viscous-drag-force technique can be used to determine the trapping force of optical tweezers (Wright et al., 1994). The maximum moving speed is determined by gradually increasing the moving speed of the cell until the cell escapes from the optical trap (Wang et al., 2011).

In applications that require fast-moving optical traps, it is beneficial to move the cell in steps of cell radius (Eriksson et al., 2007). Under this condition, Eq. (8.4) can then be modified as

$$\frac{r_c}{dt} = \frac{F_{\text{trap}}\left(q_y\right)}{6\pi\eta r_c}. \tag{8.5}$$

The movement of the target cell is shown in Fig. 8.6. An optical trap is generated at the cell position P_1. By combining the drag speed of the fluid and the trapping speed of the optical trap, the target cell quickly moves to the destination. At position P_2, the power of the optical trap is turned off, and the cell is released by the optical trap, and then moves to the collection outlet with the fluid flow.

8.2.2 Experiments

8.2.2.1 Isolation of yeast cells

The experiment of separating yeast cells from the mixture with microbeads was first conducted to evaluate the sorting performance of the proposed cell sorter. Both the sample stream and the buffer stream (deionized water) entered the microfluidic channel from two separate inlets. Yeast cells were defined as target particles and were collected in a collection reservoir. When the microbeads moved with the sample flow and passed through the ROI, they were identified as nontarget particles and flowed into the waste channel with the sample flow, as shown in Fig. 8.7A and B. When yeast cells passed

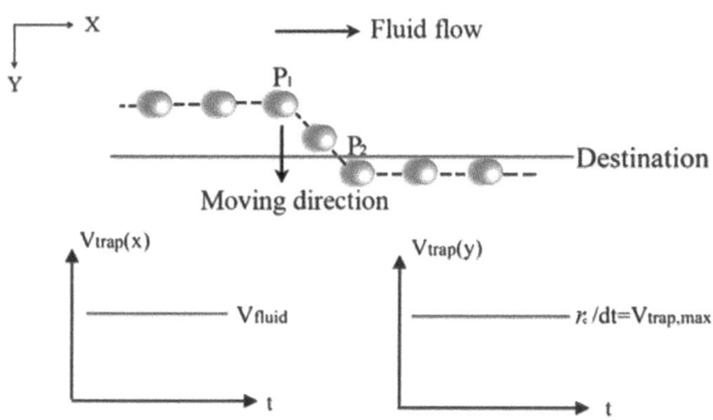

Figure 8.6 Motion analysis of the optical trap for cell transportation (Wang et al., 2011).

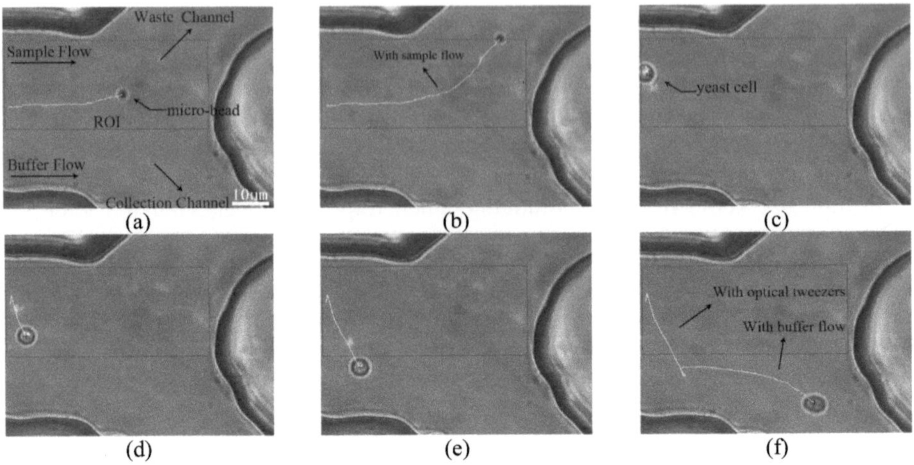

Figure 8.7 Isolation of yeast cells (Wang et al., 2011). (A, B) Trajectory of the microbead along the conjunction channel. The microbead flows into the waste channel with the sample flow. (C–F) Trajectory of the yeast cell along the conjunction channel. The yeast cell is separated from the sample flow using optical tweezers, and then flows into the collection channel with the buffer flow. (The light spot on the yeast cell is the optical trap.)

through the ROI, they were detected as target cells and moved away from the sample stream by optical tweezers. Finally, the yeast cells flowed into the collection channel driven by the buffer flow, as shown in Fig. 8.7C–F. In the experiment, the output laser power was set to 350 mW, and the yeast cells moved at a speed of 120 μm/s perpendicular to the flow direction.

To increase the throughput without affecting the purity and recovery rate, a multi-trap parallel sorting strategy can be used. In the cell sorter prototype made by Wang et al. (2011), five optical traps can be used to sort yeast cells, and two optical traps can be used to sort GFP-tagged hESCs. The maximum number of optical traps that can be used simultaneously depends on the cell type, cell concentration, and laser power limitations. The actual number of optical traps used depends on the number of target cells present in the ROI. Fig. 8.8 shows the experimental process of sorting

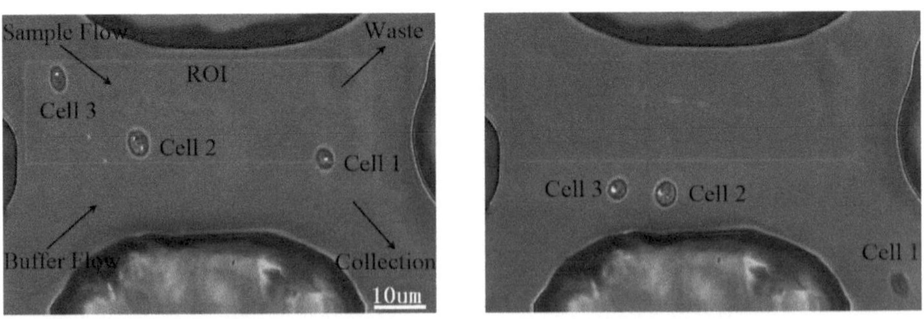

Figure 8.8 Multitrap parallel sorting (Wang et al., 2011). (The light spot on the yeast cell is the optical trap.)

multiple yeast cells using the multitrap parallel sorting strategy. In this test, three optical traps were generated at the same time to drive three yeast cells when the cells were identified in the ROI. After the yeast cells arrived in the desired destination, the optical traps were powered off so that the yeast cells were released from the optical traps and flowed into the collection channel together with the buffer.

Table 8.1 shows the results of the recovery rate and purity of yeast cells sorted using single-trap and multitrap sorting strategies in the experiments of Wang et al. (2011). A total of 438 particles (including 205 yeast cells) passed through the sorter at a throughput of 1 particle/s. A single optical trap can successfully isolate 199 of 205 yeast cells, with a recovery rate of 97%. In the collection reservoir, 199 yeast cells and four microbeads were recovered after sorting, indicating that the purity of the yeast cells was 98%. As the concentration increases, a multitrap parallel sorting strategy can be used, as shown in Table 8.1. Using multitrap parallel sorting, 1062 particles were sorted at a throughput of 5 particles/s, with a recovery rate of 94% and a purity of 96%. Although the recovery rate and purity of multitrap parallel sorting were worse than those of single-trap sorting, it can better fulfill the requirements of relatively high throughput.

8.2.2.2 Isolation of hESC

Tests were also conducted to isolate hESC from a mixture of different cells. As shown in Fig. 8.9A, the size of hESC is very similar to the sizes of other cells or particles in the mixture. Therefore, the size-dependent image-processing method cannot be used for this sorting application. In the experiment, the fluorescence-dependent image-processing method was used to identify target cells. Fig. 8.9B illustrates the target hESC with GFP. When the cells entered the ROI with the sample flow, the cell recognition process was deliberately optimized so that any target cells can be accurately identified. In the experiment, the fluorescence image was taken with a

Table 8.1 Sorting results (Wang et al., 2011).

Sample	Strategy	Concentration (particles/mL)	Total sorted particles	Recovery rate (%)	Purity (%)
Yeast cells plus microbeads	Single trap serial sorting	1.2×10^7	438	97	98
	Multitrap parallel sorting	5×10^7	1062	94	96
GFP tagged hESC plus nontagged cells	Multitrap parallel sorting	1×10^7	210	90	90

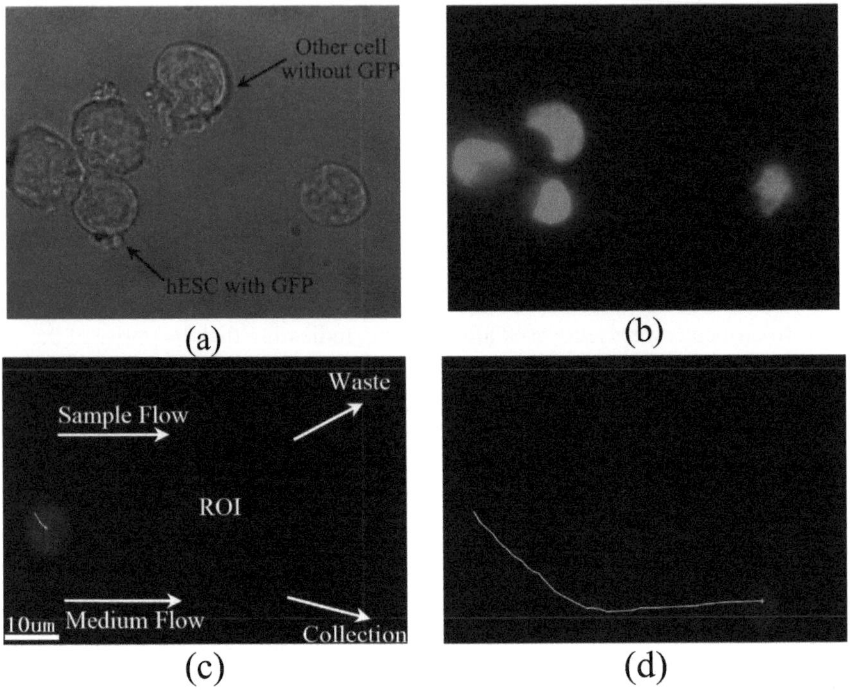

Figure 8.9 Results of hESC isolation (Wang et al., 2011). (A) Optical image of hESCs and other cells. (B) Fluorescence image of hECSs with GFP over a long exposure time (700 ms). (C) Cell recognition based on GFP. (D) hESCs with GFP are detected and driven into the collection channel, and the other cells without GFP flow into the waste channel.

short exposure time of 100 ms and the 2×2 grid merge mode was used, which can increase the acquisition rate of the CCD camera by reducing the image size. To increase the intensity of the GFP fluorescence image, a gain of 20× in the green channel was used. In this way, although the intensity of intracellular fluorescence was reduced due to the use of a short exposure time, the proposed fluorescence-dependent image processing method was still good enough for cell recognition. Given that the size of hESC (i.e., 10–15 μm) was much larger than that of yeast cells, a higher laser power (1.5 W) was used to provide sufficient trapping force to move hESC. The manipulation process was the same as in the isolation of yeast cells. As shown in Figs. 8.9C and D, hESCs with GFP were driven to the collection channel by the optical traps, and then flowed into the collection reservoir together with the medium flow. Other cells without GFP flowed into the waste channel with the sample stream. In the sorting process, two optical traps were generated simultaneously. After sorting, there were 26 hESCs with GFP and three other cells without GFP in the collection reservoir, and 178 cells without GFP and 3 hESCs with GFP in the waste reservoir. The results indicated that 90% recovery rate and 90% purity can be achieved, as shown in Table 8.1.

8.3 Cell isolation and deposition

This section introduces an automated cell manipulation tool that combines optical tweezers and a uniquely designed microwell array to identify, isolate, assemble, transport, and deposit cells of interest. The microwell array allows passive hydrodynamic docking of cells, while providing an opportunity to examine interesting cell phenotypes with high spatiotemporal resolution based on flexible image-processing techniques. In addition, dynamic and parallel cell processing in three dimensions can achieve the levitation of target cells through microwell and pattern assembly with multiple optical traps. Integrated with a programmed motorized stage, optically levitated and assembled cells can be transported and deposited into a predefined microenvironment. Therefore, this tool can facilitate the integration of other on-chip functions for further research without removing the isolated cells from the chip. Experiments with human embryonic stem cells (hESCs) and yeast cells have been performed to prove the effectiveness of the proposed cell manipulation tool.

8.3.1 Methods

The automated cell manipulation system is mainly composed of four modules: optical tweezers module, motorized stage module, computer vision module, and microfluidic chip module. The first three modules were introduced in Section 8.2. The microfluidic chip module is based on a microwell array and is manufactured by soft lithography (Xia and Whitesides, 1998). The microfluidic chip consists of two parts: the bottom microwell array layer and the top polydimethylsiloxane (PDMS, SYLGARD) fluid channel, as shown in Fig. 8.10A. A negative photoresist SU-8 (35 μm thick, 4000 rpm, SU-3050, MicroChem) is used to fabricate a microwell array on a cover glass (0.13−0.16 μm thick). Each microwell array has 80 microwells arranged in an 8×10 array. The separation distance between the two microwell arrays is 700 μm. The diameter of the microwell is designed to be 100 μm (with an interval of 100 μm) or 30 μm (with an interval of 40 μm). The master of the PDMS fluid channel is manufactured on a silicon wafer using the same SU-8 (100 μm thick, 1500 rpm). The individual microwell arrays for cell docking and cell deposition are connected by narrow channels on the PDMS fluid channel. There are five connected passages, and the length of each connected passage is designed to be 200 μm. The width of the two inlet channels for the sample flow and the specified medium is designed to be 500 μm, and the width of the other channels and connecting passage are designed to be 100 μm. By PDMS molding, the reverse structure of the master can be obtained. After punching holes at the inlets and outlets, the PDMS surface with fluid channels and the clean cover glass with microwell array are activated in oxygen plasma, and then precisely aligned and immediately bonded together to form an irreversible seal. The prototype of the microfluidic chip is shown in Fig. 8.10B.

Fig. 8.11 illustrates a schematic of a series of cell manipulation processes. The prepared suspended single cells are injected into the channel through the sample inlet and settled into the microwell array for cell docking, as shown in Fig. 8.11A. After loading,

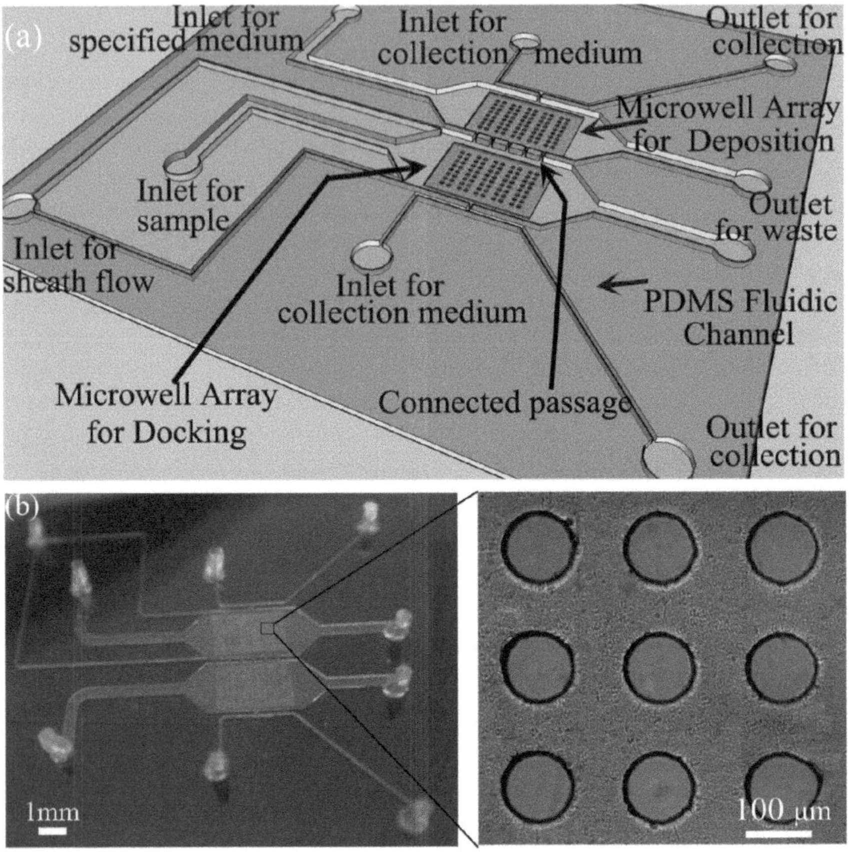

Figure 8.10 Microfluidic chip design (Wang et al., 2013). (A) The schematic design of the microwell array-based microfluidic chip. (B) The prototype of the designed microfluidic chip with microwell array.

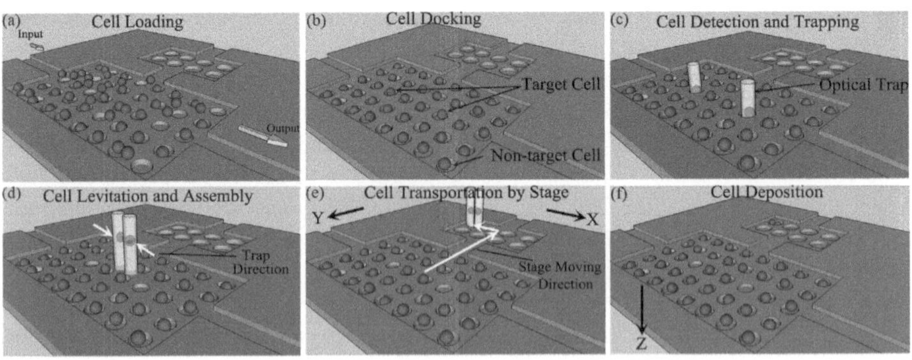

Figure 8.11 A schematic of a series of cell manipulation processes from cell loading to cell deposition (Wang et al., 2013).

the cells outside the microwells are cleared away by flowing the culture medium gently (Fig. 8.11B). After cell docking, image processing is performed for target cell detection, and optical traps are positioned on these recognized cells for cell trapping, as shown in Fig. 8.11C. Then, these optically trapped cells are levitated from the cell docking microwell by moving up the objective z stage and assembled into specific structure according to different further applications by dynamically moving multiple optical traps, as shown in Fig. 8.11D. Fig. 8.11E shows that the assembled cells are transported above the microwell array layer to the predefined target microwell by the programmed microscope x−y stage. Finally, the levitated cells with specific structure are deposited into the target microwell by moving down the objective z stage and releasing the optical traps, as shown in Fig. 8.11F.

By combining image-processing technology, the use of microwells as physical markers can accurately identify the spatial location of confined cells, which can be used as feedback to guide the automated manipulation process. In short, the first step in extracting cells in a microwell is to determine the spatial location of the microwell (Jain et al., 2009). The center of the microwell can be calculated from the outer contour of the filled microwell. According to the shape and size of the microwell, a corresponding binary microwell mask is formed in the center of the detected microwell. The bright-field image or the fluorescent image is convolved with the microwell mask, which can remove the extra part of the edge of the microwell. Then, through subsequent image processing, including thresholding to separate the cells from the background, segmentation to extract individual cells, and identification of cells with different phenotypes (external or internal features), the target cells can be detected and located in the marked microwell (Wang et al., 2011).

8.3.2 Operation procedures

A syringe pump can be used to pump the suspended cells into the microfluidic chip through the sample inlet at a flow rate of 1 μL/min. To focus the cells on the microwell array for cell docking, the medium flows through the sheath inlet at a flow rate of 0.3 μL/min. At the same time, fresh medium flows through the microwell array at a flow rate of 1 μL/min to deposit cells through the designated medium inlet. After the cells are distributed to the entire cell docking microwell array, the flow of all inlets is stopped for about 5 min to allow the cells to deposit in the cell docking microwell. Then fresh cell culture medium is pumped from all inlets at a flow rate of 0.4 μL/min to remove cells outside the cell docking microwell while still confining deposited cells in the microwell. After the cells are docked, all the liquid flowing from the injection port is stopped to perform the entire experiment in a static environment.

8.3.2.1 Cell levitation from a microwell

Although the holographic optical tweezers can perform three-dimensional cell operations, the levitated cell will be out of image focus even when the optical trap moves along the z direction only. An alternative method is introduced here, which can levitate the optically trapped cells while keeping them on the focal plane of the image for constant inspection. The operation process is divided into two steps. First, position the optical trap on the cell of interest, and the gradient force quickly drags the cell to the focus of the optical trap. Second, move the z stage of the objective lens upwards so that the optically trapped cells are levitated outside the microwell. In the experiment, the levitation distance is set to 50 μm, which is slightly larger than the height of the microwell (35 μm). Fig. 8.12A shows a schematic diagram of the levitation process of optical-trapping cells from the microwell by moving the objective *z* stage upward. As shown in Fig. 8.12B, two optical traps are used to levitate two hESCs from the microwell at the same time. On average, depending on the levitation distance and the moving speed of the objective lens z stage, it takes about 3 s to levitate the cells in the microwell.

8.3.2.2 Cell assembly by multiple optical traps

After successfully levitating the cells from the microwell, multiple optical traps are controlled to move these light-trapped cells to specific structures for further analysis or processing. To effectively transport the trapped cells without escaping from the optical trap, the optical trap should be calibrated according to the maximum moving speed of the cell and the optical trapping force under different laser powers. The maximum moving speed of the cell is defined as the speed at which the cell cannot be captured. The viscous-drag-force method can be used in a free-flowing environment to determine the maximum moving speed by gradually increasing the moving speed of the motorized stage until the cell escapes from a fixed optical trap (Wu et al., 2013; Wright et al., 1994). In the horizontal plane, the trapping force of the optical trap is equal to the drag force exerted by the laminar flow on the cell during cell movement (Hu and Sun, 2011). The drag force can be calculated using Stokes' law (Svoboda and Block, 1994).

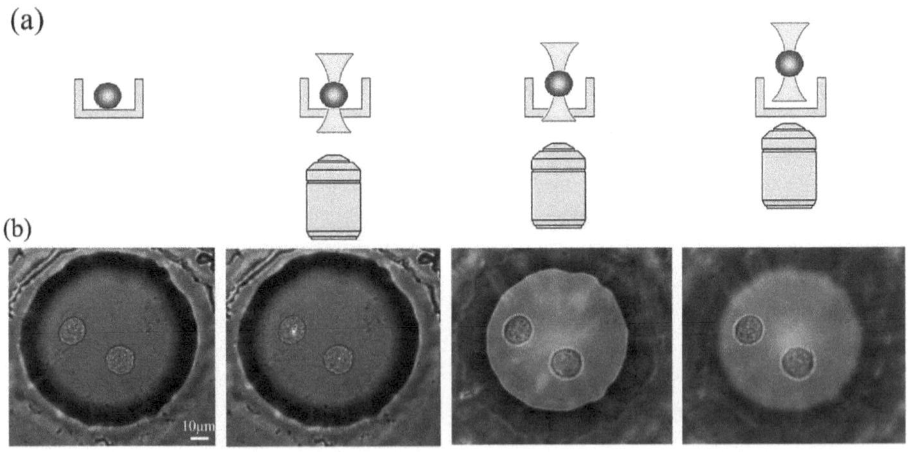

Figure 8.12 Cell levitation from the microwell (Wang et al., 2013). (A) Schematic of the cell levitation process from the microwell. (B) Levitation of two hESC cells from the microwell with two optical traps simultaneously. The levitated cells were always in the focus of the image plane for inspection, whereas the microwell became blurred after levitation.

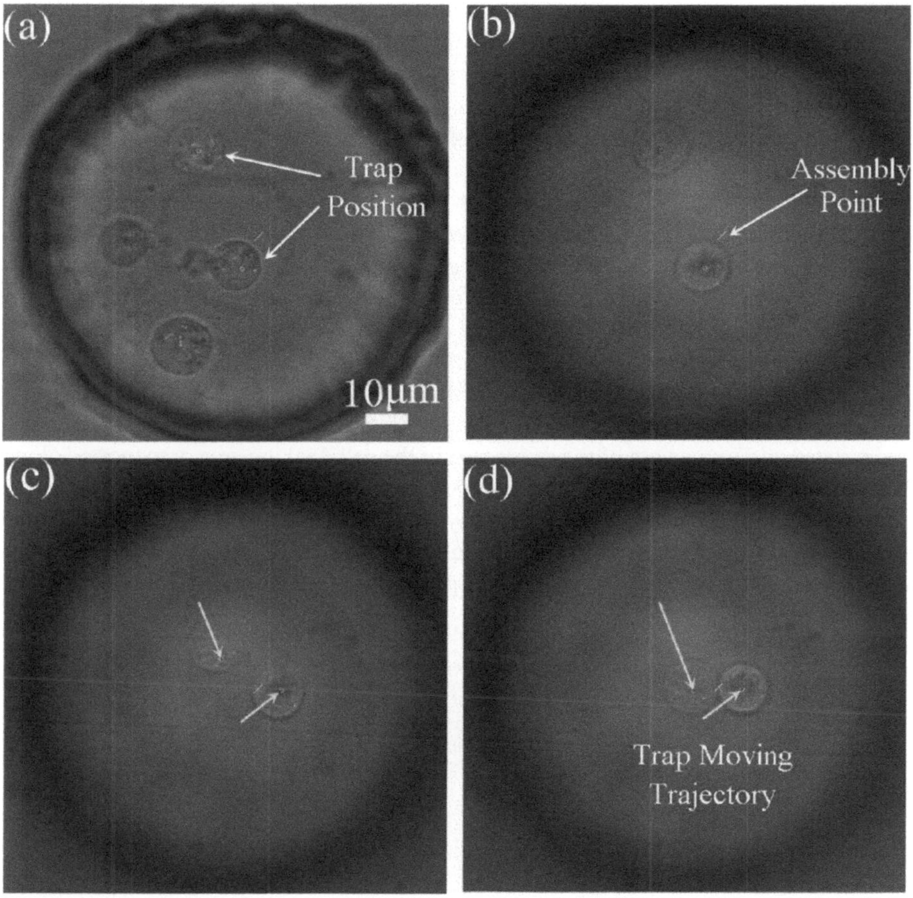

Figure 8.13 Assembly process of two hESCs into pairs after successful levitation (Wang et al., 2013). (A) Two hESCs trapped in the microwell. (B) Cells levitation from the microwell. (C) Assembly process. (D) Cells adhere to each other tightly in pairs after assembly.

Fig. 8.13 shows that the two levitated hESCs are assembled toward the assembly position at a moving speed of 30 μm/s and adhere closely to each other in pairs, which can be used for further research, such as cell fusion or cell–cell interaction. Limited by the maximum 3W laser emission power of the laser source in this experiment, a total of four optical traps can be generated simultaneously for multitrap parallel operation. Note that all the given laser emission power here is the laser output power from the laser source. During the transmission process, a large part of the actual laser power of the optical trap on the sample trap is lost. In this system, the laser power at the focal plane of the optical trap is about 15% of the original laser power emitted from the laser source.

8.3.2.3 Automated cell transportation and deposition

After the cells are successfully assembled, the next step is to accurately transfer the assembled cells to the designated microenvironment. Optical tweezers usually require a larger numerical aperture, so the movement distance is limited by the field of view. To solve this problem, the microscope x−y platform can be moved accordingly so that the optically captured cells in a no-flow environment are maintained in the field of view. After recording the position of the first microwell, the coordinates and transfer path of other microwells can be automatically calculated according to the known chip geometry. Using the cell levitation in the microwells, the assembled cells are transported to the desired location without the need for specific path planning, thereby avoiding collisions with other cells. However, the microfluidic chip may be tilted when mounted on the motorized platform, which may cause collisions between the trapped cells and the microwell array. Therefore, it is necessary to calibrate the bottom plane of the microwell array, which can be determined by using three microwells that are not on a straight line (Anis et al., 2010).

The schematic diagram of the transfer pathway is shown in Fig. 8.14A. Figs. 8.14B−D show a series of photos taken from the microscope, in which cells are levitated and moved out of the microwell in the cell docking area, transported along the transfer path, and moved to the target in the deposition area. During the entire transportation process, the pairs of cells are always in close contact. Moreover, the objective lens z stage is always adjusted to keep the relative distance between the bottom surface of the microwell array and the optical trap plane constant (50 μm). After reaching the

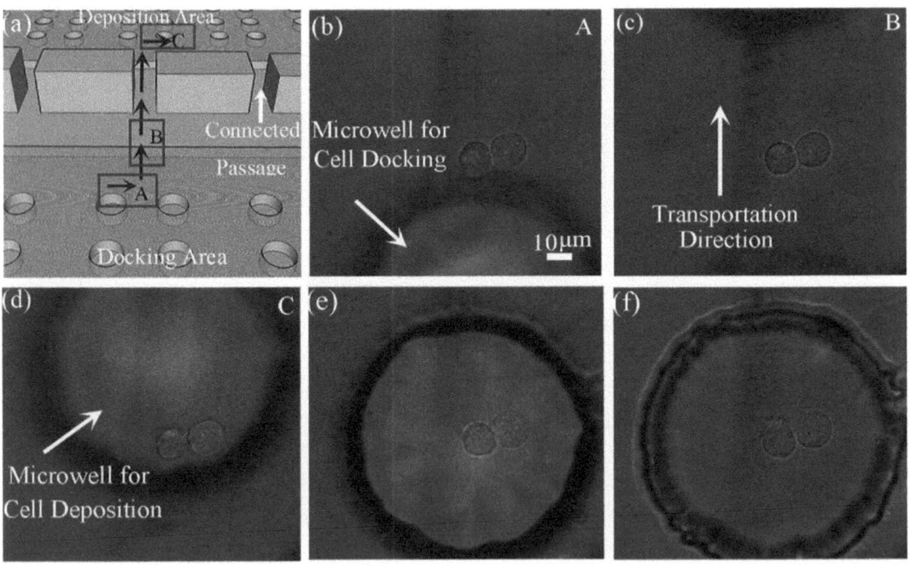

Figure 8.14 Automated cell transportation and deposition after successful assembly (Wang et al., 2013). (A) Schematic of the cell transportation from the microwell in cell docking area to the microwell in the cell deposition area along the computed transfer pathway. Black-lettered rectangles correspond to the photographs taken from the microscope presented in (B), (C), and (D). (B) Cell levitation out from the microwell in the docking area. (C) Cell transportation. (D) Reaching the target microwell in the deposition area. (E) Deposition process. (F) Successful deposition of assembled cells in the target microwell.

top of the target microwell, the objective lens z stage moves down, and the deposition distance is also set to 50 mm. Fig. 8.14E shows the deposition process, and Fig. 8.14F shows the assembled cells successfully deposited in the target microwell in a paired mode.

8.3.3 Case studies

8.3.3.1 Isolation and deposition of hESCs and yeast cells

Stem cells offer unprecedented promise, especially in regenerative medicine. However, stem cells may form tumors after being transplanted into patients without undergoing a purification process (Blum and Benvenisty, 2008). Therefore, in the clinical application of stem cell therapy, stem cell purification is very important.

In this case study, hESCs were isolated and deposited from a mixture of different cells based on fluorescent labeling. After loading the hESC lines transfected with LV-Oct4 promoter-driven GFP, hESCs with GFP and/or other cells without GFP were confined in the microwells, as shown in Fig. 8.15A. Brightfield and fluorescence images can be checked with high spatial and temporal resolution over time. As shown in Fig. 8.15B, the fluorescence-based image-processing method was used to distinguish the GFP-tagged hESCs from other unlabeled cells. Two optical traps were

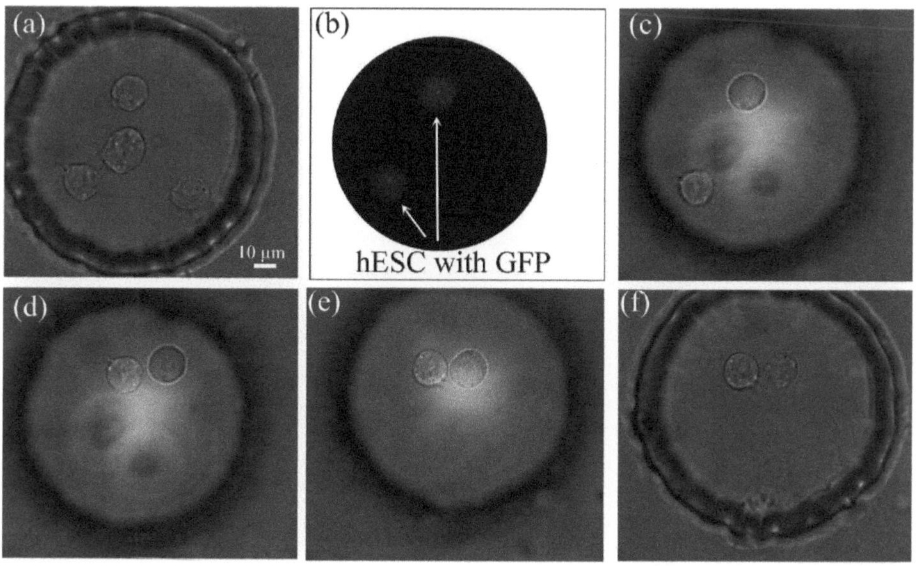

Figure 8.15 Fluorescence- based cell isolation and deposition on hESC (Wang et al., 2013). (A) Brightfield image of four cells confined in the microwell. (B) The corresponding fluorescence image of two target hESCs with GFP in the marked microwell (exposure time: 500 ms). (C) Levitation of hESCs from the microwell while leaving the other cells in the microwell. (D) Assembly of the optically trapped two hESCs into pairs. (E) Reaching the destination at the top of the desired microwell for deposition. (F) Cell deposition.

then created on the two detected hESCs to levitate them from the microwell, while the other cells without GFP were still confined in the microwell, as shown in Fig. 8.15C. In Fig. 8.15D, levitated hESCs were assembled in pairs. Finally, the paired cells were transferred to the desired position for deposition by the program-controlled motorized stage, as shown in Fig. 8.15E. Fig. 8.15F shows that hESCs were deposited in the required microwell in a paired mode.

The image-processing algorithm can be adjusted to detect and identify different target cells with different characteristics. The developed image-based cell manipulation tool can isolate cells based on external features (such as fluorescent proteins) and inherent features (such as morphological differences), and is not limited to any specific cell type. Fig. 8.16 shows the experimental results of isolating yeast cells from beads based on size characteristics and depositing in the target microwell. The manipulation process was the same as that of GFP-tagged hESCs described above.

Table 8.2 shows the statistical results of isolation and deposition of hESCs and yeast cells using the developed tool. The successful levitation rate refers to the percentage of successfully levitated cells in the total number of target cells to suspended. The successful transfer rate is defined as the ratio of the nonescaped cells from the optical trap to all levitated cells in the process. The final target cell purity after isolation is the percentage of target cells relative to all cells in the cell deposition microwells.

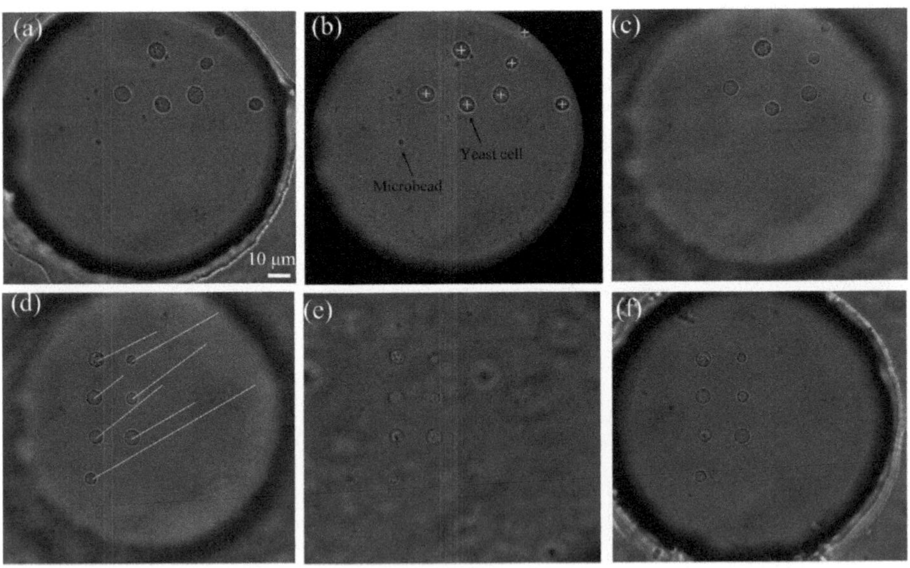

Figure 8.16 Size-based cell isolation and deposition of yeast cells from microbeads (Wang et al., 2013). (A) Brightfield image of cells and microbeads confined in the microwell. (B) Size-based image-processing technique for yeast cell identification and position in the marked microwell. (C) Levitation of seven yeast cells from the microwell while leaving the microbeads in the microwell. (D) Assembly of the optically levitated yeast cells. (E) Transportation process. (F) Cell deposition in the target microwell.

Table 8.2 Statistical results of isolation and deposition on hESC and yeast cell (Wang et al., 2013).

Cell type	Total cells (n = 4)	Initial purity before isolation	Successful levitation rate	Successful transfer rate	Final purity after isolation
hESC	2912	12.75% ± 0.96%	78.5% ± 5.4%	97% ± 1.41%	96.75% ± 1.5%
Yeast cell	1290	52.25% ± 10.27%	86.37% ± 4.75%	99.25% ± 0.95%	95.25% ± 1.89%

In these case studies, data were collected from four groups of 2912 hESCs and four groups of 1290 yeast cells. The rate of successful levitation from the microwell was affected by nonspecific surface adhesion. Due to the optimized and precise control of cell tracking during transportation, the successful transfer rate of both cell types was high. When target cells and nontarget particles were close to or adhered to each other, the impurities of the target cells in the deposited microwell were mainly caused by random trapping of nontarget particles. In general, compared to conventional flow cytometry (for example, FACS) that usually requires a large number of samples (for example, more than 100,000 cells), the proposed tool is especially effective in isolating a much smaller number of cells (for example, less than 1000) (Shapiro, 2003).

The average time required for the cell manipulation process was 27–37 s, of which was 3 s for cell suspension, 1 s for cell assembly, 20–30 s for cell transportation, and 3 s for cell deposition. The most time-consuming factor was the cell transportation process. By shortening the transportation distance between the cell docking area and the cell deposition area, the time cost can be greatly reduced. The throughput can be further increased by reducing the well-to-well distance to more densely fill the microwell array.

Maintaining cell health and viability is another important issue. Laser-induced photo damage and thermal damage are the two main effects on biological cells, which are highly dependent on the laser wavelength and applied laser power. When the wavelength is higher than 800 nm, the heating effect may cause cell damage (Zhang and Liu, 2008). In most systems, a near-infrared laser with a wavelength of 1064 nm can be selected as the laser source. In order to avoid or reduce thermal damage to the cell, a laser power as low as possible should be used according to the calibration result of the optical trap. In addition, in the most common experimental environment, the absorption of laser light by the surrounding medium rather than the particle itself contributes the most to heating (Peterman et al., 2003). In the above case studies, the trapped particles are transported in the medium, so the moving fluid can make the heat transfer more efficient.

Two methods can be used to test the viability of hESCs affected by optical traps. One is to use SYTOX orange dead cell stain, and the other is to use trypan blue, as shown in Fig. 8.17. The cells under the optical trap with 3 W laser emission power were exposed for 15 min. When using SYTOX orange nucleic acid stain, healthy cells trapped by the optical trap did not detect red fluorescence within 15 min. For

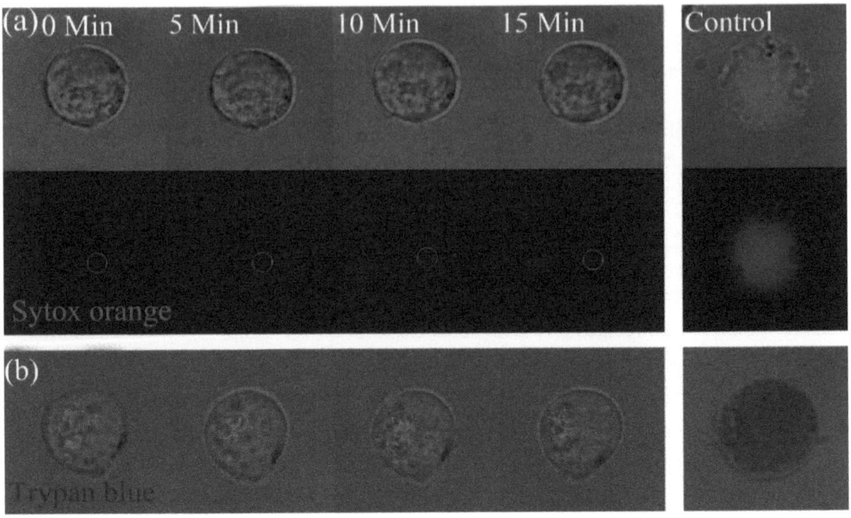

Figure 8.17 Viability test of the hESC affected by the optical trap (Wang et al., 2013). (A) Viability test using SYTOX orange dead cell stain. For healthy cells, no red fluorescence is detected with 3W laser emission power for up to 15 min. For controlled cell, red fluorescence is detected in the fluorescence image. (B) Viability test using trypan blue. No stain is observed in the healthy cells when applying the 3 W laser emission power for up to 15 min. For controlled cells, the whole cell is stained with dye as an indicator of cell death.

controlled cells, the dye was found to penetrate the dead cell membrane, and it would show red fluorescence when the cell was excited with a 488 nm laser. Similarly, when using the trypan blue exclusion test, no staining was observed in healthy cells when 3 W laser emission power was applied for 15 min. However, for the controlled cells, the entire cell was stained with dye as an indicator of cell death.

8.3.3.2 Other applications

Besides cell isolation, the developed tool can also be used for other applications, with three examples briefly introduced below.

Cell fusion on two tightly paired cells. After successful levitation from the microwell, the interesting cells are assembled by optical traps into pairs dynamically and tightly, and they are then located precisely in the desired microwell for cell fusion. Applying the optical scissors with the pulsed laser at the contact point of the paired cells, the cell fusion can be induced. The advantage of such laser-induced cell fusions lies in high selectivity and controllability, and the on-chip microwell environment will allow further manipulation or analysis on the fused cells at the predefined location without removing them from the chip.

Cell–liposome interaction for drug delivery. Liposomes are considered as well-established nanoparticles used for as a drug carrier. After cell–liposome interactions, the drug-loaded liposomes can adsorb onto the cell surface or fuse with the cell membrane, and then the encapsulated drugs can be released into the cytoplasm. The drugs can penetrate the cell membrane through micropinocytosis or be delivered by the endosome into the lysosome (Spyratou et al., 2012). With the developed cell manipulation tool, the drug amount can be well controlled by trapping different numbers of liposomes toward the cells, and multiple drugs can be delivered simultaneously by trapping liposomes encapsulated with different drugs.

Cell migration or chemotaxis assay. Specially designed microbeads contain certain soluble molecules that can be utilized as the microsources for cell stimulation, and the gradient of diffusion can be quickly generated around the microbead (Kress et al., 2009). The developed cell manipulation tool can also be used for cell migration or chemotaxis assay, with the advantage that not only can the fixed bead assay be performed under different conditions (such as different molecules from multiple different beads or different concentrations by trapping different number of beads with the same molecule), but also the free bead assay which can change the migration direction of the cells to move toward the microbeads trapped by the optical traps (Theveneau and Mayor, 2011; Gou et al., 2014).

8.4 A simplified sheathless cell separation approach

In the above sections, optical tweezers are used for high-precision small cell population sorting based on microfluidic chip technology. In addition to optical tweezers, DEP manipulation can also be combined with microfluidic technology to achieve effective cell separation. This section introduces a simplified nonsheathed cell separation method that combines the sheathless prefocusing and DEP separation methods based on gravity sedimentation. By gravitational sedimentation in tubing inserted into the inlet of the microfluidic chip, the cells can be focused into the flow in the upstream area of the microchannel before separation. The DEP force is then applied to the downstream area of the microchannel to actively separate the cells. This sheathless solution focuses a mixture of cells with different sizes and dielectric properties into a stream at a wide range of flow rates without changing the design of the microfluidic chip. The DEP method is a label-free method that can continuously separate cells according to their size or dielectric properties, so that they can be separated with great flexibility. The efficiency of the reported method has been verified by a series of experiments conducted by Luo et al. (2018).

8.4.1 Methods

8.4.1.1 Design of the DEP separator

The chip is designed to consist of platinum (Pt) electrodes and a polydimethylsiloxane (PDMS) microchannel with one inlet and two outlets, as shown in Fig. 8.18. The entire chip can be divided into three functional areas, namely the sheathless cell focusing area, the label-free DEP separation area and the outlets. The sheathless cell focusing area consists of a tube inserted into the inlet. The tubing has an appropriate steering angle θ in the flow direction (x direction in Fig. 8.18A). When flowing forward in

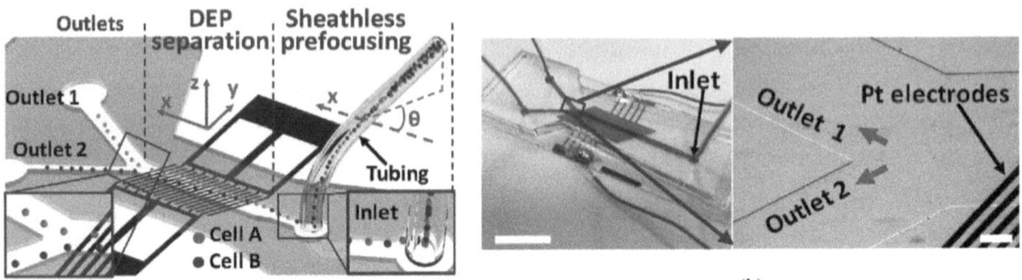

(a) (b)

Figure 8.18 Design of the microfluidic cell separator (Luo et al., 2018). (A) Schematic of the cell separator containing one inlet and two outlets. (B) Photograph of the cell separator in the microfluidic channel for visualization (scale bar = 2 cm), together with a bright-field microscopic image of the cell separation region (scale bar = 200 μm).

the tubing, the widely dispersed cells gradually sediment to the bottom wall of the tubing due to the action of gravity. This precipitation focuses the cells in the z-direction and sends the z-axis focused cells to the inlet of the downstream separation channel. In this way, before the cells flow into the DEP separation zone, the cells are focused in the separation channel along the x direction, which is usually achieved by sheath flow to achieve efficient downstream cell separation. The DEP separation zone has a microfluidic channel that is 1 mm wide and 14 mm long. The microelectrodes are composed of 40 intersecting wire pairs and aligned with the microchannel at an angle of 45 degrees (Fig. 8.18B). The width and gap of platinum (Pt) electrodes are both 50 μm. Two outlets with widths of 634 and 891 μm are used to collect separated cells. Before flowing into the DEP separation area, all cells are focused on the upper side of the channel. When passing through the DEP separation zone, cells subjected to a stronger DEP force flow into outlet 2, and cells subjected to a weaker DEP force flow into outlet 1. The DEP force F_{DEP} is given as

$$F_{\mathrm{DEP}} = 2\pi\varepsilon_m r^3 Re[K(\omega)]\nabla E^2, \tag{8.6}$$

where ε_m is the absolute permittivity of the suspending medium, r is the radius of the cell, ∇E^2 is the gradient of the square of the applied electric field E, $K(\omega)$ refers to the Clausius–Mossotti (CM) factor (Yan et al., 2017), Re denotes the real part of the CM factor, and $K(\omega)$ depends on the complex permittivity of the cell and the suspending medium, and the frequency of the external electric field. $K(\omega)$ can be given as

$$K(\omega) = \left(\varepsilon^*_{\mathrm{cell}} - \varepsilon^*_{\mathrm{medium}}\right) / \left(\varepsilon^*_{\mathrm{cell}} + 2\varepsilon^*_{\mathrm{medium}}\right), \tag{8.7}$$

where $\varepsilon^* = \varepsilon - i\sigma/\omega\left(i^2 = -1\right)$ is the complex permittivity, σ is the electrical conductivity, and ω is the frequency of the electric field. Notably, the DEP force is a function of particle size and dielectric parameters, and cells of different sizes or different dielectric properties will experience different DEP forces, allowing the cells to be successfully separated (Fig. 8.18A). The fabrication process of the DEP separator is mainly based on soft lithography and lift-off technology (Luo et al., 2018).

The 3D CFD model on COMSOL Multiphysics can be used to simulate the cell trajectory in the tubing as the flow rate and diameter of the tubing and cells change. To simplify the model and reduce the solution time, the simulation was carried out from two aspects. In the first aspect, the steady-state CFD problem was solved through the use of laminar flow physics, which excluded cells. Here multiblock structural meshes with approximately six million cells and near-wall optimization can be used. In this way, a standard Hagen–Poiseuille flow solution can be obtained for the tubing with circular cross-sections. In the second aspect, time-dependent cell trajectories were determined using the physics property of particle tracking for fluid flow. A total of 100 cells uniformly distributed at the inlet were released at 0 s. Drag force and gravity were then applied to calculate the cell trajectory. Different flow rates were used at the inlet, and zero-pressure boundary condition was set at the outlet. No slip boundary condition was applied on the channel wall. The influence of flow and geometric parameters on cell trajectories were investigated through parameterizing the flow velocity and diameters of cells and the tubing. Given the physical properties of the fluid, the density of the particle ρ_p was set to 1070 kg/m^3 (Luo et al., 2018). According to the simulated cell trajectory, the required minimum tubing length L_{min} and diameter D (Fig. 8.19A) were obtained to make the cells in the tubing sediment completely. The 3D CFD model was also used to predict the flow pattern (trajectory) of cells in the microfluidic channel. Using streamlines, the trajectories of the cells in the microchannel can be seen relative to the different steering angles of the tubing.

8.4.1.2 Experimental procedures

Experiments were performed on OCI-AML3 cells cultured in 80% alpha-MEM (Sigma, St Louis, MO) supplemented with 20% h.i. FBS (Atlanta Biological Company, Flowery Branch, GA). THP-1 cells were cultured in RPMI 1640 medium (Sigma, St Louis, MO) supplemented with 10% fetal bovine serum (Atlanta Bio, Flowery Branch, GA). Before the experiment, all cells were incubated at 37°C under a 5% CO_2 atmosphere. Immediately before the DEP experiment, OCI-AML3 and THP-1 cells were stained with fluorescent dyes, namely, CFDA-SE with green fluorescence and Hoechst 33342 with blue fluorescence. After that, the cells were washed twice with 1 mL PBS and suspended in isotonic low conductivity DEP buffer containing 8.6% w/w sucrose, 0.3% w/w glucose, and enough PBS to increase the conductivity of the solution to 400 μS/cm at pH 7.4. Before each experiment, the microfluidic chip was cleaned with ethanol and deionized water to sterilize and remove bubbles, and treated with 1% BSA (Sigma, St Louis, MO) to precoat the microchannel to prevent nonspecific adhesion of the attached cells.

The suspended cells were injected into the inlet of the microchannel through a tube connected to a syringe pump with a 1 mL syringe. The sinusoidal voltage was applied between the microelectrodes using a functional signal generator, which was connected to the electrode pads of the DEP chip. The steering angle of the tube was fixed at 30 degrees to achieve reliable cell focusing in the downstream area along the upper side of the microfluidic channel. Subsequently, the frequency and magnitude of the applied voltage were adjusted to achieve effective cell separation. A microscope with a

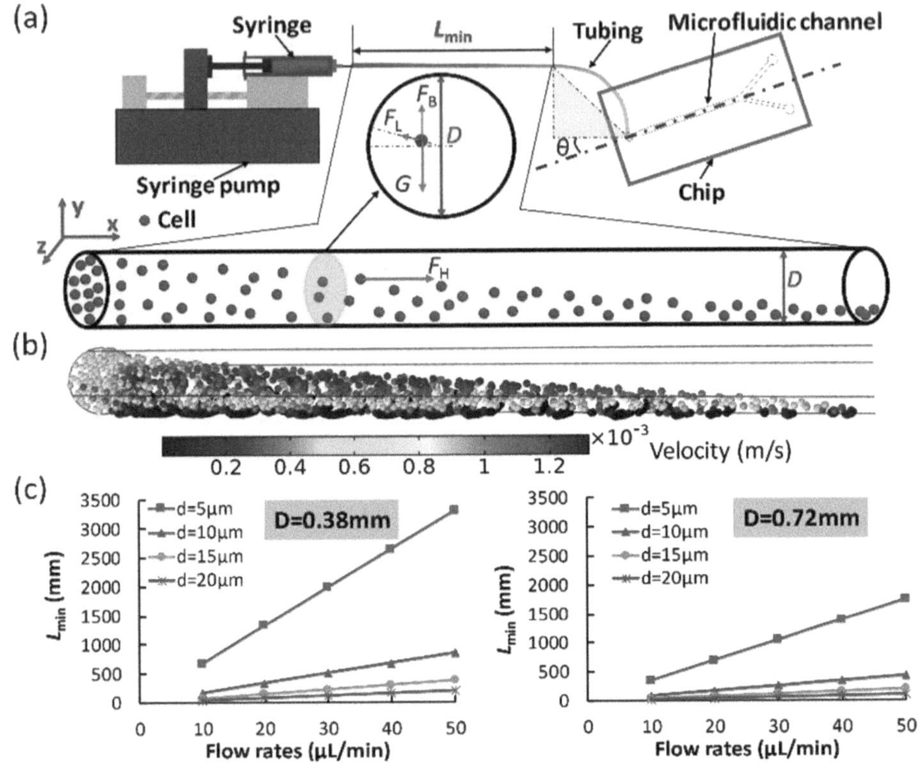

Figure 8.19 Operation principle of using gravitational sedimentation for sheathless cell focusing (Luo et al., 2018). (A) Schematic of the experimental setup for using gravitational sedimentation of cells in a tubing to achieve sheathless cell focusing in the microfluidic channel. (B) Simulated cell trajectory pattern in the tubing by using COMSOL Multiphysics software. (C) Minimum tubing length L_{min} for complete sedimentation of cells in the tubing versus the input flow rate under different d (diameter of the cell) and D (inner diameter of the tubing).

CCD camera was used to observe and record the cell trajectories. A hemocytometer was used to count the number of cells collected from the import and export for quantitative analysis.

The cells collected from the inlet and outlet were washed twice by adding 1 mL of PBS. Then, 1 mL of diluted propidium iodide (PI) was added to the staining buffer (50 μg/mL). Finally, the cells were incubated at 37°C for 5 min were analyzed by microscope images to calculate cell viability. Only dead cells showed red fluorescence. Cell viability was defined as the ratio of the number of cells that do not show red fluorescence to the total number of cells.

ImageJ (http://rsb.info.nih.gov/ij/) was used to analyze and process all recorded images. The separation efficiency was defined as the ratio of the number of one cell type collected at the expected outlet to the total number of the same type of cells collected at all outlets. Purity was defined as the ratio of the number of one type of cell collected at the outlet to the total number of all cells collected at the same outlet. All experiments were repeated at least three times.

8.4.2 Results and discussion

8.4.2.1 Gravitational sedimentation of non-neutrally buoyant cells in tubing

Cells are generally considered to be neutrally buoyant when they are suspended in a culture medium or PBS buffer. However, the density of many cells is slightly higher than the density of plasma, culture medium, and PBS buffer (Grover et al., 2011), indicating that most cells appear gravity effect when they are suspended in liquids such as culture medium and PBS buffer. Fig. 8.19A shows that the suspended cells are pumped into the microfluidic chip through the capillary tubing. The cell trajectory in the tubing is affected by buoyant force F_B, gravity G, net inertial lift F_L, and hydrodynamic drag force F_H. All the forces of F_B, G, and F_L affect the lateral motion of the cell, while F_H triggers the cell to move forward along the axis of the tubing (Fig. 8.19A). F_L can be ignored when the Reynolds (Re) number ($\rho vD/\eta$) is low (Zhang et al., 2016), where ρ is the fluid density, v is the average speed, η is the dynamic viscosity, and D is the characteristic channel size, namely, the diameter of the circular section of the tubing. Therefore, the lateral motion of cells is mainly determined by the net force of gravity and buoyancy, which is defined as $G - F_B = (\rho_c - \rho)V_c g$, where ρ_c is the cell density. The densities of THP-1, OCI-AML3, and yeast cells used in this study are 1070, 1070, and 1100 kg/m^3, respectively. V_c is the volume of a single cell, and $g = 9.8\ m/s^2$ is the acceleration due to gravity.

As the cells flow through the tubing, the cells gradually sediment. If the tubing is long enough, all cells can sediment to the bottom of the tubing. The minimum tubing length L_{min} that allows all cells to sediment to the bottom of the tubing can be obtained by CFD simulation (Fig. 8.19B). The relationship between L_{min} and other parameters (for example, the flow rate and diameter of cells and tubing) can be quantitatively characterized based on the simulation results (Fig. 8.19C). L_{min} increases linearly with the increase in input flow. The cells with smaller size require a longer length of tubing for sedimentation, and increasing the diameter of the tubing will reduce L_{min}. To make the DEP cell separation successful, the flow rate cannot exceed 30 μL/min; otherwise, the DEP force will not be large enough to deflect the cells. According to the flow rate requirement, the availability of the tubing (with a diameter of 0.38 mm) and the size distribution of the cells, the tubing length is selected as 400 mm for subsequent experiments in this study.

To visualize the sedimentation of cells in the tubing, a microfluidic chip with an inlet located in the center of the circular channel and an outlet with 360 degrees opening is designed and fabricated, as shown in Fig. 8.20A. For circular microfluidic channels, when cells sediment to the bottom of the tubing, the cells flow in a sector pattern, and the direction of the sector can be adjusted by changing the steering angle of the tubing. Fig. 8.20B shows the flow patterns of cells in the microfluidic channel at different flow

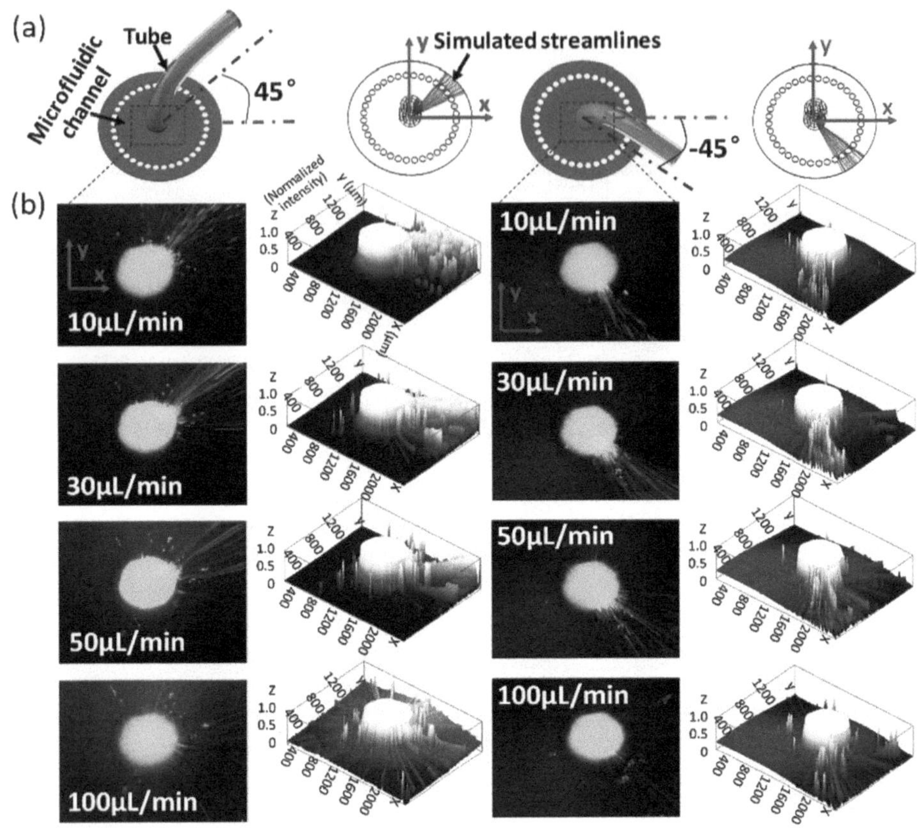

Figure 8.20 Experimental study of gravitational sedimentation of cells in the tubing (Luo et al., 2018). (A) Schematic of the experimental setup for gravitational sedimentation of cells in the tubing based on a designed microfluidic chip with an inlet and a 360 degrees-opened outlet. (B) Results for cell flow pattern under different flow rates. THP-1 cells stained with green fluorescent dye CFDA-SE are suspended in DEP buffer. The cell flow pattern is characterized by the normalized fluorescence intensity. The diameter and length of the tubing are 0.38 and 400 mm, respectively. Scale bar = 300 μm.

rates and tubing steering angles. THP-1 cells stained with the green fluorescent dye CFDA-SE and suspended in DEP buffer are used in the experiments. It can be seen that the cells flow in a sector pattern in the microfluidic channel, as predicted by the simulated streamline shown in Fig. 8.20A. The sector angle increases as the flow rate increases (Fig. 8.20B). When the flow rate is increased from 10 to 50 μL/min, most of the cells sediment to the bottom of the tubing, and the sector angle increases slightly, indicating that the proposed cell-focusing method is effective in a wide range of flow rates. When the flow rate is increased to 100 μL/min, the tubing length of 400 mm is insufficient to allow most of the cells to sediment. Therefore, the sector angle of the cell flow pattern is increased to 360 degrees. These experimental results show that gravitational-sedimentation-based sheathless cell focusing can work in a wide range of flow rates by adjusting the geometry of the tubing. Moreover, changing the angle of the tubing can correspondingly change the direction of the cell flow sector, which demonstrates the potential of using gravity sedimentation in the tubing for tunable sheathless cell focusing in microfluidic channels in various applications.

8.4.2.2 Regulating sheathless cell focusing with different tubing steering angle

Fig. 8.21 shows the different cell flow patterns at a flow rate of 10 μL/min at six different tubing steering angles of the microfluidic channel in the proposed DEP separator. THP-1 cells stained with the green fluorescent dye CFDA-SE and suspended in DEP buffer are used for this analysis. Fig. 8.21A shows a schematic diagram of different tubing steering angles, and Fig. 8.21B shows the cell trajectories predicted by CFD simulation and visualized by red streamlines. Fig. 8.21C and D illustrate six different cell flow patterns under different tubing steering angles. When the steering angle of the tubing is −30 degrees, the cells flow on the lower side of the channel;

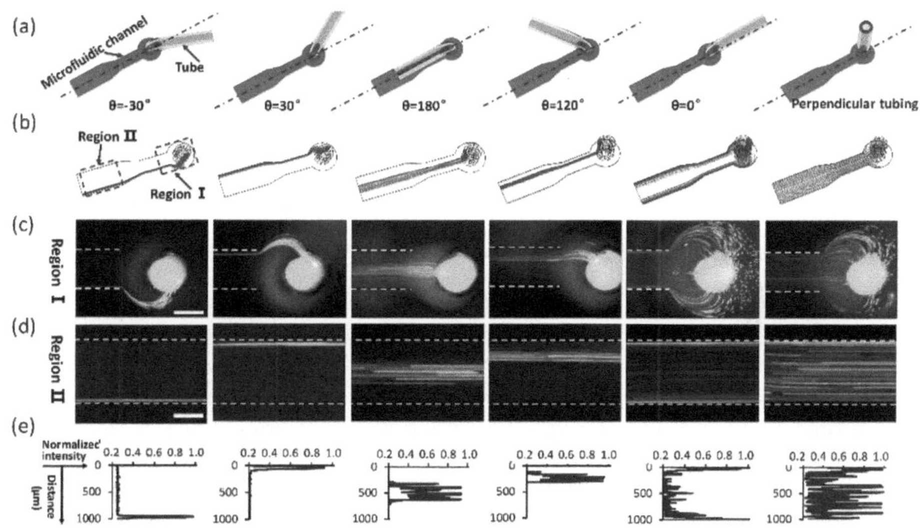

Figure 8.21 Experimental study using gravitational sedimentation of cells in the tubing for sheathless cell focusing in the microfluidic channel of the cell separator at the flow rate of 10 μL/min (Luo et al., 2018). (A) Schematic of changing the steering angle of the tubing to achieve different cell flow patterns in the microfluidic channel. (B) Predicted cell flow patterns for different steering angles of the tubing using CFD simulation. (C) Cell flow pattern results at region I of the microfluidic channel under different steering angles. THP-1 cells stained with green fluorescent dye CFDA-SE are suspended into DEP buffer. The diameter and length of the tubing are 0.38 and 400 mm, respectively. (D) Cell flow pattern results at region II of the microfluidic channel under different steering angles. (E) Illustration of cell distribution across the 1 mm wide channel at region II using normalized fluorescence intensity. Scale bar = 500 μm.

when the steering angle of the tubing is 30 degrees, the cells flow along the upper side of the channel. When the steering angle of the tubing is 180 and 120 degrees, the cells focus on the center of the channel and the position between the center and the upper side of the channel. When the steering angle of the tubing is 0 degree, most of the cells flow along the upper or lower sides of the channel, and a few cells are randomly distributed between the upper and lower sides of the channel. When the tubing is inserted into the inlet in the same direction as gravity, the cells do not sediment to one side of the channel, but evenly distribute across the entire width of the microchannel. The normalized fluorescence intensity is used to quantitatively characterize the cell distribution across the 1-mm-wide channel on region II, as shown in Fig. 8.21E.

The results in Fig. 8.21 show that the gravity sedimentation method can successfully achieve sheathless cell focusing. Different cell-focusing modes can be selected by adjusting the steering angle of the tubing. Similarly, if the smallest cell of L_{min} is used, cells of different sizes can be focused into the same stream. In some applications, cells may need to flow or be evenly distributed in the channel at a relatively low flow rate. If the tubing length cannot be shortened, a tubing with small diameter can be used, or the flow direction of the cell can be the same as gravity. If the flow path in the tubing is long enough to allow the cells to sediment completely, the bending angle of the tubing relative to the x−y plane will not affect the gravity sedimentation of the cells in the z direction. Therefore, the change in the bending angle of the tubing will have very little effect on the focusing mode of the cells in the microfluidic channel. Overall, compared with other methods such as sheath and inertial focusing methods, the gravity sedimentation-based sheathless cell focusing has unique advantages in terms of simplicity and flexibility.

8.4.2.3 Size-based separation of THP-1 cells from yeast cells

A case study of isolating THP-1 cells from yeast cells was conducted to prove the effectiveness of the proposed cell separation method based on size difference. The average diameters of yeast and THP-1 cells were approximately 6 and 13 μm, respectively. The mixed cell suspension was injected into the cell separator at a flow rate of 12.5 μL/min through a 400 mm long PE tubing with a steering angle of 30 degrees (Fig. 8.22A). All cells were focused on the upper side of the channel and flow into outlet 1, as shown in Fig. 8.22A. When a sinusoidal voltage of 5 MHz and 12 $V_{p\text{-}p}$ was applied, the cells deflected due to the combined force of the hydrodynamic resistance and the DEP force. The CM factor values of THP-1 and yeast cells were calculated based on literature data (Wei et al., 2016). Obviously, Re $[K(\omega)] > 0$ at an operating frequency of 5 MHz, which meant that all cells were subjected to a positive DEP force. Because THP-1 cells were larger, their deformation was more pronounced than that of yeast cells. Therefore, most THP-1 cells flowed into outlet 2, and most yeast cells flowed into outlet 1. In this way, two types of cells were successfully separated on the cell separator based on their different sizes, as shown in Fig. 8.22B. Fig. 8.22C shows that most yeast cells were collected at outlet 1, while most THP-1 cells were collected at outlet 2. The collection efficiency of yeast cells at outlet 1 can reach 92.7%, and the maximum secretion of THP-1 cells at outlet 2 can reach

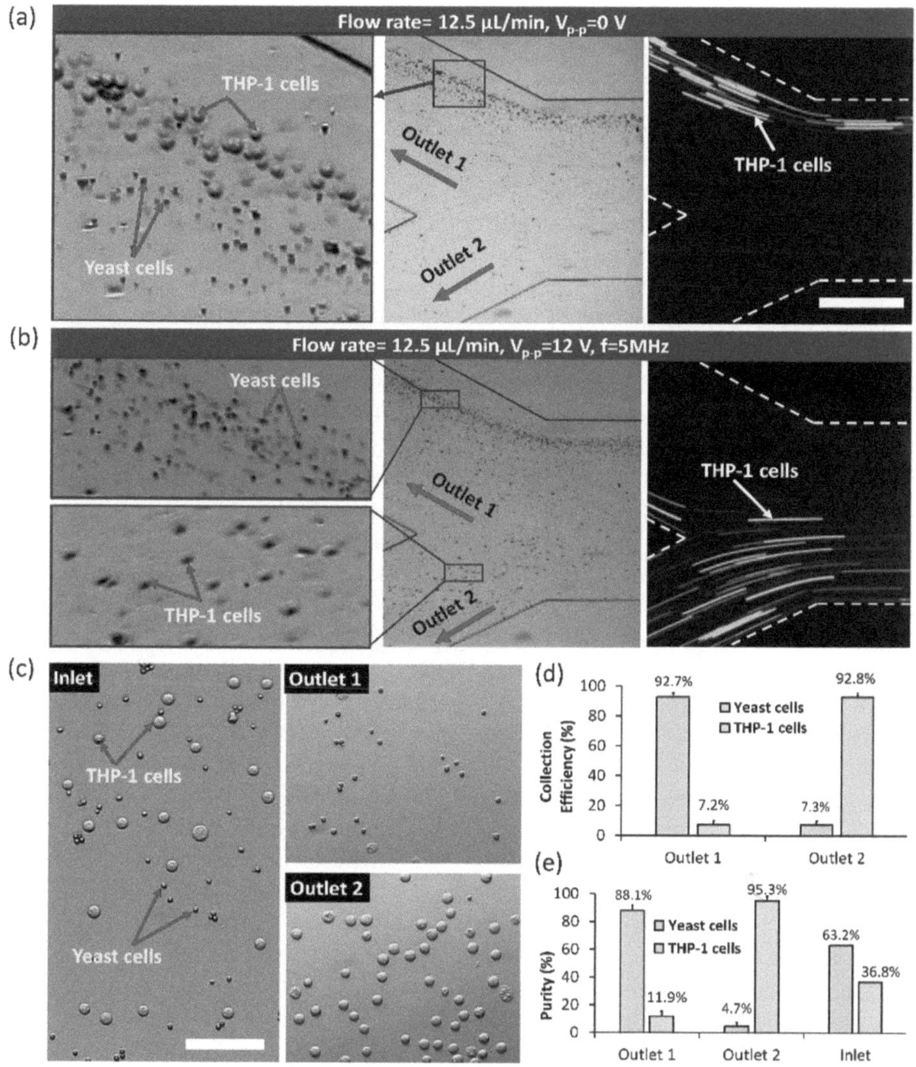

Figure 8.22 Experimental results of size-based separation of THP-1 cells from yeast cells (Luo et al., 2018). (A) All cells are focused to the upper side of the channel and flowed into outlet 1 at a flow rate of 12.5 μL/min when the electric field is off. THP-1 cells are stained with green fluorescent dye CFDA-SE. Scale bar = 500 μm. (B) Yeast cells flow into outlet 1 and THP-1 cells flow into outlet 2 when 5 MHz and 12 $V_{p\text{-}p}$ sinusoidal signal is applied to the separator. (C) Microscopic images of cells collected from the inlet and two outlets. Scale bar = 100 μm. (D) Cell collection efficiency of two outlets. (E) Purity of cells in two outlets.

92.8% (Fig. 8.22D). The purity of yeast cells at outlet 1 was 88.1%, and the purity of THP-1 cells at outlet 2 was 95.3% (Fig. 8.22E). These results proved the good separation performance of the separation method.

8.4.2.4 Dielectric property-based separation of THP-1 cells from OCI-AML3 cells

The second case study of isolating THP-1 cells from OCI-AML3 cells was conducted to prove the effectiveness of the separation method based on dielectric properties. THP-1 and OCI-AML3 cells are acute myeloid leukemia (AML) cells of similar size. They have different subtypes according to their maturity and the cell type in which the leukemia develops. According to the French–US–UK (FAB) classification, OCI-AML3 cells belong to the FAB M4 subtype, while THP-1 cells belong to the FAB M5 subtype. These two types of cells can only be separated according to their different dielectric properties, because the DEP force is related to cell diameter and dielectric properties (membrane capacitance, cytoplasmic conductivity, etc.), and the different dielectric properties are determined by the heterogeneity within the cell (Markx and Davey, 1999). In the experiment, the mixed cell suspension was injected into the cell separator through a 400 mm long PE tubing at a flow rate of 12.5 μL/min at a steering angle of 30 degrees (Fig. 8.23A). Before entering the DEP separation zone, the cells were focused on the upper side of the microfluidic channel, as shown in Figs. 8.23C and D.

As shown in Fig. 8.23A, when the applied peak-to-peak voltage $V_{p\text{-}p}$ was zero, all cells flowed into outlet 1. When a sinusoidal voltage of 5 MHz and 12 $V_{p\text{-}p}$ was applied, the cells deflected due to the combined force of the hydrodynamic resistance and the DEP force. In this study, Re $[K(\omega)] > 0$ at a working frequency of 5 MHz, which meant that both THP-1 and OCI-AML3 cells were subject to positive DEP forces. Most THP-1 cells were deflected more significantly than OCI-AML3 cells and flowed into outlet 2, while most OCI-AML3 cells flowed into outlet 1. In this way, two cell subtypes can be successfully separated. Fig. 8.23B shows that most OCI-AML3 cells were collected at outlet 1, and most THP-1 cells were collected at outlet 2. The efficiency of collecting OCI-AML3 at outlet 1 can reach 96.6%, and the conductivity of THP-1 cells at outlet 2 can reach 91.4% (Fig. 8.23C). The purity of OCI-AML3 cells from outlet 1 was 91%, and the purity of THP-1 cells from outlet 2 was 97.3% (Fig. 8.23D). The sizes of these two cell subtypes were very similar, indicating that they suffered from similar hydrodynamic drag force. Therefore, THP-1 cells must undergo considerable DEP force to separate from OCI-AML3 cells.

Note that both gravity-sedimentation-based prefocusing and dielectrophoresis separation methods are limited by low flow rates. Some methods to overcome this limitation have been reported in the literature. From the perspective of gravity-sedimentation-based prefocusing, the flow rate can be increased by using longer or larger diameter tubing, as shown in Fig. 8.19. From the perspective of dielectrophoresis separation, the flow rate can also be increased by increasing the DEP force or extending the flow path of the cells in the DEP separation area. Increasing the DEP force means generating a larger electric field, which may reduce the viability of cells. Therefore, it is preferable to extend the flow path in the DEP region. For example, a serpentine channel can be used to extend the flow path in the DEP area.

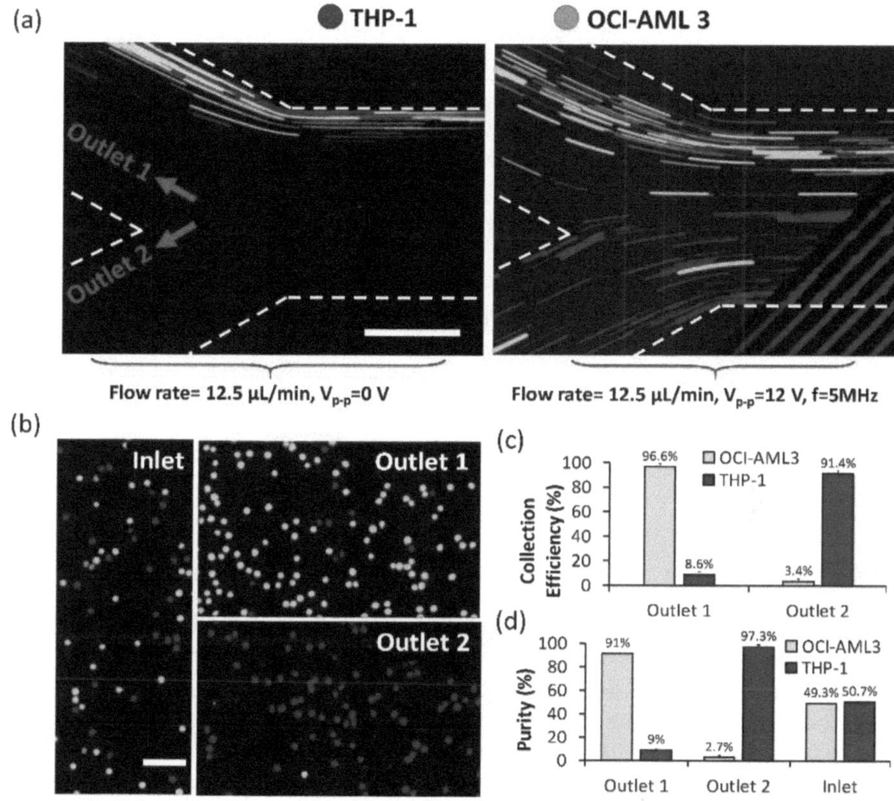

Figure 8.23 Experimental results of dielectric property-based separation of leukemic cell subpopulations (THP-1 and OCI-AML3 cells) (Luo et al., 2018). (A) Composite fluorescence images showing the trajectories of THP-1 and OCI-AML3 cells. Scale bar = 500 μm. (B) Composite fluorescence images of particles collected at the inlet and two outlets. Scale bar = 100 μm. (C) Cell collection efficiency of two outlets. (D) Purity of cells in the two outlets.

8.5 Conclusions

This chapter introduces two strategies based on microfluidic chips to solve the challenging problem of cell sorting and separation. The first strategy is to use the robot-assisted optical tweezers manipulation method to achieve high-precision cell sorting and separation of a small number of cell samples. The second strategy is to use a DEP manipulation platform to effectively separate cells not only by size but also by dielectric properties. With the first strategy, a generic single-cell manipulation tool that integrates optical tweezers, microfluidic chips, and imaging processing technology is developed. This method shows high purity and high recovery rate when processing small sample populations and is very suitable for separation and enrichment of rare cells. Multiple optical traps can be generated at the same time to realize multicell parallel sorting, and the sorter has the unique function of identifying multiple functions of the cell. With the second strategy, an automated cell separation and deposition tool combining microwell array and holographic optical tweezers technology is developed to achieve a series of cell manipulation processes, including cell docking, cell recognition and suspension, cell assembly, and cell transportation and deposition. This tool can perform cell inspection with high spatiotemporal resolution and has the ability to recognize different cell phenotypes. The isolated target cells can be accurately transported and deposited to the designated target location, showing great potential for functional integration with other chips without removing these cells from the chip. With the second strategy, the sheathless method is integrated with the DEP method to achieve the separation of cells with different sizes or dielectric properties. Sheathless cell focusing is achieved via the gravity sedimentation of cells in tubing inserted into the inlet of the microfluidic chip with an adjustable steering angle. Using the interdigital electrode array at the bottom of the microchannel, a DEP force can be generated to deflect the motion of the target cells and separate the cell mixture.

References

Anis, Y.H., Holl, M., Meldrum, D.R., 2010. Automated selection and placement of single cell using vision-based feedback control. IEEE Trans. Autom. Sci. Eng. 7, 598–606.

Beech, J.P., Peter, J., Tegenfeldt, J.O.T., 2009. Tipping the balance of deterministic lateral displacement devices using dielectrophoresis. Lab Chip 9, 2698–2706.

Blum, B., Benvenisty, N., 2008. The tumorigenicity of human embryonic stem cells. Adv. Cancer Res. 100, 133–158.

Braschler, T., Demierre, N., Nascimento, E., Silva, T., Oliva, A.G., Renaud, P., 2008. Continuous separation of cells by balanced dielectrophoretic forces at multiple frequencies. Lab Chip 8, 280–286.

Chen, H., Sun, D., 2012. Moving groups of microparticles into array with a robot-tweezers manipulation system. IEEE Trans. Robot. 28, 1069–1080.

Cheng, S.I., Huang, W.L., Chen, T.Y., Liu, C.W., Lin, Y.D., Su, W., 2015. Anitbody-free isolation of rare cancer cells from blood based on 3D lateral dielectrophoresis. Lab Chip 15, 2950–2959.

Dittrich, P.S., Tachikawa, K., Manz, A., 2006. Micro total analysis systems. Latest advancements and trends. Anal. Chem. 78, 3887–3907.

Eriksson, E., Keen, S., Leach, J., Goksör, M., Padgett, M., 2007. The effect of external forces on discrete motion within holographic optical tweezers. Opt. Express 15, 18268–18274.

Gou, X., Yang, H., Fahmy, T.M., Wang, Y., Sun, D., 2014. Direct measurement of cell protrusion force utilizing a robot-aided cell manipulation system with optical tweezers for cell migration control. Int. J. Robot Res. 33 (14), 1782–1792.

Grover, W.H., Bryan, A.K., Diez-Silva, M., Suresh, S., Higgins, J.M., Manalis, S.R., 2011. Measuring single-cell density. Proc. Natl. Acad. Sci. 108, 10992–10996.

Han, S.I., Lee, S.M., Jooc, Y.D., Han, K.H., 2011. Lateral dielectrophoretic microseparators to measure the size distribution of blood cells. Lab Chip 11, 3864–3872.

Hu, S., Sun, D., 2011. Automatic transportation of biological cells with robot-tweezer manipulation system. Int. J. Robot Res. 30, 1681–1694.

Jain, T., McBride, R., Head, S., Saez, E., 2009. Highly parallel introduction of nucleic acids into mammalian cells grown in microwell arrays. Lab Chip 9, 3557–3566.

Jen, C.P., Weng, C.H., Huang, C.T., 2011. Three-dimensional focusing of particles using negative dielectrophoretic force in a microfluidic chip with insulating microstructures and dual planar microelectrodes. Electrophoresis 32, 2428–2435.

Kanai, M., Ikeda, S., Tanaka, J., Go, J.S., Nakanishi, H., Shoji, S., 2004. The multiple sample injector using improved sheath flow to prevent sample dilution. Sens. Actuators A Phys. 111, 32–36.

Kovac, J.R., Voldman, J., 2007. Intuitive, image-based cell sorting using optofluidic cell sorting. Anal. Chem. 79, 9321–9330.

Kress, H., Park, J., Mejean, C.O., Forster, J.D., Park, J., Walse, S.S., Weiner, O.D., Fahmy, T.M., Dufresne, E.R., 2009. Cell stimulation with optically manipulated microsources. Nat. Methods 6, 905–909.

Lenshof, A., Laurell, T., 2010. Continuous separation of cells and particles in microfluidic systems. Chem. Soc. Rev. 39, 1203–1217.

Luo, T., Fan, L., Zeng, Y., Liu, Y., Chen, S., Tan, Q., Lam, R.H.W., Sun, D., 2018. A simplified sheathless cell separation approach using combined gravitational-sedimentation-based prefocusing and dielectrophoretic separation. Lab Chip 18 (11), 1521–1532.

MacDonald, M.P., Spalding, G.C., Dholakia, K., 2003. Microfluidic soring in an optical lattice. Nature 426, 421–424.

Markx, G.H., Davey, C.L., 1999. The dielectric properties of biological cells at radiofrequencies: applications in biotechnology. Enzym. Microb. Technol. 25, 161–171.

Pamme, N., Manz, A., 2004. On-chip free-flow magnetophoresis: continuous-flow separation of magnetic particles and agglomerates. Anal. Chem. 76, 7250–7256.

Park, J., Kim, B., Choi, S.K., Hong, S., Lee, S.H., Lee, K.I., 2005. An efficient cell separation system using 3D-asymmetric microelectrodes. Lab Chip 5, 1264–1270.

Park, M.C., Hur, J.Y., Cho, H.S., Park, S.H., Suh, K.Y., 2011. High-throughput single-cell quantification using simple microwell-based cell docking and programmable time-course live-cell imaging. Lab Chip 11, 79–86.

Peterman, E.J.G., Gittes, F., Schmidt, C.F., 2003. Laser-induced heating in optical traps. Biophys. J. 84, 1308–1316.

Petersson, F., Nilsson, A., Holm, C., Jönssonc, H., Laurell, T., 2005. Continuous separation of lipid particles from erythrocytes by means of laminar flow and acoustic standing wave forces. Lab Chip 5, 20–22.

Petersson, F., Aberg, L., Sward-Nilsson, A.M., Laurell, T., 2007. Free flow acoustophoresis: microfluidic-based mode of particle and cell separation. Anal. Chem. 79, 5117–5123.

Ramadan, Q., Samper, V., Poenar, D.P., Yu, C., 2006. Magnetic-based microfluidic platform for biomolecular separation. Biosens. Bioelectron. 21, 1693–1702.

Ren, Y., Liu, J., Liu, W., Lang, Q., Tao, Y., Hu, Q., Hou, L., Jiang, H., 2016. Scaled particle focusing in a microfluidic device with asymmetric electrodes utilizing induced-charge electroosmosis. Lab Chip 16, 2803–2812.

Shah, G.J., Ohta, A.T., Chiou, P.Y., Wu, M.C., Kim, C.J., 2009. EWOD-driven droplet microfluidic device integrated with optoelectronic tweezers as an automated platform for cellular isolation and analysis. Lab Chip 9, 1732–1739.

Shapiro, H.M., 2003. Practical Flow Cytometry. Wiley-Liss, New York.

Skelley, A.M., Kirak, O., Suh, H., Jaenisch, R., Voldman, J., 2009. Microfluidic control of cell pairing and fusion. Nat. Methods 6, 147–152.

Sollier, E., Go, D.E., Che, J., Gossett, D.R., Byrne, S.O., Weaver, W.M., Kummer, N., Rettig, M., Goldman, J., Nickols, N., Mccloskey, S., Kulkarni, P., Di Carlo, D., 2014. High efficiency vortex trapping of circulating tumor cells. Lab Chip 14, 63−77.

Song, H., Rosano, J.M., Wang, Y., Garson, C.J., Prabhakarpandian, B., Pant, K., Klarmann, G.J., Perantoni, A., Alvarez, L.M., Lai, E., 2015. Continuous-flow sorting of stem cells and differentiation products based on dielectrophoresis. Lab Chip 15, 1320−1328.

Spyratou, E., Makropoulou, M., Mourelatou, E.A., Demetzos, C., 2012. Biophotonic techniques for manipulation and characterization of drug delivery nanosystems in cancer therapy. Cancer Lett. 327, 111−122.

Svoboda, K., Block, S.M., 1994. Biological applications of optical forces. Annu. Rev. Biophys. Biomol. Struct. 23, 247−285.

Tan, Y., Sun, D., Wang, J., Huang, W., 2010. Mechanical characterization of human red blood cells under different osmotic conditions by robotic manipulation with optical tweezers. IEEE Trans. Biomed. Eng. 57, 1816−1825.

Theveneau, E., Mayor, R., 2011. Beads on the run: beads as alternative tools for chemotaxis assays. Methods Mol. Biol. 769, 449−460.

Wang, X., Chen, S., Kong, M., Wang, Z., Costa, K.D., Li, R.A., Sun, D., 2011. Enhanced cell sorting and manipulation with combined optical tweezer and microfluidic chip technologies. Lab Chip 11, 3656−3662.

Wang, X., Gou, X., Chen, S., Yan, X., Sun, D., 2013. Cell manipulation tool with combined microwell array and optical tweezers for cell isolation and deposition. J. Micromech. Microeng. 23 (7), 075006.

Wei, Y., Xu, Z., Cachia, M.A., Nguyen, J., Zheng, Y., Wang, C., Sun, Y., 2016. Embedded silver PDMS electrodes for single cell electrical impedance spectroscopy. J. Micromech. Microeng. 26 (9), 95006.

Wright, W.H., Sonek, G.J., Berns, M.W., 1994. Parametric study of the forces on microspheres held by optical tweezers. Appl. Opt. 33, 1735−1748.

Wu, Y., Sun, D., Huang, W., 2011. Mechanical force characterization in manipulating live cells with optical tweezers. J. Biomech. 44, 741−746.

Wu, Y., Sun, D., Huang, W., Xi, N., 2013. Dynamics analysis and motion planning for automated cell transportation with optical tweezers. IEEE/ASME Trans. Mechatron. 18 (2), 706−713.

Xia, Y., Whitesides, G.M., 1998. Soft lithography. Annu. Rev. Mater. Sci. 28, 153−184.

Yan, S., Zhang, J., Alici, G., Du, H., Zhu, Y., Li, W., 2014. Isolating plasma from blood using a dielectrophoresis-active hydrophoretic device. Lab Chip 14, 2993−3003.

Yan, S., Zhang, J., Yuan, Y., Lovrecz, G., Alici, G., Du, H., Zhu, Y., Li, W., 2015. A hybrid dielectrophoretic and hydrophoretic microchip for particle sorting using integrated prefocusing and sorting steps. Electrophoresis 36, 284−291.

Yan, S., Zhang, J., Yuan, D., Li, W., 2017. Hybrid microfluidics combined with active and passive approaches for continuous cell separation. Electrophoresis 38, 238−249.

Yao, B., Luo, G.A., Feng, X., Wang, W., Chen, L.X., Wang, Y.M., 2004. A microfluidic device based on gravity and electric force driving for flow cytometry and fluorescence activated cell sorting. Lab Chip 4, 603−607.

Zhang, H., Liu, K.K., 2008. Optical tweezers for single cells. J. R. Soc. Interface 5, 671−690.

Zhang, J., Yan, S., Yuan, D., Alici, G., Nguyen, N.T., Warkiani, M.E., Li, W., 2016. Fundamentals and applications of inertial microfluidics: a review. Lab Chip 16, 10−34.

Cell stimulation and migration control

9

9.1 Introduction

Cell migration refers to the movement of cells to a specific location in a specific direction in response to a chemoattractant stimulation, and represents the central process of a variety of biological phenomena (Haastert and Devreotes, 2004; Roussos et al., 2011). Although great progress has been made already in the study of cell migration, especially in the study of various stimuli and related proteins (Gurdon and Bourillot, 2001; Ridley et al., 2003), the understanding of cell migration mechanisms for precise and active control of cells of cell movement remains limited. During migration, cells rearrange their shapes in response to extracellular signals and extend protrusions at the leading edge (Haastert and Devreotes, 2004). The protrusion force generated by the polymerization of actin in the cell drives the cell to move toward the stimulus. Elucidating the protrusion force is very important for understanding the movement produced by actin polymerization.

The gradient of chemoattractant molecules activates the inner filament network and causes a cell chemotactic response (Gurdon and Bourillot, 2001; Amselem et al., 2012). It is important to determine the relationship between the chemoattractant gradient and cell motility quantitatively. As is well known, cells are subjected to a variety of forces (including protruding force) in the process of migration, which overcomes obstacles caused by friction and stickiness, and drives cells to move toward stimuli. Other forces on the cell are caused by the adhesion of the leading edge, the deadhesion of cell body and back, and contraction of the cytoskeleton (Ananthakrishnan and Ehrlicher, 2007). The precise estimation of the cell protrusion force has remained a challenging problem (Prechtel et al., 2002; Tan et al., 2011; Wang et al., 2013). Gou et al. (2014) proposed the use of robotically controlled optical tweezers to trap a chemoattractant-loaded biocompatible polylactic-co-glycolic acid (PLGA) microparticle, which releases chemoattractant molecules into a liquid environment and induces cell polarization and migration. The establishment of a cell manipulation tool that can artificially generate a gradient field under in vitro conditions will help to facilitate in-depth research on cell migration in vivo. Yang et al. (2015) proposed a dynamic model of cell migration in an in vitro chemoattractant environment, simulating in vivo conditions to induce cell polarization and migration. This model aims to illustrate the relationship between the chemoattractant gradient and cell force, and to reveal the cell motility capacity. Compared with other cell manipulation methods, the migration control framework of Gou et al. (2014) provides a unique platform to explore cell migration models by Yang et al. (2015) and enable automatic cell migration control.

Biological research and medical applications are in great need of cell migration control technology. This efficient technology is necessary to solve many challenges of cell

Robotic Cell Manipulation. https://doi.org/10.1016/B978-0-323-85259-3.00004-0

migration. These challenges include determining the dynamic mechanisms that guide cell migration (Gou et al., 2014) and molecular components that influence the process (Lauffenburger and Horwitz, 1996), determining the way cells establish and maintain polarity during migration, investigating the formation and dispersion of adhesions, as well as studying cellular target recognition (Ridley et al., 2003). By determining disease through migration, migration-oriented drug delivery may become more effective, and can be accelerated by an automatic induction system. Improving these cell migration studies requires the design of automated technologies for cell migration control. Yang et al. (2017) developed a robot-assisted technology for cell migration control, which can monitor the response of cells stimulated by optically trapped microsources. To achieve automatic cell migration control, the interaction among the optical tweezers manipulator, microsource beads, and target cells is well regulated. This control allows the optical tweezers to trap the microbeads well, and the beads to be confined at a suitable distance from the cell to ensure a high stimulation effect. Meng et al. (2019) further developed a dual closed-loop control strategy, which includes an inner tweezers—bead control loop and an outer bead—cell control loop. The inner loop adopts a proportional integral feedback plus a feedforward controller, and the outer loop adopts an active disturbance rejection controller, which can solve the cell migration modeling error and unknown external interference.

Electrical stimulation (ES) is also widely used to stimulate cells to treat heart disease (Dura et al., 2012; Fonseca et al., 2013) and to promote bone healing (Hannouche et al., 2001). ES can affect the distribution and ligand binding of receptors on the cell membrane to regulate transmembrane signals, thereby upregulating related mRNA expression levels and protein synthesis during bone formation (Aaron et al., 1999). Compared with medium-induced differentiation, ES-induced differentiation can provide a safer and more convenient method to induce osteogenic differentiation. Direct current (DC) and alternating current (AC) have been used in osteogenesis research (Wiesmann et al., 2001). ES may affect cell behavior through calcium ion activities (Ramezani and Akan, 2018). A DC electric field with a frequency range of 1—10 Hz can induce Ca^{2+} influx (Cho et al., 1999). In addition, low-frequency alternating current stimulation can change intracellular Ca^{2+} without causing cellular damage (Cho et al., 2002). The calcium spike pattern varies with different cell types, including undifferentiated mesenchymal stem cells (MSCs). Undifferentiated MSCs show regular calcium spike patterns, while MSCs show a reduced frequency of calcium spike patterns during osteogenic differentiation (Titushkin et al., 2010). Therefore, a new method for controlling Ca^{2+} spikes in MSCs by microsecond electric pulses has been reported (Hanna et al., 2017). Motivated by these studies, researchers have recognized the need to optimize ES conditions based on changes in calcium spike patterns. However, due to complex components, including waveform, voltage, frequency, and duty time, it is difficult to determine the appropriate parameters for the existing AC ES. Hou et al. (2019) successfully described how ES parameters affect ES-induced differentiation based on the calcium spike patterns. To verify the hypothesis that increasing the voltage and low frequency of ES can reduce the frequency of calcium spikes in MSCs, which may be related to the osteogenic differentiation process, they used a microfluidic chip with patterned indium tin oxide (ITO) microelectrodes and PDMS cell culture wells to analyze the differentiation of MSCs under different sets of ES parameters. Quantitative characterization of the effects of various ES parameters on calcium spike patterns can provide new insights into how to use cell information to improve existing knowledge of ES-based MSC osteogenic differentiation.

The remainder of this chapter introduces cell stimulation and migration from three perspectives, namely, the chemoattractant-induced cell migration model, the use of the stimulus-induced robotic manipulation system to control cell migration, and electrical stimulation to improve the osteogenic differentiation of MSCs.

9.2 Dynamic model of chemoattractant-induced cell migration

9.2.1 Model development

The optical tweezers manipulation system reported in earlier chapters can be used to manipulate the cell migration control. The system provides an intuitive user interface and allows dexterous control of the optical trap. The incubator is installed on a motorized stage to keep the cells in an atmosphere of 5% CO_2 at a temperature of 37°C. The optical trapping stiffness (k) can be calibrated through a series of experiments on trapping PLGA beads (Wu et al., 2013), which has been reported in detail in earlier chapters. The leukemia cancer Jurkat cell was selected as the sample for the cell migration test. The Jurkat cell is a kind of immortalized T lymphocyte line. Because of its relatively fast movement speed, it is suitable for the study of cell motility.

The chemoattractant concentration gradient is generated by PLGA beads manipulated by optical tweezers. PLGA beads are fabricated using solvent evaporation-spontaneous emulsification technology (Fahmy et al., 2005), which are loaded with SDF-1α chemoattractant and can stimulate the migration of leukemia cancer Jurkat cells. The radius of the beads ranges from 1 to 3 μm. The beads are trapped using optical tweezers and placed within 3–5 μm of the cell. The soluble chemoattractant molecules are released into the liquid with a relatively slow diffusion coefficient (approximately 1.7×10^{-13} m^2/s). Over a time period of 100–200 s, the PLGA beads create a concentration spherical field with a radius of approximately 4–8 μm. Fig. 9.1 illustrates the simulated gradient field generated by two microsources, which was obtained by the finite element analysis software COMSOL.

Once the cell detects the chemoattractant gradient, it generates a force that drives the cell to the chemoattractant-loaded microsource. This force is defined as the protrusion force denoted by F_p. During the migration process, the cell is resisted by viscous $F_{viscous}$ (generated by the liquid environment) and friction $F_{friction}$ (found between the cell and the substrate), as shown in Fig. 9.2A. F_p, $F_{viscous}$, and $F_{friction}$ contribute to cell movement, as described in the following dynamic equation:

$$F_c + m\ddot{q} = F_p - F_{friction} - F_{viscous}, \tag{9.1}$$

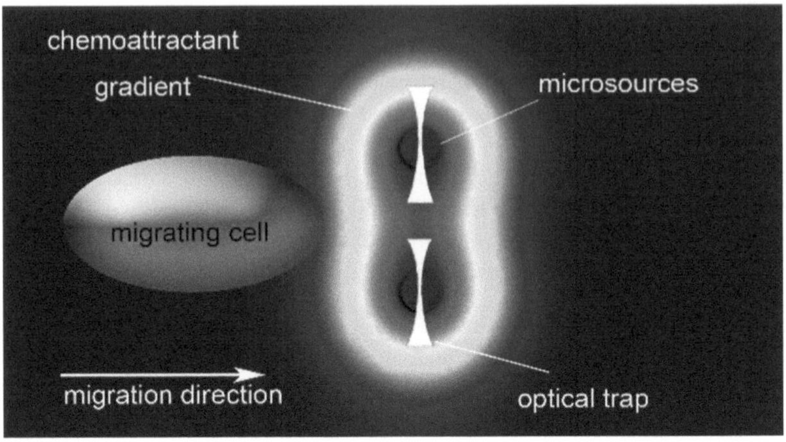

Figure 9.1 Simulated gradient generation with two microsources (Yang et al., 2015).

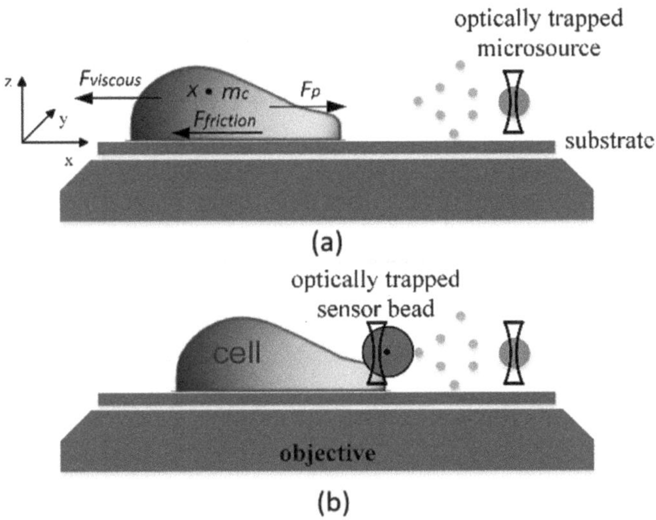

Figure 9.2 Schematic of the model for probing cell migration (Yang et al., 2015). (A) A cell stimulated by a chemoattractant-loaded PLGA microsource. (B) Use of an optically trapped bead for force sensing.

where m and q denote the mass and position of the centroid of the cell, respectively, and $m\ddot{q}$ is generally neglected in an environment with low Reynolds number. According to Svoboda and Block (1994), $F_{viscous} = \beta\dot{q}$, where β is the drag coefficient. The friction force $F_{friction}$ can be determined using the adapted Zhurkov model (Pompe et al., 2011), expressed as $F_{friction} = dA\mu^{-1}\dot{q}$, where d is defined as the area density of the ligand adhesion in effective proportion A. Specifically, d is approximately 200 μm^{-2} to 300 μm^{-2}, the ligand mobility μ ranging from 10^4 to 10^5 m/Ns (Pompe et al., 2011), and A can be experimentally determined. F_c is a term generated by the complex actin polymerization and molecular motors (Ananthakrishnan and Ehrlicher, 2007). To measure the influence of F_c, a polystyrene bead (with a radius of 1−2 μm) can be used as a force sensor and trapped by optical tweezers, placed between the cell and the microsource bead, as shown in Fig. 9.2B. When the cell moves toward the microsource, the cell pushes this sensor bead away from the focus of the trap, resulting in an optical trapping force applied to the bead. At this moment, the moving speed of the cell also drops rapidly. The trapping force applied to the bead can be estimated as $F_{trap} = kx_b$ when the bead is within the critical displacement, where x_b is the offset of the bead (Wu et al., 2011). In this method, F_c can be indirectly examined by calculating the trapping force F_{trap}, using $F_c = F_{trap} = kx_b$. Note that when the cell stops moving, F_c is measured in a static equilibrium state. Gou et al. (2014) have shown that the cell is sensitive to the external barrier, implying that the cell velocity decreases rapidly when there is a barrier present in front of the cell. This is coincident with the elastic Brownian ratchet model (Mogilner and Oster, 2003).

The substitution of $F_{viscous}$, $F_{friction}$, and F_c into Eq. (9.1) yields the relationship between the protrusion force and the velocity of the migrating cell, which can be expressed as:

$$F_p = \left(\beta + dA\mu^{-1}\right)\dot{q} + kx_b \tag{9.2}$$

Methods to explain how cells detect gradients have been reported in the literature. For example, cell use receptors and G protein-linked signaling pathways to detect gradients (Parent and Devreotes, 1999); by measuring the concentration of chemoattractants around the cell, the cell can recognize the highest concentration gradient and determine the direction of stimulation (Alex and Simon, 1994). In the studies by Gou et al. (2014) and Yang et al. (2015), the chemoattractant gradient was created by placing an optically trapped microsource near the cell, which is standardized to $g = \nabla C/g_0$, where C denotes the chemoattractant concentration, and $g_0 = 1$ mol/m^4. The concentration of chemoattractant molecules on the surface of the spherical microsource can be expressed as $C_0 = \frac{l_0 \rho_b a^2}{3M_w t_r D}$ (Kress et al., 2009), where $l_0 < 1$ is the loading ratio (the molecular mass loaded into the particle divided by the particle mass), ρ_b is the mass density of the particulate material, a is the particle radius, M_w is the molecular weight of the molecule, t_r is the release time measured when the bead is placed in the solution, and D is the diffusion coefficient of the molecule (Kress et al., 2009).

According to the Elastic Brownian Ratchet model (Mogilner and Oster, 2003), the protrusion force is generated by the filament network, and the cell migration velocity can be expressed as:

$$\dot{q} = V_{\max} \exp\left[-l\left(f a\frac{a}{w} + \frac{F_c}{w}\right) / k_B T\right] - V_{dep} \tag{9.3}$$

where l is the average length increase in the growth direction of actin filaments after one assembly f_a is the attachment force of each filament, a is the number of attached filaments, w is the number of working filaments, k_BT is thermal energy, $V_{\max}$ is the free polymerization rate, and V_{dep} is the free depolymerization rate. Notably, $a = n/\delta$ and $w = n/\kappa$, where n, δ, and κ denote the nucleation, dissociation, and capping rates, respectively.

The chemoattractant stimulation changes the number of filaments. Working filaments contribute to the cell movement, but attached filaments do not. The dissociation rate δ represents the conversion rate of attached filaments to working filaments. Therefore, a high δ value promotes cell migration. Conversely, the capping rate κ inhibits the growth of working filaments, thus hindering cell motility. Considering that attached filaments can be converted into working filaments, a high nucleation rate n value that helps attached filaments grow (Mogilner and Oster, 2003) can also promote cell motility. Therefore, when cells are stimulated by a chemoattractant, the rate of filament dissociation and nucleation may increase, while the capping rate tends to decrease.

Based on the above analysis and the excitation response of the cell (Parent and Devreotes, 1999), δ, κ, and n can be formulated as $\delta = \lambda_1 \tanh g$, $\kappa = \lambda_2/(g+1)$, and $n = \lambda_3 \tanh g$, where λ_1 denotes the maximum dissociation rate, λ_2 denotes the capping rate when $g = 0$, and λ_3 denotes the maximum nucleation rate. As a result, the number of attached and working filaments can be calculated as $a = n/\delta = \lambda_3/\lambda_1$ and $w = n/\kappa = \frac{\lambda_3}{\lambda_2}(g+1)\tanh g$, which clearly indicates that the gradient promotes the growth of working filaments, not the growth of attached filaments. Consequently, Eq. (9.3) can be modified as:

$$\dot{q} = V_{\max} \exp\left[-\frac{l}{(g+1)k_BT \tanh g}\left(\frac{\lambda_2 f_a}{\lambda_1} + \frac{\lambda_2 F_c}{\lambda_3}\right)\right] - V_{dep} \tag{9.4}$$

Eq. (9.4) explicitly reveals the relationship between the cell movement velocity and gradient. By substituting Eq. (9.4) into Eq. (9.2), the relationship between the protrusion force F_p and the gradient g can be derived as:

$$F_p = \phi \exp\left(-\xi \frac{1}{(g+1)\tanh g}\right) - \rho \tag{9.5}$$

where $\phi = \left(\beta + dA\mu^{-1}\right)V_{\max}$ (with a unit of pN) denotes the maximum force generated by cell, $\xi = \frac{l}{k_BT}\left(f_a\frac{\lambda_2}{\lambda_1} + F_c\frac{\lambda_2}{\lambda_3}\right)$ denotes the gradient effect coefficient (which is dimensionless), and $\rho = \left(\beta + dA\mu^{-1}\right)V_{dep} - kx_b$ (with a unit of pN) denotes the hinder force generated by cell.

Fig. 9.3 illustrates the prediction results of the quantitative model. As the gradient increases, the number of attached filaments (a) remains the same, while the number of working filaments (w) increases. When the gradient changes initially, the cell velocity and protrusion force increase rapidly, indicating that the cells are sensitive to external

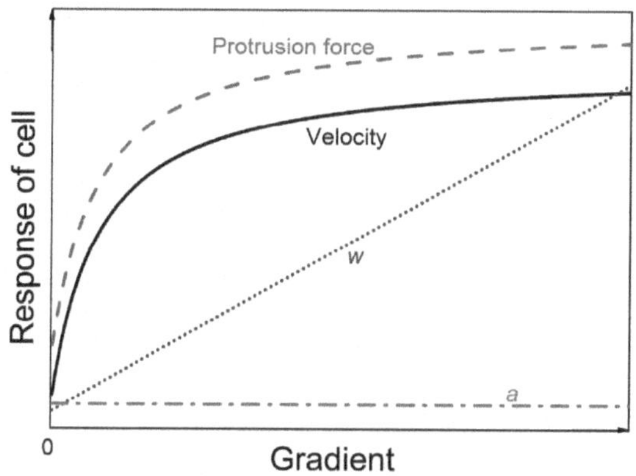

Figure 9.3 Model prediction results for filament numbers, cell velocity, and cell protrusion force as the gradient increases (Yang et al., 2015).

stimuli. The cell speed and protrusion force gradually stabilize. This result is very consistent with the known knowledge that cell receptors, proteins, and filaments can be saturated. Note that although the modeling parameters are different for different types of cells, the cell response trends of different cells should be similar.

9.2.2 Model verification

The accuracy of the models described by Eqs. (9.2), (9.4), and (9.5) was experimentally verified using migrating leukemia cancer Jurkat cells stimulated by optically manipulated SDF-1α-loaded PLGA beads. According to Merks et al. (2008), the diffusion coefficient of SDF-1α is about 1.7×10^{-13} m^2/s, and the molecular weight of SDF-1α is $M_w = 8008$. Therefore, the estimated concentration on the surface of the microsource is calculated as $C_0 = 2.5$ μM. A three-dimensional numerical model based on the experimental setup can be established by the finite element analysis software COMSOL to calculate the concentration gradient, as shown in Fig. 9.4A and B. Fig. 9.4C and D show the concentration and gradient distribution along the central axis of the microsource bead. Fig. 9.4E and F show the concentration and gradient distribution on the cell surface. The distance between the cell and the microsource bead is set as 3.5 μm. When the cell directly faces the two beads at zero degrees, as shown in Fig. 9.4F, the concentration and gradient reach the maximum.

Fig. 9.5 shows a typical experimental process, illustrating that when the cell moves toward the stimulus induced by the chemical attractant gradient, the barrier bead (as a force sensor) is pushed away from the focal point of the optical trap. Hu et al. (2013) reported that even if it is trapped directly, the trapping process will not significantly impair cell viability.

Fig. 9.6A illustrates a set of test results based on Eq. (9.2), arranged in the chronological order of F_p, $F_{friction}$, and F_c. The protrusion force F_p reaches as high as 1000 pN or more, and $F_{friction}$ closely follows F_p. When the cell is nearly stationary at 130 s, F_c

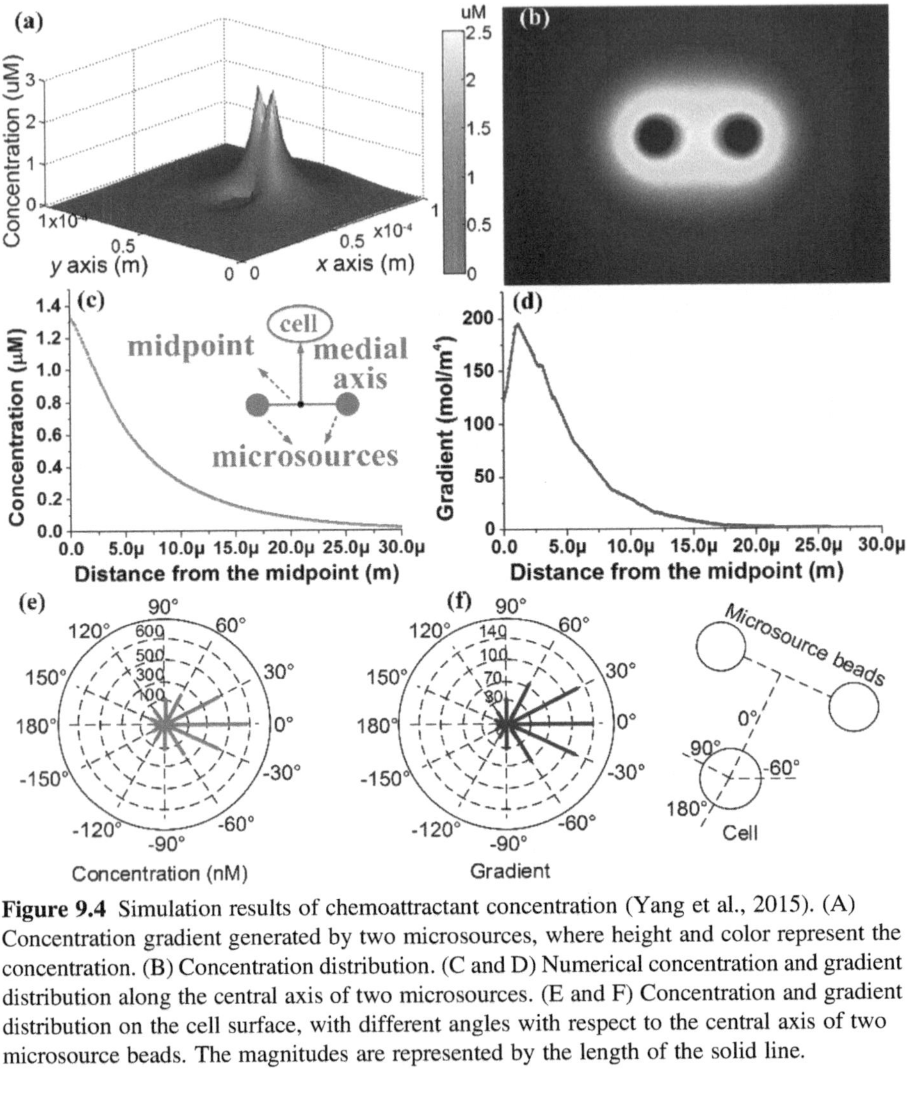

Figure 9.4 Simulation results of chemoattractant concentration (Yang et al., 2015). (A) Concentration gradient generated by two microsources, where height and color represent the concentration. (B) Concentration distribution. (C and D) Numerical concentration and gradient distribution along the central axis of two microsources. (E and F) Concentration and gradient distribution on the cell surface, with different angles with respect to the central axis of two microsource beads. The magnitudes are represented by the length of the solid line.

measures 150 pN. The viscous force of the cell is only 10^{-3} pN, calculated using $\beta = 0.7$ pNs/μm, which is too small to be shown in Fig. 9.6A. Fig. 9.6B shows the relationship between F_p and velocity $\dot{q}$, where $\dot{q}$ is measured based on image processing. Compared with F_c, the influence of $F_{friction}$ in Eq. (9.2) is more significant, which explains the approximately linear relationship between F_p and $\dot{q}$ in Fig. 9.6B. Fig. 9.6C shows the distance between the cell leading edge and the microsource beads. Fig. 9.6D shows the migration of cells along the gradient direction.

Table 9.1 provides the experimental results based on 10 cell samples. It can be seen that the range of F_c is between 100 and 300 pN, and the average protrusion force F_p is

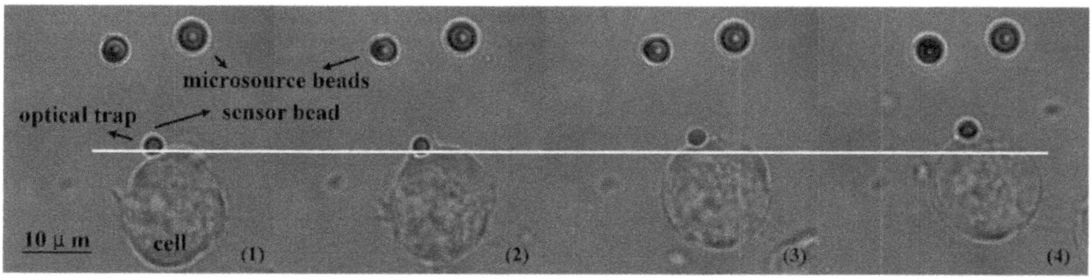

Figure 9.5 Experimental process in chronological sequence for protrusion force measurement (Yang et al., 2015).

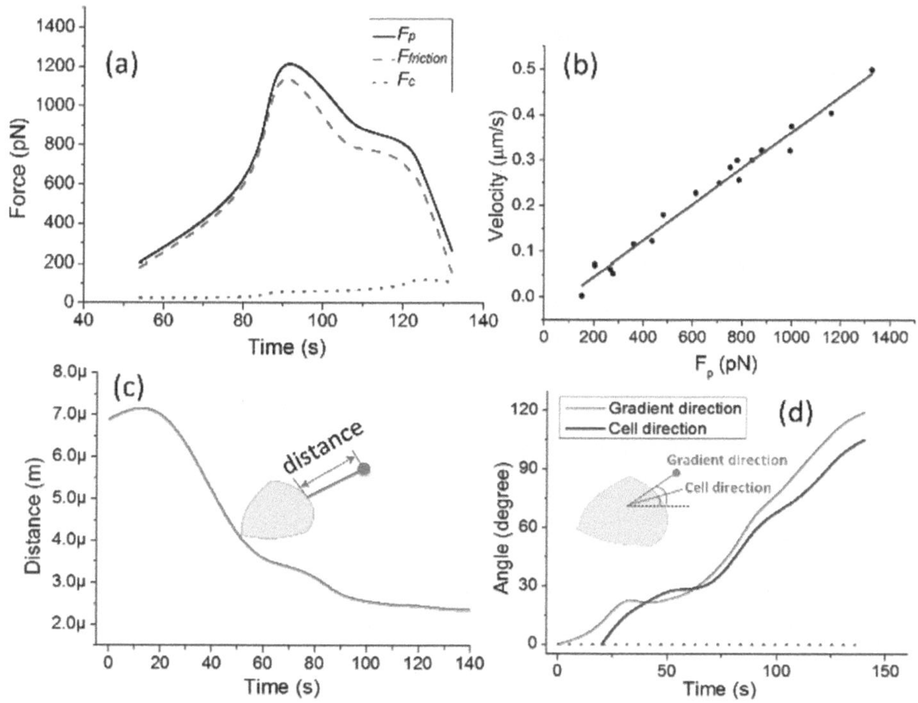

Figure 9.6 Experimental results (Yang et al., 2015). (A) Variation of the main forces experienced by the cell during migration. (B) Relationship between the protrusion force and the cell speed. (C) The distance between the cell leading edge and microsources during migration. (D) Directions of the cell migration and gradient.

about 1000 pN. The protrusion force is large enough to overcome the friction and viscous forces that drive the cell to move forward.

Fig. 9.7 illustrates F_p and $\dot{q}$ with respect to the concentration gradient g. When the gradient starts to increase, both F_p and $\dot{q}$ increase rapidly, and then both stabilize when the gradient reaches 150 mol/m^4. The solid lines are the fitting results of the protrusion

Table 9.1 Force measurement data of Jurkat cells (Yang et al., 2015).

Cell No.	Avg. F_c (pN)	Avg. F_p (pN)	Avg. $F_{friction}$ (pN)	Avg. $F_{viscous}$ (pN)
1	124.1	1000.4	938.4	0.0025
2	297.6	1124.0	808.4	0.0031
3	73.3	1254.9	1191.6	0.0042
4	36.7	896.7	865.2	0.0045
5	147.7	846.8	681.5	0.0016
6	135.8	965.7	825.6	0.0033
7	108.9	1043.6	930.8	0.0036
8	257.1	1095.4	749.8	0.0020
9	315.1	1068.2	717.3	0.0022
10	313.5	1306.5	984.2	0.0033

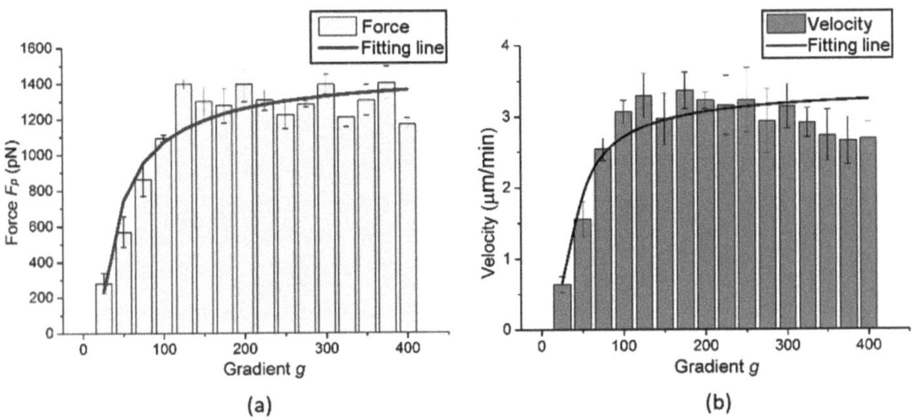

Figure 9.7 Experimental analysis of cell motility (Yang et al., 2015). (A) Protrusion force F_p and the fitting line of F_p with respect to gradient g. (B) Cell velocity and the fitting line with respect to gradient g.

force and velocity based on the actual test results, which can be mathematically modeled as:

$$F_p = 2576 \exp\left(-\frac{16}{(g+1)\tanh g}\right) - 1106 \tag{9.6}$$

$$\dot{q} = 6.4 \exp\left(-\frac{16}{(g+1)\tanh g}\right) - 2.8 \tag{9.7}$$

After fitting Eq. (9.6) to Eq. (9.5) and Eq. (9.7) to Eq. (9.4), the modeling parameters in Eqs. (9.4) and (9.5) can be extracted, as given in Table 9.2. Based on these

Table 9.2 Identified parameters (Yang et al., 2015).

Equations	Parameters						
	ϕ (pN)	ξ	ρ (pN)	V_{max} (μm/min)	V_{dep} (μm/min)	R-sq.	Adj. R-sq.
Eq. (9.5)	NA	16 ± 3	NA	6.4 ± 1.2	2.8 ± 0.5	0.801	0.762
Eq. (9.6)	2576 ± 165	16 ± 3	1106 ± 92	NA	NA	0.867	0.847

parameters, λ_1, λ_2, and λ_3 can be identified as 0.4/s, 0.8/s, and 8/s, respectively, which are close to the prediction results of δ (0.5/s), κ (0.5/s), and n (10/s) by Mogilner and Oster (2003).

The experimental results in Fig. 9.7 clearly show that both the protrusion force and the cell velocity increase with increase of the gradient, and their trends are the same as the predicted results of the model shown in Fig. 9.3, thus verifying the correctness of the proposed model. Moreover, the model given in Eqs. (9.4) and (9.5) clarify the quantitative relationship between cell motility and gradient.

Cell motility is also significantly affected by the concentration at the leading edge of the cell, denoted by C_{front}. Fig. 9.8 shows the experimental results of the relationship between F_p and the concentration at the leading edge of the cell. When the concentration is about 30 nM, the cell exhibits the highest migration ability, indicating that the motility of the cell does not necessarily increase with the increase of the concentration. This phenomenon can be attributed to the saturation and limited number of chemoattractant receptors. This finding indicates that the migration ability of each cell reaches its maximum at a concentration close to the dissociation constant (K_d). This is because,

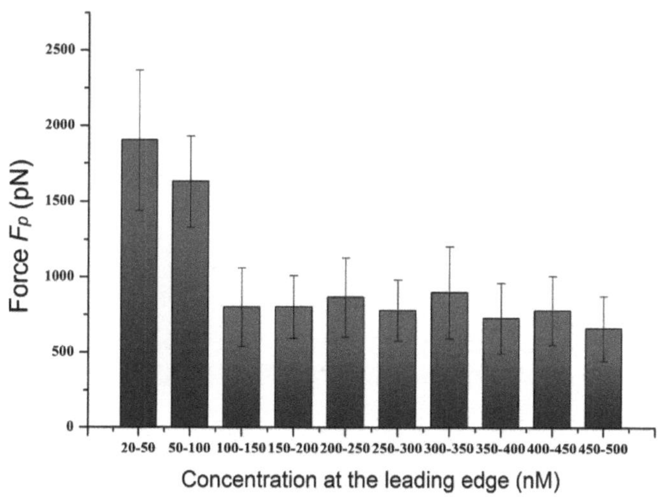

Figure 9.8 The trend of F_p as C_{front} changes (Yang et al., 2015).

according to Pelletier et al. (2000), the K_d of SDF-1α is between 20 and 40 nM, and the 30 nM concentration value at which cells exhibit the highest motility falls within this range. This finding leads to a hypothesis that both the concentration C_{front} and the gradient g considerably affect cell motility.

9.3 Cell migration control using a stimulus-induced robotic manipulation system

In this section, a robotic single-cell-migration control framework is introduced. As shown in Fig. 9.9, the chemoattractant-loaded microsource beads trapped by optical tweezers release the chemoattractant molecules into the medium to form a chemical gradient. The radius of the beads ranges from 1 to 3 μm. The cell perceives the gradient and moves toward the microsource beads. When the microbeads are moved by robotically controlled optical tweezers, the cell will migrate with the movement of the beads. Note that the cell adheres to the substrate with greater friction during the migration process, so the optical trap near the cell will not significantly affect the cell movement. PLGA beads are used here to generate a chemoattractant concentration gradient field. The PLGA beads are fabricated using a solvent evaporation−spontaneous emulsification technology (Banerjee et al., 2010), and are loaded with SDF-1α chemoattractant and can stimulate leukemic cancer cells. According to Lin and Butcher (2016), soluble chemoattractant molecules are released into the medium with a relatively slow diffusion coefficient D, which is approximately 1.7×10^{-10} m^2/s. The concentration on the surface of the beads is about 2.5 nM, and the drug can be released continuously for over 1 h (Kress et al., 2009). Under the condition that the velocity of the microbeads is sufficiently low, the concentration distribution in the region of interest around the beads can be considered to be in a stable state (Kress et al., 2009).

9.3.1 Model

9.3.1.1 Optical manipulation of the microsource beads

The microsource beads are controlled by the optical tweezer manipulators to induce cell migration. Suspended in a liquid environment, the microsource beads are trapped

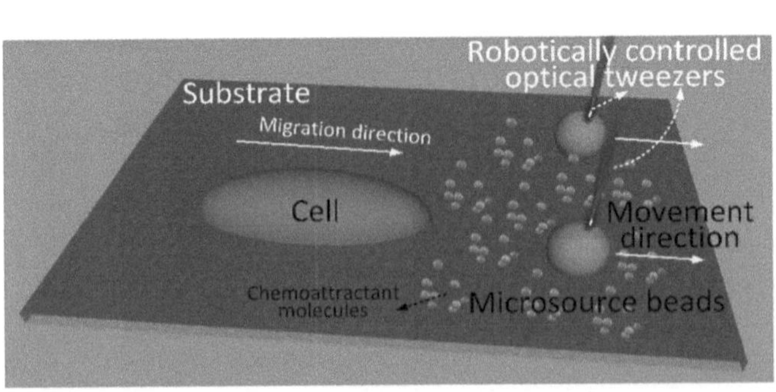

Figure 9.9 Schematic of cell migration induced by the microsource beads trapped by optical tweezers (Yang et al., 2017).

and moved along the x−y plane by the optical tweezers, and so they are regarded as multiple agents in a two-dimensional (2D) space. The microsource bead is denoted as a circle centered at $q_{bi} \in \Re^2$ with a radius of br_i, and the desired position of the micro-source bead as q_{bi}^d, where i is the index of the bead. Similarly, the optical trap is denoted as a circle centered at $l_i(t) \in \Re^2$ with a radius of or_i. The motion of the micro-source bead is mainly governed by two forces, namely the trapping force F_{trap} caused by the optical trap and the viscous drag force F_{drag} in the liquid environment, as reported in Wu et al. (2011). The dynamics of the ith microsource bead trapped by optical tweezers in a liquid environment is given by

$$m_i \ddot{q}_{bi} = F_{trap} - F_{drag} = k_t(l_i - q_{bi}) - k_d \dot{q}_{bi}, \tag{9.8}$$

where m_i denotes the mass of the ith bead, the optical trapping force $F_{trap} = k_t(l_i - q_{bi})$, $l_i - q_{bi}$ denotes the offset between the center of mass of the microsource bead and the focus of the optical trap, k_t denotes the trapping stiffness when the offset is less than the critical displacement r_0 (Wu et al., 2011), and the viscous drag force $F_{drag} = k_d \dot{q}_{bi}$, k_d denotes the viscous coefficient. To effectively manipulate the beads, the offset $l_i - q_{bi}$ should be limited to the critical offset r_0. Otherwise, the beads may escape from the optical trap during manipulation.

The trapping area of the ith microsource bead is defined as

$$C_i = \left\{ q_{bi} \middle| r_0^2 - \|l_i - q_{bi}\|^2 > 0 \right\}. \tag{9.9}$$

If $q_{bi} \in C_i$, then the bead is located inside the trapping area.

When the Reynolds number of the liquid environment is low, the inertial force $m_i \ddot{q}_i$ can be ignored. Considering that the velocity of the beads is lower than 10 μm/s, the Reynolds number ($Re < 10^{-4} << 1$) is small enough that the inertial force can be ignored. Then, the dynamics of the microsource bead is simplified to

$$\dot{q}_{bi} = \frac{k_t}{k_d}(l_i - q_{bi}). \tag{9.10}$$

Consider n beads represented by $\{q_{b1}, \ldots, q_{bn}\}$ with a radius of $br = \{br_1, \ldots, br_n\}$ and n traps applied on the beads. Their positions are represented by $l = \{l_1, \ldots, l_n\}$. Only when the center of the bead is located inside the trapping area C_i can the robot−tweezer system effectively manipulate the ith bead. Therefore, the center of the laser trap must be controlled to maintain the connection with the bead and ensure that the ith bead will not escape from the ith trap. This tweezer−bead connection is defined as the T−B coalition (Yang et al., 2017), which is similar to the concept of Li et al. (2015).

A constraint function is introduced to maintain the ith T−B coalition as follows:

$$G_i^{T-B} = \frac{1}{2}\left(r_0^2 - \|l_i - q_{bi}\|^2 \right). \tag{9.11}$$

The T−B coalition can be considered as a virtual circle defined as follows:

Definition 1 (T−B coalition): T−B coalition is defined as a virtual circle with a center of q_{bi} and radius of R_i^{T-B}, which satisfies the T−B coalition constraint $G_i^{T-B} > 0$.

9.3.1.2 Cell manipulation through microsource beads

Yang et al. (2015) demonstrated that cell motility is greatly affected by the chemoattractant concentration gradient. To promote cell migration in a chemoattractant environment, the concentration gradient around the cell should be high. On one hand, it is expected that the microsource beads are confined near the cell to create a high-gradient field. On the other hand, the beads should also maintain a safe distance from the cell to avoid contact. The area surrounding a safe distance around the cell is defined as the *high-motility area*. If the beads are confined to such a high-motility area, the resulting gradient can be high enough and there will be no collisions between the cell and the beads.

9.3.1.2.1 B−C coalition

By placing microsource beads near the cell, a bead−cell connection defined as B−C coalition is introduced. The constraint function for maintaining the ith B−C coalition is defined as follows:

$$G_i^{B-C} = \begin{cases} 1, & \text{if } l_i - q \geq r_h \\ \frac{1}{2}\left(r_i^{BC^2} - l_i - q^2\right), & \text{if } l_i - q < r_h \end{cases}, \tag{9.12}$$

where $r_i^{BC} = r_1 + br_i + r_c$, q denotes the position of the cell, and $r_h = r_1 + br_i + r_c - \rho_d$. r_1 denotes the extremity between the bead and the cell, at which the high gradient sensed by the cell can be guaranteed. r_c denotes the radius of the cell, and ρ_d is defined as the buffer distance.

The B−C coalition can also be regarded as a virtual circle, defined as follows:

Definition 2 (B−C coalition): B−C coalition is defined as a virtual circle with a center of c and a radius of $r_1 + br_i + r_c$, which satisfies the B−C coalition constraint $G_i^{B-C} > 0$.

9.3.1.2.2 Contractive coalition

At the beginning of the manipulation, the microsource beads may be far away from the cell. To transport the beads to the high-motility area to form the initial B−C coalition, preliminary manipulation of the microsource beads is required. A concept called "*contractive coalition*" is introduced. To drive the ith bead closer to the cell, a constraint function is introduced as follows:

$$G_i^{CC} = \begin{cases} \frac{1}{2}\left(r_i^{CC^2} - l_i - q^2\right), & \text{if } l_i - q \geq r_h \\ 1, & \text{if } l_i - q < r_h \end{cases}, \tag{9.13}$$

where $r_i^{CC} = \|q_{bi} - q\| + \rho_d . r_i^{cc}$ is a parameter that depends on the distance between the cell and the ith bead. $G_i^{CC} > 0$ indicates that the bead is located within the contractive coalition of the cell. The border of this coalition is set close to the bead, implying that the bead is driven away from the border and close to the cell. Once the border of the contractive coalition coincides with the B–C coalition boundary, the contractive coalition (9.13) ceases to operate and the B–C coalition (9.12) is activated. The contractive coalition can be considered as a virtual circle with varying radius, defined as follows:

Definition 3 (*contractive coalition*): Contractive coalition is defined as a virtual circle with a center of q and a radius of r_i^{cc}, which satisfies the contractive coalition constraint $G_i^{CC} > 0$.

9.3.1.2.3 B–C wall

To avoid the beads being too close to the cell, the distance between the ith bead and the cell should be greater than the threshold value r_2. Such a threshold distance is like a "wall" between the cell and the beads. The bead–cell repulsion as the B–C wall, which can be maintained by introducing the following constraint function, is defined as:

$$G_i^{B-CW} = \frac{1}{2}\left(\|l_i - q\|^2 - r_i^{BCW^2}\right), \tag{9.14}$$

where r_i^{BCW} is a variable parameter designed to gradually remove the B–C wall when the cell reaches the desired area. r_i^{BCW} is expressed as follows:

$$r_i^{BCW} = \begin{cases} r_c + br_i + r_2, & q_{bi}^d - q \geq r_c + br_i + r_1 \\ r_2 - r_1 + q_{bi}^d - q, & r_1 - r_2 < q_{bi}^d - q < r_c + br_i + r_1 \\ 0, & q_{bi}^d - q \leq r_1 - r_2 \end{cases}. \tag{9.15}$$

It is worth noting that $G_i^{B-CW} > 0$ indicates that the ith bead is not close to the cell and that the B–C wall is maintained. Through the constraint function (9.14), the B–C wall can be considered as a virtual circle defined as follows:

Definition 4 (*B–C wall*): The B–C wall is defined as a virtual circle with a center of c and a radius of r_i^{BCW}. When the bead is located outside the virtual circle, the B–C wall constraint of $G_i^{B-CW} > 0$ is satisfied.

9.3.1.2.4 High-motility area

The *high-motility area* is defined as follows:

Definition 5 (*high-motility area*): The high-motility area of the cell with respect to the ith bead is defined as the area of $G_i^{B-C} > 0 \cap G_i^{B-CW} > 0$ when $\|l_i - q\| \langle\, r_h$.

9.3.1.2.5 B−B wall

To ensure that there will be no collisions between different beads, the B−B wall is defined as no single bead will be very close to other beads. The constraint function used to maintain the *i*th B−B wall is designed as follows:

$$G_i^{B-B} = \prod_j \left(\left\| l_i - q_{bj} \right\|^2 - r_i^{BBW^2} \right) = \prod_j \beta_j \tag{9.16}$$

where $r_i^{BBW} = br_i + r_3$, $j \in \{1, \ldots, n\}$ $(j \neq i)$, representing the index for a set of microsource beads except the *i*th bead, and r_3 denotes the safety distance between two adjacent beads. $G_i^{B-B} > 0$ indicates that there is no collision between the microsource beads.

Definition 6 (*B−B wall*): B−B wall is defined as a virtual circle with a center of l_i and radius of $br_i + r_3$. Other beads are located outside the virtual circle, satisfying the B−B wall constraint $G_i^{B-B} > 0$.

Fig. 9.10A illustrates the concepts of T−B and B−C coalitions and B−C and B−B walls, and Fig. 9.10B shows the relevant parameters.

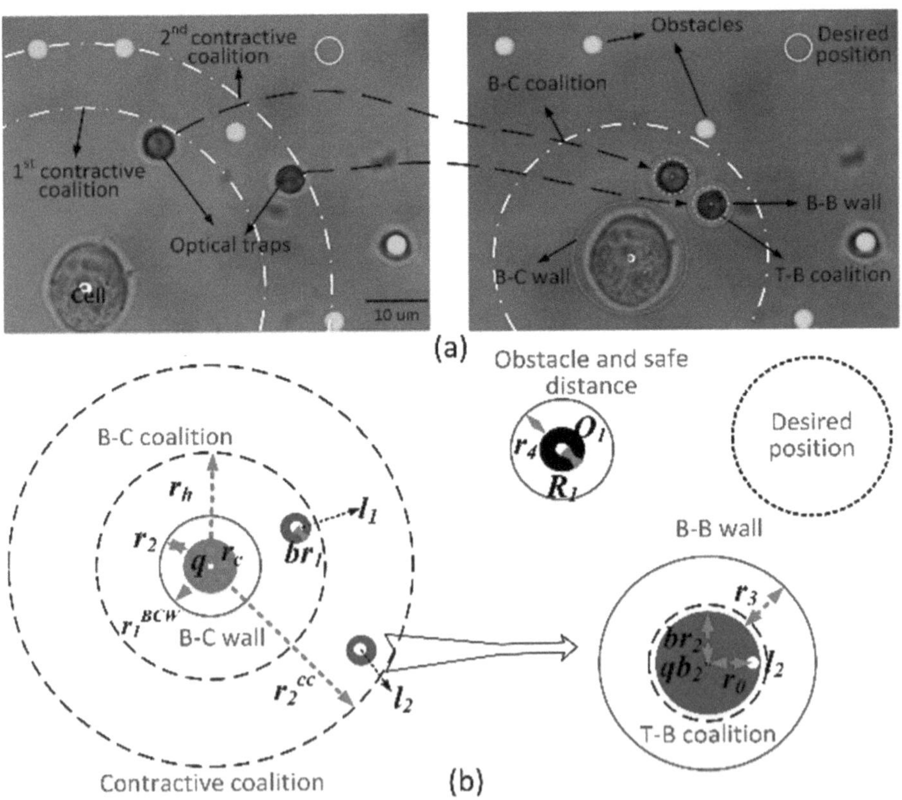

Figure 9.10 Illustration of the control framework (Yang et al., 2017). (A) Main coalitions and walls. (B) Schematic showing the different parameters.

9.3.1.3 Free coalition manipulation space

Collision between the T−B coalition and the other particles should be avoided. All particles that affect the cell migration are denoted as circular obstacles with a center of O_ς and a radius of R_ς for $\varsigma \in \{1, \cdots, m\}$. The following collision avoidance constraint function is introduced:

$$G_i^o = \prod_\varsigma \frac{1}{2}\left(l_i - O_\varsigma^2 - (br_i + R_\varsigma + r_4)^2\right) = \prod_\varsigma \alpha_\varsigma \tag{9.17}$$

where r_4 denotes the safety distance between the ith bead and the obstacles. If $G_i^o > 0$, there is no collision between the ith T−B coalition and the other particles.

By integrating all the constraint functions of the T−B and B−C coalitions, B−C and B−B walls, and obstacle avoidance, a new workspace called *free coalition manipulation space* is defined as follows:

Definition 7 (*free coalition manipulation space*):

$$F_i = \{l_i | G(l_i(t)) = G_i^{T-B} G_i^{B-C} G_i^{CC} G_i^{B-CW} G_i^{B-B} G_i^o > 0\} \tag{9.18}$$

In the *free coalition manipulation space*, the ith bead is located in the trapping area to maintain the T−B coalition. The cell is located in the high-motility area to maintain the B−C coalition and the B−C wall without collision in space.

9.3.2 Control

Denote $u_i = i_i \in R^2$ as the velocity of the ith optical trap, which is defined as the control input to the ith optical tweezer manipulator. The cell-migration control problem is formulated as follows:

Consider n microsource beads that can induce cell migration with dynamics (9.10). Under the initial configuration of $G(l_i(0)) > 0$, *determine the control input* $u = \{u_1, \ldots, u_n\}$ *of the optical tweezers manipulators that drive the microsource beads to the desired positions* $q_b^d = \{q_{b1}^d, \ldots, q_{bn}^d\}$. *This step is performed while guiding the cell to follow the beads to the desired area. Meanwhile,* $G(l_i(t)) \rangle 0, \quad \forall t > 0$.

A bounded potential field function $\phi \in [0, 1]$ is defined as follows:

$$\phi_i = \frac{\gamma(l_i)}{\left(\gamma^\delta(l_i) + G(l_i)\right)^{\frac{1}{\delta}}} \tag{9.19}$$

where δ is a positive parameter, $\gamma(l_i) = \frac{1}{2} e_i^T e_i$ is a criteria function, and $e_i = l_i - q_{bi}^d$ denotes the position error of the ith T−B coalition. The control input is designed as a negative gradient of the potential function ϕ_i, expressed by the following relation:

$$u_i = -k_i \frac{\partial \phi_i}{\partial l_i} \tag{9.20}$$

where k_i is a positive control gain.

Theorem 9.1. A microsource-induced cell migration system controlled by robotic tweezers is considered, which is subjected to dynamics Eq. (9.10). In the initial configuration of $G(l_i(0)) > 0$, the control law (9.20) gives rise to the following: (1) $G(l_i(t))\rangle 0, \forall t > 0$; (2) trapped beads confined in the optical trap and the induced cell maintained within the high-motility area; and (3) collision-free T—B coalitions.

Proof:

$\nabla_{l_i} G(l_i)$ is denoted as the gradient of $G(l_i)$ of the ith bead, where $\nabla_{l_i}(\cdot)$ denotes the partial derivative with respect to l_i. Thus, the vector $\nabla_{l_i} G(l_i)$ is perpendicular to the boundary of the free coalition space $(G(l_i) = 0)$ and toward the inside of F_i $(G(l_i) > 0)$.

The control input of the ith optical tweezers manipulator u_i can be simplified over the boundary as follows:

$$u_i = k_i \frac{\nabla_{l_i} G(l_i)}{\delta \gamma^{\delta}} \tag{9.21}$$

The inner product of the vectors u_i and $\nabla_{l_i} G(l_i)$ over the boundary are taken to produce

$$u_i \nabla_{l_i} G(l_i) = k_i \frac{(\nabla_{l_i} G(l_i))^T}{\delta \gamma^{\delta}} \nabla_{l_i} G(l_i) = \frac{k_i}{\delta \gamma^{\delta}} \nabla_{l_i} G(l_i)^2 \tag{9.22}$$

It will be shown in the following that the microsource beads can always remain in the optical trapping area, while the cell can always be located in the high-motility area. If the constraint condition (9.18) is broken and the center of the coalition is very close to the boundary of the free coalition manipulation space, then one of the following cases holds.

Case 1: The ith microsource bead almost escapes from the optical trap, and the center of the ith trap is located at the boundary of F_i formed by $G_i^{T-B} = 0$.
Case 2: The ith microsource bead almost moves outside the high-motility area of the cell when the cell is guided to the desired position. Or the microsource bead almost exceeds the contractive coalition when approaching the high-motility area. The center of the ith optical trap is located at the boundary of F_i formed by $G_i^{B-C} = 0$ or $G_i^{CC} = 0$.
Case 3: The ith microsource bead almost moves outside the high-motility area of the cell, and the center of the ith optical trap is located at the boundary of F_i formed by $G_i^{B-CW} = 0$.
Case 4: The ith T—B coalition collides with the ςth obstacle, and the center of the coalition is located at the boundary of F_i formed by $\alpha_{\varsigma} = 0$.
Case 5: The ith T—B coalition collides with the jth T—B coalition ($i \neq j$), and the center of the ith T—B coalition is located at the boundary of F_i formed by $G_i^{B-B} = 0$.

In Case 1, $G_i^{T-B} = 0$, $\|l_i - q_{bi}\| = r_0$, and

$$\nabla_{l_i} G(l_i) = -(l_i - q_{bi}) G_i^{B-C} G_i^{CC} G_i^{B-CW} G_i^{B-B} G_i^{o} \tag{9.23}$$

Substituting Eq. (9.23) into Eq. (9.22) yields

$$u_i \nabla_{l_i} G(l_i) = \frac{k_i}{\delta\gamma^\delta}\left(G_i^{B-C} G_i^{CC} G_i^{B-CW} G_i^{B-B} G_i^o r_0\right)^2 > 0 \tag{9.24}$$

Inequality (9.24) means that when the ith microsource bead is located at the boundary of F_i, the velocity direction of the optical trap is consistent with the vector $\nabla_{l_i} G(l_i)$, so that the optical trap converges to the space F inside. Therefore, $G_i^{T-B} = 0$ will not happen, implying that the boundary formed by $G_i^{T-B} = 0$ will never be reached.

In Case 2, $G_i^{B-C} = 0$ and $l_i - q = r_1$, or $G_i^{CC} = 0$ and $l_i - q = r_i^{cc}$. Then,

$$u_i \nabla_{l_i} G(l_i) = \frac{k_i}{\delta\gamma^\delta}\left(G_i^{T-B} G_i^{CC} G_i^{B-CW} G_i^{B-B} G_i^o r_1\right)^2 > 0 \tag{9.25}$$

or

$$u_i \nabla_{l_i} G(l_i) = \frac{k_i}{\delta\gamma^\delta}\left(G_i^{T-B} G_i^{B-C} G_i^{B-CW} G_i^{B-B} G_i^o r_i^{cc}\right)^2 > 0 \tag{9.26}$$

Similarly, inequalities (9.25) and (9.26) mean that $G_i^{B-C} = 0$ or $G_i^{CC} = 0$ will not happen.

In Case 3, $G_i^{B-CW} = 0$ and $l_i - q = r_2$. Then, a result similar to that in Case 2 can be obtained as follows:

$$u_i \nabla_{l_i} G(l_i) = \frac{k_i}{\delta\gamma^\delta}\left(G_i^{T-B} G_i^{B-C} G_i^{CC} G_i^{B-B} G_i^o r_2\right)^2 > 0 \tag{9.27}$$

In Case 4, $\alpha_\varsigma = 0, \ \forall \varsigma \in \{1, \ldots, m\}$. Then, a similar result can be obtained as follows:

$$u_i \nabla_{l_i} G(l_i) = \frac{k_i}{\delta\gamma^\delta}\left(G_i^{T-B} G_i^{B-C} G_i^{CC} G_i^{B-CW} G_i^{B-B} (r_1 + R_\varsigma + r_4)\right)^2 > 0 \tag{9.28}$$

Therefore, $\alpha_\varsigma = 0, \quad \forall \varsigma \in \{1, \ldots, m\}$ will not happen, and the boundary formed by $G_i^o = 0$ will never be reached.

In Case 5, $G_i^{B-B} = 0$. A result similar to that in Case 4 can be obtained as follows:

$$u_i \nabla_{l_i} G(l_i) = \frac{k_i}{\delta\gamma^\delta}\left(G_i^{T-B} G_i^{B-C} G_i^{CC} G_i^{B-CW} G_i^o (r_0 + r_3)\right)^2 > 0 \tag{9.29}$$

Therefore, the boundary of the manipulation space F_i can never be reached under controller (9.20), such that $G(l_i(t)) > 0, \quad \forall t > 0$. The microsource bead will not escape from the optical trap, and the velocity of the optical trap can be adjusted accordingly to confine the cell in the high-motility area. Collisions among the microsource beads and obstacles can also be avoided during the migration process.

Yang et al. (2017) proved that the parameter δ has a positive lower bound $\widehat{\delta}$, so that the desired position q_{bi}^{d} is the only critical point in the free coalition manipulation space F_i. Notably, the function ϕ_i is continuous and admissible, and the free workspace is compact. Therefore, the controller based on the navigation function (9.20) is naturally bounded.

As mentioned earlier, the robustness of the controller is important to allow changes in cell migration speed. For control of the T—B coalition, it can be proved in a similar way (Li et al., 2015) that any addition to the velocity control input specified below will not affect the stability of the system.

$$u_i^r = u_i + \Delta u_i = -k_i \frac{\partial \phi_i}{\partial l_i} + \Delta u_i(t) \tag{9.30}$$

In particular, in the initial configuration of $G(l_i(0)) > 0$, the control input (9.29) is the same as the controller (9.20). Both Eqs. (9.20) and (9.29) can give rise to $G(l_i(t)) > 0, \quad \forall t > 0$ for $\sup\{\Delta u_i\} < B$, where B denotes a bounded constant. Therefore, the T—B coalition control is robust to velocity alternation.

For control of the B—C coalition, the microsource beads are kept within a distance from the vicinity of the controlled cell, which has been proved by Theorem 9.1. In other words, regardless of the cell velocity, the microsource beads can always be positioned in the vicinity of the cell under the proposed control method. Therefore, the controller (9.20) is sufficiently robust to changes in cell velocity caused by various environmental disturbances.

9.3.3 Experiments

Yang et al. (2017) conducted an experiment to induce human leukemia cancer NB-4 cells to migrate to the desired location through microsource beads loaded with SDF-1α. These beads were robotically controlled by optical tweezers. Leukemia cancer NB-4 cells were selected as the sample for the cell migration test. NB-4 cells were cultured in RPMI 1640 medium containing 10% (v/v) fetal bovine serum (FBS) (Invitrogen, Carllsba, CA, United States) and incubated in a humidified atmosphere at 37°C under 5% CO_2. A 35-mm thin-bottomed Petri dish was used to culture NB-4 cells. The culture dish was first coated with fibronectin at 4°C and left overnight before the experiment. After the fibronectin was aspirated the next day, the Petri dish was rinsed with PBS and filled with RPMI 1640 medium supplemented with 10% (v/v) FBS. The cells were seeded on the fibronectin layer and incubated for 2—3 h to allow them to attach.

9.3.3.1 Single-cell-migration control with multiple beads

The experimental parameters were set as follows: the critical offset was $r_0 = 1$ μm, the maximum distance between the cell and bead was $r_1 = 10$ μm, and the minimum

Table 9.3 Experimental parameters (Yang et al., 2017).

	Index				
Position (μm)	**1**	**2**	**3**	**4**	**5**
$q(0)$	(13.0, 42.4)				
$q_{bi}(0)$	(25.1, 18.0)	(46.3, 24.7)			
O_i	(60.5, 35.9)	(36.1, 18.2)	(19.1, 5.1)	(5.7, 5.2)	(50.9, 47.7)
q_{bi}^d	(47.8, 5.7)	(53.7, 5.7)			

distance between the cell and bead was $r_2 = 1$ μm. Furthermore, the minimum distance between the beads was $r_3 = 1$ μm, the safety distance between the bead and the obstacle was $r_4 = 2$ μm, and the buffer distance of the contractive coalition was $\rho = 1$ μm. The feedback control gain was set to $k_1 = k_2 = 2000$, and the positive parameter $\delta = 6$. The initial positions of the cell, the two beads, the obstacle, and the destinations of the beads are listed in Table 9.3.

Fig. 9.11 shows the migration of the cell to the desired area by following two microsource beads. The microsource beads were trapped by two optical traps indicated by solid circles. Irrelevant particles in the workspace were marked as obstacles,

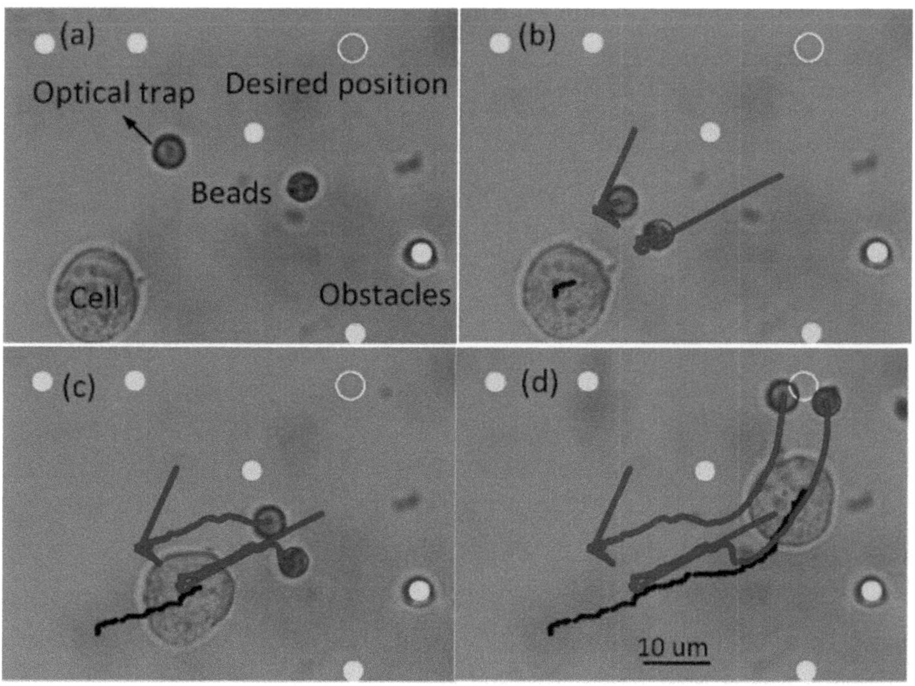

Figure 9.11 Cell-migration control experiment with two microsource beads (Yang et al., 2017). (A) Initial stage. (B) Result at $t = 9$ s. (C) Result at $t = 253$ s. (D) Result at $t = 560$ s.

represented by disks. Those very small impurities that do not affect cell migration were not marked as obstacles. Initially, the two beads were far away from the cell, as shown in Fig. 9.11A. Then, the beads were driven closer to the cell under the proposed controller and were displayed at the cell front (Fig. 9.11B). Fig. 9.11C shows that the beads bypassed the obstacle. Fig. 9.11D illustrates that the beads reached the desired positions and at the same time guided the cell to the desired position. These figures demonstrate the success of the robot-assisted cell migration control approach.

Fig. 9.12 shows the quantitative results of the control experiment. Fig. 9.12A and B show the positional errors of the two beads with respect to the desired positions in the x and y directions, respectively. Fig. 9.12C shows the distance between the cell and the desired position. Fig. 9.12D shows that the distance between the two beads was kept at a safe distance greater than $r_3 = 1$ μm. Fig. 9.12E shows that the distances between the cell and the two beads were all less than $r_1 = 10$ μm and greater than $r_2 =$ 1 μm, indicating that the cell was restricted to the high-motility area during the manipulation. It is worth noting that in the single-bead and double-bead experiments, there is a final position error of approximately 10 μm along the y-axis. This discovery was made because the maximum distance between the bead and the cell was set to 10 μm in the y-axis direction. As long as the cell reached the area within 10 μm from the bead, the control action would stop. Fig. 9.12F illustrates the velocities of the cell and beads, demonstrating that the proposed controller can always confine the beads to the high-motility area to stimulate cell migration.

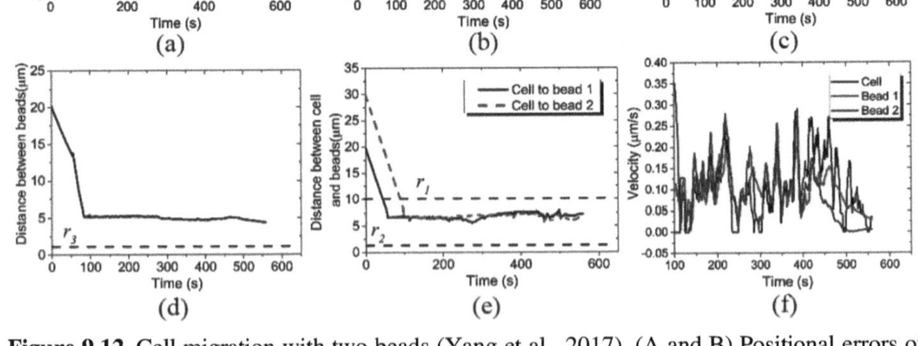

Figure 9.12 Cell migration with two beads (Yang et al., 2017). (A and B) Positional errors of the two microsource beads. (C) Positional error of the cell with respect to the desired position. (D) Distance between the two beads. (E) Distances between the two beads and the cell. (F) Velocities of the cell and beads.

9.3.3.2 *Chemoattractant analysis*

Further experiments were performed to analyze how the release of chemoattractant from the microbeads into the culture medium affects the background concentration. Addressing this issue can help clarify whether the release of accumulated chemoattractants significantly affects cell migration control.

RPMI 1640 medium with different SDF-1α background concentrations was used to provide an environment for cell migration. The initial SDF-1α was dissolved in PBS to a concentration of 1.25 μM and then diluted separately to 0.1, 0.2, 0.5, 1, 1.5, and 2 nM with RPMI. (The concentration on the surface of the beads was approximately 2.5 nM.) After the cells were attached to the bottom of the Petri dish, the supernatant medium was extracted. The media containing different concentrations of SDF-1α were added to the Petri dish. During the experiment, microsource beads were placed near the cells to stimulate cell migration, and cell velocity in different concentration environments was measured and compared.

Fig. 9.13 shows the velocities of five cell samples in media with different background concentrations. A low-background SDF-1α concentration (lower than 1.0 nM) had little effect on cell migration velocity. When the background concentration exceeded 1.5 nM, the cell velocity decreased significantly. When the background concentration reached 2.0 nM, the microbeads no longer stimulated the cell. This phenomenon occurred because too high a background concentration usually stabilized the concentration distribution near the cell. As a result, the cell could not perceive the gradient of the surrounding environment and therefore could not respond to the stimulus. This experiment quantitatively verified that low background concentrations (e.g., less than 1 nM) have little effect on cell migration. When using multiple microsource beads, the cumulative release of the chemoattractant has very little effect on the background concentration in a relatively large workspace. Therefore, the cell migration velocity was not greatly affected.

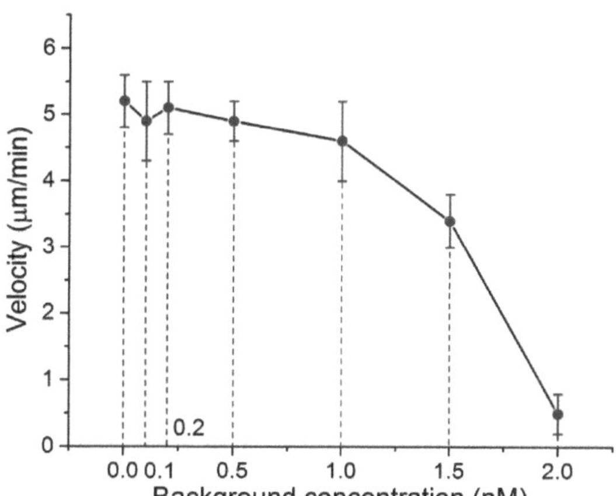

Figure 9.13 Cell-migration velocities with different background SDF-1α concentrations (Yang et al., 2017).

9.4 Electrical stimulation based on calcium spike patterns of MSCs to improve osteogenic differentiation

MSCs are multipotent cells that can be differentiated into various cell types, including osteoblasts, adipocytes, and chondrocytes, as well as myocytes and neurons. MSCs can be easily isolated from various parts of the human body, such as the bone marrow, adipose tissue, synovium, and other mesodermal tissues. The role of MSCs in the treatment of tissue trauma, musculoskeletal diseases, and immune and inflammation-mediated diseases has been extensively studied (Taketani et al., 2015; Uccelli et al., 2011). Electrical stimulation (ES) can promote bone healing and osteogenic differentiation of bone marrow mesenchymal stem cells. Direct current and alternating current (AC) are widely used to promote the osteogenic differentiation of MSCs in vivo and in vitro. However, there remains little information about making effective differentiation. Hou et al. (2019) proposed a method for optimizing ES parameters based on the calcium spike mode of MSCs. Various ES parameters through real-time monitoring of calcium spike patterns have been tested. This section introduces the osteogenic differentiation process of MSCs by using the optimal parameters of AC, including voltage, signal shapes, frequency, and duty time. The method of optimizing osteogenic differentiation can be potentially useful in clinical treatments, such as fractures.

9.4.1 Materials and methods

9.4.1.1 Cell culture and materials

Human fetal MSCs (fMSCs) were used in this study. All fMSCs were donated by the Stem Cell Bank of the Prince of Wales Hospital in Hong Kong. The surface antigen profiles of fMSCs were CD105+, CD73+, CD90+, CD45−, CD34−, CD14−, CD11b−, CD79a−, CD19−, and HLA-DR−. All the cells were cultured in a humidified incubator at 37°C in 5% CO_2, with MEM α supplemented with 10% (v/v) fetal bovine serum (FBS, Invitrogen) and 1% (v/v) antibiotic−antimycotic (Invitrogen). The cells were incubated in α-MEM supplemented with 10% FBS, 5 mM β-glycerol-phosphate (Sigma), and 25 μM ascorbic acid (Sigma) for 2 weeks to induce osteogenic differentiation.

9.4.1.2 Experimental setup

Before the experiment, fMSCs are seeded on glass-bottomed Petri dishes. The cells are washed three times with HBSS (Thermo Fisher) before observing them under a confocal microscope. Subsequently, the cells are incubated in 5 μM Fluo-4 AM staining solution (Thermo Fisher) for at least 30 min and washed thrice with HBSS. Then, the cells are added to a fresh culture medium and observed again under the microscope. The excitation wavelength is approximately 488 nm, and the emission wavelength is 512−520 nm. Fig. 9.14A shows the setup of calcium spike recording, which consists of a microchip and a Leica TCS SP8 confocal microscope. Fig. 9.14B shows the ES

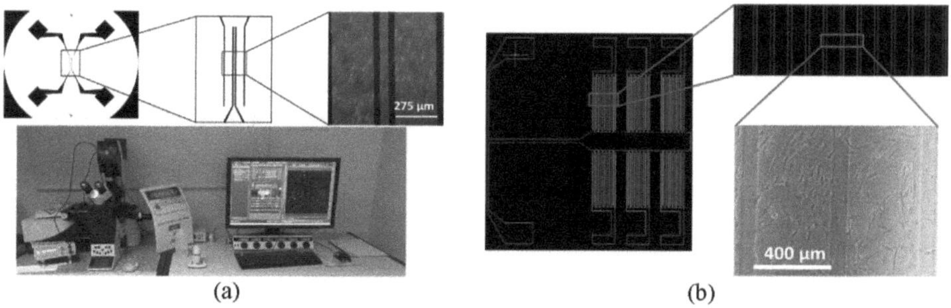

Figure 9.14 Experimental setup (Hou et al., 2019). (A) Microchip design and a Leica TCS SP8 confocal microscope for calcium spike recording. (B) Design of the chip coated with microelectrodes for long duration of ES.

system that consists of a generator and chips with patterned microelectrodes. Two types of chips with glass substrate are used here. The first chip is coated with two pairs of platinum electrodes, as shown in Fig. 9.14A. The distance between each pair of electrodes is 275 μm, to ensure real-time observation of calcium spikes in a short time. The second chip shown in Fig. 9.14B is coated with an interdigital ITO electrode array, and the distance between each pair of electrodes is 400 μm, to ensure long-time ES during cell culture.

9.4.1.3 Alizarin red staining

This process includes the following steps. First, the medium is removed from each well and washed gently with PBS. Second, 1.0 mL 4% PFA is added to each well and the well is kept at room temperature for 15 min. After washing the wells twice with PBS, 0.5 mL of Alizarin Red Working Solution (40 mM ARS, pH 4.2, Sigma–Aldrich A5533) is added to each well. After that, the wells are incubated at room temperature for 20 min. Finally, the dye solution is removed from the well and the well is gently rinsed at least four times with ddH_2O. The stained monolayer is observed through a phase microscope.

9.4.1.4 ALP staining

ALP staining is performed on the seventh day. BCIP/NBT solution (Beyotime) is prepared before staining. After removing the medium and washing with PBS, sufficient solution is added to each well. The treated cells are incubated for 30 min in the dark at room temperature. Finally, the solution is removed from the wells and the wells are washed with ddH_2O. After drying, the dyed monolayer is observed through a phase microscope.

9.4.1.5 RT-qPCR

The fold changes in the mRNA expression of three early osteoblast marker genes, namely alkaline phosphatase (ALPL), secreted phosphoprotein 1 (SPP1), and short

Table 9.4 Specific primers used in qPCR (Hou et al., 2019).

Gene	Primers sequences (5′-3′)
GAPDH	GGAGCGAGATCCCTCCAAAAT GGCTGTTGTCATACTTCTCATGG
Runx2	TGGTTACTGTCATGGCGGGTA TCTCAGATCGTTGAACCTTGCTA
SPP1	CTCCATTGACTCGAACGACTC CAGGTCTGCGAAACTTCTTAGAT
ALPL	ACCACCACGAGAGTGAACCA CGTTGTCTGAGTACCAGTCCC

DNA binding domain transcription factor (RUNX2), are analyzed. All samples are collected by centrifugation, and RNA is isolated by the phenol-chloroform extraction method. cDNA is obtained by reverse transcription of 0.2 μg total RNA using iScript cDNA Synthesis Kit (Bio-Rad). All gene expression changes are detected by the SYBR Green method (SsoAdvanced Universal SYBR Green Supermix, Bio-Rad). Glyceraldehyde 3-phosphate dehydrogenase (GAPDH) is a housekeeping gene used as a control gene to normalize mRNA levels. All primer sequences listed in Table 9.4 are from PrimerBank.

9.4.1.6 Cell viability

Cells are harvested and aliquoted up to 1×10^6 cells/100 μL into 1.5-mL tubes. After washing twice with 1 mL PBS, the cells are resuspended in 1 mL propidium iodide (PI) staining buffer (50 μg/mL) and incubated at room temperature for 15 min. Finally, all cells are transferred through a sieve to an FACS tube, and then analyzed by flow cytometry (BD Biosciences) in the presence of the dye.

9.4.1.7 Statistical analysis

All statistical tests are performed in PASW Statistics 18. First, the relationship between fluorescence intensity data and time is retrieved from the video recorded by the real-time monitoring system, which indicates the calcium ion signal of the cell. Second, the time interval of each single cell calcium spike is calculated. Third, the calculation is based on the average peak time and standard deviation of single-cell data from three independent experiments. Finally, the one-tailed Student t-test (one-tailed) is used to compare the time interval of calcium spikes under different ES parameters to statistically verify the influence of different ES parameters on the calcium spike time.

9.4.2 Results

9.4.2.1 Calcium spike pattern in fMSCs without ES

To understand the role of calcium spike osteogenic differentiation, calcium spikes in fMSCs without ES were first detected. Fig. 9.15A illustrates that the real-time concentration of calcium ions in the cytoplasm under the microscope considering that Fluo-4 AM can penetrate the cell membrane and bind calcium ion. The usual interval between calcium spikes in fMSCs without ES is about 3 min. The calcium spike interval time between the same fMSC lines with different passage numbers (P8 and P19) was tested. Fig. 9.15B and C show that the calcium spike distributions of fMSC-P8 and fMSC-P19 are almost the same. All the cells used in the following experiments are in the eighth passage.

9.4.2.2 Calcium spike frequency decreased as the differentiation process of fMSC progressed

To study the relationship between calcium spikes and osteogenic differentiation, the pattern and frequency of calcium spikes in different stages of osteogenic differentiation were tested. fMSCs were cultured in an induction medium for 7 days, and calcium

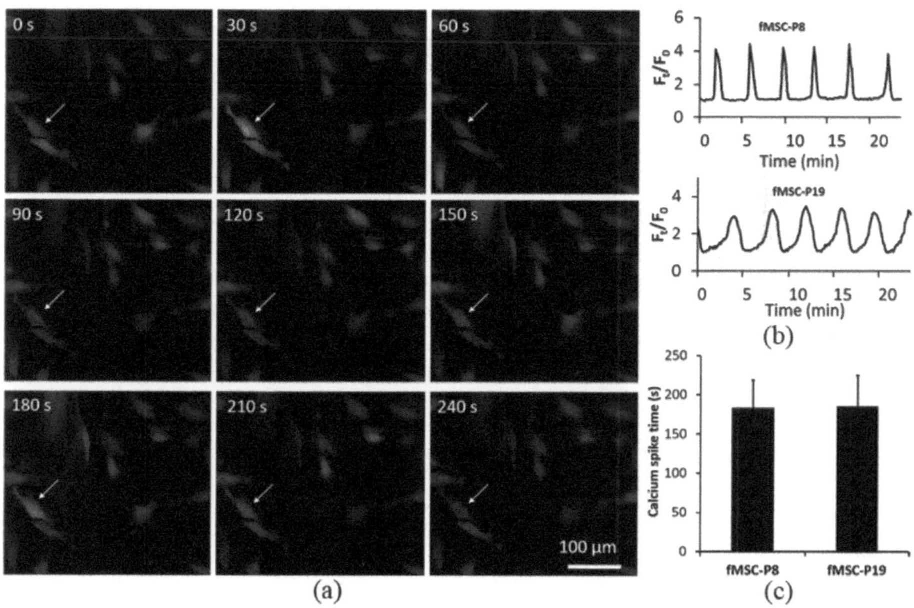

Figure 9.15 Calcium spikes of fMSCs without ES (Hou et al., 2019). (A) Real-time observation of calcium spikes of fMSC (white arrows) under fluorescence microscope. (B) Calcium spike patterns of two fMSC cells with different passage numbers. (C) Calcium spike time of fMSC cells with different passage numbers. The calcium spike time data are represented by the mean values ± standard deviations based on three independent experiments, and each is conducted on more than 11 cells.

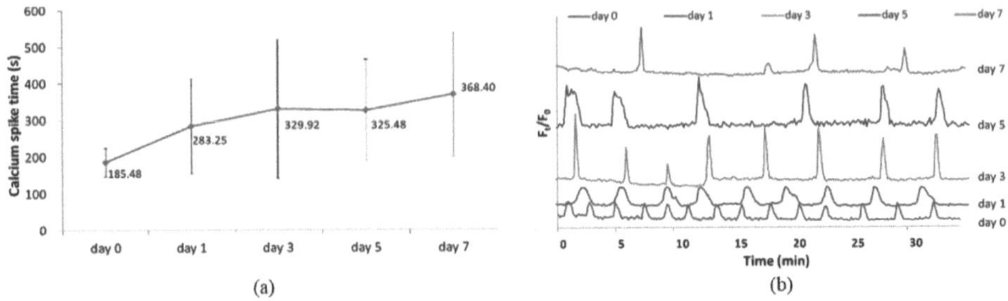

Figure 9.16 Calcium spikes of fMSC cultured under induction media (Hou et al., 2019). (A) The calcium spike time increases with the induction medium cultured time. (B) The calcium spike profiles of fMSCs at different times of induction medium culture. From bottom to top, each curve represents the calcium spike profile of a cell from days 0, 1, 3, 5, and 7 of induction of the medium culture. The calcium spike times are represented by the mean values ± standard deviations based on three independent experiments. Each experiment is conducted on more than 15 cells.

spikes were detected on days 1, 3, 5, and 7. As shown in Fig. 9.16A, as the differentiation process progresses, the frequency of calcium spikes decreases. This indicates that fMSCs in osteogenic differentiation show a decrease in the frequency of calcium spike patterns, which is consistent with previous reports (Titushkin et al., 2010). Fig. 9.16B illustrates the distribution of calcium spikes in cells at different time points. These results confirm that the calcium spike pattern can be used as an indicator of osteogenic differentiation.

9.4.2.3 Effect of different ES parameters on fMSC calcium spike

The effects of various ES parameters on the calcium spike of fMSC were characterized using the experimental setup shown in Fig. 9.14A. Fig. 9.17 shows the effect of different parameters on the time between calcium spikes. Fig. 9.17A illustrates the calcium spikes under different waveforms, sine waves and square waves, when using the same parameters (that is, the voltage is 3.64 V/cm, the ES frequency is 5 Hz, and the duty time is 50%). The results of the two groups are not significantly different,

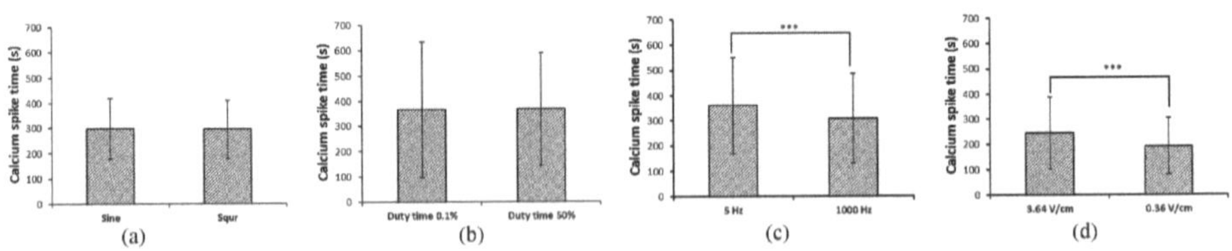

Figure 9.17 Effects of different AC parameters on calcium spikes (Hou et al., 2019). (A) Effect under different waves (sine and square). (B) Effect under high-duty time and low-duty times. (C) Effects under high and low frequencies. (D) Effects under high and low voltages. The calcium spike time data are represented by the mean values ± standard deviations based on three independent experiments, each conducted on more than 20 cells.

indicating that the waveform has no great influence on the calcium spike of fMSCs. Fig. 9.17B illustrates the calcium spike time at different operating time points (0.1% and 50%) when considering the same parameters (that is, 3.64 V/cm, 5 Hz, and sine wave). The results show that using different working hours will not cause significant changes in the calcium spike pattern. When the ES frequency of the two groups is set to 5 and 1000 Hz while using the same set of parameters (36.4 V/cm, sine wave, duty time 50%), it can be seen that the high frequency reduces the calcium spike time (Fig. 9.17C). Fig. 9.17D illustrates the calcium spike time at high voltage (3.64 V/cm) and low voltage (0.36 V/cm) using the same parameters (sine wave, 5 Hz, and duty time 0.1%). ES with high voltage (3.64 V/cm) can increase the calcium spike time or decrease the calcium spike frequency. Based on the above results, high voltage and low ES frequency may help induce osteogenic differentiation.

9.4.2.4 Long-term ES does not cause obvious cell apoptosis

The experimental setup shown in Fig. 9.14B was used to induce osteogenic differentiation through ES in a weekly timescale. Based on the findings between ES and calcium spike patterns, three sets of parameters that may lead to different abilities were selected to induce fMSC osteogenic differentiation. The parameters of the first group (ES1) are 0.25 V/cm, sine wave, 1000 Hz, and duty time 50%. The parameters of the second group (ES2) are 3.75 V/cm, square wave, 5 Hz, and duty time 0.1%. The parameters of the third group (ES3) are 2 V/cm, square wave, 500 Hz, and duty time 25%.

At different ES times, the viability of the cells collected from each group was tested by flow cytometry using PI staining. Fig. 9.18 shows that compared with the control group, the use of different ES parameters has a slight effect on cell viability, and no significant difference is observed between the three ES groups. These results indicate that these parameter sets are suitable for ES and will not cause significant apoptosis.

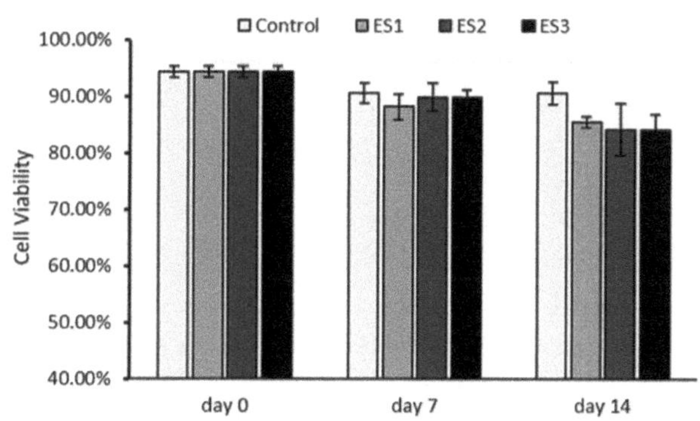

Figure 9.18 Influence of three selected sets of parameters on cell viability after culturing at different days (Hou et al., 2019).

9.4.2.5 ES-induced osteogenic differentiation

β-Glycerophosphate is essential for the maturation of osteoblasts. Therefore, the ES method using low-concentration induction medium (5 mM β-glycerophosphate and 25 μM ascorbic acid) was chosen to study the effect of ES on osteogenic differentiation. After ES 7 days (4 h/day), the expression of three osteoblast marker genes, *ALPL*, *RUNX2*, and *SPP1*, was detected. Compared with the induction medium group, the expression of these genes in the three ES groups did not increase except for *SPP1*, as shown in Fig. 9.19A. However, compared with the induction-medium-only group, the mRNA expression levels of the three genes in all ES groups showed a significant

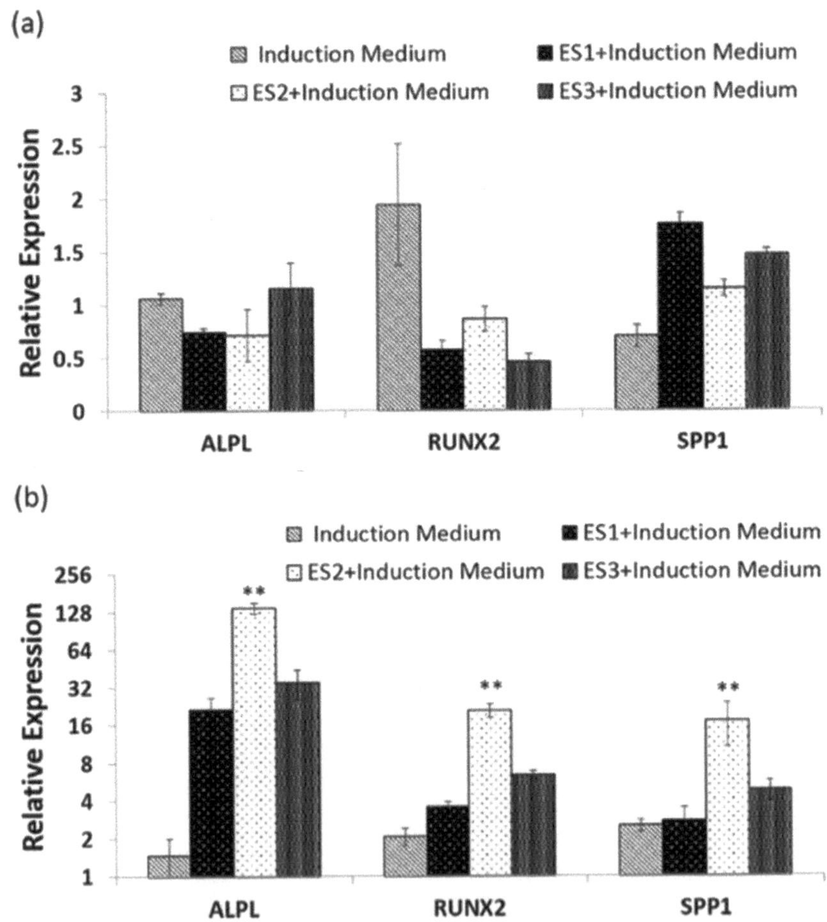

Figure 9.19 Expression of three early osteoblast marker genes at mRNA level (Hou et al., 2019). (A) At day 7, no acceleration effect was observed in all three ES groups. (B) At day 14, the osteoblast gene expressions increased in all three ES groups compared with the induction medium-only group. Data are represented as mean values ± standard deviations based on three independent experiments. $^{**}P < .01$.

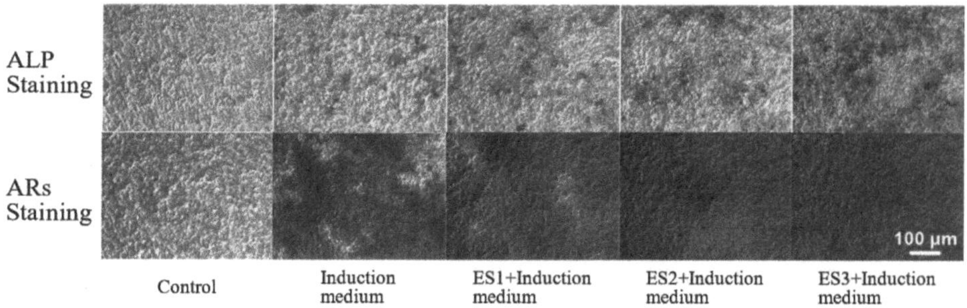

Figure 9.20 ALP (day 7) and AR (day 14) results of control group, induction medium group, and groups under ES with different sets of parameters (Hou et al., 2019).

increase on the 14th day (Fig. 9.19B). The ES2 group showed the best induction effect among all groups. The order of induction based on gene expression is ES2, ES3, ES1, and the induction-medium-only group, which indicates that the combination of ES and induction medium can effectively improve the differentiation process. This result shows that voltage plays a very important role in this process. Fig. 9.20 shows the results of ALP staining on day 7. The AR staining results on the 14th day showed a similar sequence.

9.4.2.6 Discussion

Many studies have reported the effects of ES on osteogenic differentiation, but few have quantitatively characterized the effects of different ES parameters on differentiation. Screening the ideal parameters of AC ES is challenging because multiple parameters such as voltage, frequency, duty time, and signal shape are involved in stimulation at the same time. This problem can be solved by using the cellular calcium spike pattern as an indicator of osteogenic differentiation. Calcium ions play an important role in cell activities, including cell differentiation (Gu et al., 1994). There are spontaneous calcium spikes in normal fMSCs, which usually form regular wave patterns. Hou et al. (2019) found that the frequency of calcium spikes decreased with the progress of osteogenic differentiation in their experimental study. Many studies have emphasized that calcium oscillations store information at their own frequency (Gu and Spitzer, 1995; Dolmetsch et al., 1998). Therefore, it is hypothesized that the reduced frequency of calcium spikes can be used as an indicator of cell differentiation. Hou et al. (2019) proposed searching for ideal ES conditions based on calcium peaks. A simple platinum-plated electrode chip was designed. The relationship between different AC parameters and calcium spike patterns can be found through a fluorescence microscope, and the cell calcium spikes under different AC parameters can be recorded. Comparing the results under different voltages, signal shapes, frequencies, and duty times, it is found that low frequency and high voltage can reduce the frequency of calcium spikes, suggesting that low-frequency and high-voltage AC may help induce differentiation. To test this hypothesis, another chip coated with ITO microelectrodes was designed for the long-term ES of cells. After 2 weeks of ES, the differentiation process of the cells was tested by RT-qPCR, ALP, and AR experiments. It was found that the selected parameter set (3.75 V/cm, square wave, 5 Hz, and duty time 0.1%) showed the best induction effect in three different ES parameter sets. In addition, the results indicate that voltage parameters are more important than frequency in the process of osteogenic differentiation.

9.5 Conclusions

This chapter introduced cell stimulation and migration control from three perspectives. First, a cell migration model that simulates in vivo migration by using optically manipulated chemoattractant-loaded microsource beads is proposed. This model helps to quantitatively characterize the relationship between protrusion force, cell motility, and chemoattractant gradient. Experiments on the migration of leukemia cancer Jurkat cells show that by selecting a suitable chemoattractant gradient and concentration at the cell leading edge, ideal migration ability can be obtained. Second, an automatic cell migration control method with robotically controlled optical tweezers is introduced. Chemoattractant-loaded microsource beads trapped by optical tweezers are used to release the stimulus, thereby inducing the target cells to migrate to the desired area. The dynamics of cell movement under optical tweezers manipulation are analyzed. A geometric model is established to confine the microsource beads to the effective trapping area of the optical tweezers and the high-motility area of the cell. Based on this model, a controller based on the potential field function is used to stimulate the cells to migrate to the desired area. Third, a method of using electrical stimulation (ES) to stimulate cells is proposed, and its application is used to improve the osteogenic differentiation of MSCs. ES parameters are optimized according to the calcium spike pattern of MSCs. By using the optimal parameters of AC, including voltage, signal shape, frequency, and duty time, the osteogenic differentiation process in MSCs can be effectively initiated. This method provides a new approach for optimizing osteogenic differentiation and could be potentially useful in clinical treatments, such as bone fractures.

References

Aaron, R.K., Ciombor, D.M., Keeping, H., Wang, S., Capuano, A., Polk, C., 1999. Power frequency fields promote cell differentiation coincident with an increase in transforming growth factor-β1 expression. Bioelectromagnetics 20 (7), 453−458.

Alex, L.A., Simon, M.I., 1994. Protein histidine kinases and signal transduction in prokaryotes and eukaryotes. Trends Genet. 10, 133−138.

Amselem, G., Theves, M., Bae, A., Beta, C., Bodenschatz, E., 2012. Control parameter description of eukaryotic chemotaxis. Phys. Rev. Lett. 109, 108103.

Ananthakrishnan, R., Ehrlicher, A., 2007. The forces behind cell movement. Int. J. Biol. Sci. 3, 303–317.

Banerjee, A.G., Pomerance, A., Losert, W., Gupta, S.K., 2010. Developing a stochastic dynamic programming framework for optical tweezer-based automated particle transport operations. IEEE Trans. Autom. Sci. Eng. 7 (2), 218–227.

Cho, M.R., Thatte, H.S., Silvia, M.T., Golan, D.E., 1999. Transmembrane calcium influx induced by ac electric fields. Faseb. J. 13 (6), 677–683.

Cho, M.R., Marler, J.P., Thatte, H.S., Golan, D.E., 2002. Control of calcium entry in human fibroblasts by frequency-dependent electrical stimulation. Front. Biosci. 7, a1–a8.

Dolmetsch, R.E., Xu, K., Lewis, R.S., 1998. Calcium oscillations increase the efficiency and specificity of gene expression. Nature 392, 933–936.

Dura, B., Chen, M.Q., Inan, O.T., Kovacs, G.T.A., Giovangrandi, L., 2012. High-frequency electrical stimulation of cardiac cells and application to artifact reduction. IEEE Trans. Biomed. Eng. 59 (5), 1381–1390.

Fahmy, T.M., Samstein, R.M., Harness, C.C., Saltzman, W.M., 2005. Surface modification of biodegradable polyesters with fatty acid conjugates for improved drug targeting. Biomaterials 26, 5727–5736.

Fonseca, A.V.S., Bassani, R.A., Oliveira, P.X., Bassani, J.W.M., 2013. Greater cardiac cell excitation efficiency with rapidly switching multidirectional electrical stimulation. IEEE Trans. Biomed. Eng. 60 (1), 28–34.

Gou, X., Yang, H., Fahmy, T.M., Wang, Y., Sun, D., 2014. Direct measurement of cell protrusion force utilizing a robot-aided cell manipulation system with optical tweezers for cell migration control. Int. J. Robot Res. 33 (14), 1782–1792.

Gu, X., Spitzer, N.C., 1995. Distinct aspects of neuronal differentiation encoded by frequency of spontaneous Ca^{2+} transients. Nature 375, 784–787.

Gu, X., Olson, E.C., Spitzer, N.C., 1994. Spontaneous neuronal calcium spikes and waves during early differentiation. J. Neurosci. 14 (11), 6325–6335.

Gurdon, J.B., Bourillot, P.Y., 2001. Morphogen gradient interpretation. Nature 413, 97–803.

Haastert, P.V., Devreotes, P., 2004. Chemotaxis: signalling the way forward. Nat. Rev. Mol. Cell Biol. 5, 626–634.

Hanna, H., Andre, F.M., Mir, L.M., 2017. Electrical control of calcium oscillations in mesenchymal stem cells using microsecond pulsed electric fields. Stem Cell Res. Ther. 8, 91.

Hannouche, D., Petite, H., Sedel, L., 2001. Current trends in the enhancement of fracture healing. Bone Joint Lett. J. 83 (2), 157–164.

Hou, J., Luo, T., Chen, S., Lin, S., Yang, M.M., Li, G., Sun, D., 2019. Calcium spike patterns reveal linkage of electrical stimulus and MSC osteogenic differentiation. IEEE Trans. Nanobioscience 18 (1), 3–9.

Hu, S., Gou, X., Han, H., Leung, A.Y.H., Sun, D., 2013. Manipulating cell adhesions with optical tweezers for study of cell-to-cell interactions. J. Biomed. Nanotechnol. 9, 281–285.

Kress, H., Park, J.G., Mejean, C.O., Forster, J.D., Park, J., Walse, S.S., Zhang, Y., Wu, D., Weiner, O.D., Fahmy, T.M., Dufresne, E.R., 2009. Cell stimulation with optically manipulated microsources. Nat. Methods 6, 905–909.

Lauffenburger, D.A., Horwitz, A.F., 1996. Cell migration: a physically integrated molecular process. Cell 84 (3), 359–369.

Li, X., Yang, H., Wang, J., Sun, D., 2015. Design of a robust unified controller for cell manipulation with a robot-aided optical tweezers system. Automatica 51 (5), 279–286.

Lin, F., Butcher, E.C., 2016. T cell chemotaxis in a simple microfluidic device. Lab Chip 6 (11), 1462–1469.

Meng, K., Yang, H., Wang, Y., Sun, D., 2019. Modeling and control of single-cell migration induced by a chemoattractant-loaded microbead. IEEE Trans. Cybernetics 49 (2), 427–439.

Merks, R.M., Perryn, E.D., Shirinifard, A., Glazier, J.A., 2008. Contact-inhibited chemotaxis in de novo and sprouting blood-vessel growth. PLoS Comput. Biol. 4, e1000163.

Mogilner, A., Oster, G., 2003. Force generation by actin polymerization II: the elastic ratchet and tethered filaments. Biophys. J. 84, 1591–1605.

Parent, C.A., Devreotes, P.N., 1999. A cell's sense of direction. Science 284, 765–770.

Pelletier, A.J., van der Laan, L.J., Hildbrand, P., Siani, M.A., Thompson, D.A., Dawson, P.E., Torbett, B.E., Salomon, D.R., 2000. Presentation of chemokine SDF-1 alpha by fibronectin mediates directed migration of T cells. Blood 96, 2682–2690.

Pompe, T., Kaufmann, M., Kasimir, M., Johne, S., Glorius, S., Renner, L., Werner, C., 2011. Friction-controlled traction force in cell adhesion. Biophys. J. 101, 1863–1870.

Prechtel, K., Bausch, A.R., Marchi-Artzner, V., Kantlehner, M., Kessler, H., Merkel, R., 2002. Dynamic force spectroscopy to probe adhesion strength of living cells. Phys. Rev. Lett. 89, 028101.

Ramezani, H., Akan, O.B., 2018. Impacts of spike shape variations on synaptic communication. IEEE Trans. Nanobiosci. 17 (3), 260–271.

Ridley, A.J., Schwartz, M.A., Burridge, K., Firtel, R.A., Ginsberg, M.H., Borisy, G., Parsons, J.T., Horwitz, A.R., 2003. Cell migration: integrating signals from front to back. Science 302, 1704–1709.

Roussos, E.T., Condeelis, J.S., Patsialou, A., 2011. Chemotaxis in cancer. Nat. Rev. 11, 573–587.

Svoboda, K., Block, S.M., 1994. Biological applications of optical forces. Annu. Rev. Biophys. Biomol. Struct. 23, 247–332.

Taketani, T., Oyama, C., Mihara, A., Tanabe, Y., Abe, M., Hirade, T., Yamamoto, S., Bo, R., Kanai, R., Tadenuma, T., Michibata, Y., Yamamoto, S., Hattori, M., Katsube, Y., Ohnishi, H., Sasao, M., Oda, Y., Hattori, K., Yuba, S., Ohgushi, H., Yamaguchi, S., 2015. Ex vivo expanded allogeneic mesenchymal stem cells with bone marrow transplantation improved osteogenesis in infants with severe hypophosphatasia. Cell Transplant. 24 (10), 1931–1943.

Tan, Y., Fung, T.K., Wan, H., Wang, K., Leung, A.Y.H., Sun, D., 2011. Biophysical characterization of hematopoietic cells from normal and leukemic sources with distinct primitiveness. Appl. Phys. Lett. 99 (8), 083702.

Titushkin, I., Sun, S., Shin, J., Cho, M.R., 2010. Physicochemical control of adult stem cell differentiation: shedding light on potential molecular mechanisms. J. Biomed. Biotechnol. 2010, 743476.

Uccelli, A., Laroni, A., Freedman, M.S., 2011. Mesenchymal stem cells for the treatment of multiple sclerosis and other neurological diseases. Lancet Neurol. 10 (7), 649–656.

Wang, K., Cheng, J., Cheng, S.H., Sun, D., 2013. Probing cell biophysical behavior based on actin cytoskeleton modeling and stretching manipulation with optical tweezers. Appl. Phys. Lett. 99, 083702.

Wiesmann, H., Hartig, M., Stratmann, U., Meyer, U., Joos, U., 2001. Electrical stimulation influences mineral formation of osteoblast-like cells in vitro. Biochim. Biophys. Acta 1538, 28–37.

Wu, Y., Sun, D., Huang, W., 2011. Mechanical force characterization in manipulating live cells with optical tweezers. J. Biomech. 44, 741–746.
Wu, Y., Sun, D., Huang, W., Xi, N., 2013. Dynamics analysis and motion planning for automated cell transportation with optical tweezers. IEEE/ASME Trans. Mechatron. 18 (2), 706–713.
Yang, H., Gou, X., Wang, Y., Fahmy, T.M., Leung, A.Y.H., Lu, J., Sun, D., 2015. A dynamic model of chemoattractant-induced cell migration. Biophys. J. 108 (7), 1645–1651.
Yang, H., Li, X., Wang, Y., Feng, G., Sun, D., 2017. Control of single-cell migration using a robot-aided stimulus-induced manipulation system. IEEE Trans. Mechatron. 22 (2), 815–825.

Cell patterning

10

10.1 Introduction

Cell patterning aims to arrange a group of cells in a desired position with a desired shape, and has attracted great attention due to its importance in cell and tissue applications. Cell patterning can be widely used in various biomedical applications, such as stem cell differentiation (Tang et al., 2010; Béduer et al., 2012), tissue engineering (Guillotin and Guillemot, 2011), biosensors (El-Ali et al., 2006), and cell interactions (Gou et al., 2013). Cell patterning can also be used to study cell–extracellular matrix (ECM) interactions, which are essential for determining the cell fate of many cell types (Flaim et al., 2005; Trappmann et al., 2012). The rapid progress of single-cell research also requires more accurate manipulation and positioning of single cells in various microenvironments, among which cell patterning technology plays a central role.

Various techniques for cell patterning have been developed, including photolithography, soft lithography, optical tweezers, dielectrophoresis (DEP), and microfluidics etc. Photolithography (Li and Ho, 2008) is a very versatile method that has been widely used for high-resolution cell patterning. However, photolithography is not suitable for patterning of nonplanar substrates (Kane et al., 1999). Soft lithography (Kane et al., 1999) is also called nonlithographic micromachining technology, and uses elastic materials to produce stamps and channels for pattern transfer in a simpler and cheaper way. However, due to the elastic properties of the material, the stamps undergo feature deformation (Bucknall, 2005). Therefore, the above two photolithography methods are only suitable for processing adherent cells and cannot flexibly change the cell pattern.

Optical tweezers show many advantages in cell manipulation (Banerjee et al., 2010; Hu and Sun, 2011; Chen and Sun, 2012; Li et al., 2013, 2017; Cheah et al., 2014; Yang et al., 2015). Using a strong focused beam, the optical tweezers can generate a trapping force to accurately transport the trapped object to the desired position in a noncontact manner. Yan and Sun (2015) proposed the use of robot-controlled optical tweezers for cell patterning. In this method, an overall desired region is defined so that the grouped cells can be transferred to the region first. After positioning the cells in the defined region, the cells are further controlled to accurately form the desired pattern. Using the concept based on multilevel topology (Yan et al., 2012), various cell patterns can be generated. Using a multilevel-based topology, the cells stay in the desired positions in the desired region to maintain the desired patterning, rather than random positions. An adaptive controller is developed to drive the cells to the desired region and further form the desired patterns in a level-by-level manner.

The dielectrophoresis (DEP) method (Fu et al., 2004; Cui et al., 2009) uses an uneven AC electric field to generate a force that can stably locate cells. This noncontact

Robotic Cell Manipulation. https://doi.org/10.1016/B978-0-323-85259-3.00007-6

cell manipulation technique is a useful and simple method not only for cell patterning, but also for cell sorting and separation (Cui et al., 2009). To date, most DEP research has been carried out using microfluidic chips (Pethig, 2010) as application platforms, such as sorting (Hu et al., 2005), trapping (Rosenthal and Voldman, 2005), and transporting (Hawkin et al., 2009) different biological cells. Three-dimensional (3D) porous structures called engineered scaffolds are often used to provide a template for cells to adhere to and gradually proliferate into functional tissues. Various research groups have proposed a number of engineering scaffolds (Moutos et al., 2007; Martins et al., 2014). These scaffolds are usually made of natural or synthetic polymers, such as polylactic-co-glycolic acid (PLGA), polycaprolactone (PCL), and hydrogels with different mechanical properties and geometric structures. In general, scaffolds made with traditional microprocessing techniques (such as particle leaching, gas foaming, and electrospinning) can achieve high porosity; however, pore size, pore distribution, and interconnectivity between pores are not easy to control (Levenberg et al., 2005). On the contrary, scaffolds manufactured using advanced 3D manufacturing technologies (such as rapid prototyping, laser cutting, and micromolding technologies) provide a higher degree of controllability for many design parameters, so complex scaffolding designs can be constructed to adapt to different applications (Moutos et al., 2007). However, due to limitations of manufacturing technology, the size resolution of these scaffolds is generally low, and the ability to maximize the density of cells seeded on these scaffolds with relatively large pores has become critical to ensuring the quality of the developed tissues. Chu et al. (2015) designed a scaffold structure composed of multiple layers of biocompatible materials. This structure can be combined with DEP technology to pattern cells in the 3D domain. This research extends the DEP manipulation technology beyond the lab-on-a-chip environment and studies the batch manipulation of cells to achieve active seeding and patterning of engineered scaffold structures. Extending the study of Chu et al. (2015), Huan et al. (2017) used DEP to promote cell seeding during the reconstruction of artificial bone tissue. Achieving a high-density spatial distribution of cells on a 3D scaffold is an indispensable process because it can lead to a more homogeneous extracellular matrix for cell processing and improve the quality and function of the tissue to be developed. Huan et al. (2017) automatically patterned the cells on the scaffold into a multilayer honeycomb pattern to imitate the structure and complexity of natural tissues to improve tissue culture performance.

Microfluidics have also been used for cell patterning. With the ability to manipulate and control fluids in the microliter to picoliter range, microfluidics has developed into an important platform for manipulating cells in the past few decades. It has many unparalleled advantages, such as flexible design, small volume of liquid used, high throughput, and high integration. Based on microfluidics technology, cell patterning can be used for cell coculture, which allows two or more cell types to be cultured with a certain degree of direct or indirect contact (Burmeister and Grünberger, 2020). Compared with traditional monoculture, coculture is very important for promoting the research of interactions between heterotypic cells. Traditional cell coculture strategies are mainly based on random mixing and accompanying growth of multiple cell types on Petri dishes and well plates. Differences in cell adhesion between different cell types may drive cell movement and classification, ultimately leading to spontaneous cell rearrangement (Foty and Steinberg, 2005). However, the coculture method based on the differential adhesion hypothesis has limited control over the final cell pattern. Therefore, engineering approaches that allow the patterning of multiple cell types with controlled spatial arrangement are needed. Based on the use of micropatterned surfaces (Liu et al., 2014) or physical barriers (Iwadate et al., 2019), cell printing (Tavana et al., 2010), detachable substrates (Kaji et al., 2009), electrical methods (Chu et al., 2015; Huan et al., 2017), optical methods (Chiou et al., 2005), acoustic methods (Guo et al., 2015), magnetic methods (Ino and Akira, 2007), and hydrodynamic methods (Luo et al., 2019), various patterning coculture methods have been developed. Among these techniques, micropatterning using a substrate with prepatterned adhesion molecules facilitates the generation of organized patterned coculture. However, the behavior of cells in this coculture may be affected by the heterogeneity of the substrates, which are fabricated through a highly complex process. A simple and flexible technique for patterned cocultivation of multiple cell types on a microfluidic platform is necessary. Fan et al. (2020) demonstrated the use of the gravitational sedimentation of cells in the capillary tubing to achieve a one-step pattern and coculture of multiple cell types, with adjustable spatial arrangement in the microfluidic channel.

The remainder of this chapter introduces cell patterning using optical tweezers, DEP, and microfluidic-based techniques, respectively. These cell patterning technologies can move a group of cells to a desired area for cell−cell interaction studies, enhance cell seeding to develop high-quality artificial tissues, and promote in vitro cocultivation models on microfluidic platforms for many applications, such as drug screening.

10.2 Cell patterning with robotically controlled optical tweezers

10.2.1 Multilevel-based topology

In order to manipulate a large group of cells to form the desired pattern, the target cells are driven into the overall desired region first and then controlled to construct the desired pattern. In a similar manner to Li et al. (2013b), the overall desired region is defined as being composed of many different constraint areas, which can eventually construct areas of various shapes. Denote $q_i = [x_i, y_i]^T \in R^2$ as the center position of the ith cell from a total of n target cells, and $q_o = [x_o, y_o]^T \in R^2$ as a reference point in the overall desired region. Define the mth constraint region Ω_m as follows:

$$\Omega_m : \left\{ \left[g_{m1}(Q_i(t) - q_{om1}), \ldots, g_{mL_m}(Q_i(t) - q_{omL_m}) \right]^T \right\} \leq 0, \tag{10.1}$$

where $Q_i(t) = \left[x_{Q_i}, y_{Q_i}\right]^T \in R^2$ is a time-varying transformation mapping (Hou et al., 2009), and satisfies $Q_i(t) = T(t)(q_i - q_o) + q_o$; $q_{oml} = [x_{oml}, y_{oml}]^T \in R^2$ is the lth reference point of the function $g_{ml}(Q_i(t) - q_{oml})$, where $q_{oml} = q_o + c_{ml}$. Since c_{ml} are constants for $l = 1, \ldots L_m$ (L_m is the total number of functions to form the constraint region Ω_m, and m is the index), there is $\dot{q}_{oml} = \dot{q}_o$. Notably, $g_{ml}(Q_i(t) - q_{oml})$ is a continuous scalar function with continuous partial derivative, satisfying $g_{ml}(Q_i(t) - q_{oml}) \rightarrow \infty$ as $\|Q_i(t) - q_{oml}\| \rightarrow \infty$. $g_{ml}(Q_i(t) - q_{oml})$ is chosen such that the boundedness of $g_{ml}(Q_i(t) - q_{oml})$ ensures the boundedness of $\frac{\partial g_{ml}(Q_i(t)-q_{oml})}{\partial(Q_i(t)-q_{oml})}$ and $\frac{\partial^2 g_{ml}(Q_i(t)-q_{oml})}{\partial(Q_i(t)-q_{oml})^2}$.

Define $T(t) \in R^2$ as a transformation matrix expressed by $T(t) = T_1(t) \times T_2(t)$, where $T_1(t) = \begin{bmatrix} \cos\theta(t) & -\sin\theta(t) \\ \sin\theta(t) & \cos\theta(t) \end{bmatrix}$, $T_2(t) = \begin{bmatrix} s(t) & 0 \\ 0 & s(t) \end{bmatrix}$, and $\theta(t)$ and $s(t)$ are the rotation angle and the scaling factor, respectively. Note that during the transformation process, $T(t)$ is not a unit matrix. Denote $Q_i(t)$ as the new position of the ith cell after transformation, and M as the total number of constraint regions.

If $Q_i(t) \in \Omega_m$, the ith cell is either inside or on the boundary of the mth constraint region. If $Q_i(t) \in \Omega_m$ for all $m = 1, \ldots, M$ and $i = 1, \ldots, n$, all the cells are either inside or on the boundary of the overall desired region Ω_D. For example, a desired circular region can be defined as follows:

$$\Omega_D : \left\{ g_{11}(Q_i(t) - q_{o11}) = \left(x_{Q_i} - x_{o11}\right)^2 + \left(y_{Q_i} - y_{o11}\right)^2 - \frac{1}{4} d_1^2 \leq 0 \right\}$$

where $q_{o11} = [x_{o11}, y_{o11}]^T \in R^2$ and d_1 denote the center and the diameter of the desired circular region, respectively.

In the cell manipulation method of Li et al. (2013b), the cells can successfully move to the desired region, but there is no further control after the cells enter the region, causing the cells to stay in random positions. Yan and Sun (2015) proposed a multi-level topology, as shown in Fig. 10.1, which enables cells to stay in the desired positions and form the desired pattern in the region. The reference point of the overall desired region, denoted by q_o, is defined as the center of the topology. Each circle in Fig. 10.1 represents a cell with a safety radius R. Note that R is greater than the actual radius of the cell, so each cell does not touch another cell.

Inspired by the hexagonal close packing (hcp) of atoms in the crystal structure (Bao and Cagan, 2005), the topology can be designed based on the hierarchical structure with respect to q_o. This topology represents an effective structure for cells to stay as closely together as possible. As shown in Fig. 10.1, L_1 is located at q_o, and the cells stay together with respect to q_o in a level-by-level structure, where each circle is tangent to its neighboring circle. Each level is represented as L_k, where $k = 1, 2, 3, \ldots$ is the index of a level. When the morphogenesis process occurs, this hexagonal structure has the minimal surface free energy (Bao and Cagan, 2005).

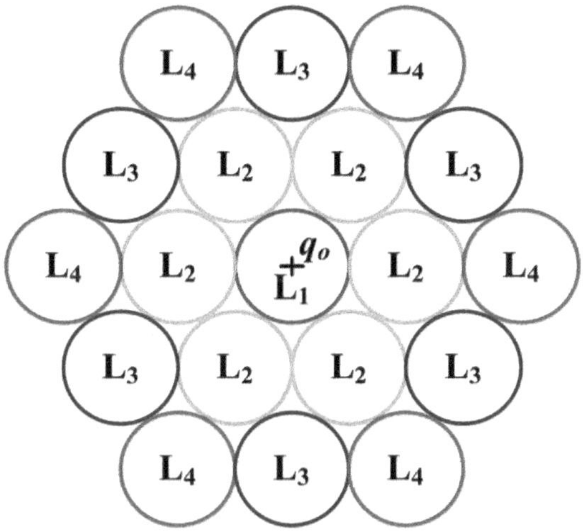

Figure 10.1 Multilevel topology (Yan and Sun, 2015).

In cell manipulations, all cells first move to the region, and then converge to the individual level starting from L_1. When the level L_k is fully filled by cells, the remaining cells will be driven to the next level L_{k+1}. In this way, the cells can be kept together while forming patterns level by level. As the number of cells increases, this multilevel-based topology expands outward.

By assigning cells in different positions at different levels, different patterns can be constructed. Each position does not necessarily have to be filled by cells. According to the requirements of the task, the position where the cell entry is prohibited is defined as the "no-to-go" position, and further treated as a "virtual obstacle" to keep the cell from approaching. Therefore, the cell can only be stopped in the allowed position according to the requirements of the desired mode.

10.2.2 Control design

10.2.2.1 Preliminary

Consider a group of n cells. Define the center position of the ith optical trap as the control input for the ith cell, denoted by $u_i \in \mathrm{R}^2$, The dynamics of the ith cell can be described as (Chen and Sun, 2012):

$$m_i\ddot{q}_i = F_{\text{trap}} - F_{\text{drag}} = k_i(l_i - q_i) - \beta_i\dot{q}_i, \tag{10.2}$$

where m_i is the mass of the ith cell; F_{trap} denotes the trapping force produced by the optical tweezers, approximated as $k_i\ (u_i - q_i)$ (Chen and Sun, 2012), where k_i is the trapping stiffness and $l_i - q_i$ is the offset between the optical trap center and the trapped cell center; F_{drag} represents the Stoke's drag force, where $\beta_i = 6\pi\mu r_{ci}$, μ is the dynamic viscosity, and r_{ci} is the radius of the ith cell.

A controller is designed to drive the cells to the desired region Ω_D and then to the desired levels without collision. Several potential field-based functions are proposed for moving cells to the desired region, positioning the cells in the desired level, and avoiding collisions among each other. The sum of these forces for the ith cell is expressed as:

$$F_i = f_{Di} + f_{ci} + \sum_{j=1, j \neq i}^{n} f_{ij}, \tag{10.3}$$

where f_{Dj}, f_{cj}, and f_{ij} denote the force to enter the desired region, locate at the desired level, and avoid collision, respectively.

Define a reference velocity $\dot{q}_{ri}$ for the ith cell:

$$\dot{q}_{ri} = \dot{q}_o - T^{-1}(t)\dot{T}(t)\Delta q_i + T^{-1}(t)F_i, \tag{10.4}$$

where $\Delta q_i = q_i - q_o$. Differentiating Eq. (10.4) with respect to time yields

$$\ddot{q}_{ri} = \ddot{q}_o - \frac{d(T^{-1}(t))}{dt}\dot{T}(t)\Delta q_i - T^{-1}(t)\ddot{T}(t)\Delta q_i - T^{-1}(t)\dot{T}(t)\Delta\dot{q}_i + \frac{d(T^{-1}(t))}{dt}F_i + T^{-1}(t)\dot{F}_i \tag{10.5}$$

A sliding vector s_i is defined for the ith cell as follows:

$$s_i = \dot{q}_i - \dot{q}_{ri} = \Delta\dot{q}_i + T^{-1}(t)\dot{T}(t)\Delta q_i - T^{-1}(t)F_i, \tag{10.6}$$

where $\Delta\dot{q}_i = \dot{q}_i - \dot{q}_o$. Differentiating Eq. (10.6) with respect to time yields:

$$\dot{s}_i = \ddot{q}_i - \ddot{q}_{ri} = \Delta\ddot{q}_i + \frac{d(T^{-1}(t))}{dt}\dot{T}(t)\Delta q_i + T^{-1}(t)\ddot{T}(t)\Delta q_i + T^{-1}(t)\dot{T}(t)\Delta\dot{q}_i - \frac{d(T^{-1}(t))}{dt}F_i - T^{-1}(t)\dot{F}_i \tag{10.7}$$

where $\Delta\ddot{q}_i = \ddot{q}_i - \ddot{q}_o$. Substituting Eqs. (10.6) and (10.7) into Eq. (10.2) yields

$$\frac{m_i}{k_i}\dot{s}_i + \frac{\beta_i}{k_i}s_i + \left(\frac{m_i}{k_i}\ddot{q}_{ri} + \frac{\beta_i}{k_i}\dot{q}_{ri}\right) = l_i - q_i, \tag{10.8}$$

which can be expressed as

$$\frac{m_i}{k_i}\dot{s}_i + \frac{\beta_i}{k_i}s_i + Y_i\left(\dot{q}_{ri}, \ddot{q}_{ri}\right)P_i = l_i - q_i, \tag{10.9}$$

where $Y_i\left(\dot{q}_{ri}, \ddot{q}_{ri}\right) = \left[\dot{q}_{ri}, \ddot{q}_{ri}\right] \in R^{2\times 2}$ is a regression matrix, and $P_i = \left[\frac{\beta_i}{k_i}, \frac{m_i}{k_i}\right]^T \in R^2$ is a parameter vector.

10.2.2.2 Region control

Define the potential field of the constraint region Ω_m for the ith cell as follows:

$$V_{mi}(Q_i(t) - q_{om}) = \sum_{l=1}^{L_m} \frac{k_{ml}}{2} (\max\{0, g_{ml}(Q_i(t) - q_{oml})\})^2, \tag{10.10}$$

where k_{ml} denotes a positive control gain for the mth constraint region.

The total potential energy of the overall desired region for the ith cell is:

$$V_{Di}(Q_i(t) - q_o) = V_{1i} \times V_{2i} \times \ldots \times V_{Mi} = \prod_{m=1}^{M} \sum_{l=1}^{L_m} \frac{k_{ml}}{2} [\max\{0, g_{ml}(Q_i(t) - q_{oml})\}]^2 \tag{10.11}$$

Define the force f_{Di} as:

$$f_{Di} = -\frac{\partial V_{Di}(Q_i(t) - q_o)}{\partial (Q_i(t) - q_o)}. \tag{10.12}$$

The force f_{Di} aims to drive cells into Ω_D. After the ith cell enters $\Omega_D, f_{Di} = 0$. Once all the cells are located in Ω_D, the task of region control is completed.

After the cells are located in Ω_D, the second force f_{ci} is activated to position the cells at the desired levels. To achieve this goal, the potential field $V_{ci}(Q_i(t) - q_o)$ and the corresponding force f_{ci} are designed as follows:

$$V_{ci}(Q_i(t) - q_o) = \frac{1}{2} k_c (\|Q_i(t) - q_o\| - R_i)^2, \tag{10.13}$$

$$f_{ci} = -\frac{\partial V_{ci}(Q_i(t) - q_o)}{\partial (Q_i(t) - q_o)}, \tag{10.14}$$

where k_c is a positive control gain, and R_i is the radius of the desired level (with respect to q_o) where the ith cell is located.

To avoid collisions, each cell should maintain a safe distance from other cells. The safety distance between cells i and j can be defined in the following way:

$$g_{ij}(Q_i(t) - Q_j(t)) = \begin{cases} 4R^2 - (Q_i(t) - Q_j(t))^2, & \text{if } L^i \geq L^j \\ 0, & \text{if } L^i < L^j \end{cases}, \tag{10.15}$$

where L^i and L^j are the desired levels for the ith and jth cells, respectively. The potential energy associated with this safe distance is defined as:

$$V_{ij}\left(Q_i(t)-Q_j(t)\right)=\frac{k_{ij}}{2}\left[\max\left\{0,g_{ij}\left(Q_i(t)-Q_j(t)\right)\right\}\right]^2, \tag{10.16}$$

where k_{ij} is a positive control gain. The interactive force between the two cells is expressed as:

$$f_{ij}=-\frac{\partial V_{ij}\left(Q_i(t)-Q_j(t)\right)}{\partial\left(Q_i(t)-Q_j(t)\right)}. \tag{10.17}$$

Notably, the force f_{ij} is activated only when $Q_i(t)-Q_j(t)<2R$ and $L^i \geq L^j$ to ensure that collision between cells i and j is avoided. To preserve the previously formed pattern, cells that are already located at their desired level should have a higher priority than cells that arrive later to stay at the current level. Therefore, if $L^j < L^i$, then $f_{ji}=0$.

The controller design of the ith cell is as follows:

$$u_i=-K_{s_i}s_i+k_F T^T(t)F_i+Y_i\left(\dot{q}_{ri},\ddot{q}_{ri}\right)\widehat{P}_i+q_i, \tag{10.18}$$

where K_{s_i} is a positive definite matrix, and k_F is a positive control gain. Define $\Delta P_i = P_i-\widehat{P}_i$, and the estimated parameter vector $\widehat{P}_i$ is updated with the following adaptation law:

$$\dot{\widehat{P}}_i=-Y_i^T\left(\dot{q}_{ri},\ddot{q}_{ri}\right)s_i. \tag{10.19}$$

Note that $\Delta\dot{P}_i=-\dot{\widehat{P}}_i$ because $\dot{P}_i=0$. Substituting the controller Eq. (10.18) into Eq. (10.9) yields the following closed-loop equation:

$$\frac{m_i}{k_i}\dot{s}_i+\frac{\beta_i}{k_i}s_i+K_{s_i}s_i+Y_i\left(\dot{q}_{ri},\ddot{q}_{ri}\right)\Delta P_i-k_F T^T(t)F_i=0, \tag{10.20}$$

Yan and Sun (2015) have proved that the controller (10.18) can guarantee the convergence of $s_i\rightarrow 0$ and $F_i\rightarrow 0$ for all $i=1,2,\ldots,n$, as $t\rightarrow\infty$. To prove this, the following Lyapunov function candidate can be defined

$$\begin{aligned}V=\sum_{i=1}^{n}\Bigg[&\frac{m_i}{2k_i}s_i^T s_i+\frac{1}{2}\Delta P_i^T\Delta P_i+k_F V_{Di}(Q_i(t)-q_o)\\&+k_F V_{ci}(Q_i(t)-q_o)+\frac{k_p}{2}k_F\sum_{j=1,j\neq i}^{n}V_{ij}\left(Q_i(t),Q_j(t)\right)\Bigg],\end{aligned} \tag{10.21}$$

where $k_p = \begin{cases} 2, & \text{if } \dot{Q}_j(t) = 0 \\ 1, & \text{otherwise} \end{cases}$. Yan and Sun (2015) have proven that $\dot{V} \leq 0$ and $\ddot{V}$ is bounded. Then, Barbalat's lemma shows that $s_i \to 0$ and $F_i \to 0$ as $t \to \infty$, and the same is true for all cells.

10.2.2.3 Pattern regulatory control force

When $F_i \to 0$, $\alpha_i f_{Di} + \beta_i f_{ci} + \gamma_i \sum_{j=1, j \neq i}^{n} f_{ij} \to 0$. Assume that there are no obstacles in the environment and there is enough space in the desired region to accommodate all target cells. When $\dot{T}(t) \to 0$, if $f_{Di} \neq 0$, some cells must be outside of Ω_D, so $V_{Di}(Q_i(t) - q_o)\rangle 0$ for these cells. Then these cells will be driven by the force f_{Di} to move toward Ω_D, resulting in $\Delta\dot{q}_i \neq 0$ for these cells. This contradicts the conclusion that $\Delta\dot{q}_i \to 0$ for all cells when $\dot{T}(t) \to 0$. Therefore, $f_{Di} = 0$, and the following result can be obtained:

$$\beta_i f_{ci} + \gamma_i \sum_{j=1, j \neq i}^{n} f_{ij} \to 0, \tag{10.22}$$

Based on Eq. (10.22), when $f_{ci} = 0$, $\sum_{j=1;j \neq i}^{n} f_{ij} = 0$, which indicates that all cells are located at the desired level within Ω_D. However, when $f_{ci} \neq 0$, $\sum_{j=1;j \neq i}^{n} f_{ij} \neq 0$, indicating that f_{ci} and $\sum_{j=1;j \neq i}^{n} f_{ij}$ are equal in magnitude but opposite in direction. In this case, the cells will stop in the unwanted positions. As shown in Fig. 10.2, the cell denoted by the dash-dot line tries to converge to its desired level L_3, but stops at an undesired position because the two forces in Eq. (10.22) cancel out each other. That is why the cell stops at an undesired position. Such a problem can be solved by adding a pattern regulatory control force f_{si} to the controller, as shown here:

$$u_i = -K_{s_i} s_i + k_F T^T(t) F_i + Y_i\left(\dot{q}_{ri}, \ddot{q}_{ri}\right)\widehat{P}_i + f_{si} + q_i, \tag{10.23}$$

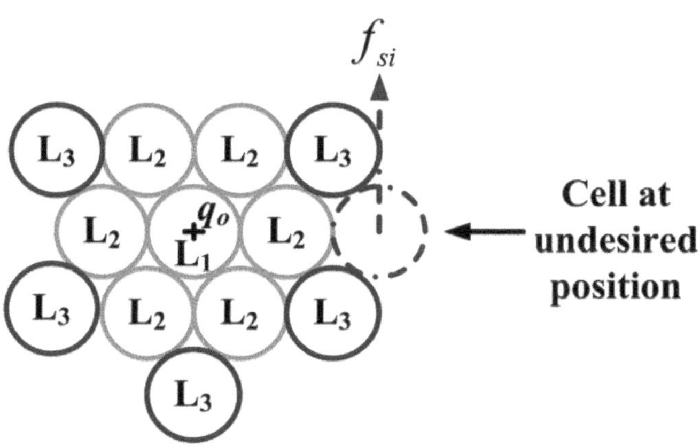

Figure 10.2 Special case: the cell stops at an undesired position (Yan and Sun, 2015).

where

$$f_{si} = k_s T_s \frac{Q_i(t) - q_o}{\|Q_i(t) - q_o\|}. \tag{10.24}$$

In Eq. (10.24), k_s is a positive control gain, $T_s = \begin{bmatrix} \cos\phi & -\sin\phi \\ \sin\phi & \cos\phi \end{bmatrix}$ is a rotation matrix, $\phi \in (0 \text{ degree}, 90 \text{ degree}]$ is a constant rotation angle, and $\frac{Q_i(t)-q_o}{\|Q_i(t)-q_o\|}$ is a unit vector. If $\|Q_i(t) - q_o\| = 0$, the cell is on L_1, which is not a stuck situation. Therefore, $\|Q_i(t) - q_o\| \rangle 0$. As can be seen in Fig. 10.2, f_{si} becomes a tangent force when ϕ is set to 90 degree.

The pattern regulatory control force f_{si} only works when the cell stops at an undesired position, otherwise it is zero. If a cell stops at a position that is not at its desired level, the cell is considered to be at an undesired position. Consequently, f_{si} is activated to drive the cell counterclockwise from its current position. During this process, the cell may be pushed to other cells to take over their positions. Then the other cells repeat the same actions until they all leave the unwanted positions. Notably, the force f_{si} is only activated to move stuck cells out of undesired locations. Once the cell moves away from the unwanted location, it becomes zero.

Using the controller Eq. (10.23), the cells can be driven to the desired region. Then, the cells converge to their desired level and finally form the desired pattern.

10.2.3 Experiments

Experiments were performed on yeast cells to demonstrate the effectiveness of the proposed control approach to cell patterning. The desired circular region Ω_D was defined as follows:

$$\Omega_D : \left\{ g_{11}(Q_i(t) - q_{o11}) = (x_{Q_i} - x_{o11})^2 + \left(y_{Q_i} - y_{o11}\right)^2 - \frac{1}{4}d_1^2 \leq 0 \right\}$$

where $q_{o11} = [x_{o11}, y_{o11}]^T$ is the center of the image obtained from the CCD camera, and $d_1 = 460$ pixels. The control parameters were set to $K_{si} = \text{diag}\{1, 1\}$, $k_F = 1$, $k_{11} = 10$, $k_c = 20$, $k_{ij} = 500$, $k_s = 100$, and $\phi = 90$ degrees. The estimated parameters were initially set to be $\widehat{P}_i = [0, 0]^T$ for all cells. Note that in order to avoid conflicts among cells, the control gain k_{ij} was set to a relatively large value. The parameter k_s for the pattern regulation control force f_{si} was chosen appropriately so that the cell can quickly move away from undesired positions. The safety radius R for each cell was set to $R = 36$ pixels, which was greater than the actual diameter of the cell.

In the first experiment, HOT was used to manipulate the cells to form a hexagonal pattern inside Ω_D. No transformation was required during the formation process, and the matrix T was set to $T = \begin{bmatrix} 1 & 0 \\ 0 & 1 \end{bmatrix}$. As shown in Fig. 10.3A, the centers of six yeast

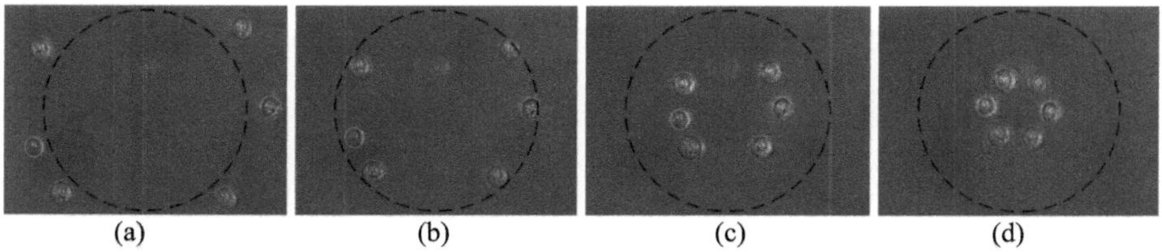

Figure 10.3 Hexagon patterning experiment: (A) $t = 0$ s; (B) $t = 1$ s; (C) $t = 2$ s; (D) $t = 7$ s (Yan and Sun, 2015).

cells were initially located outside Ω_D, then moved into Ω_D after 1 s (Fig. 10.3B), and finally converged to their desired level (Fig. 10.3C). After 7 s, the cells formed a hexagonal pattern (Fig. 10.3D).

Fig. 10.4A shows the sum of the absolute values of all cell velocities in the process, which finally converged to zero, indicating that all cells stopped at the desired positions. The sum of the total potential force $\|F_i\|$ and the sum of $\|s_i\|$ are shown in Fig. 10.4B and C, respectively. Fig. 10.4D illustrates the sum of $\|\Delta Q_i - R_i\|$, which represents the total force acting on the cell, and the sum of the absolute position error.

In the second experiment, 12 cells were manipulated according to the initial position shown in Fig. 10.5A. Eight yeast cells (cell numbers 1–8) initially trapped by the

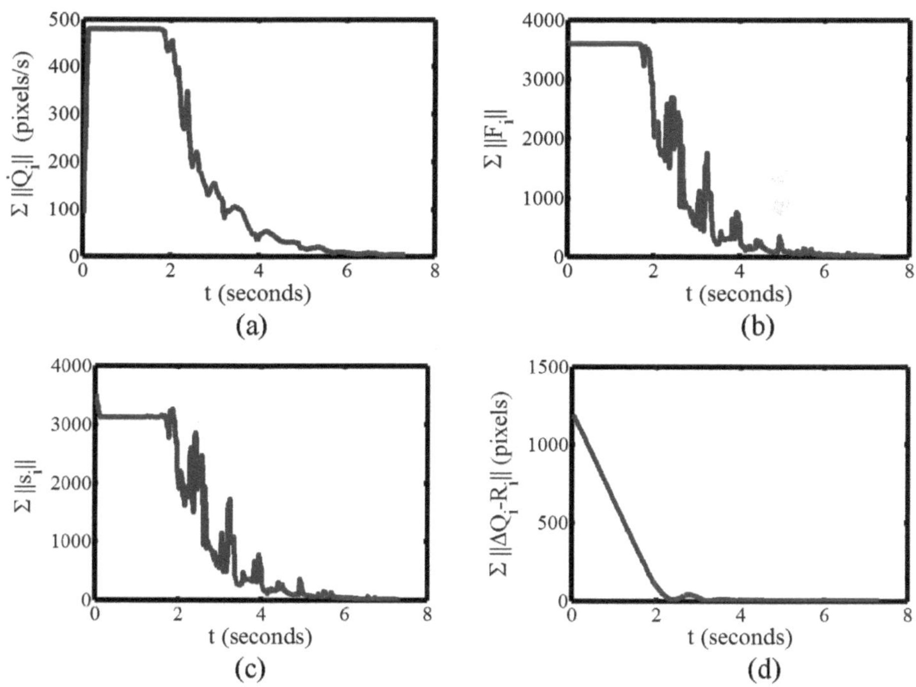

Figure 10.4 Hexagon patterning experiment results (Yan and Sun, 2015). (A) Sum of cell velocities of the hexagon patterning experiment. (B) Sum of the absolute value of F_i. (C) Sum of the absolute value of s_i. (D) Sum of the cell position error with respect to the desired level.

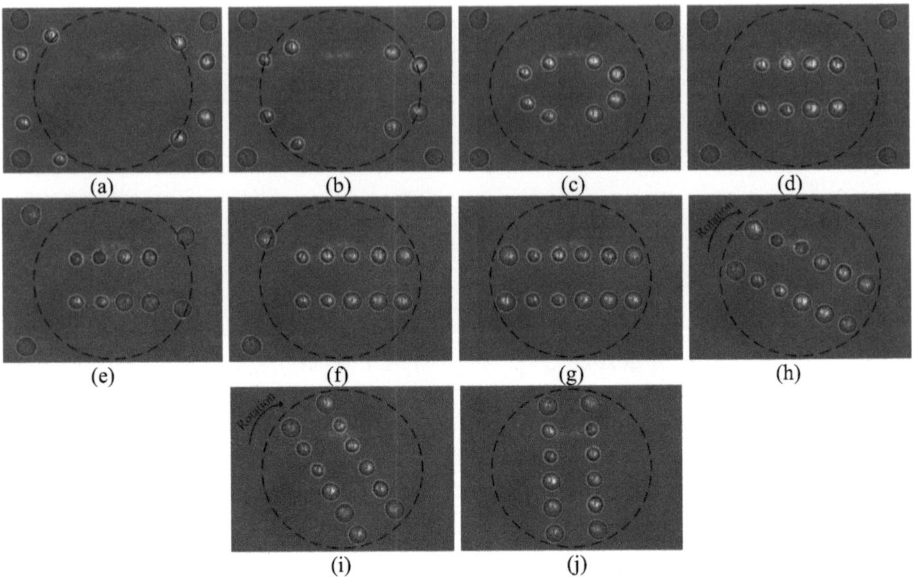

Figure 10.5 Rectangular array experiment (Yan and Sun, 2015): (A) $t = 0$ s; (B) $t = 1$ s; (C) $t = 2$ s; (D) $t = 4$ s; (E) $t = 7$ s; (F) $t = 8$ s; (G) $t = 11$ s; (H) $t = 15$ s; (I) $t = 17$ s; (J) $t = 20$ s.

HOT system were used to form a 2×4 rectangular array. The transformation matrix T was initially set as the identity matrix. After 1 s, the eight cells were located inside Ω_D in terms of their center positions, as shown in Fig. 10.5B–C. The eight cells formed a 2×4 array after 4 s, as shown in Fig. 10.5D. After 5 s, the other four cells (cell numbers 9–12) outside Ω_D were driven to Ω_D, as shown in Figs. 10.5E–F. The cells finally formed a 2×6 rectangular array after 11 s, as shown in Fig. 10.5G. Then the cell group rotated, as shown in Fig. 10.5H–I, and the transformation matrix was set to $T = \begin{bmatrix} \cos\theta(t) & -\sin\theta(t) \\ \sin\theta(t) & \cos\theta(t) \end{bmatrix}$, where the desired rotation angle is $\theta_d = -\frac{\pi}{2}$, and the angular velocity was $\dot{\theta}(t) = -\frac{\pi}{15}$. After 20 s, the cell group stopped rotating and formed a 6×2 array.

Similar to the first experiment, Fig. 10.6 shows the sum of the experimental results during the whole process to demonstrate the convergence performance of the controller. All these results confirm the effectiveness of the cell patterning control approach.

10.3 Cell patterning using a dielectrophoresis-based multilayer scaffold structure

This section introduces the use of multilayer engineered scaffolds to perform 3D cell manipulation and patterning (Chu et al., 2015). This scaffold structure uses

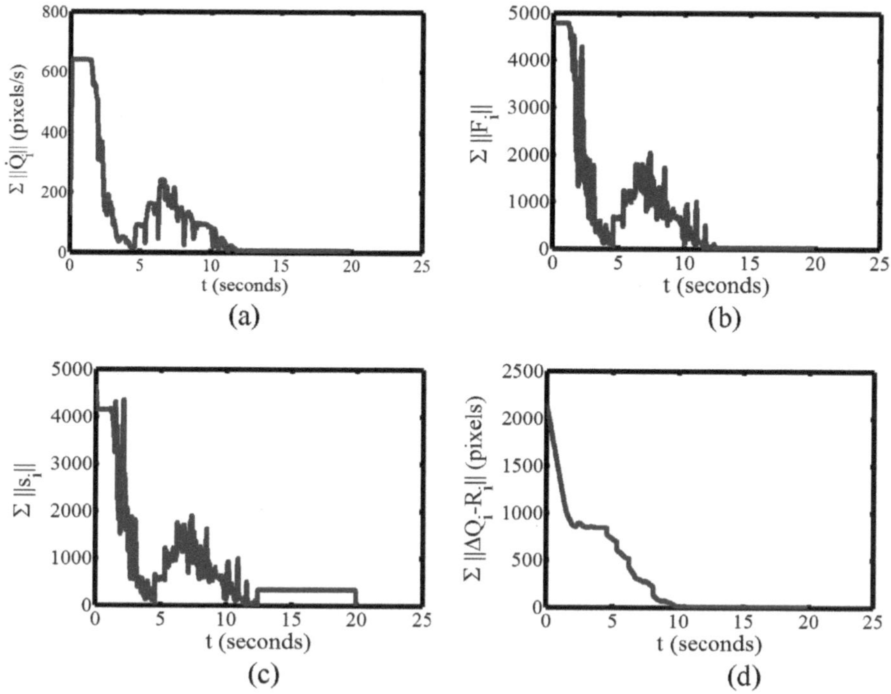

Figure 10.6 Rectangular array experiment results (Yan and Sun, 2015). (A) Sum of cell velocities of the rectangular array experiment. (B) Sum of the absolute value of F_i. (C) Sum of the absolute value of s_i. (D) Sum of the cell position error with respect to the desired level.

dielectrophoresis as a noncontact mechanism to manipulate cells in the 3D domain. By establishing an electric field through the multilayer structure, the cells in the medium are polarized and attracted to the inside of the structure, thereby forming a 3D cellular pattern.

10.3.1 Dielectrophoresis manipulation on a multilayer scaffold structure

10.3.1.1 Multilayer scaffold structure design

The multilayer scaffold structure is designed to automatically manipulate cells through dielectrophoresis, as shown in Fig. 10.7A. Each layer of the structure has two main purposes: to provide a platform for cell adhesion, and as an electrode to generate an electric field. The size of each layer is 15 mm × 15 mm, and the thickness is 500 μm. To prevent direct electrical contact between layers, the bottom inside of each layer is coated with a 100 μm thick insulating material. Trenches 800 μm wide are cut from each layer to construct multiple 800 μm wide parallel microelectrodes for cell attachment. To generate the required electric field in the 3D spatial domain, an AC voltage is provided to adjacent layers of the structure. After stacking multiple

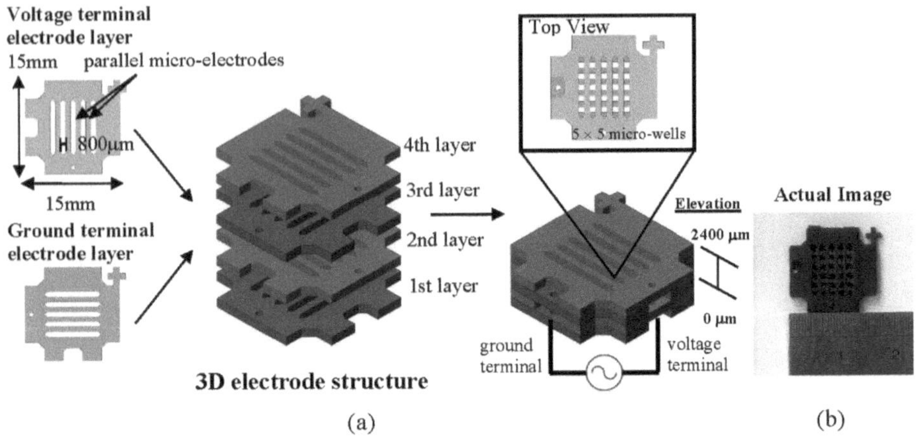

Figure 10.7 A multilayer scaffold (Chu et al., 2015): (A) schematic; (B) photograph of the multilayer scaffold structure for 3D cell manipulation.

layers together, a 5 × 5 interconnected rectangular microwell (pore) array is established in the scaffold structure for cell attachment and nutrient exchange, as shown in Fig. 10.7B.

When a droplet of cell medium is pipetted onto the scaffold, DEP force will be generated on the cells, thereby constructing a 3D cellular pattern on the entire multilayer scaffold, as shown in Fig. 10.8A and B. To perform effective cell manipulation

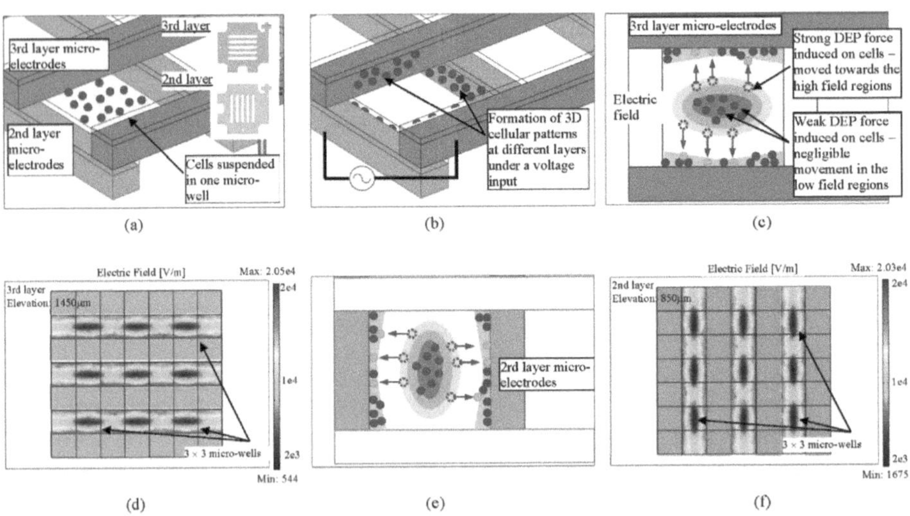

Figure 10.8 DEP cell manipulation by the multilayer scaffold (Chu et al., 2015). (A) Cells in one microwell. (B) Formation of 3D cellular pattern. (C) Cell manipulation at the third layer due to the electric field. (D) Electric field simulation of the third layer at 10 V voltage input. (E) Cell manipulation at the second layer due to the electric field. (F) Electric field simulation of the second layer at 10 V voltage input.

by positive dielectrophoresis, the electric field strengths along the parallel microelectrodes must be higher than the surrounding medium. The finite element analysis (FEA) software COMOSL can be used to simulate the electric field distribution under a voltage supply. The simulation results show that through this multilayer configuration, a highly nonuniform electric field can be generated between the parallel microelectrodes in each layer. As shown in Fig. 10.8C−F, relatively weak DEP force is induced on the biological cells located near the center of the microwell (blue area [dark gray in print version]), and the movement of these cells is negligible. In contrast, cells closer to the microelectrode will produce stronger DEP forces. Therefore, these cells are polarized and manipulated toward the high electric field (red area [light gray in print version]), forming cell patterns in different layers along the electrode surface (Fig. 10.8C and E).

Conductive biocompatible polymer composites, such as polydimethylsiloxane (PDMS) elastomer (Sylgard 184, Dow Corning), can be selected as the structural material to fabricate the multilayer scaffold. PDMS is a common biocompatible material used in pharmaceutical and biomedical applications, and has been widely used to fabricate 3D scaffolds for culturing different types of biological cells. To synthesize this biological material, approximately 5 g of PDMS base material are first mixed with a curing agent in a 10:1 ratio, and then degassed in a vacuum desiccator to remove any trapped air bubbles. To provide conductivity, a conductive filler, carbon black (CB) nanopowder (VXC72R, Cabot), is added to the mixture in an amount of 30% (by weight). Nanocarbon powder is chosen because it is less toxic than other carbon-based conductive fillers such as single-walled or multiwalled carbon nanotubes (Martins et al., 2014). The CB-PDMS paste is thoroughly shear-mixed and sonicated in an ultrasonic bath for 1 h. Then, the CB-PDMS paste is cast onto a metal mold to form a 500 μm thick 10 mm × 10 mm sheet. The CB-PDMS sheet is cured in an oven at 70°C for 1 h. To develop an insulating coating, 1 g of PDMS is poured onto the sheet, and an insulating layer about 100 μm thick is formed on one side of the CB-PDMS sheet. Then the sheet is heated to 70°C again and maintained at this temperature for 1 h to fully cure the double-layer sheet. Subsequently, a commercial CO_2 laser cutting machine is used to cut the CB-PDMS double-layer board into a stent layer array. The processed voltage and ground scaffold layers are finally stacked and bonded together by a plasma bonding machine.

Fig. 10.9 illustrates the setup for experimental testing. The multilayer scaffold structure is first bonded onto the 35 mm Petri dish of the stage-top incubator of the system. A functional generator is connected to an in-house amplifier circuit to amplify the sinusoidal voltage output to a maximum of 60 Vpp at a frequency of 0−300 kHz. Before the experiments, each structure is sterilized in a 70% ethanol solution for 30 min and then coated with poly-L-lysine (Sigma Aldrich) to enhance the affinity of the surface for cell attachment. A low-conductivity DEP buffer (5% sucrose solution) is prepared as a temporary medium to perform DEP manipulation on various biological cells examined in this work. Before the experiment, the scaffold structure is first rinsed with the DEP buffer, and then a droplet of cell-containing medium is transferred to the structure for cell seeding and patterning. This experiment considered three different types of mammalian cells, namely 3T3, 293FT, and human foreskin

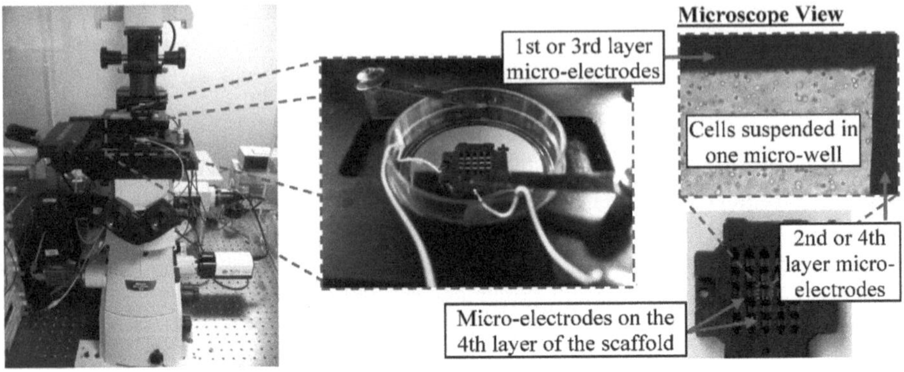

Figure 10.9 The experimental setup (Chu et al., 2015).

fibroblasts (HFFs) (Chu et al., 2015). 3T3 cells are mouse cells derived from mouse embryo tissue, while 293FT and HFF are human cells derived from embryonic kidney and foreskin, respectively. The 3D models of these cells cultured on the scaffold may be used to facilitate cell-based assays such as drug discovery (Garg et al., 2012) and transfection studies (Xie et al., 2004). The concentration of each type of cell is adjusted to approximately 1.2×10^6 cells/mL for seeding experiments.

10.3.1.2 Cell patterning experiments

The seeding and patterning performance of 3TC cells were evaluated using the experimental setup shown in Fig. 10.9. In order to enhance the contrast between the background and the cell pattern, 3T3 cells were stained with MitoTacker Red. The power supply voltage was set to 20 V. At the elevations near the first and second layers, images of the scaffold structure with a 4× objective lens were captured, as shown in Fig. 10.10.

Observed through a microscope, a similar 3D rectangular pattern can be seen in all 25 microwells, therefore the DEP mechanism can be used to automatically inoculate this multilayer scaffold. The fluorescence image in Fig. 10.10C shows that the cell

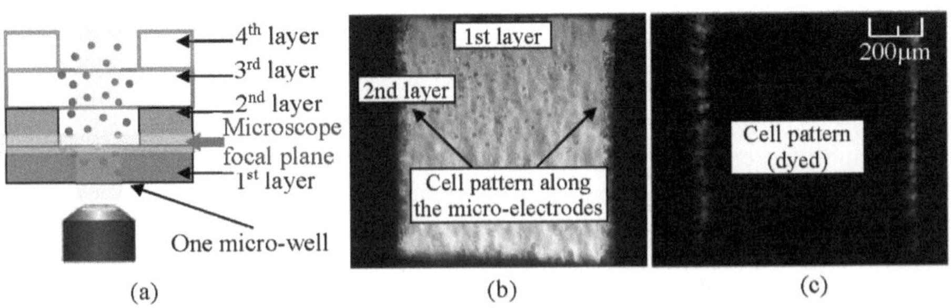

Figure 10.10 3D pattern constructed from 3T3 cells (Chu et al., 2015): (A) schematic; (B) brightfield image; (C) fluorescent image.

pattern on the first layer (horizontal line) of the structure has a lower cell density than the other layers (vertical line). This can be explained by the medium flow conditions of different layers. In the current setup, the first layer was bonded onto the surface of the Petri dish; therefore, the additional wall shear from this boundary can change the flow of the medium around the first layer from laminar to turbulent, which was due to corner eddies (Angelescu, 2011).

The reported engineering scaffold was then tested with different voltage inputs to determine their influence on cell viability after DEP manipulation. A higher voltage input can reduce the time for cellular pattern formation, but as a trade-off, this may reduce the survival rate. Several research papers have reported that the use of electric fields above 40 kV/m can cause problems such as Joule heating and cell damage (Markx, 2008; Menachery and Pethig, 2005). Therefore, the electric field generated by the structure was simulated by COMSOL, and the maximum electric field at different heights of the structure is summarized in Table 10.1. The simulation results showed that the operating structure at 10 V was relatively nondestructive to the cells. In contrast, voltages of 20 V or above may not be suitable for cell patterning, because the electric field strength generated in most areas may exceed 50 kV/m, posing a serious threat to the survival of cells.

To evaluate viability through experiments, trypan blue was used to detect the dead cells after DEP manipulation. Droplets of medium containing 3T3 cells were added to the four scaffolds, and the input voltage of each scaffold was set to 0 V (control), 5 V, 10 V, and 20 V for 30 min. Two sets of tests were performed for each voltage input to help evaluate the repeatability of the results. The cells patterned within the structure were separated from the structure for assay. The collected cell medium was dyed with 0.4% trypan blue for 5 min, and then small droplets were dispensed onto a glass slide for inspection.

Table 10.1 Maximum electric field at different heights of the scaffold structure (Chu et al., 2015).

	Electric field (kV/m)		
Elevation (μm)	**5 V**	**10 V**	**20 V**
Second layer			
601	42.6	85.2	170.3
725	12.6	25.2	50.4
850	9.2	18.5	36.9
975	18.7	37.5	74.9
1100	68.7	137.4	274.7
Third layer			
1201	43.1	86.3	172.6
1325	12.4	24.9	49.8
1450	9.5	18.9	37.8
1575	19.8	39.7	79.4
1700	77.4	154.9	309.7

To quantify the cell survival rate, the average number of dead cells in the stained cell culture medium was checked at 10 locations for each voltage input. The results obtained from the 0 and 20 V cell measurements are shown in Fig. 10.11A and B, and the survival rate under different voltage inputs is plotted in Fig. 10.11C. After 30 min of patterning DEP cells with an input voltage of less than 10 V, the cell viability was high. The cell viability of DEP cell patterning under 5 and 10 V input was approximately 78.4% ± 5.6% and 76.7% ± 5.4%, respectively; the achieved survival rate was comparable to the 79.7% ± 5% rate of the control (0 V). When the voltage was further increased to 20 V, the survival rate dropped to 70.5% ± 3.7%. According to these results, using a voltage input of 10 V or lower would not cause significant cell damage or death during DEP operation and patterning using the proposed structure.

As mentioned above, the results of the COMSOL simulation predicted that the use of a voltage input of 20 V and above may cause a significant decrease in cell viability due to the high electric field generated. It can be seen from this experiment that when the input voltage was increased to 20 V, the detrimental effect of the DEP field on cell viability was greater. The difference between the simulation prediction and the experiment can be explained by the material properties of the structure used. When the scaffold structure used a material with lower conductivity as the electrode, due to the high internal resistance of the material, the voltage drop on the scaffold layer can be expected, which would result in a weak electric field generated by the structure.

10.3.2 Patterning on an engineering scaffold for tissue engineering

Using the idea of multilayer structure design, Huan et al. (2017) developed a scaffold that can automatically seed cells into a multilayer honeycomb pattern for bone tissue engineering applications. The scaffold incorporates dielectrophoresis for noncontact manipulation of cells, and the inherent honeycomb structure is integrated in each scaffold layer. When a voltage is applied to the stacked scaffold layers to generate a 3D electric field, the cells are manipulated to form a honeycomb cell pattern for subsequent culture.

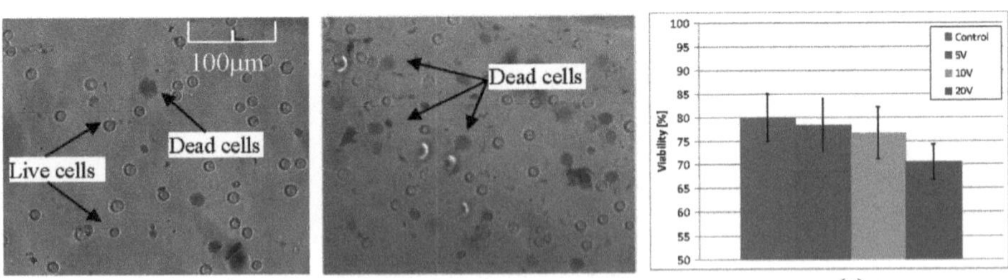

Figure 10.11 Viability test on the manipulated cells after (A) 0 V input (control), (B) 20 V input, and (C) viability of cells at different voltage inputs (Chu et al., 2015).

10.3.2.1 Scaffold design and fabrication

To allow cell attachment and tissue ingrowth, scaffolds used for tissue repair or regeneration usually have a porous structure and interconnected pores (Nouri-Felekori et al., 2015; Cox et al., 2015). Depending on the fabrication technique, the pores can be randomly distributed or precisely controlled. A large number of studies have shown that compared with traditional scaffolds, scaffolds with a honeycomb structure can more effectively improve cell proliferation, viability, and survival (Zhu et al., 2011). The honeycomb structure can more effectively simulate the morphology of natural bone tissue, while providing good mechanical stability to guide tissue formation (Itoh et al., 2001; Sato et al., 2003).

Huan et al. (2017) designed a prototype of a 3D honeycomb scaffold composed of five independent layers. In order to use DEP for cell patterning, a voltage opposite to the adjacent layer is applied to each layer to form an electrode pair, thereby generating an uneven electric field for DEP cell manipulation. Fig. 10.12 illustrates a schematic of the scaffold. The scaffold layers connected to the positive terminal of the sine function generator are displayed in red (dark gray in print version), while the scaffold layers connected to the ground terminal are displayed in blue (black in print version).

Fig. 10.13 shows the working principle of the cell patterning technology on the scaffold layer. When the cell droplet is pipetted onto the scaffold, the pores of the scaffold are filled with randomly distributed cells, as shown in Fig. 10.13A. When voltage is supplied to the scaffold, an uneven electric field is established in the microenvironment, where the gradient at the border of the honeycomb pattern is the highest. The suspended cells are polarized and manipulated toward the electrode layer to form a honeycomb pattern, as shown in Fig. 10.13B.

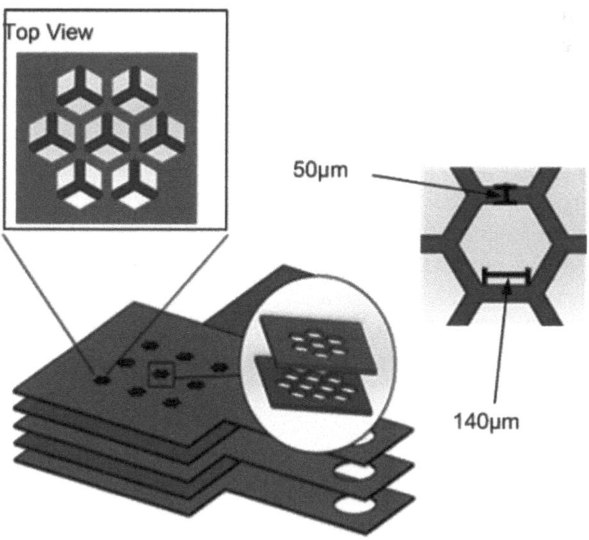

Figure 10.12 Schematic of the multilayer scaffold (Huan et al., 2017). (A) The pores of the scaffold are filled with randomly distributed cells. (B) The suspending cells are polarized and manipulated toward the electrode layer to form honeycomb patterns.

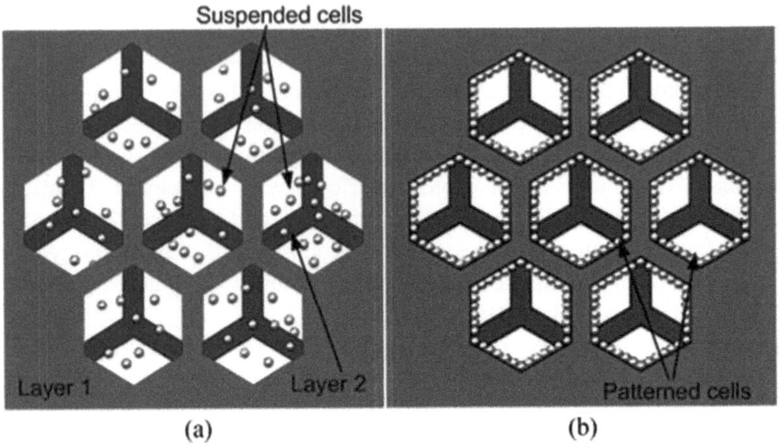

Figure 10.13 Operation principle of cell patterning (Huan et al., 2017). (A) The pores of the scaffold are filled with randomly distributed cells. (B) The suspending cells are polarized and manipulated toward the electrode layer to form honeycomb patterns.

Polymer scaffolds are widely used in tissue engineering due to their good biocompatibility, easy manufacturing, and controllable mechanical properties. Metal materials have relatively high strength and can withstand the compressive loads of daily activities after implantation, and so they can be used for hard tissue engineering (Liu et al., 2015). The metal scaffold also exhibits high conductivity, which can minimize Joule heating and voltage drop. Medical stainless steel can be chosen to fabricate multilayer scaffold because of its mechanical properties, biocompatibility, and corrosion resistance. The conductivity of stainless steel is 1.4×10^4 s/cm.

To construct a multilayer scaffold, a rectangular 10 mm × 10 mm scaffold layer is cut from stainless steel. Multiple honeycomb patterns are cut into each layer, and the positioning accuracy is 5 μm. The length and width of the honeycomb pattern are 140 and 50 μm, respectively, and the average pore size is 140 μm. Studies have shown that the average pore size ranges from 96 to 150 μm to facilitate optimal adhesion in bone tissue engineering (Murphy et al., 2010). The thickness of the material is 50 μm to reduce processing errors in the laser cutting process. Through plasma-enhanced chemical vapor deposition, each layer is coated with 1-μm-thick silicon dioxide to provide electrical insulation between the stacked layers to form a 3D scaffold. This coating can also enhance cell adhesion during seeding. Fig. 10.14A and B show the microscope image and scanning electron microscope (SEM) image of the stacked multilayer scaffold, respectively.

10.3.2.2 Experimental results

Experiments were carried out to prove the performance of using 3D honeycomb scaffolds for cell manipulation through DEP. Three types of cells, namely MC3T3-E1 cells, leukemia OCI-AML3 cells, and HFF cells, were used in the experiments. To ensure the maximum DEP force for cell manipulation through p-DEP, operating frequencies of

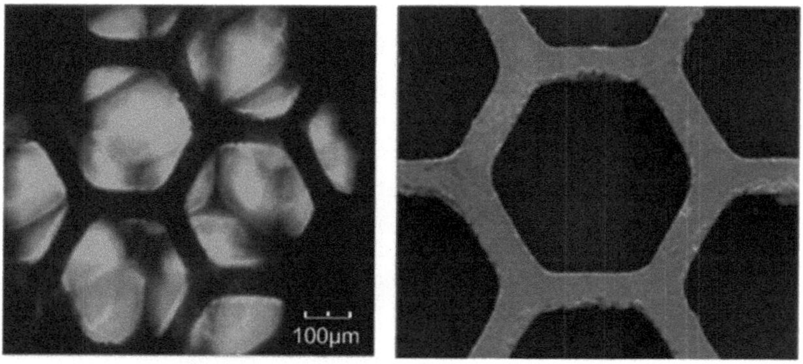

(a) (b)

Figure 10.14 A multilayer scaffold prototype (Huan et al., 2017). (A) Microscope image. (B) SEM image of the fabricated scaffold structure.

100 kHz and 1 MHz were used (Huan et al., 2017). A higher frequency input can weaken the DEP force, while a lower frequency input can change the DEP effect from positive to negative. The voltage frequency used in the experiment was 500 kHz.

To pattern cells by DEP, the cells were suspended in a sucrose medium for a period of time, resulting in cell lysis. In addition, exposure of biological cells to an electric field would cause power dissipation in the cell membrane and an increase in temperature. Fig. 10.15 illustrates the assessment results of MC3T3-E1 cells from mice using the scaffold design. The patterned cells were collected from the scaffold and the cell viability was determined using 0.4% trypan blue solution. The input voltages of 0 V (without DEP) and 10 V (with DEP) and 500 kHz for 10 min were selected as the two control groups. In the first set of experiments, input voltages of 5, 10, and 20 V were considered, and the results showed that for input voltages of 10 V or lower, more than 90% cell viability can be achieved. However, as the input voltage increased to 20 V, the cell viability dropped to 60%, as shown in Fig. 10.15A. The effect of patterning time was then studied, and the DEP patterning time was set to 5, 10, and 20 min, respectively. After 5 min of DEP patterning, the cell viability was equivalent to that of the control group (see Fig. 10.15A). When the DEP patterning was extended to 10 min, the cell viability decreased but remained above 90%. When this process lasted for 20 min, the cell viability dropped to only 50% (see Fig. 10.15B). Finally, the influence of the operating voltage frequency was checked and no significant change was discovered in cell viability, as shown in Fig. 10.15C. According to the results, the optimal setting for the DEP pattern should be around 10 V and 10 min to minimize cell death.

Fig. 10.16 illustrates the patterns of MC3T3-E1 cells, formed from three different cell concentrations by DEP force. For each test, a 10 V voltage with a frequency of 500 kHz was applied for 10 min. When the medium with low cell concentration (4.5×10^4 cells/mL) was pipetted onto the scaffold, the structure was not completely covered by cells after DEP patterning (see Fig. 10.16A). When a higher cell concentration of culture medium (1.25×10^6 cells/mL) was pipetted, more cells were manipulated by DEP to construct cell patterns (see Fig. 10.16B). Cells adhered along the edges of the structure to build a

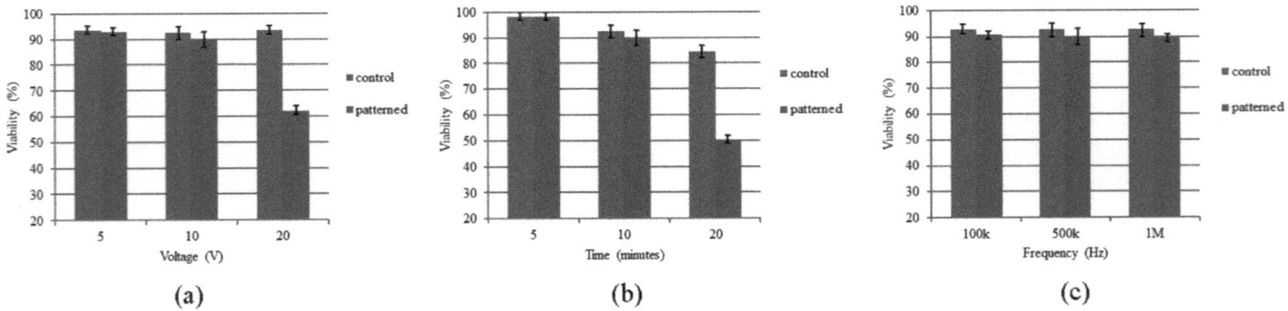

Figure 10.15 Assessment of MC3T3-E1 cell viability after DEP patterning with different (A) voltages, (B) times, and (C) frequencies (Huan et al., 2017).

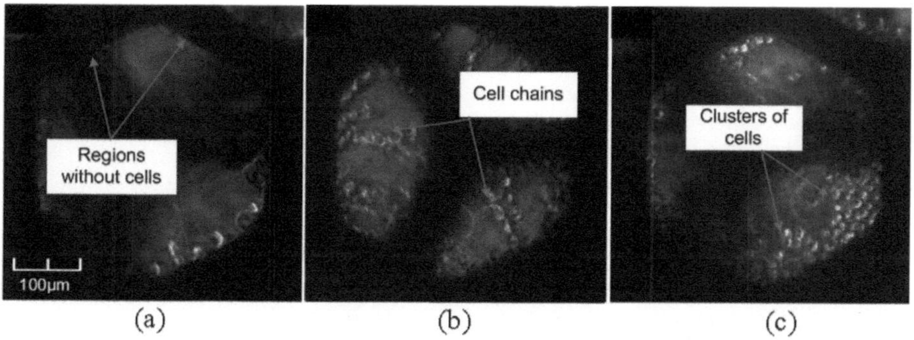

Figure 10.16 Cell patterns on the second scaffold layer with different cell concentrations (Huan et al., 2017): (A) 4.5 × 10^4 cells/mL; (B) 1.25 × 10^6 cells/mL; (C) 5 × 10^6 cells/mL.

more uniform honeycomb cell pattern. Under the DEP effect, cell chains were formed and cell patterns were formed on the adjacent layers (out of focus). Increasing the concentration to 5 × 10^6 cells/mL resulted in a denser cell pattern. The excess cells piled up on the honeycomb cell pattern and formed a pattern (see Fig. 10.16C). These extra cells did not adhere to the scaffold and could be washed away due to the exchange of medium. Therefore, an appropriate cell concentration should be used to minimize the use of cells when forming the necessary cell pattern.

To examine the effect of cell size on pattern formation, three types of cells with approximately the same concentrations (1.25 × 10^6 cells/mL) were manipulated by DEP with the multilayer scaffold. These cells were labeled with MitoTracker Red to enhance the contrast between the background and the cell pattern. Ten V voltage input is provided to the scaffold and the cell pattern observed after 10 min, as shown in Fig. 10.17A–F. Among the three types of cells, HFF has the largest diameter and smallest number of patterned cells. One possible reason for this phenomenon is that these cells exhibit enough increased resistance to reach the inside of the scaffold through the interconnected pores. As a result, fewer cells appeared in the pores to construct the patterns. As the diameter of the cell type decreases, more cells pass through to form a pattern on the scaffold, which is confirmed by the intensity of the fluorescent images. Leukemia OCI-AML3 cells with the smallest size can achieve a more uniform honeycomb pattern. Therefore, the cell size can directly affect the formation of cell patterns. For cells with larger diameters, the geometric design of interconnected pores should be adjusted accordingly.

10.4 Cell patterning using a gravitational sedimentation-based microfluidic approach

This section introduces a gravitational sedimentation-based approach that can realize cell patterning coculture on a microfluidic platform, where multiple cell types can be patterned simultaneously to form a well-organized cell coculture. Unlike many other

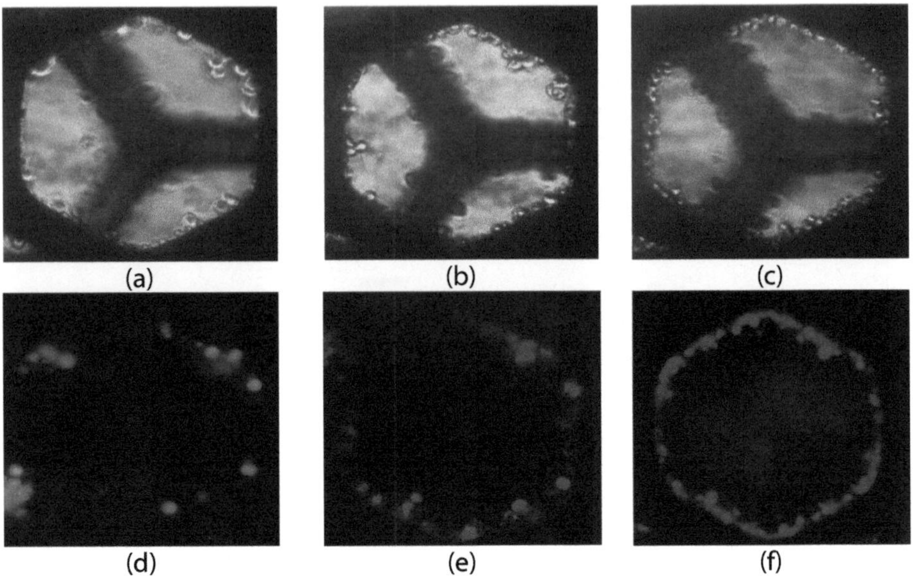

Figure 10.17 Cell patterns on the third scaffold layer with different types of cells (Huan et al., 2017). (A) Brightfield images for HFF cells. (B) Brightfield images for MC3T3-E1 cells. (C) Brightfield images for OCI-AML3 cells. (D) Fluorescent images for HFF cells. (E) Fluorescent images for MC3T3-E1 cells. (F) Fluorescent images for OCI-AML3 cells.

methods, this approach allows rapid and flexible patterning of multiple cell types in microfluidic channels without the use of sheath flow and prepatterned functional surfaces (Fan et al., 2020). This function greatly simplifies the experimental setup, operation, and chip fabrication.

10.4.1 Principle of cell patterning coculture based on gravity sedimentation

Fig. 10.18 illustrates the principle of one-step and flexible cell patterning using gravitational sedimentation in a microfluidic channel. As shown in Fig. 10.18A, the three-in-one-out microfluidic chip is used to pattern and coculture the three types of cells. A syringe pump can be used to simultaneously introduce three types of cells into the microchannel to form three cell strips with gaps between adjacent strips for cell proliferation. Note that the pattern of cell strips with gaps of different widths can be determined by the direction of the inlet tubing. As shown in Fig. 10.18B, by applying the tubing direction at the 10, 3, and 8 o'clock positions, three cell strips can be placed along the upper side wall, central axis, and lower side wall of the microchannel. With this ability, the position of the cell strip can be adjusted flexibly and independently without the need to redesign the microfluidic chip or reconfigure the multichannel flow control, which is usually required by other methods, such as microstructure and sheath flow-based hydrodynamic approach. Therefore, different

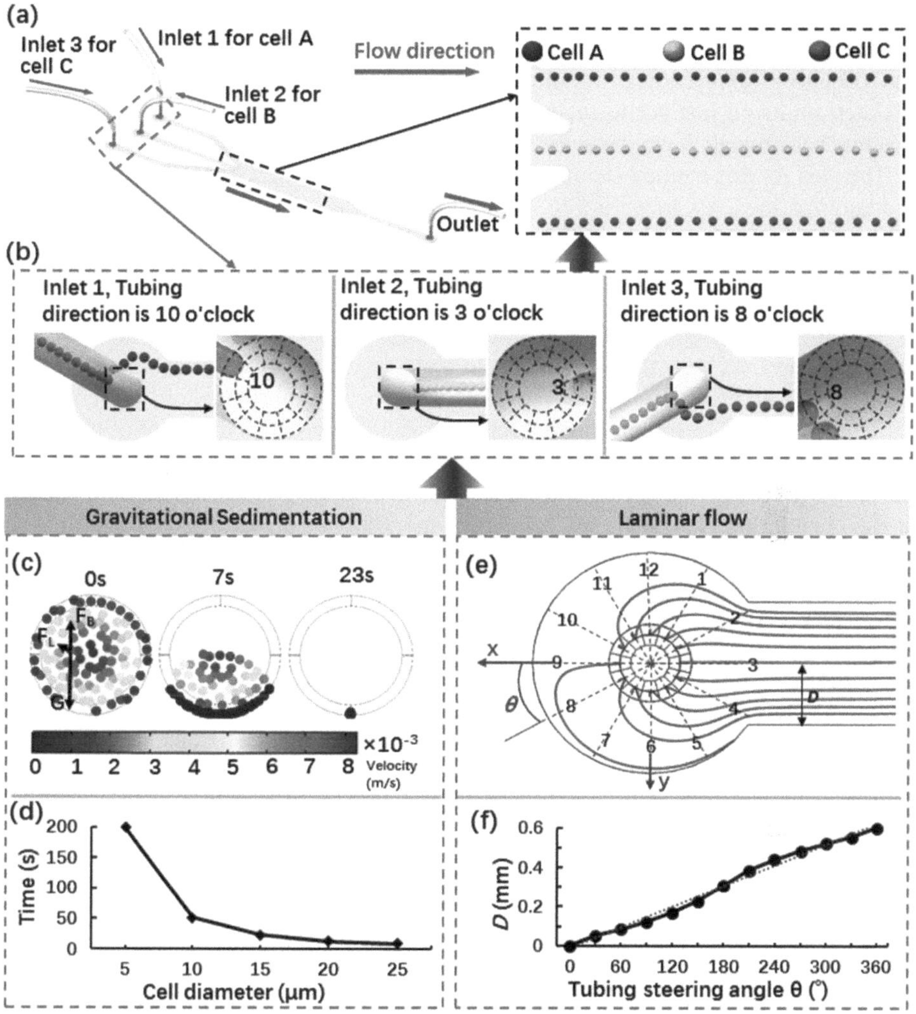

Figure 10.18 Principle of using gravitational sedimentation for one-step and flexible cell patterning in a microfluidic channel (Fan et al., 2020). (A) Schematic of patterning multiple cell types in the microfluidic channel by using gravitational sedimentation. (B) Top view of the inlets for the visualization of the tubing direction and the corresponding cell patterning. Cell A can be focused into the upper side of the channel with a tubing direction of 10 o'clock. Cell B can be focused into the center of the channel with a tubing direction of 3 o'clock. Cell C can be focused into the lower side of the channel with a tubing direction of 8 o'clock. (C) Simulated gravitational sedimentation of cells in the tubing. Sedimentation of cells to the bottom of the tubing is affected by gravity *G*, buoyant force F_B, and inertial lift force F_L. (D) Minimum time to complete cell sedimentation in the tubing versus cell diameter, indicating that the larger cells take less time to compete sedimentation. (E) Distribution of streamlines for the fluid from different inlet parts. With the increase in the tubing steering angle, streamline moves to the upper side of the channel. *D* value is distance between a streamline and the lower side of the channel. (F) Cell strip positions versus tubing steering angles. This shows that cells flow along the corresponding streamline and can be patterned to different positions after sedimentation under different tubing steering angles.

cell patterns can be easily implemented in the same microfluidic chip for various researches, such as short-distance and long-distance cell-to-cell communication. This method allows expansion of the number of inlets of the microfluidic chip by using one-step multicell loading to increase the patterned cell types. A one-step operation ensures that all cells have the same starting point for physiological-related research.

The idea for this method stems from the combination of gravitational sedimentation and laminar flow. As shown in Fig. 10.18C, the motion of the cell in the tubing cross-section is affected by gravity G, buoyant force F_B, and inertial lift force F_L. When the Reynolds number is small, the inertial lift force F_L can be ignored, so the combined force of G and F_B dominates the cell motion in the tubing cross-section. The density of cells is usually slightly higher than that of liquids, such as cell culture media and plasma. Therefore, cells form sediments in these media along the direction of gravity. Fig. 10.18C shows the simulated sedimentation process (approximately 23 s) of a cell with a diameter of 15 μm in a cross-section of the tubing with a diameter of 0.38 mm, which is approximately the size of the tubing in this case. The density of water is similar to the density of cell culture medium, and water is used as the fluid sample in this simulation. The cells will gather at the bottom of the tubing. According to the simulation results, the relationship between complete sedimentation time and cell diameter is shown in Fig. 10.18D, indicating that the time required for complete sedimentation of large cells is relatively short. The minimum tubing length required for complete cell sedimentation can be roughly calculated by multiplying the sedimentation time by the average flow rate. By using sufficient tubing length, cells of different sizes can reliably settle to the bottom of the tubing. In this way, the shortcomings of other high cell selectivity methods based on inertial and acoustic technology can be overcome.

After the cells settle at the bottom of the tubing, they finally flow into the microchannel of the microfluidic chip. The flow pattern of the cells in the microchannel completely depends on the distribution of laminar flow lines. Fig. 10.18E shows the simulation result of some streamline distribution of fluid flow at different parts of the inlet with an inner diameter of 0.38 mm, which is the same as the diameter of the inserted tubing. The outer contour refers to the microchannel, and the central structure corresponds to the inlet. It can be considered that the inlet is composed of 12 sectors and a concentric circle. The directions of these 12 sectors match the "clock time." The steering angle θ of the tubing between the centerline of each sector and the x axis represents the direction of the tubing. As shown in Fig. 10.18E, the streamline originating from each sector has its own unique trajectory, parallel to the microchannel wall. The sedimented cells from tubing flow into a sector and then flow forward along its streamline, forming a band of cells parallel to the side wall. Cells can also be directed to different sectors, and then flow along different streamlines in the microchannel by applying different steering angles of the tubing. Therefore, by simply changing the direction of the tubing, the cell pattern can be flexibly adjusted in real time, making the proposed method versatile. Fig. 10.18F shows the relationship between the steering angle of the tubing and the position of the patterned cell strips. When the tubing steering angle increases from 0 to 360 degrees, the cell strips move from the lower side wall of the microchannel to the upper side wall.

10.4.2 Multifunctional cell patterning in microfluidic channels

10.4.2.1 Cell patterning with different sizes

In the in vivo area, diseased organs and healthy organs are composed of different tissues, which contain multiple cell types and together maintain organ function (Nelson et al., 2006; Gupta and Massagu'e 2006). Different cell types have different characteristics, such as different cell sizes and growth rates. Three different cell types were used in the test, such as yeast (6 μm), NB-4 (15 μm), and HeLa-GFP cells (20 μm). Yeast and NB-4 cells can be stained with red fluorescent dye and blue fluorescent dye, respectively, to improve visualization. Fig. 10.18D shows that small cells require longer tubing to completely undergo sedimentation at a fixed flow rate of 10 μL/min. Therefore, a tubing length of 300 mm is sufficient for complete sedimentation of the thecell types.

The ability of the method to simultaneously pattern different cell types on different microchannel positions was first demonstrated. These three types of cells were suspended in supplemented Dulbecco's modified eagle medium (DMEM) and loaded onto the chip via a syringe pump. HeLa-GFP cells were introduced into the chip through tubing inserted into the upper inlet, and yeast and NB-4 cells were introduced into the chip from the tubing inserted into the lower and middle inlets, respectively. As shown in Fig. 10.19A, the red fluorescently labeled yeast cells were focused and patterned on the underside of the microchannel at a tubing steering angle of 30 degrees.

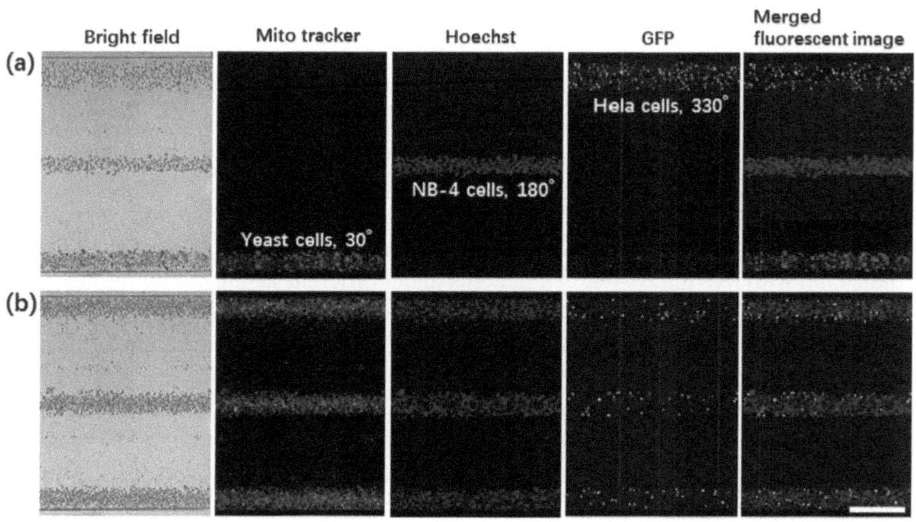

Figure 10.19 Patterning cells with different sizes in the same microfluidic chip simultaneously (Fan et al., 2020). (A) Patterning different cell types on different microchannel positions. The red yeast cells are patterned to the lower side with a tubing steering angle of 30 degrees. The blue NB-4 cells are patterned to the center with a tubing steering angle of 180 degrees. The green HeLa cells are patterned to the upper side with a tubing steering angle of 330 degrees. (B) Patterning different cell types on the same microchannel position. Cell mixtures are patterned to the lower, central, and upper sides of the channel with tubing steering angles of 30, 180, and 330 degrees simultaneously. Scale bar = 500 μm.

At the same time, NB-4 cells formed patterns along the central axis of the microchannel, and HeLa-GFP cells formed patterns on the upper side of the microchannel at 180 and 330 degrees tubing steering angles, respectively.

Then, the ability of the method to simultaneously pattern different cell types at the same location of the microchannel was demonstrated. After the three cell types were uniformly mixed and resuspended in DMEM, the cell mixture was loaded into the chip with the same tubing configuration. Fig. 10.18B shows that the cell mixture was patterned into three cell strips. These experimental results show that the method based on gravitational sedimentation has nothing to do with cell size. In view of this advantage, the gravitational sedimentation-based method shows great potential in applications that require patterning and cocultivation of different cell types on microfluidic chips without redesigning the chip structure.

10.4.2.2 Cell patterning under different tubing configurations

Cell patterning experiments under different tubing configurations were conducted to demonstrate the flexibility of the gravitational sedimentation-based method. In this experiment, NB-4 cells stained with CFDA-SE green fluorescent dye and suspended in RPMI 1640 medium were used. Fig. 10.20A shows the pattern of three cell strips using a microfluidic chip with three inlets. The cell patterns under different tubing configurations were predicted by CFD simulation, which used colored streamlines to visualize the predicted cell patterns. The experimental image in Fig. 10.20A shows that three parallel cell strips formed patterns on different microchannel positions, and the cell pattern was the same as the pattern predicted by the CFD simulation. When θ_3 increased from 30 degrees to 330 degrees, the cell strip representing the cells loaded from the lower inlet moved upward and approached the middle cell strip. This result clearly showed that the cell pattern can be flexibly adjusted by simply changing the direction of the tubing, thereby eliminating the inconvenience of redesigning and fabricating new microfluidic chips. The other two tubing steering angles θ_1 and θ_2 can also be changed to achieve different cell patterns for specific applications. Fig. 10.20B shows the patterns of five cell strips using a microfluidic chip with five inlets. The cell patterns under different tubing configurations were predicted by CFD simulation, and then verified by experimental results. Similar to the cell patterning in a microfluidic chip with three inlets, the position of each cell strip can be adjusted by changing the corresponding tubing steering angle. Unlike sheath flow-based approaches, this method showed that increasing the inlet of the microfluidic chip to pattern other cell types in the microchannel did not complicate flow control. The ability to adjust cell patterns can also facilitate many other studies, such as the construction of cell strips with different gap distances for the simultaneous study of short- and long-distance cell-to-cell communication in the same microenvironment.

10.4.2.3 Cell patterning with different flow rates and cell concentrations

The central inlet of the microfluidic chip with three inlets was used, while the other two inlets were blocked to characterize the proposed cell patterning method at different flow rates and cell concentrations. NB-4 cells stained with green fluorescence were loaded into the microchannel through tubing inserted into the central entrance. Here, the tubing length

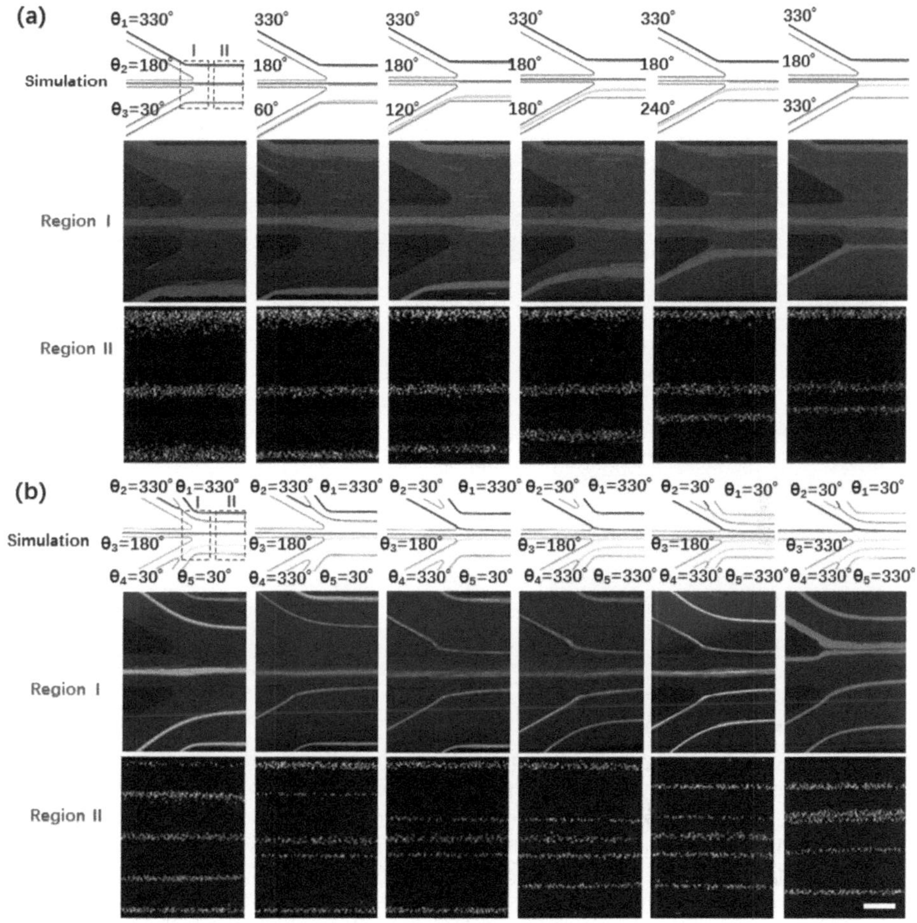

Figure 10.20 Cell patterning with different tubing steering angles (Fan et al., 2020). (A) Six different patterns of three NB-4 cell strips. The NB-4 cells from inlet 3 approaches the central cell strip when the tubing steering angle θ_3 is increased from 30 to 330 degrees. (B) Six different patterns of five NB-4 cell strips under different tubing direction configurations. The position of each cell strip and the width of the gap between two cell strips can be adjusted flexibly. Scale bar = 500 μm.

was 60 mm, and the cell concentration was set to 10^6 cells/mL to study the effect of flow rate on the cell pattern. As shown in Fig. 10.21A, when the flow rate was increased from 10 to 50 μL/min, the width of the cell strip became wider, which meant that the cells could not completely sediment to the bottom of the tubing before flowing into the microchannel. When the flow rate reached 50 μL/min, the distribution of cells in the microchannel was almost uniform, indicating that the length of the 60 mm tubing was not sufficient to achieve cell focusing at such a high flow rate. Cell focusing at high flow rates can be improved by just using long tubing. Considering the cell focusing performance in the flow rate experiment, a flow rate of 20 μL/min was selected for the cell patterning

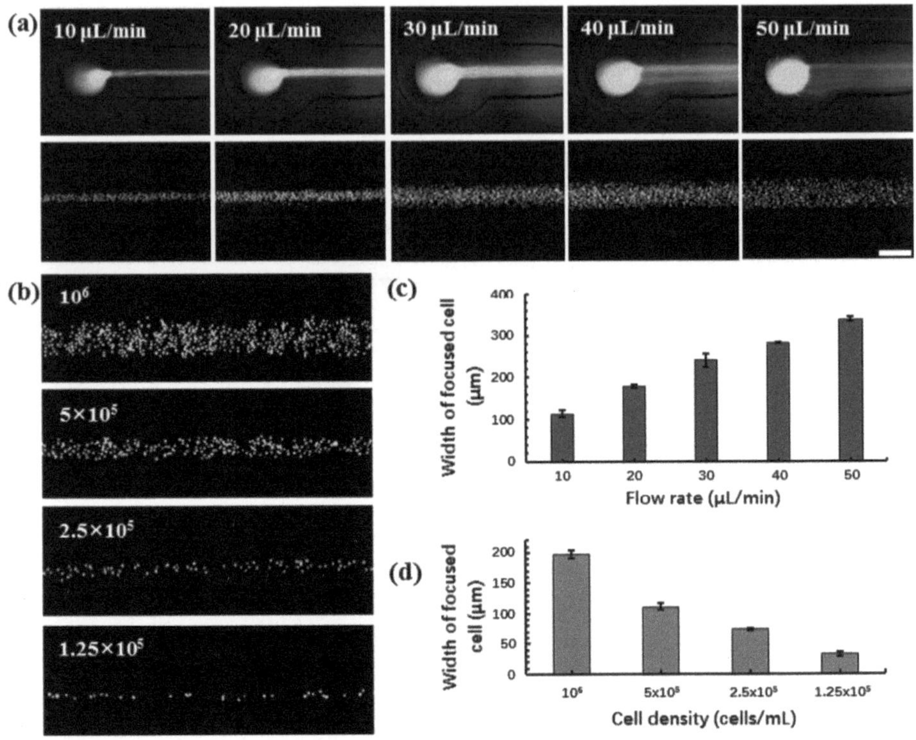

Figure 10.21 Cell patterning with different flow rates and cell concentrations (Fan et al., 2020). (A) Cell patterning in a microchannel when the flow rates increase from 10 to 50 μL/min. (B) Cell patterning in a microchannel when the cell concentration decreased from 10^6 cells/mL to 1.25×10^5 cells/mL. (C) The width of patterned cell strip versus flow rates. The width of the cell strip broadens when the flow rate increases from 10 to 50 μL/min. (D) The width of patterned cell strip versus cell concentrations. The width of each cell strip can be adjusted by changing the concentration of loaded cells. Scale bar = 400 μm.

experiment under different cell concentrations. As shown in Fig. 10.21B, as the cell concentration decreased, the width of the cell strips also decreased. The quantitative characterization of the influence of flow rate and cell concentration on the width of patterned cell strips is shown in Fig. 10.21C and D. The results in Fig. 10.21 showed that the width of all cell strips can be adjusted by changing the flow rate, and the width of a single cell strip can be selectively adjusted by changing the corresponding cell concentration, which further proved the flexibility of this method.

10.4.3 A case study of the patterned coculture of multiple cell types

Fig. 10.22A illustrates a gradient generator in the shape of a "Christmas tree" designed to integrate with a cell pattern microfluidic chip with three inlets, and to verify easy integration of the reported cell patterning method based on gravity sedimentation

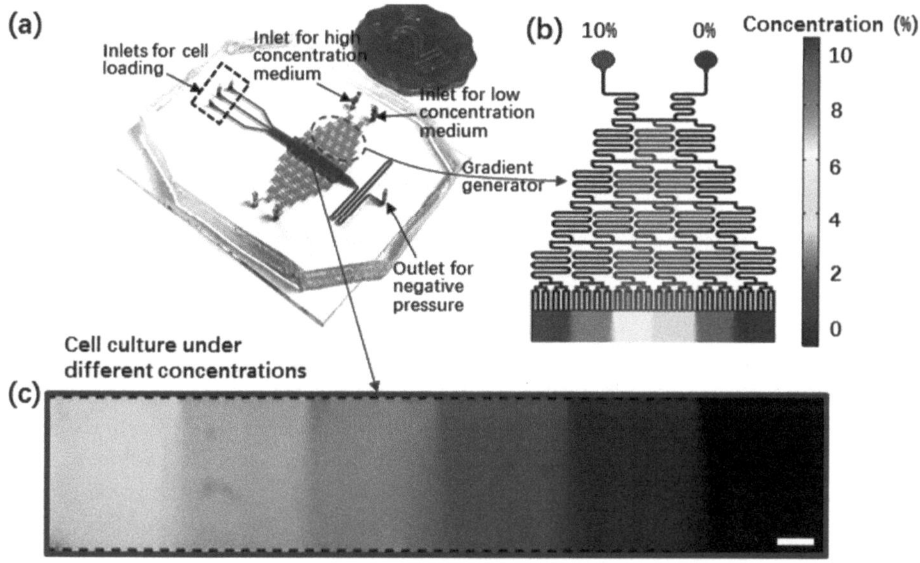

Figure 10.22 Cell patterning coculture chip integrated with gradient generation (Fan et al., 2020). (A) Fabricated cell patterning coculture chip integrated with two gradient generators. (B) Simulated result of the gradient generation in the microfluidic chip. (C) FITC gradient generation in the cell coculture region of the designed microfluidic chip, illustrating that the designed chip can generate six drug concentrations in the coculture region. Scale bar = 500 μm.

with other microfluidic functions. Fig. 10.22B illustrates the simulation results of gradient generation. When two medium concentrations of 10% and 0% were provided through the two gradient generator inlets, six concentrations were generated in six different parts of the cell coculture channel, namely 10%, 8%, 6%, 4%, 2%, and 0%. Fluorescein isothiocyanate (FITC)-dextran (10 μM, MW 10,000) with a molecular weight similar to some drugs, such as growth factor (GF) or FBS, was used in experiments to confirm that the gradient generator can be used for the fabricated microfluidic chip. Two solutions with and without FITC-dextran were injected into the inlet of the gradient generator at the same flow rate using two syringe pumps. For the gradient generation test, the inlet and outlet of the cell patterning were blocked, and the two inlets of another gradient generator were opened to allow the fluid to flow out. Fig. 10.22C shows that there were six FITC-dextran concentrations in the cell patterning coculture area, and the generated FITC-dextran gradient distribution matched well with the simulation results. The flow direction of the FITC-dextran solution during perfusion was perpendicular to the flow direction of the cell pattern, indicating that the gradient was parallel to the patterned cell strips. The integration of gradient generation and the cell patterning based on gravitational sedimentation can facilitate the study of the response of different cell behaviors to different biological/chemical stimuli under patterning coculture conditions.

A case study was conducted on the patterned HeLa-GFP cells and a mixture of human umbilical vein cell line (EA.hy926) and normal human dermal fibroblasts (HDFn) to demonstrate the feasibility and unique advantages of the reported method in the study of the interaction between cancer cells and normal stromal cells under well-organized coculture conditions. The syringe pump connected to the outlet of the chip was set to aspirate the cells into the chip during the cell patterning process. Tubing steering angles of 30, 180, and 330 degrees were used, and the inlets of the gradient generator were blocked during the cell patterning process.

Fig. 10.23A shows that HeLa-GFP cells were patterned into two cell strips (the left and middle cell strips). The mixture of EA.hy 926 and HDFn cells was patterned into the right cell strip. DMEM supplemented with 10% FBS was introduced from the inlet of the gradient generator beside the mixed cells and flowed out from the outlet of the other gradient generator at a flow rate of 0.25 μL/min. Bright and fluorescent images of cells were captured from 0 to 48 h, with a step length of 12 h to record cell proliferation. Fig. 10.23A shows that the cells adhered to the bottom surface of the microchannel, and the mixed cells occupied most of the space in the right gap after 12 h of

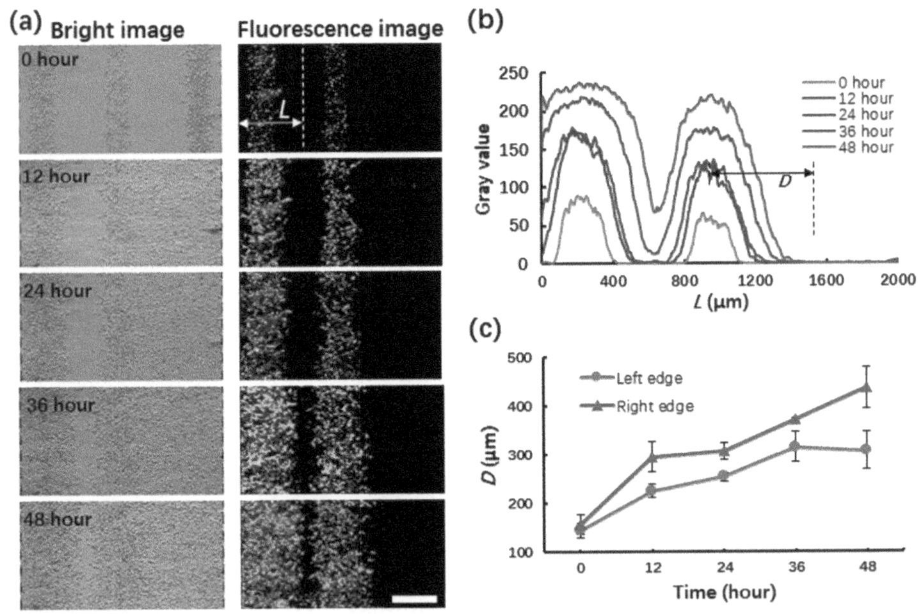

Figure 10.23 Patterning coculture of HeLa-GFP and HDFn+EA.hy926 cells (Fan et al., 2020). (A) Representative images of the cocultured cells from 0 to 48 h. The left and central strips are HeLa-GFP cells. The right strip is the mixture of HDFn and EA.hy 926 cells. *L* is the distance from the left side of channel. (B) Distribution of the HeLa-GFP cells represented by the fluorescence profiles at different times. *D* value refers to the distance from the right and left edges of middle HeLa-GFP cell strip at different times to the central position of the middle cell strip at 0 h. (C) Relationship between *D* value and time. This indicates that the cells migrated further to the right than the left. Scale bar = 500 μm.

coculture. The HeLa-GFP cells in the center tended to migrate to the side of the mixed cells, which can be seen in the fluorescence photographs in Fig. 10.23A. The GF secreted by HDFn and EA.hy 926 cells may induce the directional migration of the central HeLa-GFP cells.

Fig. 10.23B illustrates the quantitative analysis based on the fluorescence distribution profile. The distance from the left and right edges of the middle HeLa-GFP cell strip at different times to the center of the HeLa-GFP cell strip at 0 h can be seen in Fig. 10.23C. From the data in Fig. 10.23B, the gray value of the first position was selected to be less than 1, and the position of the right edge of the central HeLa-GFP cell strip was retrieved at different times. The cell strips at 0, 12, and 24 h on the left edge of the middle HeLa-GFP were also retrieved from the data in Fig. 10.23B, using threshold 1 as the gray value. After 36 h of coculture, the border between the left and central HeLa-GFP cell strips was blurred. Therefore, the left edges of the middle HeLa-GFP cell strip of 36 and 48 h were defined as the positions of the troughs.

Fig. 10.23C shows that the cells in the middle HeLa-GFP cell strip migrated further to the right than to the left, demonstrating the directional migration of HeLa-GFP cells to endothelial cells and fibroblasts under the coculture conditions. The patterning coculture of multiple cell types can also be performed under gradient generation.

All the results in Fig. 10.23 once again proved that the reported method has great simplicity and flexibility in constructing cell coculture models for various applications, such as drug screening and studying cell—cell interactions.

10.5 Conclusions

This chapter introduces cell patterning using optical tweezers, DEP, and microfluidic-based technology. First, a robotically controlled HOT is used to pattern multiple cells into a multilevel topology, where the cells form a desired pattern in a desired region instead of remaining in random positions. A potential function-based controller with a pattern regulatory control force is used to drive the cells to form the required pattern without collision. Second, DEP technology is used to polarize cells to build 3D cell patterns on multilayer structures with high cell density. The method is further applied to form honeycomb cell patterns on different layers of the tissue engineering scaffold. Studies have shown that cell pattern technology based on integrated DEP can enhance cell seeding to develop high-quality artificial tissues. Third, a method for patterning coculture of multiple cell types on a microfluidic platform is introduced. This method is based on the use of gravitational sedimentation, which has great simplicity and flexibility. Multiple cell types can be patterned in the microfluidic channel without complicated hardware setup or sophisticated chip design and fabrication. This method does not require external fields, such as acoustic and electrical fields, to help arrange the cells in the microchannel, thereby achieving cell patterning, without introducing any stimuli that may affect normal cell behavior.

References

Angelescu, D.E., 2011. Highly Integrated Microfluidics Design. Artech House, Norwood, MA.

Banerjee, A.G., Pomerance, A., Losert, W., Gupta, S.K., 2010. Developing a stochastic dynamic programming framework for optical tweezer-based automated particle transport operations. IEEE Trans. Autom. Sci. Eng. 7 (2), 218–227.

Bao, S., Cagan, R., 2005. Preferential adhesion mediated by Hibris and Roughest regulates morphogenesis and patterning in the *Drosophila* eye. Dev. Cell 8 (6), 925–935.

Béduer, A., Vieu, C., Arnauduc, F., Sol, J.C., Loubinoux, I., Vaysse, L., 2012. Engineering of adult human neural stem cells differentiation through surface micropatterning. Biomaterials 33 (2), 504–514.

Bucknall, D.G., 2005. Nanolithography and Patterning Techniques in Microelectonics. Woodhead Publishing, Cambridge, U.K.

Burmeister, A., Grünberger, A., 2020. Microfluidic cultivation and analysis tools for interaction studies of microbial co-cultures. Curr. Opin. Biotechnol. 62, 106–115.

Cheah, C.C., Li, X., Yan, X., Sun, D., 2014. Observer-based optical manipulation of biological cells with robotic tweezers. IEEE Trans. Robot. 30 (1), 68–80.

Chen, H., Sun, D., 2012. Moving groups of microparticles into array with a robot-tweezers manipulation system. IEEE Trans. Robot. 28 (5), 1069–1080.

Chiou, P.Y., Ohta, A.T., Wu, M.C., 2005. Massively parallel manipulation of single cells and microparticles using optical images. Nature 436, 370–372.

Chu, H.K., Huan, Z., Mills, J.K., Yang, J., Sun, D., 2015. Three-dimensional cell manipulation and patterning using dielectrophoresis via a multilayer scaffold structure. Lab Chip 15, 920–930.

Cox, S.C., Thornby, J.A., Gibbons, G.J., Williams, M.A., Mallick, K.K., 2015. 3D printing of porous hydroxyapatite scaffolds intended for use in bone tissue engineering applications. Mater. Sci. Eng. C 47, 237–247.

Cui, H.H., Voldman, J., He, X.F., Lim, K.M., 2009. Separation of particles by pulsed dielectrophoresis. Lab Chip 9 (16), 2306–2312.

El-Ali, J., Sorger, P.K., Jensen, K.F., 2006. Cells on chips. Nature 442 (7101), 403–411.

Fan, L., Luo, T., Guan, Z., Chow, Y.T., Chen, S., Wei, T., Shakoor, A., Lam, R.H.W., Sun, D., 2020. Gravitational sedimentation-based approach for ultra-simple and flexible cell patterning co-culture on microfluidic device. Biofabrication 12 (3), 035005.

Flaim, C.J., Chien, S., Bhatia, S.N., 2005. An extracellular matrix microarray for probing cellular differentiation. Nat. Methods 2 (2), 119–125.

Foty, R.A., Steinberg, M.S., 2005. The differential adhesion hypothesis: a direct evaluation. Dev. Biol. 278, 255–263.

Fu, L.M., Lee, G.B., Lin, Y.H., Yang, R.J., 2004. Manipulation of microparticles using new modes of traveling-wave-dielectrophoretic forces: numerical simulation and experiments. IEEE/ASME Trans. Mech. 9 (2), 377–383.

Garg, T., Singh, O., Arora, S., Murthy, R.S.R., 2012. Scaffold: a novel carrier for cell and drug Delivery. Crit. Rev. Ther. Drug Carrier Syst. 29 (1), 1–63.

Gou, X., Han, H.C., Hu, S., Leung, A.Y.H., Sun, D., 2013. Applying combined optical tweezers and fluorescence microscopy technologies to manipulate cell adhesions for cell-to-cell interaction study. IEEE Trans. Biomed. Eng. 60 (8), 2308–2315.

Guillotin, B., Guillemot, F., 2011. Cell patterning technologies for organotypic tissue fabrication. Trends Biotechnol. 29 (4), 183–190.

Guo, F., Li, P., French, J.B., Mao, Z., Zhao, H., Li, S., Nama, N., Fick, J.R., Benkovic, S.J., Huang, T.J., 2015. Controlling cell-cell interactions using surface acoustic waves. Proc. Natl. Acad. Sci. U.S.A. 112, 43–48.

Gupta, G.P., Massagùe, J., 2006. Cancer metastasis: building a framework. Cell 127, 679–695.

Hawkin, B.G., Gleghorn, J.P., Kirby, B.J., 2009. Dielectrophoresis for cell and particle manipulations. In: Zahn, J.D. (Ed.), Methods in Bioengineering: Biomicrofabrication and Biomicrofluidics. Artech House, Norwood, MA, pp. 133–181.

Hou, S.P., Cheah, C.C., Slotine, J.E., 2009. Dynamic region following formation control for a swarm of robots. In: Proc. IEEE Int. Conf. Robot. Autom., pp. 1929–1934. Kobe, Japan.

Hu, X., Bessette, P.H., Qian, J., Meinhart, C.D., Daugherty, P.S., Soh, H.T., 2005. Marker-specific sorting of rare cells using dielectrophoresis. Proc. Natl. Acad. Sci. U.S.A. 102 (44), 15757–15761.

Hu, S., Sun, D., 2011. Automatic transportation of biological cells with a robot-tweezer manipulation system. Int. J. Rob. Res. 30 (14), 1681–1694.

Huan, Z., Chu, H.K., Yang, J., Sun, D., 2017. Characterization of a honeycomb-like scaffold with dielectrophoresis-based patterning for tissue engineering. IEEE Trans. Biomed. Eng. 64 (4), 755–764.

Ino, K., Akira, I.H.H., 2007. Cell patterning using magnetite nanoparticles and magnetic force. Biotechnol. Bioeng. 97, 1309–1317.

Itoh, H., Aso, Y., Furuse, M., Noishiki, Y., Miyata, T., 2001. A honeycomb collagen carrier for cell culture as a tissue engineering scaffold. Artif. Organs 25, 213–217.

Iwadate, H., Yamada, M., Kimura, N., Hashimoto, R., Yajima, Y., Utoh, R., Seki, M., 2019. PDMS microstencil plate-supported fabrication of ultra-thin, condensed ECM membranes for separated cell co-culture on both surfaces. Sensor. Actuator. B 287, 486–495.

Kaji, H., Yokoi, T., Kawashima, T., Nishizawa, M., 2009. Controlled co-cultures of HeLa cells and human umbilical vein endothelial cells on detachable substrates. Lab Chip 9, 427–432.

Kane, R.S., Takayama, S., Ostuni, E., Ingber, D.E., Whitesides, G.M., 1999. Patterning proteins and cells using soft lithography. Biomaterials 20 (23–24), 2363–2376.

Levenberg, S., Rouwkema, J., Macdonald, M., Garfein, E.S., Kohane, D.S., Darland, D.C., 2005. Engineering vascularized skeletal muscle tissue. Nat. Biotechnol. 23 (7), 879–884.

Li, N., Ho, C.M., 2008. Photolithographic patterning of organosilane monolayer for generating large area two-dimensional B lymphocyte arrays. Lab Chip 8 (12), 2105–2112.

Li, X., Sun, D., Yang, J., 2013a. Bounded controller for multirobot navigation while maintaining network connectivity in the presence of obstacles. Automatica 49 (1), 285–292.

Li, X., Cheah, C.C., Hu, S., Sun, D., 2013b. Dynamic trapping and manipulation of biological cells with optical tweezers. Automatica 49 (6), 1614–1625.

Li, X.J., Liu, C., Chen, S., Wang, Y., Cheng, S.H., Sun, D., 2017. In vivo manipulation of single biological cells with an optical tweezers-based manipulator and a disturbance compensation controller. IEEE Trans. Robot. 33 (5), 1200–1212.

Liu, N., Liang, W., Liu, L., Wang, Y., Mai, J.D., Bin, L.G., Li, W.J., 2014. Extracellular-controlled breast cancer cell formation and growth using non-UV patterned hydrogels via optically-induced electrokinetics. Lab Chip 14, 1367–1376.

Liu, H., Wang, R., Chu, H.K., Sun, D., 2015. Design and characterization of a conductive nanostructured polypyrrole-polycaprolactone coated magnesium/PLGA composite for tissue engineering scaffolds. J. Biomed. Mater. Res. 103, 2966–2973.

Luo, T., Fan, L., Zhu, R., Sun, D., 2019. Microfluidic single-cell manipulation and analysis: methods and applications. Micromachines 10, 1–31.

Markx, G.H., 2008. The use of electric field in tissue engineering. Organogenesis 4 (1), 11–17.

Martins, A.M., Eng, G., Caridade, S.G., Mano, J.F., Reis, R.I., Vunjak-Novakovic, G., 2014. Electrically conductive chitosan/carbon scaffolds for cardiac tissue engineering. Biomacromolecules 15, 635–643.

Menachery, A., Pethig, R., 2005. Controlling cell destruction using dielectrophoretic forces. IEE Proc. Nanobiotechnol. 52 (4), 145–149.

Moutos, F.T., Freed, L.E., Guilak, F., 2007. A biomimetic threedimensional woven composite scaffold for functional tissue engineering of cartilage. Nat. Mater. 6, 162–167.

Murphy, C.M., Haugh, M.G., O'Brien, G.J., 2010. The effect of mean pore size on cell attachment, proliferation and migration in collagen–glycosaminoglycan scaffolds for bone tissue engineering. Biomaterials 31, 461–466.

Nelson, C.M., Bissell, M.J., 2006. Of extracellular matrix, scaffolds, and signaling: tissue architecture regulates development, homeostasis, and cancer. Annu. Rev. Cell Dev. Biol. 22, 287–309.

Nouri-Felekori, M., Mesgar, A.S.M., Mohammadi, Z., 2015. Development of composite scaffolds in the system of gelatin–calcium phosphate whiskers/fibrous spherulites for bone tissue engineering. Ceram. Int. 41, 6013–6019.

Pethig, R., 2010. Review article – Dielectrophoresis: status of the theory, technology, and applications. Biomicrofluidics 4 (2), 02811.

Rosenthal, A., Voldman, J., 2005. Dielectrophohoretic traps for single-particle patterning. Biophys. J. 88 (3), 2193–2206.

Sato, M., Asazuma, T., Ishihara, M., Kikuchi, T., Masuoka, K., Ichimura, S., Kikuchi, M., Kurita, A., Fujikawa, K., 2003. An atelocollagen honeycomb-shaped scaffold with amembrane seal (ACHMS-scaffold) for the culture of annulus fibrosus cells from an intervertebral disc. J. Biomed. Mater. Res. **64**, 248–256.

Tang, J., Peng, R., Ding, J., 2010. The regulation of stem cell differentiation by cell-cell contact on micropatterned material surfaces. Biomaterials 31 (9), 2470–2476.

Tavana, H., Mosadegh, B., Takayama, S., 2010. Polymeric aqueous biphasic systems for non-contact cell printing on cells: engineering heterocellular embryonic stem cell niches. Adv. Mater. 22, 2628–2631.

Trappmann, B., Gautrot, J.E., Connelly, J.T., Strange, D.G.T., Li, Y., Oyen, M.L., Stuart, M.A.C., Boehm, H., Li, B., Vogel, V., Spatz, J.P., Watt, F.M., Huck, W.T.S., 2012. Extracellular-matrix tethering regulates stem-cell fate. Nat. Mater. 11 (7), 642–649.

Xie, Y., Yang, S.T., Kniss, D.A., 2004. Three-dimensional cell-scaffold constructs promote efficient gene transfection: implications for cell-based gene therapy. Tissue Eng. 7 (5), 585–598.

Yan, X., Sun, D., 2015. Multilevel-based topology design and cell patterning with robotically controlled optical tweezers. IEEE Trans. Control Syst. Technol. 23 (1), 176–185.

Yan, X., Chen, J., Sun, D., 2012. Multilevel-based topology design and shape control of robot swarms. Automatica 48 (12), 3122–3127.

Yang, H., Gou, X., Wang, Y., Fahmy, T.M., Leung, A.Y.H., Lu, J., Sun, D., 2015. A dynamic model of chemoattractant-induced cell migration. Biophys. J. 108 (7), 1645–1651.

Zhu, Y., Sheng, R., Luo, T., Li, H., Sun, J., Chen, S., Sun, W., Cao, A., 2011. Honeycomb-structured films by multifunctional amphiphilic biodegradable copolymers: surface morphology control and biomedical application as scaffolds for cell growth. ACS Appl. Mater. Interfaces 3, 2487–2495.

Cell adhesion

11

11.1 Introduction

According to their natural portfolio, cell adhesion is a process in which cells come into contact with each other or with their substratum through specialized protein complexes. Intercellular adhesion can be mediated by adhesion junctions, tight junctions, and desmosomes, while cells can interact with extracellular matrix molecules through adhesion plaques. The study of cell—cell interactions can be achieved through use of the synergy of adhesion molecules fixed on the cell membrane and the exchange of intercellular diffusion factors (Hynes, 1992; Wijnhoven et al., 2000; Hirohashi and Kanai, 2003). Understanding the basic principles of this process is of great significance for the development of new therapeutic strategies. Traditional adhesion and transwell tests have been used to identify the role of adhesion molecules and chemokines in cell interactions. These assays extract average information from a large number of cells, but fail to obtain cellular information at the single-cell level. To gain insights into cell—cell interactions, the use of cytokines and adhesion molecules to clarify cell adhesion usually plays a key role. For example, to study the interaction between leukemia cells and stromal cells in the bone marrow microenvironment, stromal-derived factor 1 (SDF-1) and its cognate receptor CXCR4 were found to connect stromal cells and leukemia cells and to be involved in cancer treatment (Domanska et al., 2012; Lane et al., 2009). Therefore, there is a great need for an effective tool that can manipulate and control individual cells to explore the functional mechanisms of adhesion molecules and chemokines.

Several techniques have been developed to manipulate cell adhesion to study cell—cell interaction processes. Atomic force microscopy (AFM) has been developed to measure cell adhesion force (Puech et al., 2006). Microfluidics technology has been introduced to design coculture systems for characterizing cell—cell interactions (Ma et al., 2010). Optical tweezers have been used to study adhesion strength in receptor—ligand interactions (Litvinov et al., 2002), and as a force probe to observe the formation and maturation of cell adhesion (Schwingel and Bastmeyer, 2013). Among these methods, optical tweezers have the advantages of noninvasive operation and precise control of individual cells.

Through cell adhesion manipulation based on optical tweezers, Hu et al. (2013) studied the interaction between leukemia and stromal cells, and further characterized the specific adhesion characteristics of leukemia cells to bone marrow stromal cells. Leukemia cells, like their normal hematopoietic counterpart, hematopoietic stem/progenitor cells (HSPC), are affected by bone marrow stromal cells. It has been found that stromal cells produce many factors that affect the survival, proliferation, and apoptosis of leukemia cells (Mudry et al., 2000). Elucidating the mechanism of leukemia cell and stromal cell adhesion and adhesion-mediated interactions can provide promising new

Robotic Cell Manipulation. https://doi.org/10.1016/B978-0-323-85259-3.00012-X

paradigms for the development of specific targeted therapies (Robak and Wierzbowska, 2009; Krause and Van Etten, 2007).

Guo et al. (2013) proposed a cell adhesion manipulation method combining optical tweezers and a fluorescence microscope to probe the mechanism of cell interaction. In particular, the adhesion-mediated interaction between leukemia and bone marrow stromal cells was studied. After characterizing the adhesion characteristics of leukemia cells to bone marrow stromal cells under different manipulating forces, the adhesion mechanism was characterized using specific drug treatments to regulate the expression of adhesion molecules on the cell membrane. The fluorescence intensity was then used as a marker to study the Wnt signaling pathway of single cells and the interaction between cells was further explored.

In addition, Gou et al. (2015) used optical tweezers-based cell manipulation tools to control cell adhesion by assembling individual cells to detect the initial interactions between cells. This method was validated by specific studies on the interaction between leukemia cancer cells and stromal cells. The adhesion state of leukemia cells on stromal cells was first characterized based on different force manipulations. In order to study the effect of adhesion molecules on the interaction, optical tweezers were used to assemble leukemia cells at different points in the stromal cell layer. The tweezers applied a small trapping force to keep the cells in contact for several minutes. Using specific drugs to block the signal pathways involved in these processes, the function of chemokines in cell–cell interactions has been studied. In a case study, the role of stromal-secreted chemokine SDF-1 and its cognate receptor CXCR4 in the interaction of leukemia/bone marrow cells was specifically studied. The research shows that adhesion molecules can affect the adhesion of leukemia cells to stromal cells to a large extent, and can induce leukemia cells to migrate on the stromal cell layer, which depends on the tight adhesion and activation triggered by SDF-1.

The remainder of this chapter introduces the use of optical tweezers combined with fluorescence microscope to study cell–cell interactions through single-cell adhesion manipulations. As a case study, the interaction between leukemia cells and stromal cells is specifically reported. The conclusion is that single-cell adhesion manipulation provides new opportunities for studying cell–cell interactions. Unlike other traditional methods that rely on a large number of cells, the method of cell adhesion manipulation can be applied to a single cell, which makes the manipulation of rare and expensive cells possible. These advantages will make it possible to explore the heterogeneity and spatiotemporal information in the study of cell interaction.

11.2 Manipulating cell adhesion with optical tweezers

The basic approach of using optical tweezers to manipulate cell adhesion for cell–cell interaction study at the single-cell level is introduced first. Investigations into the adhesion between leukemia cells and bone marrow stromal cells have been reported as follows. Hu et al. (2013) reported the use of the human myeloid leukemia cell line K562, the mouse stromal cell line M210B4, and the human bone marrow stromal cell line

HS5 in their study. K562 and M210B4 cells were cultured in RPMI 1640 supplemented with 10% (v/v) fetal bovine serum (FBS), and HS5 was maintained in DMEM containing 10% (v/v) FBS. All cell cultures were incubated in a humidified incubator at 37°C and 5% CO_2.

11.2.1 Optical trapping

To evaluate the feasibility of using optical tweezers to study the interaction between leukemia and stromal cells and to establish safe optical trapping conditions to maintain the viability of the trapped cells, propidium iodide (PI) was used as a nucleic acid stain to access the optical damage to the trapped leukemia cells. PI is a fluorescent molecule commonly used in cell identification and viability studies (Harris and McConnell, 2008). When PI is applied to the culture medium at a low concentration (μg/mL), it is membrane-impermeable and is usually excluded from healthy cells. However, PI can quickly penetrate damaged cells, creating a sharp contrast between healthy and damaged cells, which can be immediately distinguished by fluorescence imaging. In the following test, eight leukemia K562 cells were trapped using 3 W laser power for more than 5 min and imaged at 1-min intervals to assess cell viability.

To determine the force exerted by the optical trap on the cell at a given laser power, a preliminary force calibration is required. The basic principle of the viscous-drag-force calibration method has been reported in the literature (Tan et al., 2010, 2011; Wu et al., 2011). In the calibration test, K562 cells were trapped at a constant distance from the bottom of the petri dish used in the experiment. Since the entire petri dish was driven at a specific speed by the electric stage, the fluid flow exerted viscous drag force on the trapped cells. When the flow rate increased to the critical value for the cells to escape the optical trap, the cells reached equilibrium, that was, the trapping force was equal to the viscous drag force. Fig. 11.1 shows the results of force calibration for 10 cells with different laser powers. The data represent the mean ± standard error based on two independent experiments. It can be seen that the relationship between the trapping force and the laser power is close to linear, which is consistent with the results reported in the literature.

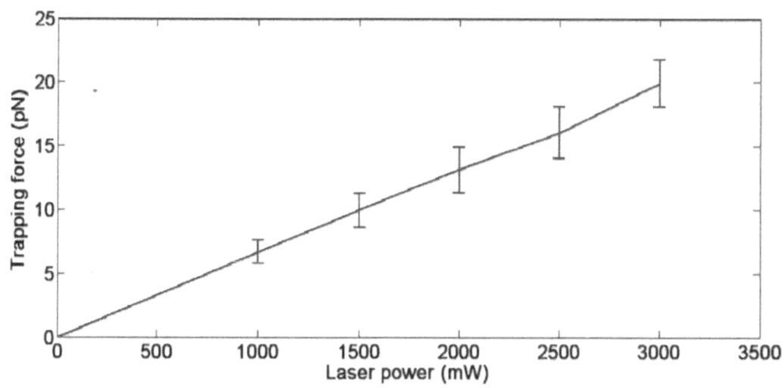

Figure 11.1 Calibration results of the trapping force versus laser power on K562 cells (Hu, 2011).

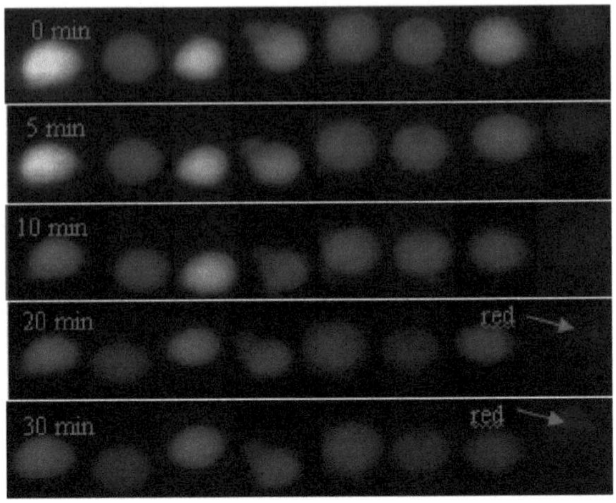

Figure 11.2 Results of short-term cell viability studies using PI as a cell damage indicator (Hu, 2011).

The viability of K562 cells was evaluated after optical trapping. Fig. 11.2 shows a series of fluorescence images of the trapped cells at intervals. It can be seen that the PI fluorescence signal (red) only appeared on one cell after 20 min of trapping, and increased as the cell membrane was damaged. This indicates that the trapping process will not immediately impair cell viability during this time. It is worth noting that the usual practical applications will not require such a long trapping time or such a high laser power. For example, it usually takes less than a minute to perform an adhesion assay on a cell. Therefore, it has been concluded that the optical damage to the viability of the trapped leukemia cells was small, and it was feasible to use optical tweezers to manipulate the adhesion between leukemia cells and stromal cells for interaction studies (Hu, 2011).

11.2.2 Adhesion of leukemia cells and bone marrow stromal cells

The adhesion properties of leukemia cells K562 to mouse bone marrow stromal cells M210B4 and human bone marrow stromal cells HS5 were characterized using optical tweezers (Hu, 2011). The binding of leukemia cells to stromal cells can be assessed by spreading suspended leukemia cells K562 in 1.5 mL medium on the stromal cell confluence layer in a 35-mm thin-bottomed culture dish. In order to form stable stromal cell monomers, stromal cells were grown to confluence and irradiated with 20 Gy (HS-5) or 80 Gy (M2-10B4) using a gamma radiator. After irradiation, the culture with fresh medium was replaced and incubated for at least 24 h before adding K562. After incubating for 2 h at 37°C, optical tweezers was used to trap and move K562 cells to check whether they were able to adhere to stromal cells. A laser power of 2.5 W can be used, in this case the corresponding trapping power was about 16 pN. Finally, heparin was used to determine the specificity of adhesion, where K562 cells were preincubated with 100 μg/mL heparin for 1 h before the adhesion test.

Optical traps were created to trap and move leukemia cells to check whether the cells adhere to the monolayer of stromal cells. The state of leukemia cells can be divided into tight adhesion, loose adhesion, or free suspension. The definitions of these three states are as follows: "tight adhesion" means that leukemia cells are tightly adhered to stromal cells and cannot be moved by the optical trap; "loose adhesion" means that leukemia cells can be moved by the optical trap, but when the optical trap is removed, the cells will return to their original position; "free suspension" means that leukemia cells can move freely through the optical trap, and will not return to their original position after the optical trap is removed.

Fig.11.3 illustrates the adhesion characteristics of K562 cells to M210B4 cells and HS5 cells under optical-trapping forces of 4 and 16 pN, respectively. There was not much difference in the adhesion state under the two forces, indicating that the adhesion force between K562 and stromal cells was greater than 16 pN. In subsequent experiments, a laser power of 0.5 W was used to reduce the potential optical damage caused by the optical trap.

One question to be answered is whether the observed adhesion is due to specific receptor–ligand binding or just nonspecific binding. Nonspecific binding often exists on living cells, which may be due to ambiguous protein–protein interactions, electrostatic double-layer forces, van der Waals forces, etc. (Leckband, 2000). In order to prove the effectiveness of this method and use it to further study cell–cell interactions, it is necessary to verify the specific receptor–ligand binding force, rather than optical trapping or unknown force, which mainly contributes to the observed adhesion.

The adhesion of K562 cells cannot be readily accounted for by integrins, or members of Ig or the selectin family (Bendall et al., 1997). It is not easy to directly block the

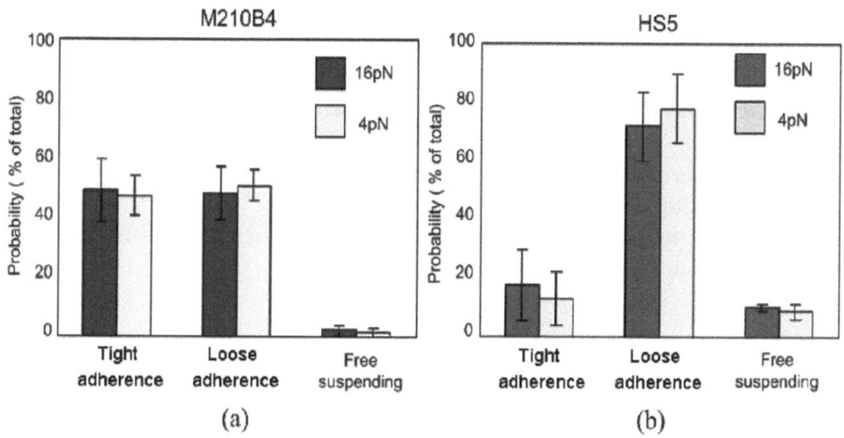

Figure 11.3 Adhesion properties of K562 on M210B4 and HS5 (Gou et al., 2013). (A) Adhesion properties of K562 on M210B4 at optical trapping forces of 16 and 4 pN. (B) Adhesion properties of K562 on HS5 at optical trapping forces of 16 and 4 pN. The adhesion data are represented by the mean values ± standard errors from three independent experiments performed on more than 300 cells.

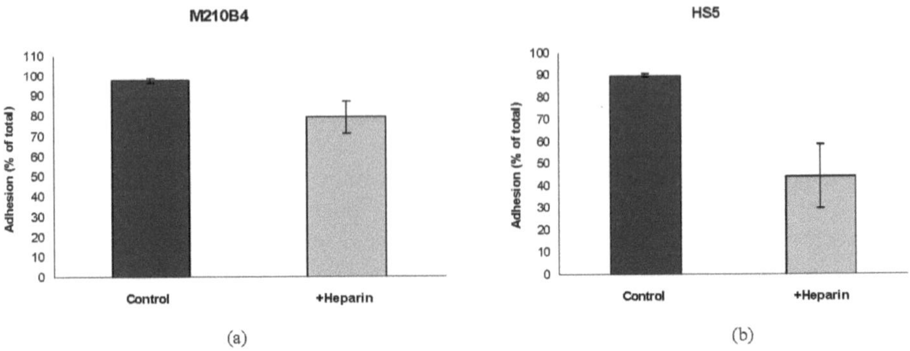

Figure 11.4 Percentages of adherent K562 cells with and without the pretreatment of heparin (Hu, 2011). Data represent mean values ± standard errors from three independent experiments performed on more than 300 cells, respectively. (A) Adhesion of K562 cells to M210B4 cells. (B) Adhesion of K562 cells to HS5 cells.

receptor—ligand interaction with one or several specific antibodies. Heparin is a highly sulfated glycosaminoglycan that can bind to a variety of adhesion molecules, such as integrin, type I collagen, and fibronectin (Yuan et al., 2003). Therefore, heparin may prevent these adhesion molecules from adhering to other binding partners, and be used to preliminarily elucidate the biological relevance and identify the adhesion mechanism. Heparin may inhibit some K562 membrane proteins and reduce the adhesion of K562 cells to stromal cells. In the test, K562 cells were preincubated with 100 μg/mL heparin, and then the adhesion test was performed. Fig. 11.4 shows the percentage of adherent K562 cells with and without heparin pretreatment. It was found that heparin pretreatment can reduce the adhesion of K562 cells to stromal cells. This finding identified the adhesion mechanism to a certain extent.

In conclusion, the method introduced above provides a new opportunity for studying the interaction process at the single-cell level. Combined with microscopy, this method can control and visualize the dynamic interaction process by manipulating the relative position of living cells and using clever markers and indicators of the interaction process. This method can be used to study the potential mechanisms of cell—cell interactions, for example, how the adhesion conditions such as physical contact or only soluble factors are involved in cell interactions, by comparing the different adhesion states of cells which have different phenotypes.

11.3 Adhesion-mediated cell—cell interaction

This section details the adhesion-mediated interaction between leukemia cancer cells and bone marrow stromal cells (Gou et al., 2013). The combined use of optical tweezers and fluorescence microscopy technology has been proven to provide a new opportunity for detecting dynamic signaling pathways in cell—cell interactions. The method can potentially be extended to other different cell types.

11.3.1 Methods

Cell interaction occurs due to the secretion of diffusible factors and direct cell–cell contact. Information on how physical contact or adhesion molecules affect specific signaling pathways helps to understand the interaction process. Whether and how adhesion is involved in specific cell–cell interactions is investigated here.

As shown in Fig. 11.5, one type of cell (such as leukemia cancer cells) is transfected with a reporter gene detection kit to fluorescently label specific proteins. The activation of targeted signaling pathways can be studied by observing changes in the number of proteins. The dynamic changes in fluorescence intensity reflect the changes in the number of specific proteins in the cell. The transfection process can be used to study single-cell signals under a fluorescence microscope. The cells are then cocultured with other types of cells (such as stromal cells). Changes in fluorescence are visualized and recorded from time to time for further analysis. After observing the cells for about 2 h, single cells are trapped with optical tweezers to identify the adhesion state between the two cells. The mechanism of interaction can be further characterized by adding specific drugs to block adhesion. In this process, optical tweezers act as a manipulation tool to clarify whether the interaction between the two cells is caused by a specific adhesion.

To prove the above ideas, the first issue to be studied is whether optical tweezers can effectively characterize the adhesion characteristics between the two types of cells, and the second is whether single-cell fluorescence imaging detects signaling pathway activation reliably. Case studies conducted on leukemia cancer cells and bone marrow

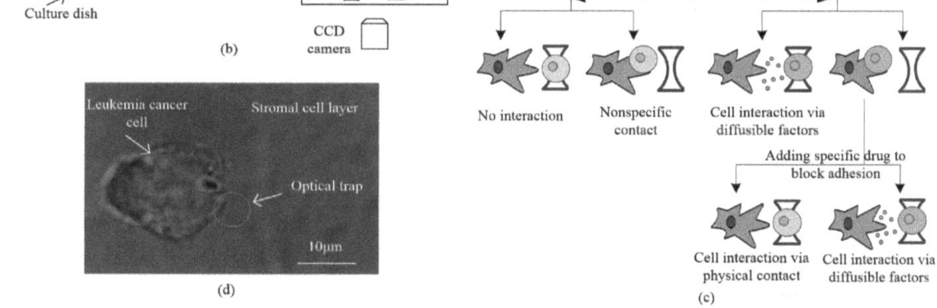

Figure 11.5 Principle of cell adhesion manipulation (Gou et al., 2013). (A) Cells are transfected with a specific reporter. (B) Coculture of the two types of cells on the motorized stage. (C) Schematic of the proposed method for study cell interactions through optical tweezers manipulation. (D) Measurement of adhesion of leukemia cancer cells to stromal cells in experiments.

stromal cells can prove the feasibility of this approach. The adhesion properties of leukemia cells to stromal cells have been characterized under the manipulation of different forces, and specific drugs were used to downregulate the expression of adhesion molecules. The Wnt signaling pathway was examined to demonstrate the reliability of fluorescence imaging.

The single-cell-based cell−cell interaction assay manipulation system combines the use of holographic optical tweezers and a fluorescence microscope. The optical tweezers system has been introduced in earlier chapters and so is not discussed here. The optical trapping force was calibrated to obtain the relationship between the laser power and the trapping force, so that the trapping force can be indirectly known according to the actual laser power in practical applications. Fig. 11.1 shows a viscous drag force calibration method in the trapping of K562 cells.

As reported in the literature, As_2O_3 can downregulate the expression of adhesion molecule β1 integrin and reduce the adhesion of K562 cells to primary bone marrow stromal cells (Wang et al., 2010). AMD3100 is a bicyclin molecule that can selectively antagonize the binding of SDF-1 to CXCR4 and preferentially mobilize leukemia blasts into the peripheral circulation (Nervi et al., 2009). Here, As_2O_3 and AMD3100 were used to determine the specificity of adhesion.

Cignal T-cytokine/lymphoid enhancer factor (TCF/LEF) reporter gene (green fluorescent protein, GFP) assay kit (CCS-018G) was used to monitor the activity of the Wnt signal transduction pathway in leukemia cells. GSK-3β inhibitor 6-bromoindirubin-3_oxime (BIO) (Merck, Darmstadt, Germany) was added to the medium 24 h after cell transfection to induce β-catenin stabilization.

11.3.2 Results

Specific drugs were used to downregulate the expression of adhesion molecules. Among them, As_2O_3 and AMD3100 were used to illustrate the biological relevance and to prove whether the changes in the adhesion state between the two types of cells can be observed by optical tweezers manipulation. Before the adhesion test, K562 cells were preincubated with 2.5 μM As_2O_3 for 24 h and/or with 10 μM AMD3100 for 2 h. Fig. 11.6 shows the percentage of adherent K562 cells with and without As_2O_3 and/or AMD3100 pretreatment. Both tightly adherent and loosely adherent cells were considered adherent cells. In Fig. 11.6A, pretreatment with As_2O_3 and AMD3100 cannot reduce the adhesion of K562 cells to M210B4. In Fig. 11.6B, pretreatment with As_2O_3 and AMD3100 can reduce the adhesion of K562 cells to HS5 stromal cells. When using As_2O_3 or AMD3100 alone, the adhesion between K562 and stromal cells did not change significantly. However, when As_2O_3 and AMD3100 were used together, the number of adherent cells decreased. This result may be because multiple receptors were involved in the adhesion of K562 cells. When only one factor was used to downregulate the expression of adhesion molecules, the adhesion state of the cells could not be changed.

The Wnt signaling pathway has become a key regulator of stem cells and many cancers (Reya and Clevers, 2005; Takebe et al., 2011). The activation of the Wnt signaling pathway may lead to the stability of β-catenin (Wang et al., 2009). The literature shows

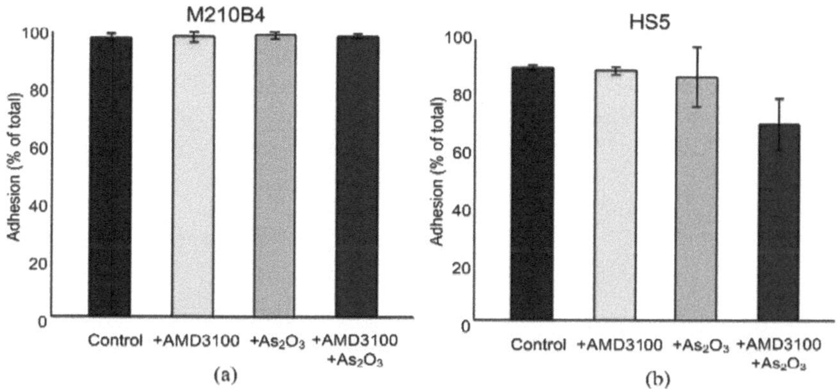

Figure 11.6 Cell adhesion after specific drug treatment (Gou et al., 2013). (A) Percentages of adherent K562 cells with and without pretreatment of As_2O_3 and AMD3100 on M210B4 cells. (B) Percentages of adherent K562 cells with and without pretreatment of As_2O_3 and AMD3100 on HS5 cells. The adhesion data are represented by the mean values ± standard errors from three independent experiments performed on more than 300 cells.

that fluorescence imaging was one of the most useful methods for studying protein localization (Sirinakis et al., 2012). The study of single-cell fluorescence imaging aims to evaluate whether single-cell fluorescence imaging can reliably detect the activation of the Wnt signaling pathway. BIO was used to induce the stability of β-catenin signal in K562 cells. The basic and induced levels of β-catenin signal in K562 cells can be evaluated by traditional flow cytometry analysis and single-cell fluorescence imaging for comparison.

Under the T-016 program (Amaxa, Cologne, Germany), a total of 1 million K562 cells were transfected with the TCF/LEF reporter gene using the nucleofector, and β-catenin was labeled with green fluorescence. 24 h after transfection, 1 million K562 cells were divided equally into two groups to study the stability of β-catenin. One group of K562 cells was cultured in 2 μM BIO medium, and the other group of K562 cells was cultured in normal medium. As shown in Fig. 11.7, GFP positive cells were gated by flow cytometry analysis. 2 μM BIO treatment for 24 h increased the proportion of GFP-positive cells, indicating the stability of β-catenin in K562 cells. The cell culture dish was observed under a microscope, and fluorescence images were acquired from time to time to record the dynamic changes of GFP in each cell. Fig. 11.8A and B show a series of fluorescence images of K562 cells. Fig. 11.8E and F shows the calculated fluorescence intensity analysis of single cells. The fluorescence intensity of K562 cells in the control group decreased with time, while the fluorescence intensity of K562 cells treated with BIO increased slightly during the 2 h observation period. Single-cell imaging results showed that BIO treatment induced the stability of β-catenin in K562 cells, which was consistent with flow cytometry analysis.

The Wnt signaling pathway between leukemia cancer cells and stromal cells was further studied. One million transfected K562 cells were divided evenly into three groups. One group was cultured in normal medium as a control group, and the other

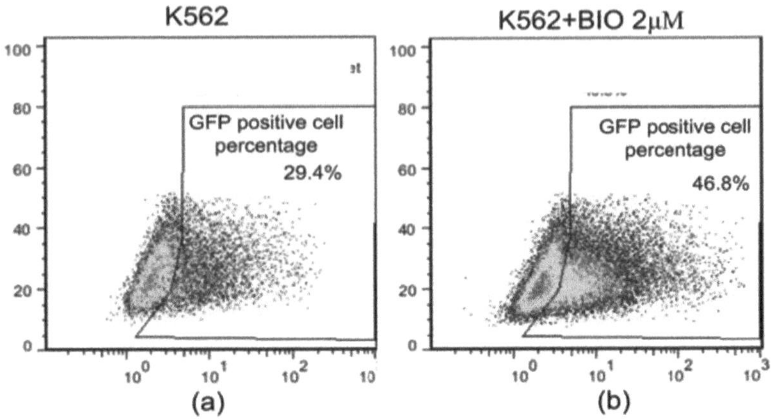

Figure 11.7 Flow cytometry analysis of K562 with and without treatment of BIO after transfection with TCF/LEF reporter (Gou et al., 2013). (A) Percentage of GFP-positive cells 48 h after transfection. (B) Percentage of GFP-positive cells after 24 h of transfection and 24 h of treatment with 2 μM BIO. The K562 cells in the two groups were divided from one group of transfected K562 cells. All the experiments have repeated for three times.

two groups were cocultured with stromal cells M210B4 and HS5. As shown in Fig. 11.9, GFP positive cells were gated by flow cytometry analysis. The percentage of GFP-positive cells in the coculture group was not much different from that in the control group, indicating that the coculture of K562 cells with M210B4/HS5 did not activate the Wnt signaling pathway.

11.4 A case study of cell adhesion characterization

This section introduces a case study describing the cell adhesion and migration mediated by the stroma-secreted chemokine SDF-1 and its cognate receptor CXCR4 at the single-cell level. The role of SDF-1 and CXCR4 in the interaction of leukemia/bone marrow cells will be specifically studied. It will show that adhesion molecules can affect the adhesion of leukemia cells to stromal cells to a large extent, and can induce leukemia cells to migrate on the stromal cell layer, depending on the tight adhesion and activation triggered by SDF-1. This method will provide a new way to characterize and control cell adhesion and explore the mechanism of cell-cell interaction.

11.4.1 Methods

11.4.1.1 Cell culture and materials

The leukemia cell line Molm13 and the stromal cell line M210B4 are commonly used model systems for leukemia cell-bone marrow interactions. They were cultured in a humidified incubator at 37°C and 5% CO_2. Both cell lines were maintained in

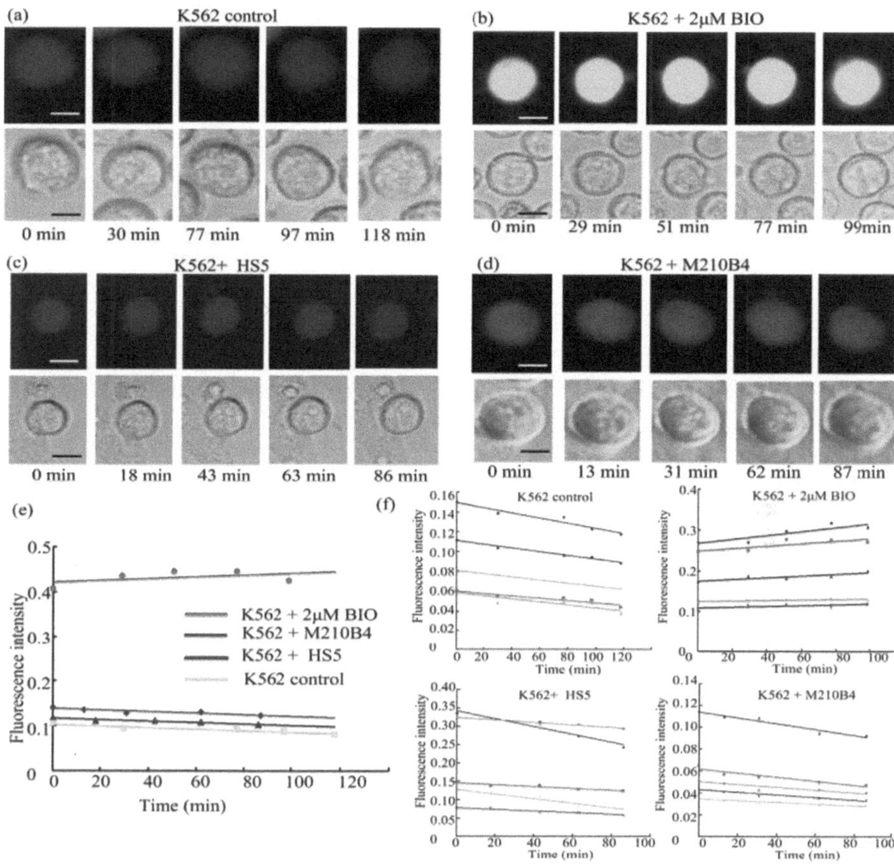

Figure 11.8 Real-time fluorescence imaging of K562 cells at different environment 24 h after transfection (Gou et al., 2013). (A) K562 cells in a normal medium. (B) K562 cells in a 2 μM BIO medium. (C) K562 cells cocultured with HS5. (D) K562 cells cocultured with M210B4. Scale bar is 10 μm. (E) Fluorescence intensity of each cells in (A)−(D). (F) Single cell samples analysis in the previously mentioned four environments. More than 80 single cells have been tested in normal and 2 μM BIO medium, respectively. About 40 single cells have been test in coculture with HS5 and M210B4, respectively.

RPMI 1640 medium supplemented with 10% (v/v) FBS (Invitrogen). AMD3100 is a widely used drug that can selectively antagonize the binding of SDF-1 to CXCR4 and preferentially mobilize leukemia blasts into the peripheral circulation, and is selected for the treatment of leukemia cells. Polyclonal goat anti-VCAM-1 antibody (Santa Cruz) was used in combination with donkey anti-goat (Invitrogen) to label the VCAM-1 protein on leukemia cells. SDF-1 protein expressed by stromal cells was stained with rabbit polyclonal SDF-1 antibody (Santa Cruz) and goat anti-rabbit IgG-CFL 488 secondary antibody (Santa Cruz). The nucleus was visualized with DAPI.

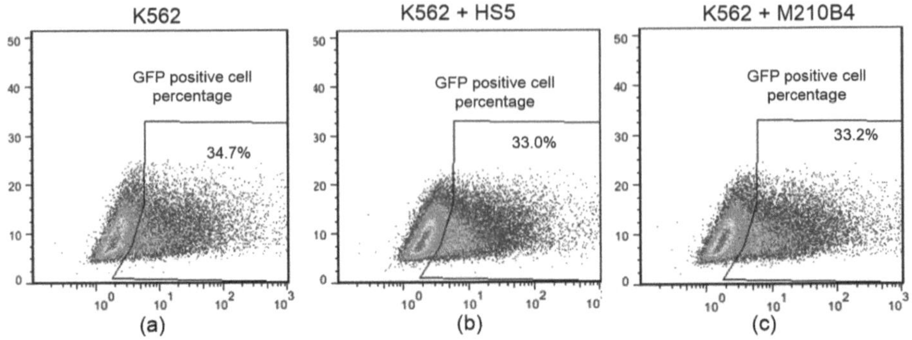

Figure 11.9 Flow cytometry analysis of K562 cells coculture with or without stromal cells (Gou et al., 2013). (A) Percentage of GFP-positive cells 48 h after transfection. (B) Percentage of GFP-positive cells after 24 h of transfection and 24 h of coculture with HS5. (C) Percentage of GFP-positive cells after 24 h of transfection and 24 h of coculture with M210B4. The K562 cells in the three groups are transfected at the same time. The K562 cells in the three groups are divided from one group of transfected K562 cells. All the experiments are repeated for three times.

11.4.1.2 CXCR4 expression flow cytometry

For CXCR4 expression studies, the leukemia cancer cell line was adjusted to a density of 0.5×10^6/mL in the culture medium. The cells were washed with 20-fold volume of ice-cold buffer without FBS, stained with a saturated concentration of phycoerythrin-conjugated anti-CXCR4 antibody at 4°C, and then analyzed by flow cytometry.

11.4.1.3 Fluorescent staining confocal microscopy

Polyclonal goat anti-VCAM-1 antibody (Santa Cruz) was used in combination with donkey anti-goat (Invitrogen) to label the VCAM-1 protein on leukemia cells. SDF1 protein expressed by stromal cells was stained with rabbit polyclonal SDF1 antibody (Santa Cruz) and goat anti-rabbit IgG-CFL 488 secondary antibody (Santa Cruz). The nucleus was visualized with DAPI.

The cells were washed twice with $1 \times$ PBS and fixed in 3.7% formaldehyde for 10 min at room temperature. Then, the cells were washed three times and permeabilized with 0.5% Triton X-100 in PBS. After 5 min, the cells were washed again and blocked with 5% goat serum in PBS for 20–30 min. The cells were incubated with the antibody for 1 h at 37°C, washed three times with PBS, and incubated with the secondary antibody for 45 min at 37°C. The nuclei were stained with DAPI for 5 min at room temperature. Then, the cells were washed three more times and observed under a laser scanning confocal microscope.

11.4.1.4 Retrograde flow assay

The dynamics of retrograde flow in stromal cells lamellipodia was characterized by tracking the motions of microparticles at the cell leading edge. Microparticles were prepared as reported (Tan et al., 2010) and positioned by optical tweezers to adhere to the leading edge of stromal cells. Then, the optical tweezers were turned off and the positions of the microparticles were measured over a 5-min period. The retrograde transmission speed of the microparticles was analyzed through image processing.

11.4.2 Results

11.4.2.1 Characterization of adhesion property

First, optical tweezers with different laser powers were used to move the leukemia cells, and the adhesion state of the leukemia cells on the stromal cells was identified according to the difficulty of the movement. As described earlier, the adhesion state was divided into tight adhesion, loose adhesion, and free suspension. When the laser power was increased from 0 to 3 W, the "tightly adhered" cells could not be removed, which corresponded to a trapping force of 0–20 pN, as shown in Fig. 11.10A. "Loosely adherent" cells can be moved away from their original positions. The displacement of these cells was defined as the maximum distance that leukemia cells can be moved away from their original adhesion site by optical tweezers, which increased with the increase of laser power. When the laser power exceeded 2.25 W, the displacement increased moderately. The maximum displacement occurred at a laser power of about 2.25 W, which corresponded to a trapping force of 16 pN. When the laser power exceeded 2.5 W, the cells were able to move at least 5 μm from their original adhesion site. Cells that did not adhere to the stromal cell layer were classified as "free suspension" cells.

To characterize the adhesion properties of the cells, the percentage of leukemia cancer cells that adhere to the stromal cells under two laser powers of 0.5 and 2.5 W was examined. Fig. 11.10B shows that 44% of Molm13 cells adhered to M210B4 cells under 0.5 W laser power, and 23% of these cells adhered tightly to stromal cells. Under

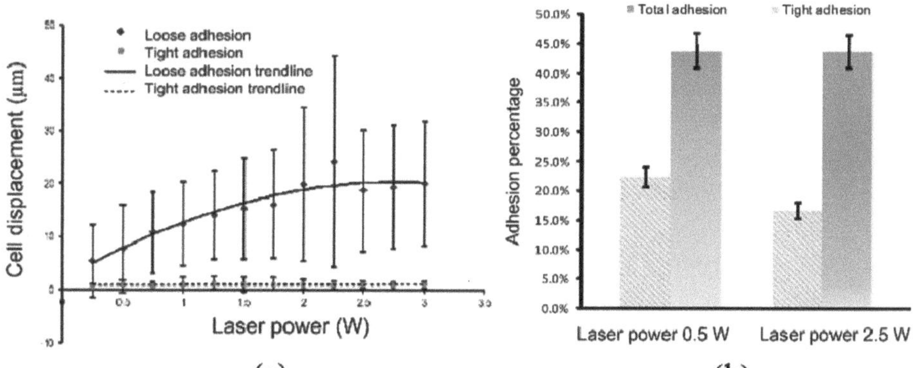

(a) (b)

Figure 11.10 Adhesion states of leukemia cells (Gou et al., 2015). (A) Characterization of tightly and loosely adherent cells under varied laser powers. (B) Adhesion characterization of leukemia cells on stromal cells.

2.5 W laser power, the adhesion percentage did not change significantly, but the number of tightly adhered cells was reduced to 18%. These results indicate that a larger trapping force can better distinguish tightly adherent and loosely adherent cells. The characterization of cell adhesion state can help determine the cell adhesion ability after the cells were treated with drugs or assembled at different sites.

11.4.2.2 Characterization of the influence of the SDF-1/CXCR4 signaling pathway in cell adhesion

Second, whether blocking the SDF-1/CXCR4 signaling pathway would affect the adhesion between leukemia and stromal cells was verified. According to the literature, SDF-1 is one of the most important chemokines, which can induce adhesion and migration by inducing integrin activation (Burger et al., 2006). The SDF-1 protein on M210B4 cells can be analyzed by fluorescent staining. M210B4 cells express high levels of SDF-1 protein, which can stimulate the adhesion and migration of cancer cells expressing CXCR4. Fig. 11.11A shows a 3D confocal microscope image of SDF-1 staining on M210B4 stromal cells in the X−Y plane, showing that SDF-1 molecules were distributed throughout the stromal cells. The fluorescence of stromal cells showed high intensity near the nucleus, and low intensity at the nucleus and cell leading edge. The expression of CXCR4 on Molm13 cells was also analyzed, as shown in Fig. 11.11B. It can be seen that compared with the isotype control cells, the fluorescence intensity of the anti-CXCR4 treated cells has changed, indicating that Molm13 cells express CXCR4 molecules on the cell membrane.

The effect of the SDF-1/CXCR4 signaling pathway on the adhesion of Molm13 cells to M210B4 stromal cells was further characterized, and AMD3100 was used as an inhibitor to inhibit the expression of CXCR4. Before the adhesion test, Molm13 cells were preincubated with 1 μM AMD3100 for 2 h. Fig. 11.11C and D show that CXCR4 expression was significantly reduced at the mRNA and protein levels after AMD 3100 treatment. Fig. 11.11E shows the percentages of Molm13 cells adhered to M210B4 cells after AMD3100 drug treatment and without AMD3100 drug treatment, in which tightly adherent cells and loosely adherent cells were both classified as having an operating force of 16 pN. Clearly, the number of adherent Molm13 cells decreased after pretreatment with 1 μM AMD3100, which was consistent with the results of other studies (Ngo et al., 2008). These results indicate that blocking the SDF-1/CXCR4 signaling pathway through drug therapy can successfully affect the adhesion of leukemia cells to stromal cells.

11.4.2.3 Control of adhesion contact sites

The effect of the adhesion contact site on cell adhesion and interaction was analyzed. In the experiment, Molm13 leukemia cells were assembled on the M210B4 stromal cell layer and kept in contact by applying a small trapping force of 500 fN to the leukemia cells for 5 min. Fig. 11.12A−D illustrate the displacement of leukemia cells relative to the trapping center of the optical tweezers. The deviation of free-suspending cells from the capture center due to Brownian motion was

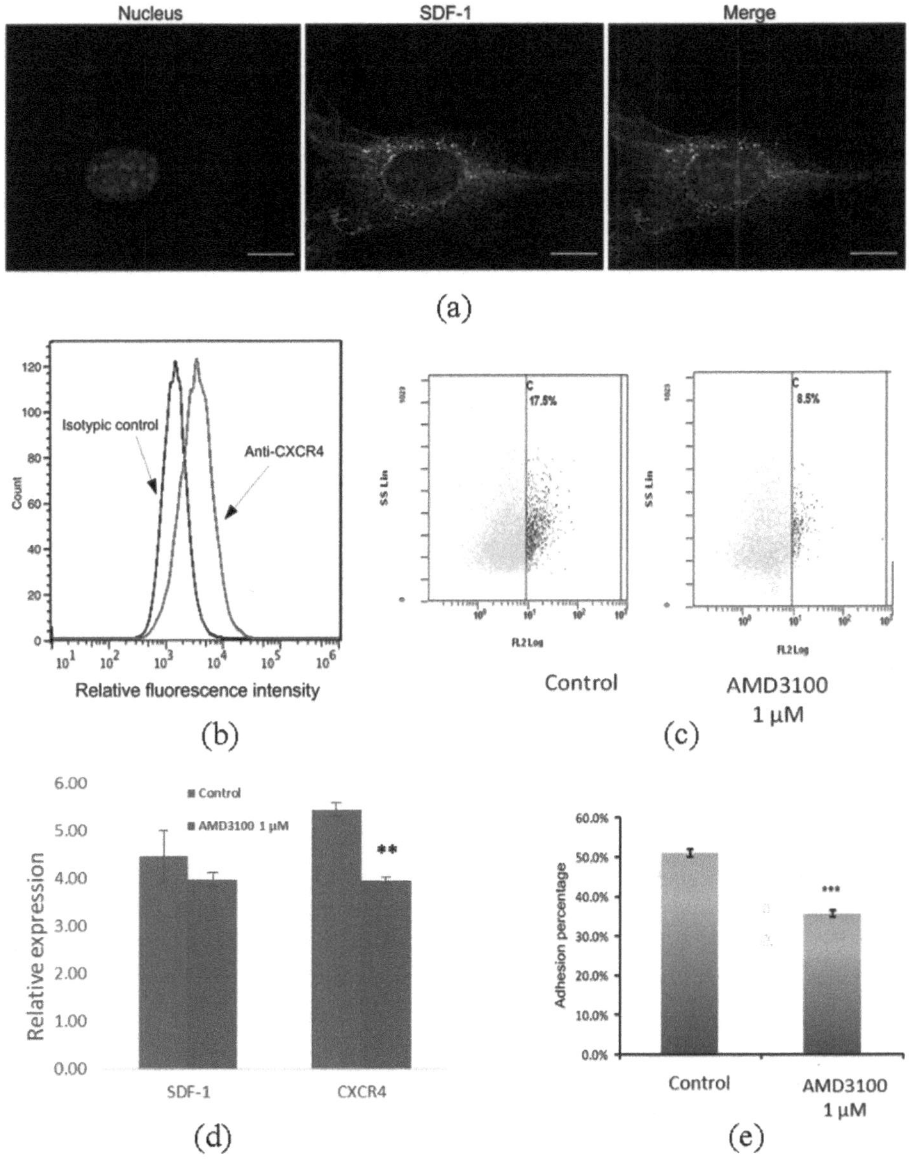

Figure 11.11 Results of SDF-1/CXCR4 signaling pathway in cell adhesion (Gou et al., 2015). (A) 3D confocal images of SDF-1 staining on M210B4 stromal cells in the X–Y plane. The scale bar is 10 μm. (B) Surface expression of CXCR4 on Molm13 cells. Molm13 cells were incubated with anti-CXCR4 and labeled with an FITC conjugate. Controls received equivalent concentrations of isotype-matched IgG. Washed cells were analyzed by flow cytometry, in which accumulated events were gated against the isotype control. (C) A flow cytometer was used to test the expression of CXC4 in molm13 cells. The CXCR4 expression cells decreased after 1 μM AMD3100 treated. (D) Expression of *sdf-1* had no significant difference after 1 μM AMD3100 treated in M210B4 cells. *Cxcr4* expression significantly decreased after AMD3100 treatment ($P < .05$). (E) Characterization of adhesion of Molm13 cells on M210B4 cells with and without drug treatment. Molm13 cells were treated with 1 μM AMD3100 for 2 h before experiments. Experiments were repeated eight times. $*P < .05$. $***P < .001$.

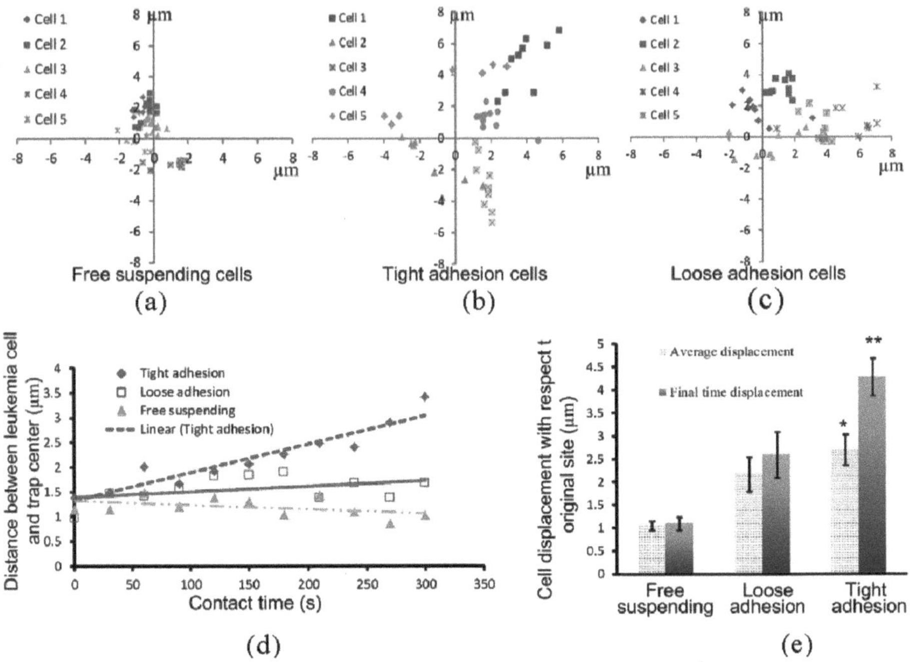

Figure 11.12 Controlled cell adhesion contact with optical tweezers (Gou et al., 2015). (A–D) Analysis of distance between the leukemia cell and trap center. (E) Leukemia cell displacements with respect to the initial contact sites. $*P < .05$. $**P < .01$.

very small. The closely adherent cells were slightly away from the trapping center, indicating that the directional migration may be induced by the activation of the SDF-1/CXCR4 signaling pathway. Loosely adherent cells exhibited mobility performance between those of free suspension and tightly adherent cells. These results indicated that the small trapping force acting on Molm13 cells can successfully maintain the cells at the initial contact site before the cells adhered closely to the stromal cells. The displacement of leukemia cells relative to their original position was also quantitatively analyzed. Fig. 11.12E illustrates the average displacement of Molm13 cells based on the measured data during the first 5 min (data collected every 30 s), and the final displacement measured at 5 min. For free-suspended cells, the final displacement and the average displacement were almost the same, indicating that no directional migration occurred. For tightly adherent cells, the final displacement was greater than the average displacement, indicating that tightly adherent cells migrate from the trapping center. For loosely adherent cells, the final displacement was different from the average displacement, but the difference was not as large as for tightly adherent cells. These results indicated that the migration ability of leukemia cells in the stromal cell layer was affected by the adhesion state, and tightly adhered cells had more opportunities for migration.

Then, the vascular cell adhesion molecule 1 (VCAM-1) on the surface of stromal cells was stained with a specific antibody and the confocal microscope image was analyzed to check the distribution of adhesion molecules. VCAM-1 is constitutively expressed in bone marrow stromal cells and is considered to be a key protein that regulates the adhesion of α4β1-integrin (the receptor of VCAM-1) expressed by leukemia cells (Young et al., 2004). Fig. 11.13A shows that VCAM-1 adhesion molecules were mainly distributed in the stromal cell body and the leading edge of the cell, and a small amount of VCAM-1 protein was found on the membrane around the nucleus.

Finally, the influence of the contact site on cell adhesion characteristics was studied. The nucleus of the stromal cell M210B4 was stained with DAPI, and the distance between the leukemia and stromal cell was calculated by image processing. Leukemia cells gathered in three different positions of stromal cells, namely the nucleus, cell body, and cell leading edge. The distances between the center of the leukemia cell

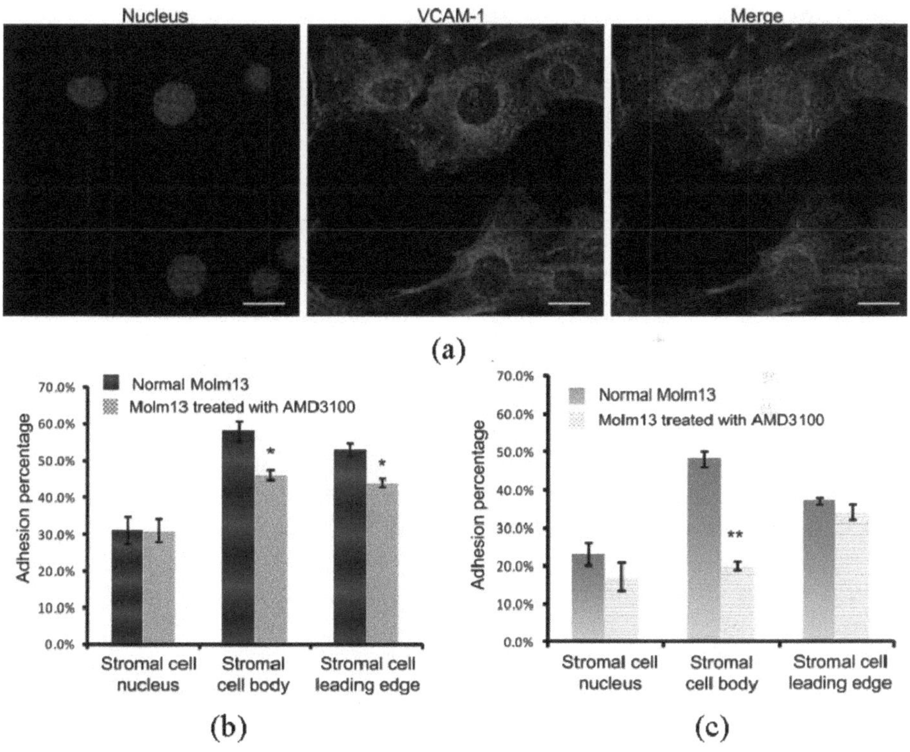

Figure 11.13 Results of adhesion molecule distribution (Gou et al., 2015). (A) Confocal images of VCAM-1 staining on M210B4 stromal cells. The scale bar is 20 μm. (B) Total adhesion percentage of Molm13 cells assembled at different positions of M210B4 cells. Two groups of Molm13 cells, namely, the normal group and group treated with 1 μM AMD3100 for 2 h before experiments. (C) Tight adhesion percentage of Molm13 cells assembled at different positions of M210B4 cells. Two groups of Molm13 cells, namely, the normal group and group treated with 1 μM AMD3100 for 2 h before experiments were studied. $*P < .05$. $**P < .01$.

and the center of the stromal cell nucleus was 8 ± 1, 19 ± 1, and 35 ± 4 μm, respectively. For the cell group assembled on the stromal cell nucleus, approximately 31 ± 11% Molm13 cells adhered to the M210B4 stromal cell layer (Fig. 11.13B), of which 23 ± 9% Molm13 cells adhered tightly to the stromal cells (N = 3, n = 59) (Fig. 11.13C). For the cell group adhered to the stromal cell body, 58 ± 9% of Molm13 cells adhered to the stromal cell layer, and about 48 ± 6% of the cells adhered tightly (N = 3, n = 55). For the cell group adhered to the leading edge of stromal cells, the percentage of adherent cells reached 53 ± 5%, and 35 ± 3% adhered tightly to stromal cells (N = 3, n = 78).

In addition, Molm13 cells pretreated with 1 μM AMD3100 for 2 h were assembled on the stromal cell layer. Fig. 11.13B shows that when Molm13 cells were placed near the nucleus of stromal cells (N = 3, n = 69), there was no significant change in the adhesion characteristics of the cells before and after drug treatment. When Molm13 cells were placed on the stromal cell body (N = 3, n = 44) or the leading edge (N = 3, n = 93), the adhesion percentage of Molm13 cells decreased. These results indicated that AMD3100 can reduce the adhesion ability of Molm13 cells to stromal cells, and when Molm13 cells were placed on the stromal cell body and leading edge with higher VCAM-1 content, the effect was more significant. Therefore, it was concluded that the number and distribution of adhesion molecules can affect cell adhesion to a large extent.

11.4.2.4 Migration of leukemia cell on stromal cell layer

It has been reported that the SDF-1 chemokine, which binds to CXCR4, regulated the trafficking of $CXCR4^+$ leukemia cells (Shen et al., 2001; Lapidot and Kollet, 2002). To verify whether SDF-1 secreted by M210B4 bone marrow stromal cells caused the directional migration of Molm13 cells expressing CXCR4, the relative movement between tightly adherent leukemia cells and stromal cells was examined. Fig. 11.14B illustrates the distance between the center of leukemia cells and the center of stromal cells, indicating that Molm13 cells on the leading edge of stromal cells have undergone directional migration to the nucleus of stromal cells. However, the Molm13 cells on the stromal cell body and nucleus did not show directional migration, which was consistent with the expression of SDF-1 in Fig. 11.11A, where SDF-1 was the highest in the stromal cell body. The gradient field from the stromal cell body to the leading edge of the stromal cell may be the reason why the leukemia cells on the leading edge of the stromal cell can migrate to the stromal cell body.

It has also been studied that the migration of leukemia cells on the leading edge of stromal cells was caused by the remodeling and shape changes of stromal cells (Schwingel and Bastmeyer, 2013), rather than the retrograde flow of stromal cells. To verify this, the movement of stromal cells and leukemia cells was quantitatively examined. The velocity of the nucleus of the stromal cell was measured to be 0.44 ± 0.06 μm/min, and the retrograde velocity of the leading edge of the stromal cell was 0.34 ± 0.02 μm/min. The velocity of the leukemia cell moving in the leading edge of the stromal cell was 1.19 ± 0.09 μm/min, which was much higher than the retrograde flow of stromal cells. This verified the cell migration induced by SDF-1.

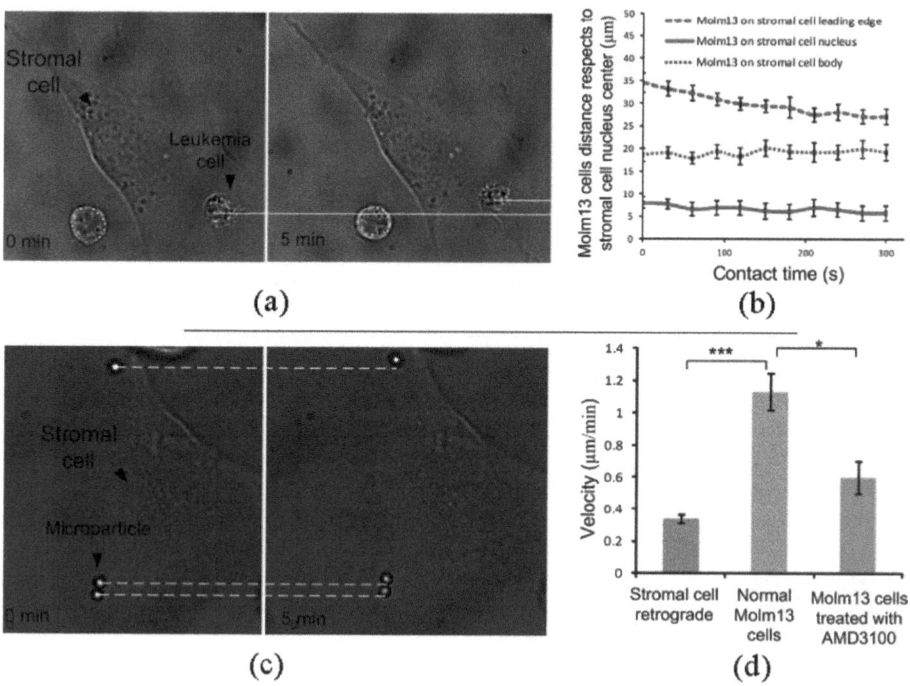

Figure 11.14 Migration results (Gou et al., 2015). (A) Experimental images show that Molm13 cells migrate on the M210B4 cell leading edge toward the stromal cell nucleus. (B) Distance of Molm13 cells with respect to the nucleus center of M210B4 cells under tight adhesion. (C) Experimental images show the retrograde flow of M210B4 cells. (D) Velocities of retrograde flow of M210B4 cells and migration velocity of Molm13 cells on M210B4 with or without AMD3100 treatment.

The migration of Molm13 cells after pretreatment with AMD3100 was further examined. According to the literature, AMD3100 can block the signal pathway (Donzella et al., 1998). The result of Fig. 11.14D showed that the migration speed of leukemia cells dropped to 0.62 ± 0.08 μm/min after treatment, indicating that AMD3100 weakened the migration ability of leukemia cells.

11.5 Conclusions

This chapter discusses the use of optical tweezers to manipulate cell adhesion for cell–cell interaction study at the single-cell level. Intercellular interactions are important for regulating various cell activities, such as proliferation, differentiation, and apoptosis. By characterizing the adhesion characteristics of leukemia cells on stromal cells and analyzing the fluorescence intensity used as a marker for the Wnt signaling pathway of leukemia cells, a case study of the interaction between leukemia cancer cells and bone marrow stromal cells was specifically studied. According to the adhesion characteristics of leukemia cells K562 to mouse stromal cells M210B4 and human HS5, three types of adhesion are defined: tight adhesion, loose adhesion, and free suspension. Through comparison with traditional flow cytometry analysis, the reliability of fluorescence imaging is confirmed. The unique cell adhesion method will provide a new way to study other inaccessible mechanisms of cell–cell interaction.

References

Bendall, L.J., Kirkness, J., Hutchinson, A., Bianchi, A., Makrynikola, V., Bradstock, K., Gottlieb, D.J., 1997. Antibodies to CD44 enhance adhesion of normal $CD34^+$ cells and acute myeloblastic but not lymphoblastic leukemia cells to bone marrow stroma. Br. J. Haematol. 98 (4), 828–837.

Burger, J.A., Kipps, T.J., 2006. CXCR4: a key receptor in the crosstalk between tumor cells and their microenvironment. Blood 107, 1761–1767.

Domanska, U.M., Timmer-Bosscha, H., Nagengast, W.B., Munnink, T.H.O., Kruizinga, R.C., Ananias, H.J.K., Kliphuis, N.M., Huls, G., De Vries, E.G.E., De Jong, I.J., Walenkamp, A.M.E., 2012. CXCR4 inhibition with AMD3100 sensitizes prostate cancer to docetaxel chemotherapy. Neoplasia 14, 709–718.

Donzella, G.A., Schols, D., Lin, S.W., Este, J.A., Nagashima, K.A., Maddon, P.J., Allaway, G.P., Sakmar, T.P., Henson, G., De Clercq, E., Moore, J.P., 1998. AMD3100, a small molecule inhibitor of HIV-1 entry via the CXCR4 co-receptor. Nat. Med. 4, 72–77.

Gou, X., Han, H., Hu, S., Leung, A.Y.H., Sun, D., 2013. Applying combined optical tweezers and fluorescence microscopy technologies to manipulate cell adhesions for cell-to-cell interaction study. IEEE Trans. Biomed. Eng. 60 (8), 2308–2315.

Gou, X., Wang, R., Lam, S.Y., Hou, J., Leung, A.Y.H., Sun, D., 2015. Cell adhesion manipulation through single cell assembly for characterization of initial cell-to-cell interaction. Biomed. Eng. Online 14 (114).

Harris, J., McConnell, G., 2008. Optical trapping and manipulation of live T cells with a low numerical aperture lens. Opt. Express 16, 14036.

Hirohashi, S., Kanai, Y., 2003. Cell adhesion system and human cancer morphogenesis. Cancer Sci. 94, 575–581.

Hu, S., 2011. Study for cell positioning and cell-to-cell interactions with robot-tweezer manipulation system (Ph.D. Thesis). City University of Hong Kong.

Hu, S., Gou, X., Han, H., Leung, A.Y.H., Sun, D., 2013. Manipulating cell adhesions with optical tweezers for study of cell-to-cell interactions. Biomed. Nanotech. 9 (2), 281–285.

Hynes, R.O., 1992. Integrins-versatility, modulation, and signaling in cell-adhesion. Cell 69, 11–25.

Krause, D.S., Van Etten, R.A., 2007. Right on target: eradicating leukemic stem cells. Trends Mol. Med. 13, 470.

Lane, S.W., Scadden, D.T., Gilliland, D.G., 2009. The leukemic stem cell niche: current concepts and therapeutic opportunities. Blood 114 (6), 1150–1157.

Lapidot, T., Kollet, O., 2002. The essential roles of the chemokine SDF-1 and its receptor CXCR4 in human stem cell homing and repopulation of transplanted immune-deficient NOD/SCID and NOD/SCID/B2m(null) mice. Leukemia 6, 1992–2003.

Leckband, D., 2000. Measuring the forces that control protein interactions. Annu. Rev. Biophys. Biomol. Struct. 29, 1–26.

Litvinov, R.I., Shuman, H., Bennett, J.S., Weisel, J.W., 2002. Binding strength and activation state of single fibrinogen-integrin pairs on living cells. Proc. Natl. Acad. Sci. USA 99, 7426–7431.

Ma, H.P., Liu, T.J., Qin, J.H., Lin, B.C., 2010. Characterization of the interaction between fibroblasts and tumor cells on a microfluidic co-culture device. Electrophoresis 31, 1599–1605.

Mudry, R.E., Fortney, J.E., York, T., Hall, B.M., Gibson, L.F., 2000. Stromal cells regulate survival of B-lineage leukemic cells during chemotherapy. Blood 96, 926.

Nervi, B., Ramirez, P., Rettig, M.P., Uy, G.L., Holt, M.S., Ritchey, J.K., Prior, J.L., Piwnica-Worms, D., Bridger, G., Ley, T.J., DiPersio, J.F., 2009. Chemosensitization of acute myeloid leukemia (AML) following mobilization by the CXCR4 antagonist AMD3100. Blood 113, 6206–6214.

Ngo, H.T., Leleu, X., Lee, J., Jia, X., Melhem, M., Runnels, J., Moreau, A.S., Burwick, N., Azab, A.K., Roccaro, A., Azab, F., Sacco, A., Farag, M., Sackstein, R., Ghobrial, I.M., 2008. SDF-1/CXCR4 and VLA-4 interaction regulates homing in Waldenstrom macroglobulinemia. Blood 112, 150–158.

Puech, P.H., Poole, K., Knebel, D., Muller, D.J., 2006. A new technical approach to quantify cell–cell adhesion forces by AFM. Ultramicroscopy 106, 637–644.

Reya, T., Clevers, H., 2005. Wnt signaling in stem cells and cancer. Nature 434, 843–850.

Robak, T., Wierzbowska, A., 2009. Current and emerging therapies for acute myeloid leukemia. Clin. Ther. 31, 2349.

Schwingel, M., Bastmeyer, M., 2013. Force mapping during the formation and maturation of cell adhesion sites with multiple optical tweezers. PLoS One 8, e54850.

Shen, W., Bendall, L.J., Gottlieb, D.J., Bradstock, K.F., 2001. The chemokine receptor CXCR4 enhances integrin-mediated in vitro adhesion and facilitates engraftment of leukemic precursor-B cells in the bone marrow. Exp. Hematol. 29, 1439–1447.

Sirinakis, G., Ren, Y., Gao, Y., Xi, Z., Zhang, Y., 2012. Combined versatile high-resolution optical tweezers and single-molecule fluorescence microscopy. Rev. Sci. Instrum. 83 (9), 093708.

Takebe, N., Harris, P.J., Warren, R.Q., Ivy, S.P., 2011. Targeting cancer stem cells by inhibiting Wnt, Notch, and Hedgehog pathways. Nat. Rev. Clin. Oncol. 8, 97–106.

Tan, Y., Sun, D., Wang, J., Huang, W., 2010. Mechanical characterization of human red blood cells under different osmotic conditions by robotic manipulation with optical tweezers. IEEE Trans. Biomed. Eng. 57 (7), 1816–1825.

Tan, Y., Fung, T.K., Wan, H., Wang, K., Leung, A.Y.H., Sun, D., 2011. Biophysical characterization of hematopoietic cells from normal and leukemic sources with distinct primitiveness. Appl. Phys. Lett. 99 (8), 083702.

Wang, L.D., Heidt, D.G., Lee, C.J., Yang, H., Logsdon, C.D., Zhang, L.Z., Fearon, E.R., Ljungman, M., Simeone, D.M., 2009. Oncogenic function of ATDC in pancreatic cancer through Wnt pathway activation and betacatenin stabilization. Cancer Cell 15, 207–219.

Wang, G., Chen, X., Geng, Q., Li, J., Lin, G., Lu, Y., 2010. Arsenic trioxide overcomes cell adhesion-mediated drug resistance through down-regulating the expression of β1-integrin in K562 chronic myelogenous leukemia cell line. Leuk. Lymphoma 5, 1090–1097.

Wijnhoven, B.P.L., Dinjens, W.N.M., Pignatelli, M., 2000. E-cadherin-catenin cell-cell adhesion complex and human cancer. Br. J. Surg. 87, 992–1005.

Wu, Y., Sun, D., Huang, W., 2011. Mechanical force characterization in manipulating live cells with optical tweezers. J. Biomech. 44, 741–746.

Young, F.M., Felgar, R.E., Eyssallenne, A.P., Bottaro, A., Bushnell, T.P., 2004. VCAM-1 expression in B-lymphopoiesis and leukemia. Blood 104, 886A–887A.

Yuan, L., Geng, J.G., Xu, Q., 2003. N-desulfated heparin improves concanavalin A-induced liver injury partly through inhibiting T lymphocyte adhesion. Inflamm. Res. 52 (9), 383–389.

Cell fusion

12

12.1 Introduction

Cell fusion is a cellular process of combining two or multiple cells to form a single entity. Currently, fusion with stem cells is used to induce somatic cell nuclear reprogramming and to study cell reprogramming mechanisms (Ficz and Reik, 2013). Cell fusion is also a fast and effective method to induce pluripotent stem cells. The ability of somatic cells to acquire homologous characteristics and transform into pluripotent cells with minimal modification has been demonstrated by stem cell fusion (Ferrand et al., 2011; Piccolo et al., 2013; Yamanaka and Blau, 2010).

Spontaneous cell fusion naturally occurs in the process of myoblast fusion, producing polynucleated muscle cells or in the process of in vivo egg—sperm fusion fertilization. Artificially induced cell fusion in vitro has become a promising method of monoclonal antibody production (Köhler and Milstein, 1975), somatic cell reprogramming (Tada et al., 1997), cancer immunotherapy (Sukhorukov et al., 2006), and tissue regeneration (Vassilopoulos et al., 2003). Most existing in vitro cell fusion methods are either by virus induction or chemical induction. For mass production, these methods usually lead to single-cell level heterogeneity and reduced spatiotemporal resolution. In contrast, electrofusion is a technique that targets individual cells with potential specificity and precision (Zimmermann, 1982); however, it needs complex electric field geometries and usually requires integration with microfluidic chips (Skelley et al., 2009). Another possible solution is to use pulsed lasers to disrupt cell membranes and subsequently induce fusion (Wiegand et al., 1987).

Generally, most cell fusion methods are carried out in a large-scale production manner on random cell pairings, with poor cell-to-cell contact and no control during the fusion process. These methods often result in unwanted cell fusion products and low cell fusion yields. Therefore, these traditional methods are rarely used for the fusion of rare cells such as stem cells or primary cells. Artificially induced cell fusion usually is accompanied by isolation of fused cells from unfused cells. However, existing cell manipulation methods have the disadvantage of low reliability and so cannot overcome this challenge. Chen et al. (2013) achieved specific cell fusion at the single-cell level using continuous-wave optical tweezers to trap and transport cells, and then using optical scissors with pulsed lasers to cut the cells. However, most of the cell fusion operations using optical tweezers are performed manually in cell culture dishes without automation.

Microfluidics-based cell fusion methods (Yang et al., 2010) can integrate different microcomponents in the microfluidic chip, such as suction tube arrays (Cui et al., 2011), weir microstructure arrays (Skelley et al., 2009), and micro-orifices (Gel et al., 2010), to achieve cell-to-cell tightness through efficient cell capture and

Robotic Cell Manipulation. https://doi.org/10.1016/B978-0-323-85259-3.00005-2

pairing, thereby facilitating cell fusion. However, due to the lack of selectivity of these methods, cells must be of high purity before entering the fusion chamber from different inlets. Roundabout pretreatment of cell sorting is required, which reduces the flexibility to fuse different cell pairs at the same time. Therefore, precise cell manipulation in a well-controlled manner during the fusion process is necessary to achieve a specific single-cell fusion. Carbon fiber microelectrodes can fuse individually selected cells with a high-precision positioning micromanipulator for electrofusion (Strömberg et al., 2000). This method requires physical contact and can easily cause damage to living cells. As fusion in a sealed environment becomes difficult (Luo et al., 2007), a highly controllable microfluidic method for the electrofusion of individually selected cells is proposed, which uses dielectrophoresis and AC voltage pulses to perform cell pairing and fusion without physical contact (Kirschbaum et al., 2012), however electrofusion methods involving microfluidic chips usually require complex electric field geometry and need to overcome buffer incompatibility (for example, conductivity).

Wang et al. (2013) proposed a laser-induced cell fusion method, which uses a microfluidic chip with a microwell array to achieve high selectivity and controllability. Using this method, on-chip cell isolation is performed to preprocess the cells of interest for subsequent cell fusion, thereby providing the feasibility of simultaneous fusion of multiple pairs of different cells. Robotically controlled optical tweezers can automatically trap and pair cells, and optical scissors with pulsed lasers can be precisely positioned in three dimensions (3D) to induce cell fusion. The program-controlled motorized stage is used for high-precision cell levitation, transportation, and deposition.

Research has found that stem cells can reprogram somatic cells through cell fusion. Chen et al. (2013) used optical tweezers and pulsed UV laser to achieve effective fusion of human embryonic stem cells (hESCs) and somatic cells. The results indicate that two or more hESCs can be fused with high efficiency ($>50\%$) by pulsed UV laser irradiation. This targeted laser-induced cell fusion method could be an effective tool for studying stem cell differentiation, maturation, and reprogramming.

Hepatocellular carcinoma (HCC) is the most common primary liver cancer and is a leading cause of cancer-related deaths worldwide. New treatment strategies for liver cancer have been extensively discussed and explored in both academic research and clinical medicine. Stem cell therapy provides a potential strategy for liver cancer treatment (Forbes and Newsome, 2012). Examples of these methods include injection of stem cells for damage repair (Sakaida et al., 2004), liver regeneration (Furst et al., 2007), and hepatocyte differentiation (Newsome et al., 2003). Wang et al. (2016) proposed a study on the engineering fusion of stem cells and cancer cells to explore the mechanism in which cancer stem cells may have a potential impact on stem cell therapy for liver cancer. With laser-induced fusion between single hepatocellular carcinoma cells (HepG2) and hESCs, they found that the fused cells acquired stemness and cancer-like characteristics. The fused cells showed increased tumorigenicity and resistance to drug treatments. Gene expression analysis showed that the fusion cells are highly similar to tumor stem cells (TSCs) or tumor-initiating cells (TICs). TICs are important in tumorigenesis, aggravation, metastasis, and recurrence (Visvader and Lindeman, 2008); liver TICs and their markers have been identified

(Yamashita and Wang, 2013; Yamashita and Kaneko, 2014). Gene expression analysis and quantitative PCR detection showed that liver TIC markers such as CD133, CD44, and ALDH1 showed significantly high expression in fusion cells. However, this was not observed in HepG2 cells. The assay of in vivo tumorigenicity and drug resistance also showed that the fusion of cancer cells and stem cells results in cancer cells that are highly similar to cancer stem cells. These results indicate the potential risk of stem cell therapies for cancer treatment.

Cell fusion can also be used for many other applications. Kong et al. (2017) reported a fusion method to increase the physical size and nucleation status of human pluripotent stem cell-derived ventricular cardiomyocytes (hPSC-VCMs), which were an unlimited source of donor cells for potential cardiac regeneration therapies. However, hPSC-CMs are immature. The body size of hPSC-CM is only one-tenth of its adult counterpart; most are mononuclear rather than dual- or multinucleated, which is an evolutionary adaptability characteristic of metabolically active cells (such as adult CM). Through fusion, a multinucleated hPSC-VCM fusion syncytium can be created.

The remainder of this chapter introduces the basic working principles of laser-induced cell fusion with optical tweezers, Then, the combination of optical tweezers and microwell array technology and a case study of transforming liver cancer cells into tumor-initiating cells through cell fusion are introduced.

12.2 Laser-induced fusion with optical tweezers

A cell manipulation platform with holographic optical trapping (HOT) system (BioRyx 200, Arryx) was introduced in Chapter 11. A 1064 nm continuous wave (Nd: YAG laser) is emitted from the laser source and transmitted through the optical fiber and HOT device, which can split the beam and generate multiple optical tweezers simultaneously. The platform also includes laser scissors with a diffraction-limited spot diameter of 0.36 μm. The focus controller guides the position of a lens in the telescope, and then adjusts the height of the cutting spot relative to the image plane. The microscope is customized by installing a two-dimensional X−Y motorized stage, carrying an environment-controlled chamber that provides a temperature of 37°C and a CO_2 concentration of 5%. The excitation light generated by the fluorescent illuminator passes through the filter combination in the filter cube and excites the fluorescence in the fluorescent protein-labeled cells. All fluorescent images are captured by a cool charge-coupled device (CCD) camera.

hESCs have been used as fusion sample cells. hESC was cultured on a commercially available serum-free, feeder-independent system supplemented with BD Matrigel hESC Qualified Matrix (BD). Primary human dermal fibroblasts (HDFns, Gibco) were cultured on 24-well culture plates (BD Falcon) and maintained in Dulbecco's modified Eagle medium containing 20% fetal bovine serum (FBS). Before the fusion experiment, single cells were obtained by treatment with 0.05% trypsin-EDTA. After proper neutralization, the cells suspended in mTeSR1 were temporarily stored at 4°C.

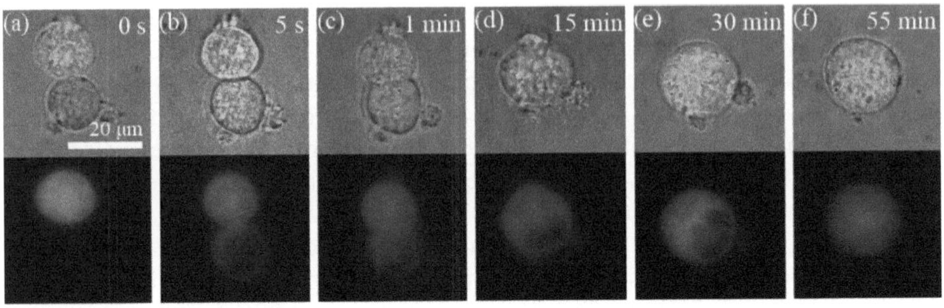

Figure 12.1 Laser-induced cell fusion of two suspended hESCs (Chen et al., 2013). (A) A GFP-labeled cell and an unlabeled cell form a cell pair before laser cutting. (B) After laser cutting, GFP transfers from the GFP-labeled cell to the unlabeled cell. (C)–(F) Time lapse images showing the fusion process (C) 1 min, (D) 15 min, (E) 30 min, and (F) 55 min after laser cutting. Scale bar is 20 μm.

Fig. 12.1 shows the laser-induced cell fusion of two suspended hESCs (Chen et al., 2013). After enzymatic digestion, green fluorescent protein (GFP)-labeled and unlabeled hESCs were mixed with 200 μL mTeSR1 and suspended in a 35-mm glass-bottomed Petri dish. An additional 500 μL of mTeSR1 was loaded into the edge of the Petri dish to compensate for evaporation of the medium. At 37°C and 5% CO_2 in the air, this dish was kept in an environment-controlled chamber. The objective lens was adjusted to focus on the cell, and the bottom of the glass scanned line by line by controlling the X–Y motorized stage. A GFP-labeled cell and an unlabeled cell were trapped by optical tweezers and manipulated to form a cell pair, and then transferred to a spot for laser scissors cutting (Fig. 12.1A). The working frequency of the laser scissors is 10 Hz, the duration of each pulse is 1 ns, and five pulses are emitted per treatment. Laser scissors cut the cell membrane at the contact point between the two cells. After cutting with laser scissors, the cytoplasmic GFP immediately transferred from GFP-labeled cells to unlabeled cells (Fig. 12.1B), indicating the start of cell fusion. Then the contact point was expanded where the fusion began, and a tunnel was formed in the contact area within the first minute (Fig. 12.1C). The two spherical cells gradually became a single larger elliptical cell, while their cytoplasm continued to mix. The fused cells gradually became round after about 15 min (Fig. 12.1D), and spherical after 30 min (Fig. 12.1E). The dark shadow in the fused cell corresponds to the nucleus of the original unlabeled cell. Their cytoplasmic mixing continued until the nucleus of the unlabeled cells became invisible, because the GFP level in the fused cells became uniform after about 55 min (Fig. 12.1F).

It has been further examined whether this technique can be used to induce multicell fusion. As shown in Fig. 12.2, under the manipulation of multiple optical tweezers, the GFP-labeled hESC was fused with two unlabeled hESCs. The cell–cell connection between the GFP-labeled hESC and the two unlabeled hESCs was cut by a pulsed laser. After each cut, GFPs transferred from the green cell to the adjacent unlabeled cell, and the three cells finally exchanged cytoplasm. The results prove the successful multicell fusion through the laser-induced engineering method.

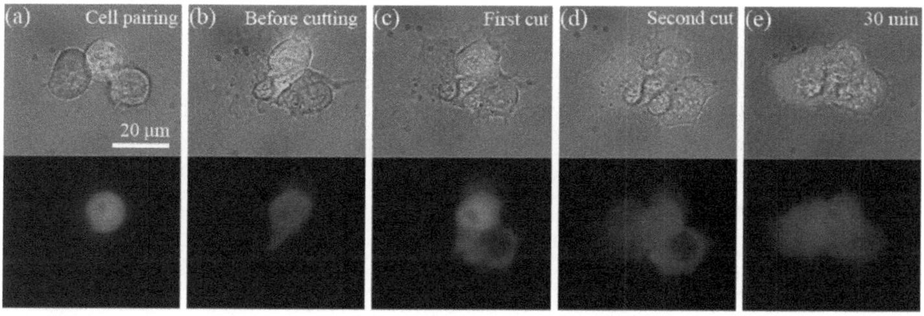

Figure 12.2 Laser-induced cell fusion of three adherent cells (Chen et al., 2013). (A) Three cell form cell pairs. (B) Three cells attach to cover glass in cell pair shape. (C) A GFP-labeled cell (middle) fuse with unlabeled cell (right) after the first cut. (D) The binucleated hESC is then fused with another unlabeled cell (left) by the second cut. (E) 30 min after laser cutting, three cells become a single cell. Scale bar is 20 μm.

The fusion efficiency of hESCs is then analyzed in different energy ranges of UV laser irradiation. Here, successful fusion is defined as the merging of two cells into one -cell within the first hour. Fusion efficiency is evaluated based on the percentage of successful fusion operations in total fusion operations. Fig. 12.3 shows the relationship between fusion efficiency and laser energy. In an experiment by Chen et al. (2013), the energy threshold for inducing cell fusion was determined to be approximately 14.47 μJ per pulse. Above 14.45 μJ, the fusion efficiency increased as the laser energy increased. The achievable maximum fusion efficiency was above 60%, and the pulse energy was about 18 μJ. The fusion efficiency decreased with a further increase in energy. It has been observed that the use of higher laser energy will cause greater damage to the fused cells, rather than prolonging the survival time. The long-term survival rate was checked by incubating the fused cells in a medium containing 0.5 μM SYTOX Orange dye for 10 min. SYTOX Orange dye can easily penetrate apoptotic cells with damaged

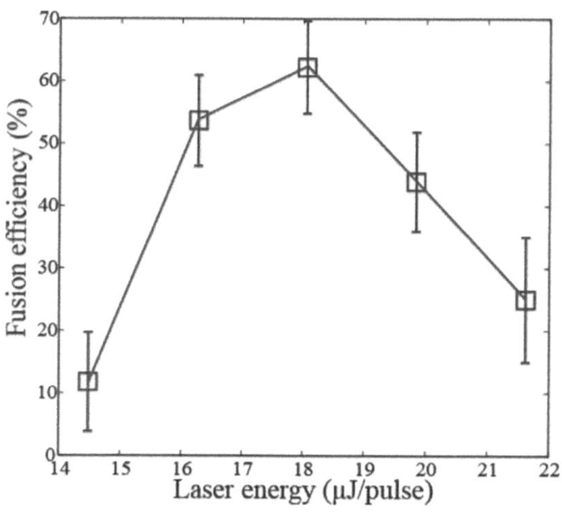

Figure 12.3 Fusion efficiency data for the cutting of n > 200 cell pairs using a pulsed UV laser. Each point represents the mean ± standard error of at least four experiments (Chen et al., 2013).

plasma membranes, but will not penetrate healthy cell membranes. When the fusion cells were cultured in mTeSR1 at 37°C and 5% CO_2, 90% of the fusion cells can survive more than 2.5 h, and 40% of the fusion cells can survive more than 10 h (n = 20). Fig. 12.4A shows that no apoptosis was detected in the fused cells 12 h after cell fusion. The fused cell has two nuclei, as shown by the specific nuclear fluorescent protein (Fig. 12.4C). The results indicate that if the optimal laser energy is used, viable multinucleated cells can be obtained.

Finally, hESC is fused with somatic HDFns, as shown in Fig. 12.5. HDFns labeled with mCherry fluorescent protein were mixed with unlabeled hESC immediately after enzymolysis (Fig. 12.5A). After laser cutting the membrane, the two cells begin to fuse, as shown by the transfer of red fluorescence from HDFn to unlabeled hESC (Fig. 12.5B). Similar to hESC fusion, the dark area representing the hESC nucleus was observed immediately after laser cutting. This area moved toward HDFns within the first minute, and then disappeared when the cytoplasm was further mixed (Fig. 12.5C). The fusion was completed in about 10 min (Fig. 12.5D), and the fused cells attached to the coverslip showed a similar morphology to the surrounding cells (Fig. 12.5E). These results prove the effectiveness of laser-induced cell fusion technology in fusing stem cells with somatic cells.

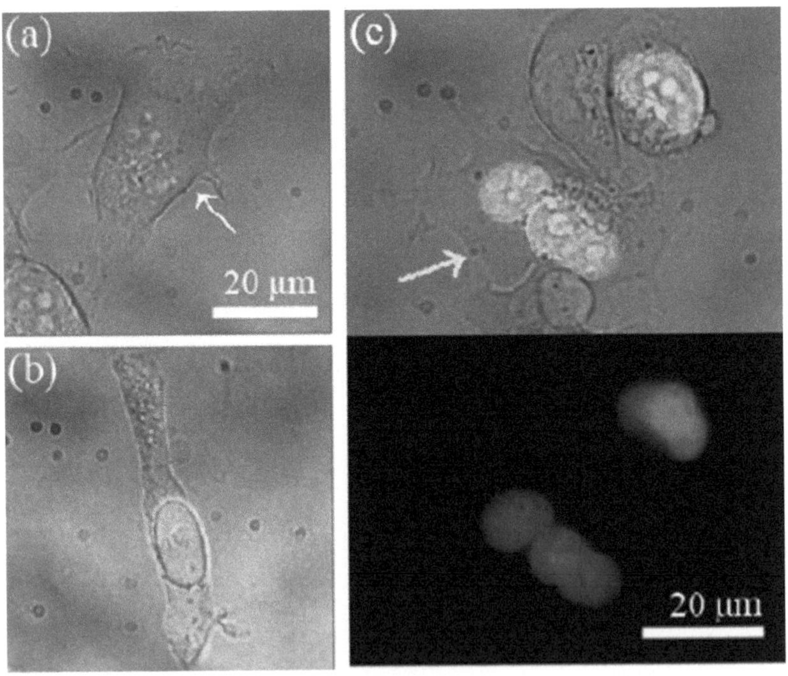

Figure 12.4 Cell surviving results after fusion (Chen et al., 2013). (A) The fused cell (*arrow*) is viable and no apoptotic signal is detected, as indicated by negative SYTOX Orange staining 12 h after fusion. (B) A hESC fixed by 4% paraformaldehyde is positively stained with SYTOX Orange staining. (C) The fused cell has two normal nuclei structures. Arrows indicate fused cells. Scale bar is 20 μm.

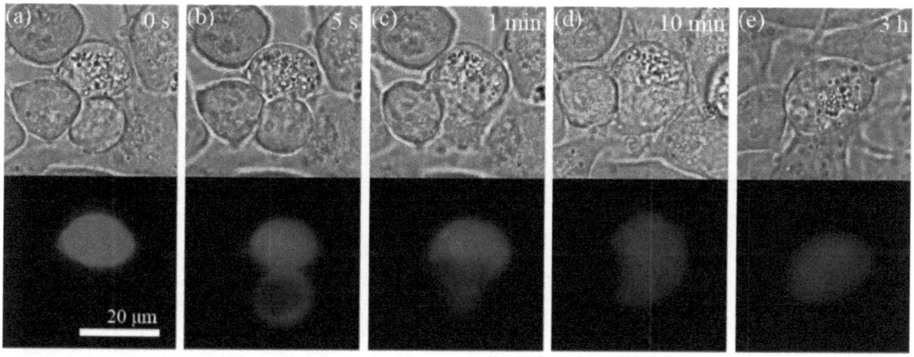

Figure 12.5 Laser-induced fusion of hESC and HDFn (Chen et al., 2013). (A) Image of an mCherry-labeled HDFn; (B) the red HDFn is fused with a transparent hESC after pulsed laser cutting. (C) The fused cell gradually rounds up during the first minute. (D) Ten minutes after laser cutting. (E) Three hours after laser cutting, the fused cell shows similar morphology to the surrounding cells. Scale bar is 20 μm.

The above study has successfully proved that the targeted laser-induced cell fusion technology using 355 nm pulsed UV laser can fuse two or multiple stem cells, and can also fuse stem cells with somatic cells. The laser-induced stem cell fusion produces viable multinucleated cells. This specific and accurate technology could be used to create multinucleated mature cells by fusing stem or progenitor cells to facilitate the study of cell fusion-driven differentiation and maturation.

12.3 Cell fusion with combined optical tweezers and microwell array technology

In this section, laser-induced cell fusion is combined with a microfluidic chip based on a microwell array to achieve highly selective and controllable cell fusion.

12.3.1 Microwell array design for cell fusion

Fig. 12.6 illustrates a schematic of the operational principle of the cell fusion process based on the microwell array. Suspended single cells and cell culture medium are injected from the sample inlet and buffer inlet, respectively. The two-phase laminar flow can only confine cells in the cell docking microwells through fluid dynamics. The cells outside the docking microwells are removed by flowing cell culture medium after 5 min of sedimentation, as shown in Fig. 12.6A. Image processing is performed to detect specific cells in the microwells, and the physical mark serves as feedback to guide the entire manipulation process with high precision. After detection, the optical trap is immediately positioned on the cell of interest for cell capture. By moving the objective lens Z stage upwards, these optically trapped cells are levitated vertically from the cell docking microwells, as shown in Fig. 12.6B. Levitated cells are

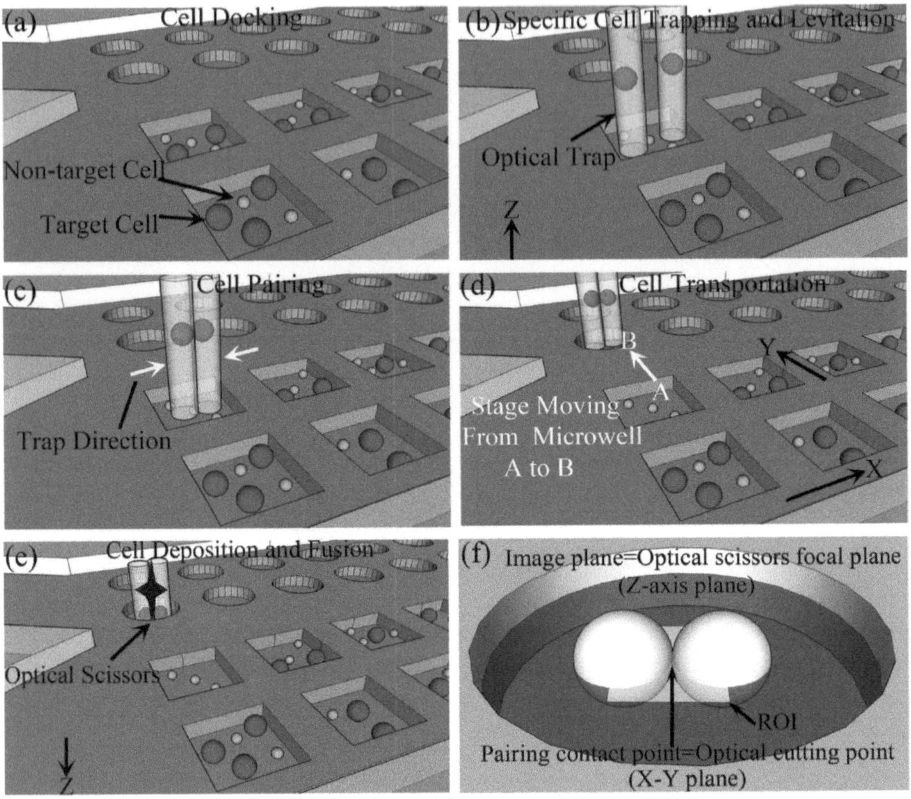

Figure 12.6 Schematic of the operational principle for the laser-induced cell fusion process with high selectivity and controllability (Wang et al., 2013). (A) Moving the targeted cells into the docking microwells. (B) Levitating the optically trapped cells. (C) Assembly of the levitated cells in pairs by dynamically moving the corresponding optical traps. (D) Transporting the paired cells to the microwells. (E) Depositing the paired cells into the microwells for cell fusion. (F) Releasing the optical traps from the fused cells.

assembled in pairs by dynamically moving the corresponding optical traps, as shown in Fig. 12.6C. Fig. 12.6D shows that the paired cells are transported above the microwell array layer to the predefined cell fusion microwells through the programmed motorized X−Y platform. After reaching the target position, the paired cells are deposited into the cell fusion microwells by moving the objective lens Z stage downwards, and then fused by optical scissors, as shown in Fig. 12.6E. Finally, the optical traps are released from the fused cells, so that the cells in the cell fusion microwells can be further analyzed or manipulated with high spatiotemporal resolution.

Successful laser-induced cell fusion largely depends on three factors: the parameters of the applied pulsed laser, the membrane gap of the paired cells, and the 3D focus position of the optical scissors. Peak power and irradiation time are the main parameters of focused pulse laser induced cell fusion. By optimizing the distance between the two optical traps, close membrane contact with paired cells with very narrow spaces (less than 50 Å) can be achieved (Wojcieszyn et al., 1983). Precise positioning of the membrane cutting point in 3D is also critical for manipulating optical scissors for cell cutting, as shown in Fig. 12.6F. When paired cells are deposited in the microwells, an autofocus algorithm based on fast Fourier transform can be used to determine the focal plane of the image, which is also the focal plane of the optical scissors (Wu et al., 2013). To accurately position the laser cutting point on the focal plane, the contact point of the two paired cells is set to coincide with the fixed cutting point of the optical scissors. Only a small region of interest (ROI) centered on the contact point is treated to ensure high autofocus processing speed.

The experimental study was conducted on the fusion of hESC and Jurkat cells by Wang et al. (2013). HESC HES2 (NIH code: ES02) from ES Cell International (ESI) (passages 40–60) was used for experimental research. The detailed cell culture, cell transfection, and single-cell processing of hESC have been reported in Wang et al. (2011). Jurkat cells were cultured in RPMI-1640 medium supplemented with 10% FBS. Before the experiment, the channels of the microfluidic chip were filled with 70% ethanol for sterilization. The channel was rinsed with phosphate-buffered saline (PBS) and then filled with PBS containing 10 mg/mL bovine serum albumin (BSA). The chip was dried at room temperature and kept at 4°C for 2 days until the plasma effect was eliminated, which prevented cells from adhering to the channel. The channel was washed twice with cell culture medium, and air bubbles were removed from the microwells by placing the chip in a vacuum chamber. Then, the microfluidic chip was oriented and fixed on the motorized stage to ensure that the upper side of the microwell array was orthogonal to the left side of the image, which helps with the accurate positioning of each microwell and the preciseness of the motorized stage control. The desktop humidified incubator was installed on the electric stage to maintain the cell survival environment at 5% CO_2 and 37°C.

To keep the target cells on the image focal plane for continuous inspection during the levitation process, another method is to use the objective lens Z platform to levitate these optically trapped cells. During the cell-pairing process, the optically trapped cells must be confined in the optical trap. The maximum moving velocity of the cell under a certain laser power can be determined by the viscous drag force method (Wu et al., 2013). To move the paired cells to the target microwell without being restricted by distance, while keeping them in the field of view, a robotic motorized stage control is used during transportation. A more detailed description of cell trapping, levitation, assembly, transportation, and deposition in microwells has been introduced in Chapter 11. This tool can realize a set of manipulation tasks with high spatiotemporal resolution, and realize dynamic and parallel cell manipulations. The two optical traps are generally considered to be independent. However, when the optical traps are in close contact or adjacent, the perturbation of each optical trap cannot be ignored (Ling et al., 2011). When the two cells trapped by the two optical traps are close to each other, the cell in each optical trap receives the optical force from the two optical traps simultaneously, causing the two cells to approach each other. Therefore, the minimum distance between the two optical traps should not be less than the cell diameter.

12.3.2 Results of cell fusion on the chip

A series of experiments were performed with different laser powers for specific irradiation time to determine the appropriate parameters for laser-induced cell fusion. The frequency of the optical scissors is set to 10 Hz, and the irradiation time of each pulse is set to 1 ns. Five pulses per cut are applied in each round of cell fusion. The next cut is applied when no fusion occurs. The time interval between each cut is 1 min. Fig. 12.7 shows that under a laser energy of 18 mJ (before transmitting through the objective lens), the fusion efficiency can be as high as 62%.

First, two paired GFP-labeled hESCs were deposited in the cell fusion microwell. Fig. 12.8A shows that before the pulsed laser was applied at t = 0 min, the two paired cells had clear circular contours and visible membrane contact areas. After using laser scissors for the first cut, the membranes began to fuse and the contact area became blurred. After the second cut at t = 1 min, the membrane in the contact area disappeared and the two cells were connected to each other. The mixed fusion cells became

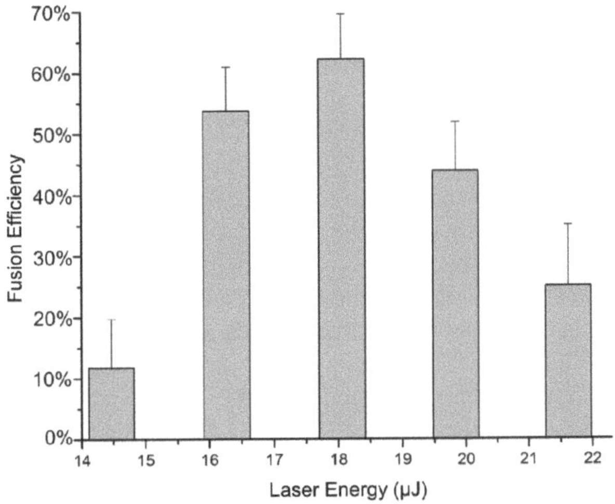

Figure 12.7 Fusion efficiency at different laser powers before transmitting through the objective lens (Wang et al., 2013).

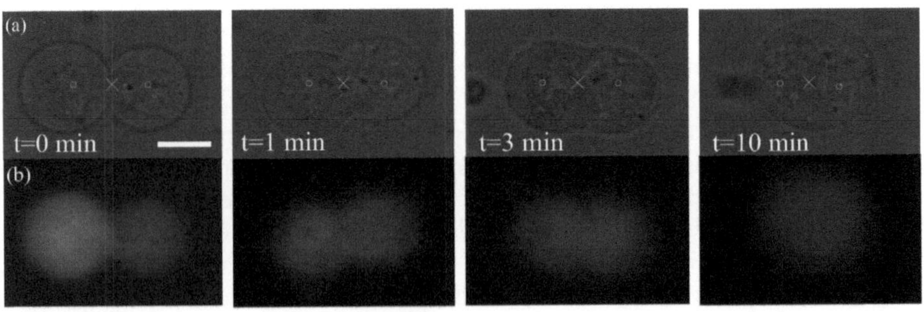

Figure 12.8 Fusion process of paired hESCs (Wang et al., 2013). (A) Brightfield image of cell fusion at different times. (B) Corresponding fluorescence image. Scale bar is 10 μm.

an elliptical cell at t = 3 min. The fused cell became round and formed a spherical cell with two nuclei after 10 min. Fig. 12.8B shows the fluorescence distribution at different times during the cell fusion process. The paired cells both have Oct4-GFP before fusion, indicating that these cells are hESCs. The fluorescence intensity of the left hESC is higher than that of the right hESC. After fusion, the fluorescence diffuses from the hESC on the left to the hESC on the right through the exchange of cytoplasm, resulting in an almost uniform fluorescence distribution. Finally, GFP is evenly distributed in the spherical fusion cell.

Second, the fusion of the nonadherent Jurkat cells stained with MitoTracker red dye for mitochondria labeling was performed to verify whether the optimized laser-induced cell fusion approach is cell-type specific. Mitochondria are mainly located around the nucleus of normal Jurkat cells. The optically trapped Jurkat cells were paired with optical tweezers and cut by optical scissors. The fusion process of Jurkat cells is similar to that of hESC, as shown in Fig. 12.9A. As shown in Fig. 12.9B, the two nuclei were separated by a membrane before fusion; after cell fusion, the two nuclei touched each other and remained intact.

The cytoplasmic exchanges between the two fused cells were also examined. The cytoplasmic exchange between hESC-hESC fusions was slow. It usually took a long time to form a hybrid cell with two nuclei. The cytoplasmic exchange in the Jurkat–Jurkat fusion occurred rapidly, immediately after cell cutting, and lasted only a few seconds. Fig. 12.10 illustrates the movement of cytoplasm with mitochondria and nuclei from one cell to another. Nuclear transfer is marked by a dotted circle in the

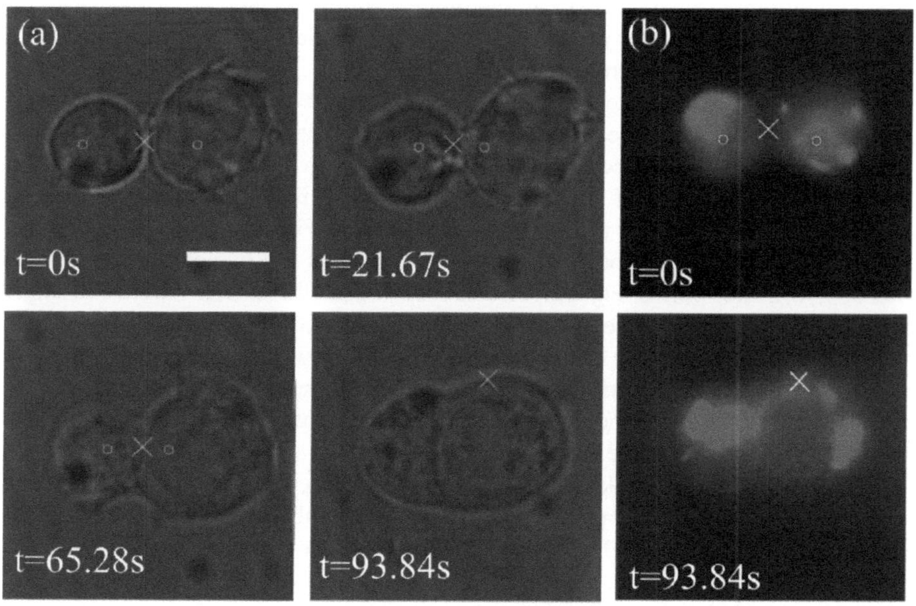

Figure 12.9 Fusion process of paired Jurkat cells with GFP (Wang et al., 2013). (A) Fusion of paired Jurkat cells at different times. (B) Fluorescence image showing the relative position of the two nuclei before and after fusion. Scale bar is 10 μm.

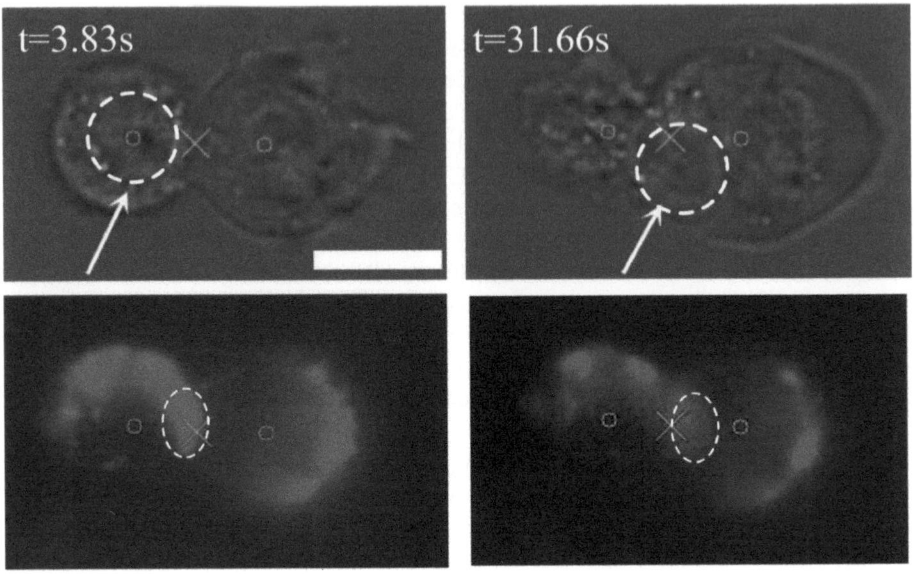

Figure 12.10 Transfer process of cytoplasm with mitochondria and nucleus from the left Jurkat cell to the right Jurkat cell during cell fusion (Wang et al., 2013). Scale bar is 10 μm.

brightfield image, and mitochondrial transfer is marked by a dotted ellipse in the fluorescent image with RFP. The relative transfer distance can be visualized based on the fixed cutting point (the cross mark in the figure). Different cytoplasmic exchange behaviors may be determined by the cytoplasm content or membrane composition, which varies greatly between different cell types.

Fusion of two different cell types was further verified. By using a microwell array chip designed with high selectivity and controllability, specific cells with the phenotype of interest can be selected for fusion. HESC with GFP and Jurkat cells with RFP were mixed in a ratio of 1:1. Fig. 12.11A shows the hESC–Jurkat cell pair, where the left cell is hESC and the right cell is the Jurkat cell. Fig. 12.11B and C show each cell with GFP and RFP, respectively. Fig. 12.11D shows that two cells fused together after applying three pulses. Fig. 12.11E and F show that GFP and RFP were exchanged between the two cells after cell fusion. Considering that GFP is distributed in the cytoplasm, fluorescence transfer can be detected within a few seconds after applying the pulsed laser. The GFP distribution in the fused cell showed uniformity. However, because RFP is located in the mitochondria, relatively low diffusion and nonuniform distribution will occur in the fused cells.

Fig. 12.12 illustrates the laser-induced fusion efficiency of different pairs of hESC and Jurkat cells at different optical cutting times. Thirty hESC–ESC pairs, 67 Jurkat–Jurkat pairs, and 14 hESC–Jurkat pairs were tested. After the first cut was applied at $t = 0$ min, the second, third, and fourth cuts were applied with 1-min intervals until fusion occurred. Here, successful fusion was defined as the merging of two cells into one cell and the start of the fluorescence transfer process. The ratio of successful fusion pairs to total pairs was used to express the fusion efficiency in the study.

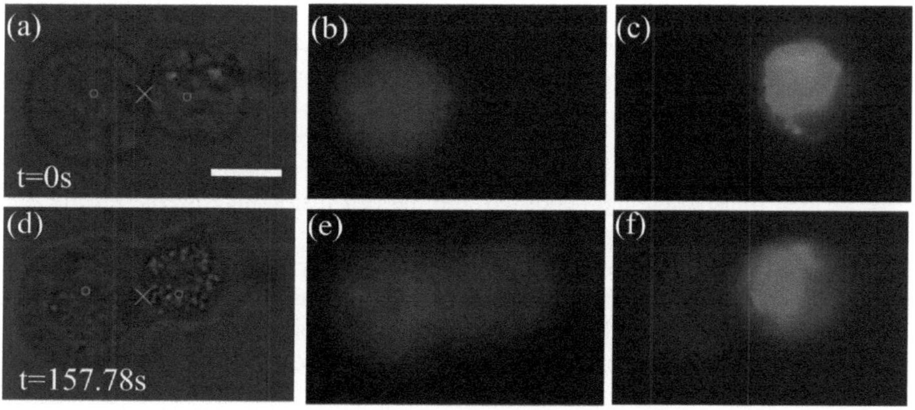

Figure 12.11 Fusion of hESC with GPF and Jurkat cell with RFP and fluorescence distribution before and after fusion (Wang et al., 2013). (A) The hESC (left)-Jurkat (right) cell pair. (B) hESC with GFP. (C) Jurkat cell with RFP. (D) Fusing process of the two cells after applying three pulses. (E-F) GFP and RFP were exchanged between the two cells after cell fusion. Scale bar is 10 μm.

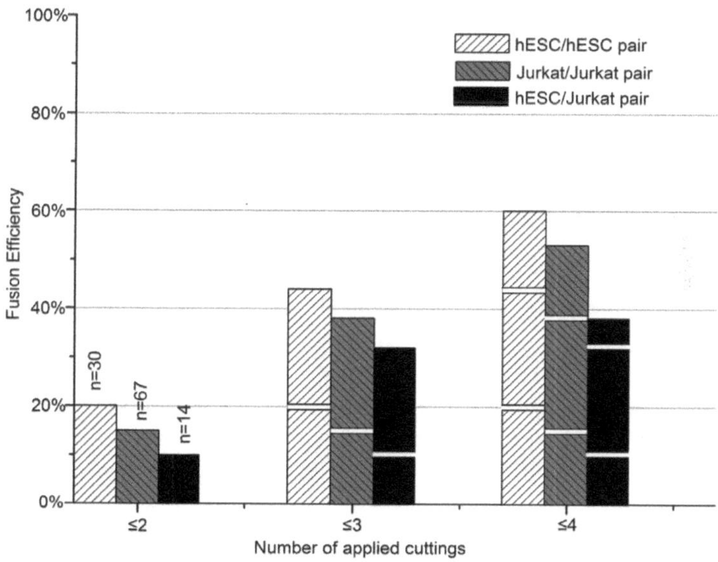

Figure 12.12 Fusion efficiency of different pairs of hESC and Jurkat cells at different optical cutting times (Wang et al., 2013).

Fig. 12.12 illustrates the fusion efficiency accumulated along the time of applying laser cutting. A longer cutting time led to higher fusion efficiency, but at the same time caused more damage to the fused cells. In addition, the results of the three groups (different cutting times) showed that the fusion efficiency of homologous cell pairs was higher than that of heterologous cell pairs.

In summary, this section introduces cell fusion combining optical tweezers and microwell array technology to achieve high selectivity and controllability. Target cells with a specific phenotype are preselected with optical tweezers from the cell mixture in the cell docking microwells through the on-chip cell isolation method. The selected cells are then levitated and paired with the indispensable tight membrane contact. The contact point coincides with the cutting point of the optical scissors. The paired cells are then transported and deposited into the cell fusion microwells. Finally, the deposited cell pairs are fused by applying laser scissors with optimized parameters. This method enables a series of cell manipulations from cell trapping to cell fusion, and provides the opportunity to fuse different cell pairs simultaneously, thereby improving the flexibility of the operation. The fused cells enclosed in the microwells can be further analyzed or manipulated at high spatiotemporal resolution without being removed from the chip.

12.4 A case study of transforming liver cancer cells into tumor initiating-like cells by cell fusion

This section introduces a case study of the engineered fusion of a stem cell and a cancer cell, and exploration of the mechanism by which cancer stem cells may have a potential impact on stem cell therapy for liver cancer. The fused cell through laser-induced fusion of a single hepatocellular carcinoma cell (HepG2) and hESC can obtain both stemness and carcinoid characteristics, and exhibits increased tumorigenicity and resistance to drug treatment. Fusion cells are highly similar to tumor stem cells (TSCs) or tumor-initiating cells (TICs). TICs are important in tumorigenesis, aggravation, metastasis, and recurrence (Visvader and Lindeman, 2008). Liver TICs and their markers have been identified in the literature (Yamashita and Wang, 2013; Yamashita and Kaneko, 2014). According to the results of gene expression analysis and quantitative PCR detection, Wang et al. (2016) found that some liver TIC markers such as CD133, CD44, and ALDH1 showed significant high expression in fusion cells; however, this situation was not observed in HepG2 cells. In vivo tumorigenicity assays and drug resistance assays also prove that the fusion of cancer cells and stem cells results in cancer cells that are highly similar to cancer stem cells. These results indicate that when certain stem cell therapies are used in cancer therapy risks maybe incurred. In the following, a case study by Wang et al. (2016) is described in detail.

12.4.1 Methods

12.4.1.1 Cell culture

The hESC line HES2 (NIH code: ES02) from ES Cell International (generations 60–84) was cultured on a commercially available, serum-free, feeder-independent system and supplemented with BD Matrigel hESC qualified substrate (BD Catalog No. 354277). The genetically labeled Oct4-GFP$^+$ hESCs were produced by transduction (MOI = 5), and the lentiviral vector carried a cassette of Oct4 promoter-driven GFP. HepG2 cells were stored in DMEM (Gibco, Catalog No. 11965-092), supplemented with 10% FBS (Gibco, Catalog No. 10270-106), 100 U/mL penicillin, and 100 U/mL streptomycin (Invitrogen, Catalog No. 15240-062) at 37°C in a humidified atmosphere of 5% CO_2.

12.4.1.2 Cell fusion

Before the fusion experiment, the obtained single cells were passaged by enzyme treatment. After proper neutralization, the single cell suspension in the culture medium was temporarily stored at 4°C. To distinguish hESCs from HepG2, hESCs were labeled with Oct-GFP, and HepG2 cells were stained with red mitochondrial selective probe. For mitochondrial staining, single HepG2 cells were incubated in a 40 nM Mito-Tracker probe for 15 min and washed three times. The stained cells were resuspended in DMEM containing 10% FBS.

Fusion experiments were performed as described in Section 12.1. A GFP-labeled hESC and a mitochondrial stained HepG2 cell were trapped and manipulated with optical tweezers to form a cell pair. The working frequency of the laser scissors was 10 Hz, and the duration of each pulse was 1 ns, which was able to cut the cell membrane at the contact point between two cells. Successful fusion was verified by observing the transfer of cytoplasmic GFP from hESC to HepG2 cells, as shown in Fig. 12.13. The fused cells were attached to the bottom of the coverslip and were able to survive.

12.4.1.3 Cell isolation and colony formation

A total of 24 h after fusion, the fused cells were collected after trypsin-EDTA treatment and diluted in a low-density single-cell suspension (6−10 cells/mL). In each well of a 96-well plate, 100 μL of cell suspension was seeded. After 24 h of incubation, the plate was inspected under a microscope and wells containing single cells were selected. The cells were fed with new DMEM medium every 2 days. After 1 week of cultivation, colonies were formed in the labeled wells. These colonies showed different morphologies from HepG2, and were gradually replanted into 35 mm Petri dishes for further characterization.

12.4.1.4 Flow cytometry

FACS tests were performed on HepG2, fusion cells, and hESC. The cells were detached from the culture dish and suspended in 100 μL buffer and human serum (1: 1) at 4°C for 15 min. The cells were then incubated with AFP primary antibody (Santa Cruz Biotechnology, Catalog No. sc-8399) and CD133-PE (Miltenyi Biotec, Catalog No. 130-098-829) for 45 min. The cells were washed with FACS buffer and incubated with the secondary antibody (Santa Cruz Biotechnology, Catalog No. sc-2856) for 30 min at 4°C. FACSVerseTM (BD Pharmingen) was used to detect cell markers. The flow cytometry results were analyzed using BD FACSuite software.

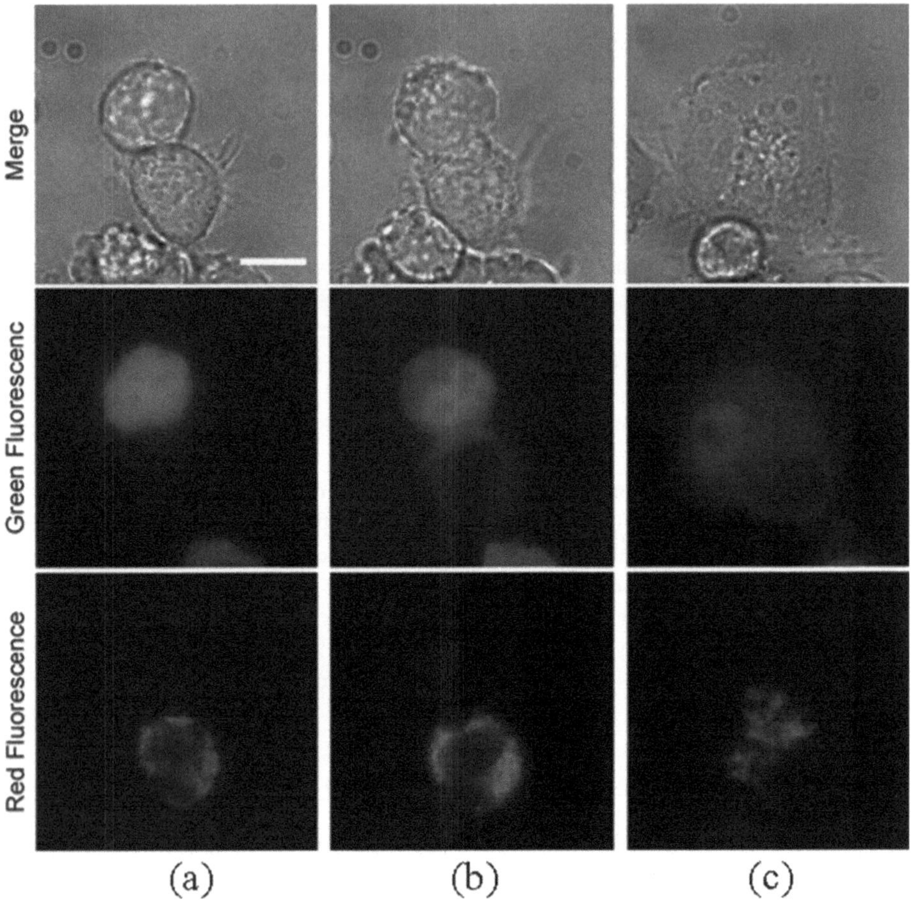

Figure 12.13 Laser-induced cell fusion of hESC and HepG2 (Wang et al., 2016). (A) GFP-labeled hESC and mitochondria-labeled HepG2 forming a cell pair before laser cutting. (B) GFP transfer from the hESC cell to the HepG2 cell after laser cutting. (C) The fused cell attaches to the cover glass surface and exhibits adherent cell morphology about 25 min after laser cutting. Scale bar is 20 μm.

12.4.1.5 Quantitative RT-PCR

Using the method provided by the manufacturer, Trizol reagent was used to extract total RNA from the cells. iScriptTM cDNA Synthesis Kit (Bio-Rad, Catalog No. 170-8890) was used to generate reverse-transcribed cDNA. SsoAdvanced SYBR Green supermix kit (Bio-Rad, Catalog No. 1725260) was used for real-time quantitative PCR amplification in the CFX96 real-time system (Bio-Rad, United States). The specific primers used in the analysis are listed in Table 12.1. CD133 and CD44 primers were described in Wagner et al. (2004) and Mima et al. (2012). The other primer sequences were from the primer library (Wang and Seed, 2003).

Table 12.1 Specific primers used in qPCR (Wang et al., 2016).

Gene	Forward primer (5′-3′)	Reverse primer (5′-3′)
AFP	AGACTGAAAACCCTCTTGAATGC	GTCCTCACTGAGTTGGCAACA
CD133	ACATGAAAAG ACCTGGGGG	GATCTGGTGTCCCAGCATG
CD44	TCCCAGACGAAGACAGTCCCTGGAT	CACTGGGGTGGAATGTGTCTTGGTC
ALDH1A1	CTGCTGGCGACAATGGAGT	CTGCTGGCGACAATGGAGT
ABCB1	GGGAGCTTAACACCCGACTTA	GCCAAAATCACAAGGGTTAGCTT
EpCAM	AATCGTCAATGCCAGTGTACTT	TCTCATCGCAGTCAGGATCATAA
Bcl-2	GACTGAATCGGAGATGGAGACC	GCAGTTCAAACTCGTCGCCT
β-actin	CATCCTCACCCTGAAGTACCC	AGCCTGGATAGCAACGTACATG

12.4.1.6 Drug resistance

The fused cells and HepG2 were first incubated in a six-well plate for 15 h. After this step, 0.1, 0.2, and 0.5 μm DOX was added to the medium, with three parallel samples per group. The cells were then incubated for another 48 h. The cell viability was determined by the trypan blue exclusion test.

12.4.1.7 In vivo tumorigenicity assay

HepG2 cells and fusion cells (5×10^4, 1×10^5, and 1×10^6 cells in 100 μL DMEM) were injected subcutaneously into the right scapula of each nude mouse (BALB/c nu/nu, 4–6 weeks old). Four nude mice were prepared for each group. Tumor growth in nude mice was measured every 7 days for 6 weeks. Nude mice were sacrificed at 6 or 7 weeks. The tumor was fixed with formaldehyde solution and stained with hematoxylin-eosin (H&E).

12.4.1.8 Statistical analysis

RT-PCR results and drug resistance data are expressed as mean ± SD. Data from in vivo tumor experiments are expressed as mean ± SEM. A two-tailed Student's t-test was used for statistical analysis. Differences with $P \leq .05$ were considered significant.

12.4.2 Results

12.4.2.1 Gene expression of fusion cells is different to HepG2 cells

Fig. 12.14 illustrates the morphology of HepG2, fusion cells, and hESC, respectively. It can be seen from this figure that the isolated fusion cells did not show a conspicuous spindle shape, which is different from the morphology of HepG2 cells and hESC. Fig. 12.15 shows the detection results of the marker protein and gene expression of the fusion cell and its parent cell. The results indicate that both HepG2 and hESC can affect fusion cells. To determine the functional differences between fusion cells and HepG2 cells, pairwise comparisons were performed to examine significantly different molecular functions, biological processes, and cellular components [gene ontology (GO)]. As shown in Table 12.2, the immune response, immune system process, and apoptosis regulation of differentially expressed genes are improved. Similar to CD133, CD44 showed different expression in fusion cells and HepG2 cells in the analysis. Then qPCR tests were performed on related genes. The results showed that, compared with HepG2 cells, several liver tumor-initiating cell markers in fusion cells, including AFP, CD133, CD44, and EpCAM (Yamashita and Wang, 2013), were not regulated (Fig. 12.15B). CD133 is an important stem biomarker in normal stem cells and TICs. It can help maintain tumorigenic properties and affect the growth of tumor cells (Yao et al., 2009). The CD44 invariant regulates redox status, which affects tumor initiation, tumorigenesis, and metastasis (Patrawala et al., 2007). CD133 and

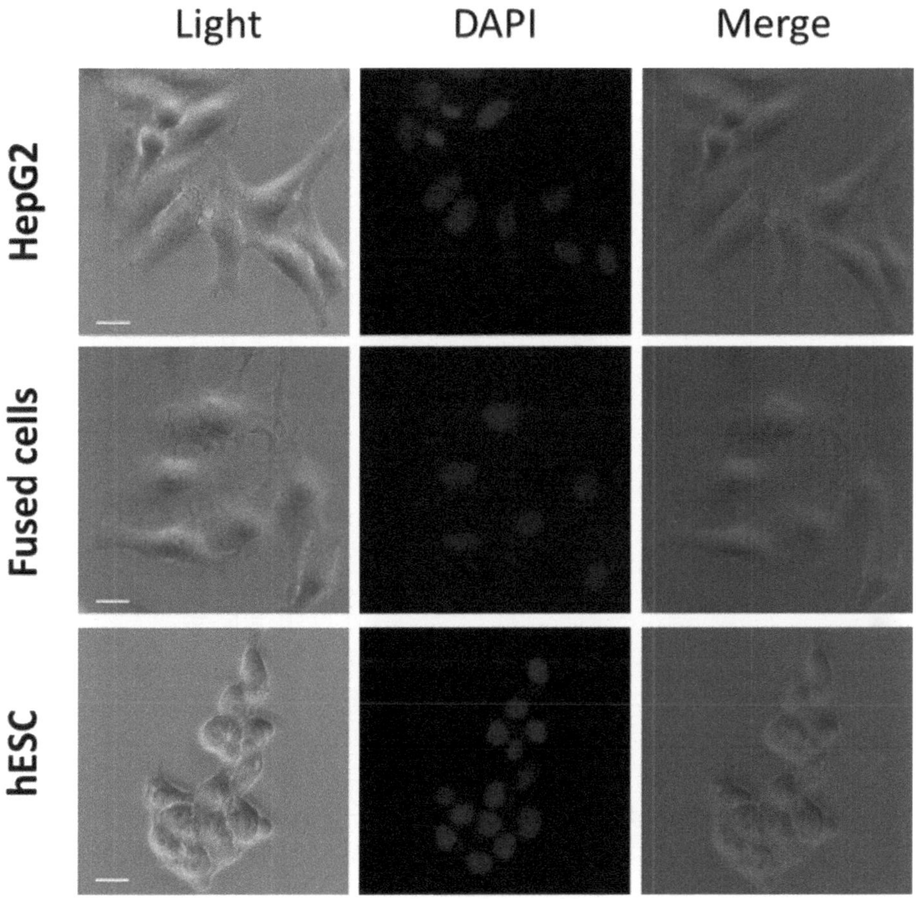

Figure 12.14 Morphology of HepG2, fused cells, and hESC. Morphology of the fused cells differs from that of HepG2 cells and hEScs. Scale bar is 20 μm (Wang et al., 2016).

CD44 are rarely expressed in normal cancer cells. EpCAM is a key protein that activates the Wnt signaling pathway and is related to tumorigenesis, invasion, and resistance to drug therapy. The high expression of EpCAM enhances the chemoresistance of cells (Ji et al., 2009; Gostner et al., 2011).

12.4.2.2 Fusion cells show increased drug resistance

The drug resistance of the fused cells was examined and the results are shown in Fig. 12.16. Fusion cells and HepG2 were treated with different concentrations of doxorubicin (DOX) for 48 h. Fig. 12.16A shows that the survival rate of fusion cells is significantly higher than that of HepG2, and with the increase of DOX concentration, the survival rate of fusion cells and HepG2 decreases. In this study, the survival rate was defined as the number of live cells after DOX treatment divided by the number

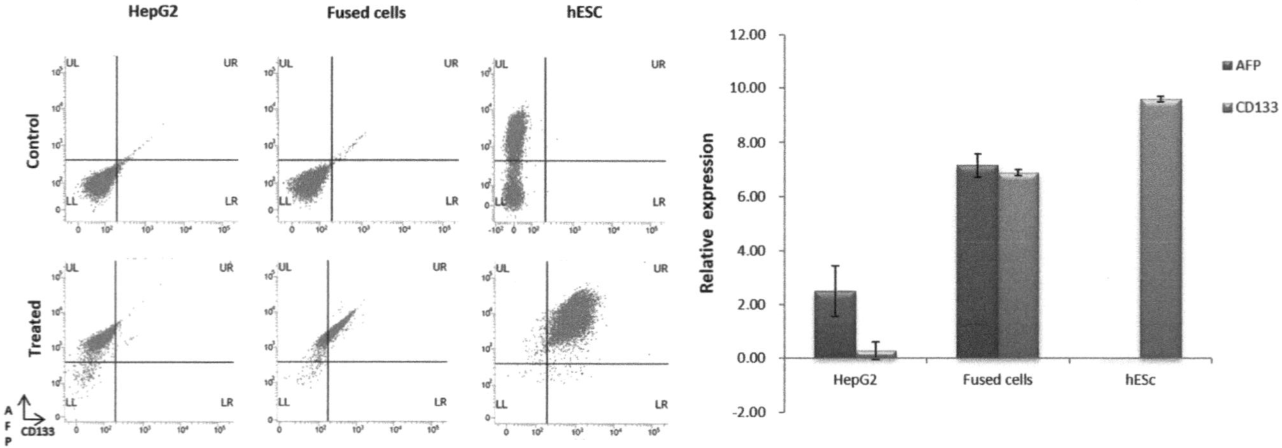

Figure 12.15 Representative gene marker expression in HepG2 and fusion cells (Wang et al., 2016). (A) Flow cytometer analysis for the expression of marker protein AFP and CD133 in HepG2, fusion cells, and hESCs. Cells in the control group are not antibody incubated, while cells in the treated group are incubated with AFP and CD133 antibody. As hESCs are labeled with GFP, hESCs from both the control and treated groups are green-positive populations. (B) Gene marker expression analysis shows that both AFP and CD133 are expressed in the fused cells, indicating that both HepG2 and hEScs affect the gene expression in fusion cells.

Table 12.2 Significantly enriched GO terms in DEGs (Wang et al. 2016).

Gene ontology term	Cluster frequency (%)	Genome frequency of use (%)	Corrected *P*-value
Immune response	10.2	4.9%	2.74e-07
Immune system process	12.4	6.8	3.77e-06
Response to virus	2.6	0.8	0.00138
Regulation of apoptosis	7.8	4.3	0.00508
Regulation of programmed cell death	7.8	4.4	0.00840
Regulation of cell death	7.8	4.4	0.00888

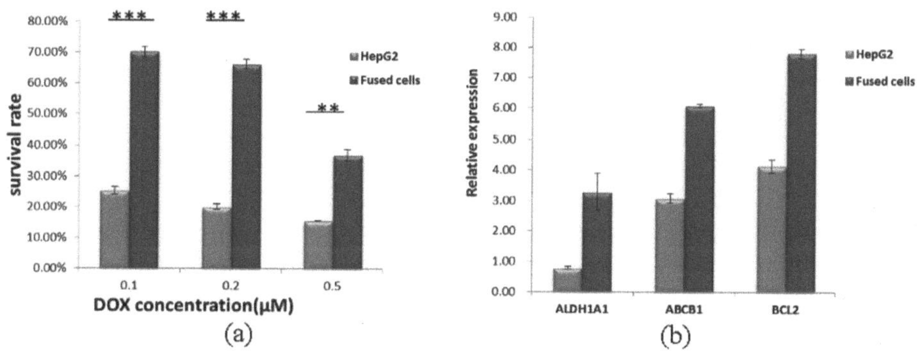

Figure 12.16 Drug resistance and related gene expression analysis (Wang et al., 2016). (A) Drug resistance of HepG2 and fusion cells examined with different DOX concentrations (n = 4 for three independent experiments). ***$P < .01$, **$P < .05$. Statistical significance was determined using a two-tailed Student's t-test. (B) Drug resistance-related gene expressed significantly in fusion cells compared with HepG2.

of live cells without DOX treatment. The results showed that compared with the donor HepG2 cells, the fusion cells showed higher drug resistance.

The qPCR results showed that CD133 (Fig. 12.15B), ALDH1A1, ATP binding cassette subfamily B member 1 (ABCB1), and B-cell lymphoma 2 (Bcl-2) (Fig. 12.16B) were highly expressed in fusion cells. The high expression of CD133 is related to the drug resistance and recurrence of a variety of solid tumors. ALDH is an effective detoxification enzyme, and the high expression of ALDH can provide a way for tumors to resist chemotherapy. The expression of ABCB1 has the ability to actively repair DNA and resist apoptosis (Dean et al., 2005; Houthuijzen et al., 2012). The antiapoptotic protein Bcl-2 has been shown to cause resistance to cancer treatment by forming heterodimers with many proapoptotic proteins (Abdullah and Chow, 2013). Bcl-2 also contributes to the development of resistance to multiple chemotherapeutic drugs (Siddique et al., 2013). The expression of CD133, ABCB1, Bcl-2, and ALDH1A1 in fusion cells explained the increased drug resistance of fusion cells (Ji and Wang, 2012), indicating that cancer cells will acquire drug resistance through cell fusion with stem cells.

12.4.2.3 Fusion cells are highly tumorigenic

To analyze the tumor initiation ability, nude mice were transplanted with different numbers of fusion cells. The same number of HepG2 cells was used as a control. The tumor volume was measured weekly. Compared with HepG2 cells, fusion cells can lead to the gradual growth of tumors in nude mice, with fewer cells. As shown in Fig. 12.17, the injection of 5×10^4 fusion cells promoted the progressive growth of tumors in nude mice, while injection of 5×10^4 HepG2 cells did not induce this effect. When the injected dose of fusion cells was increased to 1×10^5, the incidence of tumors increased. However, mice injected with the same number of HepG2 cells still did not form tumors. When the number of injected cells was increased to 1×10^6, both fusion cells and HepG2 cells promoted tumor growth in nude mice. Fusion cells induced 100% tumor incidence, while HepG2 cells only induced 50% tumor incidence. Fusion cells had higher tumorigenicity and faster tumor growth than HepG2 cells, as shown in Table 12.3.

Fig. 12.17 illustrates that in mice injected with fusion cells or HepG2 cells, xenograft tumors show similar histological features, indicating that the tumor tissue is not a teratoma induced by hESCs. The results of in vivo tumorigenicity determined by qPCR are shown in Fig. 12.18, indicating that the fused cells exhibit increased tumorigenicity in vivo. Highly expressed CD133 (Fig. 12.15), CD44, and EpCAM can illustrate the mechanism of enhanced tumorigenicity (Fig. 12.18A). The expression of two tumor growth factors, proliferating cell nuclear antigen (PCNA) and ki67, were also tested. The qPCR results showed that PCNA and Ki67 were relatively highly expressed in the fusion cells (Fig. 12.18B). The high expression of PCNA indicates

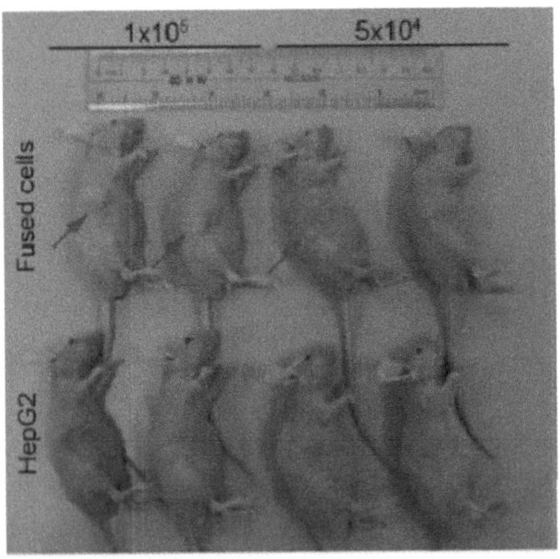

(a)

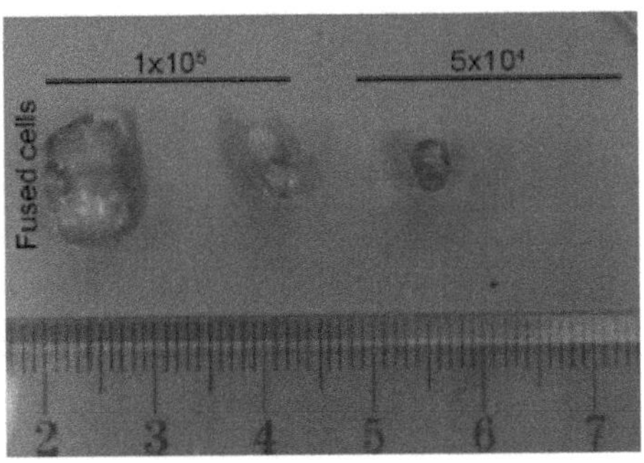

(b)

Figure 12.17 The in vivo test for tumorigenicity of fusion cells (Wang et al., 2016). (A) Mice injected with fusion cells (*top line*) and HepG2 (*bottom line*) in quantities of 5×10^4 and 1×10^5. *Arrows* indicate the tumors from the fused cell, whereas in the control group, no tumor is found. (B) Tumors stripped from the corresponding mice.

Table 12.3 In vivo tumor development experiments of HepG2 cells and fusion cells in nude mice (Wang et al., 2016).

Cell type	Cell numbers injected	Tumor incidence[a]	Latency (days)[b]
HepG2	5×10^4	0/4	
	1×10^5	0/4	
	1×10^6	1/2	14
Fused cells	5×10^4	2/4	14
	1×10^5	3/4	14
	1×10^6	4/4	12

[a]Number of tumors detected/number of injections.
[b]Approximate number of days from tumor cell injection to appearance of a tumor.

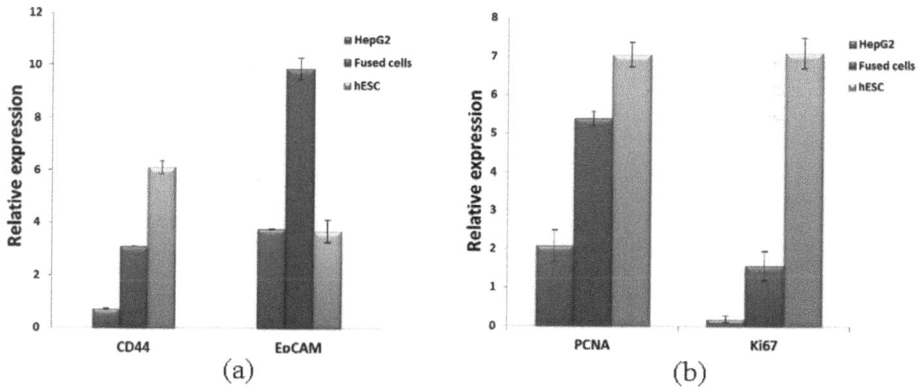

Figure 12.18 Tumorigenicity-related gene expression analysis (Wang et al., 2016). Tumorigenicity-related gene expressions were detected by qPCR. (A) CD44 is a cell surface molecule that affects tumorigenesis. EpCAM is the activator of the WNT pathway, which is important in cancer cells. (B) PCNA and Ki67 are tumor proliferation cell nuclear antigens. All of these genes are highly expressed in fusion cells ($P < .05$).

a high risk of cancer. Ki67 is a nuclear antigen expressed in a variety of solid malignant tumors, and its expression level is significantly higher than that of normal tissues. Ki67 is closely related to the occurrence, metastasis, and prognosis of malignant tumors (Inwald et al., 2013).

12.4.2.4 Discussion

Using engineered laser-induced single-cell fusion technology, fusion cell lines can be successfully produced. The fused cell line combined the gene expression information of parental cells (hepatocellular carcinoma cells) and maternal cells (stem cells). Experimental results confirmed that compared with donor hepatocellular carcinoma cells, the fused cells have a high degree of tumorigenicity and chemoresistance. The fusion of stem cells and cancer cells allows hybrids to exhibit characteristics of stem cells and cancer. Traditionally, the epigenetic modification of the somatic pluripotency gene is considered to be a key factor during stem cell fusion-induced reprogramming of somatic cells, which has been explained as one of the parental cells dominates the phenotype (Lluis and Cosma, 2010). Epigenetic modifications include chromatin remodeling, histone modification, and DNA demethylation (Silva et al., 2006). However, the mechanism of the fusion of cancer cells and stem cells has been rarely elaborated on.

The study of artificial fusion of stem cells and liver cancer cells demonstrates the possible mechanism of tumor-initiating cell generation in humans. After stem cell injection or transplantation, the fusion of stem cells can occur spontaneously in the body, which may explain the risk of liver cancer induced by stem cell therapy. On the one hand, some stem cell therapies may produce cancer stem cell-like cells and exacerbate cancer, rather than cure the disease. On the other hand, artificially generated tumor-initiating cells can be used to generate malignant cells for cancer stem cell drug screening and research into its mechanism.

12.5 Conclusions

This chapter introduced a laser-induced cell fusion method through manipulation with optical tweezers. First, the basic working principle of hESCs-based fusion was introduced, in which cells are manipulated by optical tweezers and fused under 355 nm pulsed UV laser irradiation. Green fluorescent protein transfer indicates the success of fusion. The effect of laser pulse energy on fusion efficiency has been studied also. The successful fusion of hESC with somatic cells was also demonstrated. Second, laser-induced cell fusion with high selectivity and controllability are achieved by using a microfluidic chip with a microwell array. Specific cells with the characteristics of high spatial and temporal resolution are preselected from the mixture by the on-chip isolation method before pairing. The paired cells are then transported, deposited, fused, and released at the desired location in a highly controlled manner. The biophysical analysis of the fused cells shows that the fusion efficiency of homotype pairs is higher than that of heterologous pairs obtained based on different combinations of sample cells, such as human embryonic stem cells and Jurkat cells. Finally, a case study of artificial fusion of HepG2-hESC cell pairs with fusion cell line isolation was reported. The results of genetic analysis show that the fusion of cancer cells and stem cells results in cancer cells being more tumorigenic and showing higher chemoresistance. The results also show that the fusion cells are highly similar to tumor-initiating cells in biological processes or cell compartments. The expression of related genes in fusion cells, such as CD133, CD44, and EpCAM, also supports this conclusion. As a unique method, cell fusion will give a great deal of support to many important studies into cell differentiation, maturation, and reprogramming.

References

Abdullah, L.N., Chow, E.K., 2013. Mechanisms of chemoresistance in cancer stem cells. Clin. Transl. Med. 2 (1), 3.

Chen, S., Cheng, J., Kong, C.W., Wang, X., Cheng, S.H., Li, R.A., Sun, D., 2013. Laser-induced fusion of human embryonic stem cells with optical tweezers. Appl. Phys. Lett. 103, 033701.

Cui, S., Liu, Y., Wang, W., Sun, Y., Fan, Y., 2011. A microfluidic chip for highly efficient cell capturing and pairing. Biomicrofluidics 5, 032003.

Dean, M., Fojo, T., Bates, S., 2005. Tumour stem cells and drug resistance. Nat. Rev. Cancer 25 (4), 275–284.

Ferrand, J., Noel, D., Lehours, P., Prochazkova-Carlotti, M., Chambonnier, L., Menard, A., Mégraud, F., Varon, C., 2011. Human bone marrow-derived stem cells acquire epithelial characteristics through fusion with gastrointestinal epithelial cells. PLoS One 6 (5), e19569.

Ficz, G., Reik, W., 2013. Reprogramming by cell fusion: boosted by Tets. Mol. Cell 49 (6), 1017–1018.

Forbes, S.J., Newsome, P.N., 2012. New horizons for stem cell therapy in liver disease. J. Hepatol. 56 (2), 496–499.

Furst, G., Schulte am Esch, J., Poll, L.W., Hosch, S.B., Fritz, L.B., Klein, M., Godehardt, E., Krieg, A., Wecker, B., Stoldt, V., Stockschläder, M., Eisenberger, C.F., Mödder, U., Knoefel, W.T., 2007. Portal vein embolization and autologous CD133+ bone marrow stem cells for liver regeneration: initial experience. Radiology 243 (1), 171–179.

Gel, M., Kimura, Y., Kurosawa, O., Oana, H., Kotera, H., Washizu, M., 2010. Dielectrophoretic cell trapping and parallel one-to-one fusion based on field constriction created by a micro-orifice array. Biomicrofluidics 4 (2), 022808.

Gostner, J.M., Fong, D., Wrulich, O.A., Lehne, F., Zitt, M., Hermann, M., Krobitsch, S., Martowicz, A., Gastl, G., Spizzo, G., 2011. Effects of EpCAM overexpression on human breast cancer cell lines. BMC Cancer 11 (45).

Houthuijzen, J.M., Daenen, L.G., Roodhart, J.M., Voest, E.E., 2012. The role of mesenchymal stem cells in anti-cancer drug resistance and tumour progression. Br. J. Cancer 106 (12), 1901–1906.

Inwald, E.C., Klinkhammer-Schalke, M., Hofstadter, F., Zeman, F., Koller, M., Gerstenhauer, M., Ortmann, O., 2013. Ki-67 is a prognostic parameter in breast cancer patients: results of a large population-based cohort of a cancer registry. Breast Cancer Res. Treat. 139 (2), 539–552.

Ji, J., Wang, X.W., 2012. Clinical implications of cancer stem cell biology in hepatocellular carcinoma. Semin. Oncol. 39 (4), 461–472.

Ji, J., Yamashita, T., Budhu, A., Forgues, M., Jia, H.L., Li, C.L., Deng, C., Wauthier, E., Reid, L.M., Ye, Q.H., Qin, L.X., Yang, W., Wang, H.Y., Tang, Z.Y., Croce, C.M., Wang, X.W., 2009. Identification of MicroRNA-181 by genome-wide screening as a critical player in EpCAM-positive hepatic cancer stem cells. Hepatology 50 (2), 472–480.

Kirschbaum, M., Guernth-Marschner, C.R., Cherré, S., de Pablo Peña, A., Jaeger, M.S., Kroczek, R.A., Schnelle, T., Mueller, T., Duschl, C., 2012. Highly controlled electrofusion of individually selected cells in dielectrophoretic field cages. Lab Chip 12, 443–450.

Köhler, G., Milstein, C., 1975. Continuous cultures of fused cells secreting antibody of pre-defined specificity. Nature 256, 495–497.

Kong, C.W., Chen, S., Geng, L., Shum, A.M.Y., Sun, D., Li, R.A., 2017. Increasing the physical size and nucleation status of human pluripotent stem cell-derived ventricular cardiomyocytes by cell fusion. Stem Cell Res. 19, 76–81.

Ling, L., Zhou, F., Huang, L., Guo, H., Li, Z., Li, Z., 2011. Perturbation between two traps in dual-trap optical tweezers. J. Appl. Phys. 109, 083116.

Lluis, F., Cosma, M.P., 2010. Cell-fusion-mediated somatic-cell reprogramming: a mechanism for tissue regeneration. J. Cell Physiol. 223 (1), 6–13.

Luo, C., Li, H., Xiong, C., Peng, X., Kou, Q., Chen, Y., Ji, H., Ouyang, Q., 2007. The combination of optical tweezers and microwell array for cells physical manipulation and isolation in microfluidic device. Biomed. Microdevices 9, 573–578.

Mima, K., Okabe, H., Ishimoto, T., Hayashi, H., Nakagawa, S., Kuroki, H., Watanabe, M., Beppu, T., Tamada, M., Nagano, O., Saya, H., Baba, H., 2012. CD44s regulates the TGF-beta-mediated mesenchymal phenotype and is associated with poor prognosis in patients with hepatocellular carcinoma. Cancer Res. 72 (13), 3414–3423.

Newsome, P.N., Johannessen, I., Boyle, S., Dalakas, E., McAulay, K.A., Samuel, K., 2003. Human cord blood-derived cells can differentiate into hepatocytes in the mouse liver with no evidence of cellular fusion. Gastroenterology 124 (7), 1891–1900.

Patrawala, L., Calhoun-Davis, T., Schneider-Broussard, R., Tang, D.G., 2007. Hierarchical organization of prostate cancer cells in xenograft tumors: the CD44(+)alpha 2 beta 1(+) cell population is enriched in tumor-initiating cells. Cancer Res. 67 (14), 6796–6805.

Piccolo, F.M., Bagci, H., Brown, K.E., Landeira, D., Soza-Ried, J., Feytout, A., Mooijman, D., Hajkova, P., Leitch, H.G., Tada, T., Kriaucionis, S., Dawlaty, M.M., Jaenisch, R., Merkenschlager, M., Fisher, A.G., 2013. Different roles for Tet1 and Tet2 proteins in reprogramming-mediated erasure of imprints induced by EGC fusion. Mol. Cell 49 (6), 1023–1033.

Sakaida, I., Terai, S., Yamamoto, N., Aoyama, K., Ishikawa, T., Nishina, H., Okita, K., 2004. Transplantation of bone marrow cells reduces CCl4-induced liver fibrosis in mice. Hepatology 40 (6), 1304–1311.

Siddique, H.R., Parray, A., Tarapore, R.S., Wang, L., Mukhtar, H., Karnes, R.J., Deng, Y., Konety, B.R., Saleem, M., 2013. BMI1 polycomb group protein acts as a master switch for growth and death of tumor cells: regulates TCF4-transcriptional factor-induced BCL2 signaling. PLoS One 8 (5), e60664.

Silva, J., Chambers, I., Pollard, S., Smith, A., 2006. Nanog promotes transfer of pluripotency after cell fusion. Nature 441 (7096), 997–1001.

Skelley, A.M., Kirak, O., Suh, H., Jaenisch, R., Voldman, J., 2009. Microfluidic control of cell pairing and fusion. Nat. Methods 6, 147–152.

Strömberg, A., Ryttsen, F., Chiu, D.T., Davidson, M., Eriksson, P.S., Wilson, C.F., Orwar, O., Zare, R.N., 2000. Manipulating the genetic identity and biochemical surface properties of individual cells with electric-field-induced fusion. Proc. Natl. Acad. Sci. U.S.A. 97, 7–11.

Sukhorukov, V.L., Reuss, R., Endter, J.M., Fehrmann, S., Katsen-Globa, A., Gessner, P., Steinbach, A., Muller, K.J., Karpas, A., Zimmermann, U., Zimmermann, H., 2006. A biophysical approach to the optimisation of dendritictumour cell electrofusion. Biochem. Biophys. Res. Commun. 346, 829–839.

Tada, M., Tada, T., Lefebvre, L., Barton, S.C., Surani, M.A., 1997. Embryonic germ cells induce epigenetic reprogramming of somatic nucleus in hybrid cells. EMBO J. 16, 6510–6520.

Vassilopoulos, G., Wang, P.R., Russell, D.W., 2003. Nature 422, 901–904.

Visvader, J.E., Lindeman, G.J., 2008. Cancer stem cells in solid tumours: accumulating evidence and unresolved questions. Nat. Rev. Cancer 8 (10), 755–768.

Wagner, W., Ansorge, A., Wirkner, U., Eckstein, V., Schwager, C., Blake, J., Miesala, K., Selig, J., Saffrich, R., Ansorge, W., Ho, A.D., 2004. Molecular evidence for stem cell function of the slow-dividing fraction among human hematopoietic progenitor cells by genome-wide analysis. Blood 104 (3), 675–686.

Wang, R., Chen, S., Li, C., Ng, T.P., Kong, C.W., Cheng, J., Cheng, S.H., Li, R.A., Lo, C.M., Man, K., Sun, D., 2016. Fusion with stem cell makes the hepatocellular carcinoma cells similar to liver tumor-initiating cells. BMC Cancer 16 (56), 1–9.

Wang, X., Chen, S., Kong, M., Wang, Z., Costa, K.D., Li, R.A., Sun, D., 2011. Enhanced cell sorting and manipulation with combined optical tweezer and microfluidic chip technologies. Lab Chip 11, 3656–3662.

Wang, X., Chen, S., Chow, Y.T., Kong, C.W., Li, R.A., Sun, D., 2013. A microengineered cell fusion approach with combined optical tweezers and microwell array technologies. RSC Adv. 3, 23589–23595.

Wang, X.W., Seed, B., 2003. A PCR primer bank for quantitative gene expression analysis. Nucleic Acids Res. 31 (24), e154.

Wiegand, R., Weber, G., Zimmermann, K., Monajembashi, S., Wolfrum, J., Greulich, K., 1987. Laser-induced fusion of mammalian cells and plant protoplasts. J. Cell Sci. 88 (2), 145–149.

Wojcieszyn, J., Schlegel, R., Lumley-Sapanski, K., Jacobson, B.L.A., 1983. Studies on the mechanism of polytheylene glycol-mediated cell fusion using fluorescent membrane and cytoplasmic probes. J. Cell Biol. 96, 151–159.

Wu, Y., Sun, D., Huang, W., Xi, N., 2013. Dynamics analysis and motion planning for automated cell transportation with optical tweezers. IEEE/ASME Trans. Mechatron. 18 (2), 706–713.

Yamanaka, S., Blau, H.M., 2010. Nuclear reprogramming to a pluripotent state by three approaches. Nature 465 (7299), 704–712.

Yamashita, T., Wang, X.W., 2013. Cancer stem cells in the development of liver cancer. J. Clin. Invest. 123 (5), 1911–1918.

Yamashita, T., Kaneko, S., 2014. Orchestration of hepatocellular carcinoma development by diverse liver cancer stem cells. J. Gastroenterol. 49 (7), 1105–1110.

Yang, J., Zhao, L.P., Yin, Z.Q., Hu, N., Chen, J., Li, T.Y., Svir, I., Zheng, X.L., 2010. Chip-based cell electrofusion. Adv. Eng. Mater. 12, B398–B405.

Yao, J., Zhang, T., Ren, J., Yu, M., Wu, G., 2009. Effect of CD133/prominin-1 antisense oligodeoxynucleotide on in vitro growth characteristics of Huh-7 human hepatocarcinoma cells and U251 human glioma cells. Oncol. Rep. 22 (4), 781–787.

Zimmermann, U., 1982. Electric field-mediated fusion and related electrical phenomena. Biochim. Biophys. Acta 694 (3), 227–277.

Cell navigation and delivery in vivo

13

13.1 Introduction

Cell-based therapies have shown great potential to treat diseases (Segers and Lee, 2008; Aijaz et al., 2018). Compared with passive chemical methods such as those described by Felfoul et al. (2016) and Wen et al. (2019), cells can dynamically sense and respond to diseases, with fewer side effects experienced by the host (Labanieh et al., 2018). However, navigating and delivering therapeutic cells (such as stem cells) to the diseased site in vivo is a challenge. In cancer research, cancer cells are usually separated from the primary tumor and then transported to living animals by limiting dilution. An extreme challenge in conducting such research is the inability to accurately track individual cells in the body. These limitations hinder the further development of metastasis research (Oskarsson et al., 2014).

In earlier chapters, optical tweezers have been extensively used to manipulate single cells in vitro for various biomedical applications. However, there are few studies on precise cell manipulation in vivo. Zhong et al. (2013) demonstrated the use of optical tweezers for in vivo cell manipulation, in which red blood cells (RBCs) from living mice were transported to produce or eliminate thrombosis. Johnson et al. (2016) reported the optical manipulation of nanoparticles and cells in living zebrafish. The feasibility of using optical tweezers to trap nanoparticles adhered to cells in vivo to analyze the adhesion properties and membrane deformation was also been confirmed in animal models in their report. Jun et al. (2014) calibrated optical tweezers for force measurement in vivo. Compared with other manipulation tools, such as magnetic tweezers (Arcese et al., 2013), electron microscopes (Fukuda et al., 2009), and atomic force microscopes (Xie et al., 2009), optical tweezers have no special requirements for materials of the manipulated particles, and can provide a powerful noncontact force on cells with a size of 10 microns. Robot-assisted optical tweezers have been widely used in various cell manipulation tasks, such as cell transportation (Hu and Sun, 2011), cell pairing (Xie et al., 2014), cell sorting (Wang et al., 2011), and cell assembly (Yan et al., 2015). However, there are few reports in the literature on the application of robot-assisted optical tweezers in automated cell manipulation in vivo. Most optical trapping applications reported in in vivo studies are manually operated (such as Zhong et al., 2013 and Johansen et al., 2016). Manual manipulation of biological particles in the complex in vivo environment is restricted and affected by various disturbances and uncertainties. Using manual control, once the cells escape from the optical tweezers, it is difficult for the operator to retrieve the cells. This is because the cells quickly move away from the bloodstream, and it is almost impossible for a human operator to quickly find the missing cells.

Li et al. (2017b) studied the use of a robot-assisted optical tweezers manipulation system to automatically transport a single red blood cell (RBC) to the desired

Robotic Cell Manipulation. https://doi.org/10.1016/B978-0-323-85259-3.00008-8

destination in live zebrafish. Zebrafish represents a common cancer model and has been widely used in cancer research (Evensen et al., 2016). Using the concept of disturbance observer-based control (Pan et al., 2016; Li et al., 2018) designed an enhanced disturbance compensation controller to navigate cells in vivo. The controller treats the influence of blood flow as disturbance, which can be observed and compensated. When the trapped cell collides with other particles and deviates from its desired direction, the controller can switch the cell back to its original trajectory, thereby increasing the success rate of cell transportation. The steady-state error of cell motion can also be minimized by compensating for the disturbance caused by blood flow.

Compared to single-cell in vivo manipulation, multicell in vivo delivery is more meaningful and challenging for precision cell therapy. It is increasingly believe that the problem of multicell in vivo delivery can be solved by using specially designed microcarriers that allow cells to preferentially stay in the vascular circulation and retain cell function (Nelson et al., 2010; Stephan et al., 2015; Tang et al., 2018). The use of microrobots can enable the therapeutic dose of cells to access difficult-to-reach tissues or human cavities, making various medical treatments possible and minimally invasive (Li et al., 2017a). To ensure that these cell-loaded microrobots can be accurately guided to the desired location, in vivo imaging technology is required to visually track the cell-loaded microrobots during tissue routing (Medina-Sánchez and Schmidt, 2017). After performing tasks in vivo, these microrobots should ideally be removed or degraded (Sitti, 2018).

Microrobots can be driven by different power supply methods (Ceylan et al., 2017; Park et al., 2016; Williams et al., 2014; Palagi et al., 2016). Among them, the magnetic field method has the advantages of insensitivity to biological tissues and noncontact precise positioning. Several microtransporters have been developed to efficiently manipulate and transport cells (Yasa et al., 2019; Tottori et al., 2012), which include 3D porous microstructures designed to improve the ability to carry cells (Jeon et al., 2019), and the use of 3D porous structure microrobots to deliver cells in vivo through a gradient magnetic field has been reported (Li et al., 2018). It is worth noting that many microrobots developed use biocompatible but nondegradable materials (Steager et al., 2013). Some microrobots are made of synthetic composite materials or extracts and have undergone in vitro degradability tests (Wang et al., 2018; Yan et al., 2017; Ceylan et al., 2019). Despite these progresses, research on degradable microrobots for in vivo applications remains in its infancy.

Traceability is another challenging problem for real-time tracking and precise navigation of microrobots in vivo. Fluorescence imaging allows the visibility of decorative microrobots, but this method is only applicable to shallow tissues (Hong et al., 2017). Magnetic resonance imaging can image microrobots, but the driving and imaging magnetic fields must be separated, and the real-time imaging speed may not be fast enough (Lu et al., 2017). The use of radiation imaging techniques (such as X-ray computed tomography) to track macroscopic structures has been studied, but long-term ionizing radiation is carcinogenic (Iacovacci et al., 2019). Ultrasound (US) imaging is affected by strong interference signals from the background (Ahmed et al., 2017). Photoacoustic (PA) imaging detects optical absorption contrast at high resolution (Liba and de la Zerda, 2017), and has recently been used to detect the movement of microrobots in the intestines of mice (Wu et al., 2019).

Wei et al. (2020) reported the development of a degradable and image-guided microrobot to realize automatic navigation in vascular tissue for cell delivery, driven by an external gradient magnetic field actuation system. The microrobot has a burr-like porous spherical structure and is made of synthetic composite materials with degradability, mechanical strength, and magnetic actuation ability. Through the use of unique PA imaging technology, microrobots can be seen in tissues up to a few centimeters in depth. Preclinical tests on nude mice with orthotopic liver tumor have shown that the engineered stem cells released from microrobots on-site can significantly reduce tumor growth. This study revealed the use of degradable microrobots to transport and deliver therapeutic cells to the target site, and demonstrated their therapeutic effect on orthotopic liver tumors in mice.

The remainder of this chapter introduces the three main approaches to cell navigation and delivery in vivo. The first approach is to use optical tweezers-based manipulators and a disturbance compensation controller to transport single cells in vivo (Li et al., 2017b). The second approach is to develop magnetic microrobots for carrying and delivering cells in vivo (Li et al., 2018). The third approach is to use magnetic and image-guided degradable microrobots to accurately deliver engineered stem cells for cancer treatment applications (Wei et al., 2020).

13.2 In vivo navigation of single cells with an optical tweezers-based manipulator

In this section, a robot-assisted optical tweezers-based manipulation technology is introduced, which can transport a single biological cell in vivo. An enhanced disturbance compensation controller is used to minimize the influence of fluid (such as blood flow) on cells. This method has the advantages of online adjustment of cell tracking trajectory and the ability to minimize steady-state errors and eliminate overshoot.

13.2.1 Manipulation system for in vivo cell navigation

The earlier chapters introduced the cell manipulation system equipped with holographic optical tweezers (HOT). The system consists of three modules: execution, sensing, and control. Fig. 13.1 shows a schematic of the entire manipulation system, in which a 30-h postfertilization (hpf) zebrafish is used for in vivo testing. The target cells in the zebrafish can be imaged by the microscope of HOT and a CCD camera, and the image is transmitted to a computer for visual processing. The program can identify and detect moving cells in the body through a series of image-processing steps. The expected position of the optical trap can be calculated by the controller based on the measured cell position, and then transmitted to the spatial light modulator (SLM) to generate the optical trap.

Accurate measurement of cell position is necessary for the in vivo control system. In contrast to in vitro applications, the images showing the in vivo environment are chaotic, so it is difficult to extract cells from a single frame. Fig. 13.2 illustrates the extraction of RBCs from the blood vessel background.

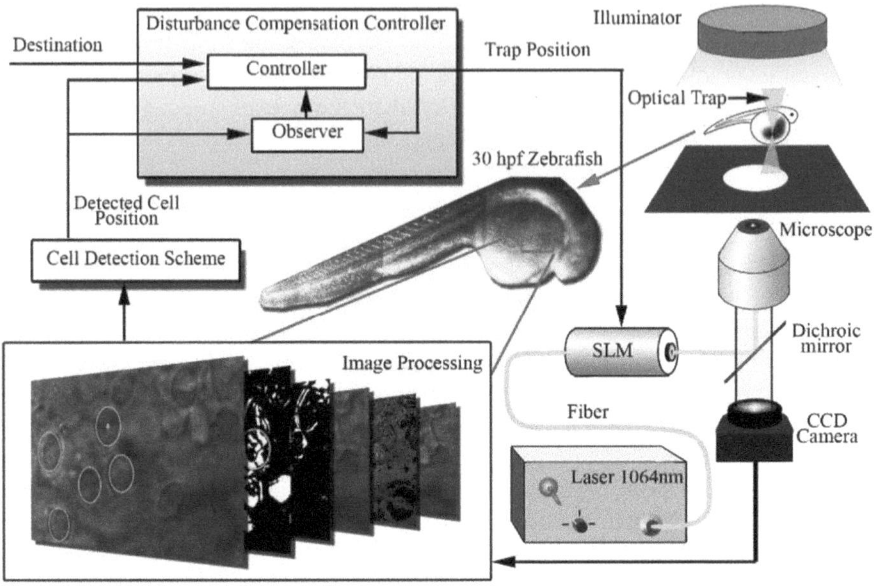

Figure 13.1 Schematic of the entire manipulation system (Li et al., 2017b).

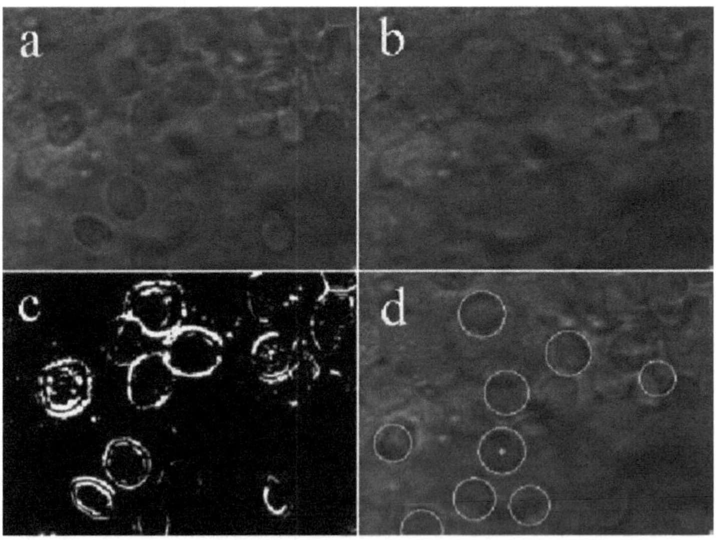

Figure 13.2 Image processing steps (Li et al., 2017b). (a) The cell image obtained by the CCD camera. (b) Image background. (c) The image of moving cells. (d) The cell position identified by the Hough transform technique.

The cell image obtained by the CCD camera is shown in Fig. 13.2A, which can be expressed as a matrix $O(k) \in \mathbb{R}^{W \times H \times 3}$ constituted by $W \times H$ vector elements $o_{x,y}(k) \in \mathbb{R}^{1 \times 3}$, which represents the red–green–blue intensity value of the pixel located at

(x, y). $k \in \mathbb{N}$ is the frame number. W and H are the width and height of the image, respectively. The image background in Fig. 13.2B can be expressed as $B(k) \in \mathbb{R}^{W \times H \times 3}$, and the vector elements can be expressed as:

$$b_{x,y}(k) = \begin{cases} \tau b_{x,y}(k-1) + (1-\tau) o_{x,y}(k), \\ \left\| o_{x,y}(k) - o_{x,y}(k-1) \right\| \leq T_b \\ \quad b_{x,y}(k-1), \\ \left\| o_{x,y}(k) - o_{x,y}(k-1) \right\| > T_b \end{cases} \tag{13.1}$$

where T_b is the positive threshold, and $0 \leq \tau < 1$ is the proportional coefficient. The background is usually initialized with $B(0) = 1$.

The comparison between the original image $O(k)$ and the background $B(k)$ shows that the image of moving cells in Fig. 13.2C can be denoted as $N(k) \in \mathbb{R}^{W \times H \times 1}$, and the vector elements can be obtained as follows:

$$n_{x,y}(k) = \begin{cases} \left\| b_{x,y}(k) - o_{x,y}(k) \right\|, & \left\| b_{x,y}(k) - o_{x,y}(k) \right\| \geq T_c \\ 0, & \left\| b_{x,y}(k) - o_{x,y}(k) \right\| \geq T_c \end{cases}, \tag{13.2}$$

where T_c is the positive threshold.

Furthermore, the cell position in Fig. 13.2D can be identified by the Hough transform technique. In the experiments, the blood flow velocity is less than 6×10^{-5} m/s, and the capture rate is 20 Hz. The cell movement distance between two adjacent frames is less than 3 μm, which is slightly smaller than the radius of the tracked cell, that is, 4–5 μm. Therefore, cells can be easily tracked by finding the nearest cell in the next frame. As the velocity of blood flow increases, the method can still be used by increasing the capture rate.

13.2.2 Controller design

Based on Chapter 12, the force equilibrium equation of the trapped cell can be expressed as follows:

$$0 = F_{\text{trap}} - F_{\text{drag}}, \tag{13.3}$$

where F_{trap} is the optical trapping force, and F_{drag} is the viscous drag force. According to Stokes' law, the drag force exerted on the cell can be calculated as

$$F_{\text{drag}} = \beta\left(\dot{q} - v_b\right), \tag{13.4}$$

where β is the drag coefficient and defined in Chapter 5, q and $\dot{q}$ denote the position and velocity of the cell, and v_b is the blood velocity. When the cell is located within the optical trap, the trapping force is appropriately described as

$$F_{\text{trap}} = kd_o, d_o \leq r_0, \tag{13.5}$$

where k is the stiffness of the optical trap, $d_o = l - q$ represents the deviation (or offset) of the cell from the center of the trap, $l \in R^{2\times 1}$ is the position of the optical trap, trap, and r_0 is the critical offset when the trapping force is maximum. Substituting Eqs. (13.4) and (13.5) into Eq. (13.3) yields the following equation:

$$\dot{q} = \frac{k}{\beta} d_o + v_b. \tag{13.6}$$

If the disturbance is defined as an equivalent offset of the optical trap caused by the blood flow, it can be expressed as $\varepsilon = \overline{\beta} v_b$, where $\overline{\beta} = \frac{\beta}{k}$. Then, Eq. (13.6) can be expressed as

$$\dot{q} = \frac{1}{\overline{\beta}}(d_o + \varepsilon). \tag{13.7}$$

The measured cell position is denoted as $\widetilde{q} \in \mathbb{R}^{2\times 1}$. Taking the measurement noise in the imaging process into account, $\widetilde{q}$ includes the true value and error, expressed as

$$\widetilde{q} = q + \omega, \tag{13.8}$$

where $\omega \in \mathbb{R}^{2\times 1}$ is the measurement error.

To reduce the influence of measurement error ω on the observer while ensuring the convergence speed of the observer, an observer with variable parameter is proposed as follows:

$$\begin{cases} \dot{x} = Ax + Bu \\ \widetilde{\varepsilon} = x + Du \end{cases} \tag{13.9}$$

where

$$\begin{cases} A = -\alpha I \\ B = \left[(\alpha - \alpha^2 \overline{\beta}) I \quad -\alpha I \right] \\ D = \left[\alpha \overline{\beta} I \quad 0 \right] \end{cases} \tag{13.10}$$

$$\alpha = \alpha_0 e^{-\gamma / \left\| \widetilde{\varepsilon} + \boldsymbol{d}_o - \overline{\beta} \dot{q} \right\|} \tag{13.11}$$

$$u = \begin{bmatrix} \widetilde{q} \\ l \end{bmatrix} \tag{13.12}$$

Note that x in Eq. (13.9) represents the observer status, and $\widetilde{\varepsilon}$ is the observer output representing the estimated value of the disturbance ε. α is a variable parameter, and it will decrease as the disturbance estimate $\widetilde{\varepsilon}$ approaches the true value ε. α_0 and γ are positive real numbers. In addition, the choice of the parameters α_0 and γ affects the performance of the observer and the trajectory of cell transportation. The larger the parameter α_0, the faster the convergence speed of the observer. A large parameter γ will help reduce the steady-state error of the observer.

The observer state can be initialized at the beginning of the operation, as follows:

$$x = \widetilde{\varepsilon}_0 - \alpha \overline{\beta} \widetilde{q} \tag{13.13}$$

where $\widetilde{\varepsilon}_0$ is the initial value of the estimated disturbance and is usually given as:

$$\widetilde{\varepsilon}_0 = b \overline{\beta} v_b \tag{13.14}$$

where b is a positive real number. Parameter b affects the observer's initial value, which in turn affects the initial direction of the trajectory, and can be selected within the range of $[1, 5]$.

Li et al. (2017b) has proved that the disturbance observer Eq. (13.9) gives rise to $\widetilde{\varepsilon} \to \varepsilon$ as time $t \to \infty$, under the condition that the observation error ω is zero and the blood flow velocity v_b is a constant vector. The case of $\omega \neq 0$ will be discussed in the remainder of this chapter. In the real in vivo environment, the blood flow velocity v_b changes significantly in the arteries, but does not change much in the veins and capillaries. Therefore, this condition can be valid if cells are transported in veins and capillaries.

When the offset d_o is greater than the critical value r_0, the cell can easily escape from the optical trap during the manipulation (Hu and Sun, 2011). To ensure that $d_o \leq r_0$, the following nonlinear saturation function is introduced:

$$f_\sigma(x) = \frac{\|x\| + \sigma - \left| \|x\| - \sigma \right|}{2\|x\|} x \tag{13.15}$$

where $x \in \mathbb{R}^{2\times 1}$ is the argument of the saturation function, and σ is the upper bound of $\|f_\sigma(x)\|$. Based on Eq. (13.15), the enhanced disturbance compensation controller is designed as follows:

$$\widetilde{l} = \widetilde{q} + f_{r_0}\left(f_{r_0}\left(\widetilde{e}\right) - f_{\phi r_0}\left(\widetilde{\varepsilon}\right)\right) \tag{13.16}$$

$$\widetilde{e} = q^d - \widetilde{q} = e - \omega \tag{13.17}$$

where $\widehat{l}$ denotes the expected position of the optical trap, $e = q^d - q$ denotes the error between the desired and actual positions of the cell, $\widetilde{e}$ denotes the estimated value of the error e, and $\phi \geq 1$ is a positive real number.

Li et al. (2017b) have proved that the controller Eq. (13.17) gives rise to $e \rightarrow 0$ as time $t \rightarrow \infty$, provided that the observation error $\omega = 0$, the observer output $\widetilde{\varepsilon} = \varepsilon$, and the disturbance $\|\varepsilon\| \langle r_0$.

13.2.3 Experiments

Experiments were performed to track RBCs in 30 hpf zebrafish to demonstrate the effectiveness of the proposed controller. The RBCs of zebrafish before 48 hpf are regularly spherical, and easy to identify and control. Fig. 13.3 shows the venous sinuses (depth range from 10 to 60 μm) of zebrafish undergoing cell movement experiments. Since zebrafish are transparent, the depth limit of optical tweezers can reach ~120 μm, which is greater than the depth limit of mice (~60 μm) (Zhong et al., 2013). Therefore, cell transport in zebrafish is not affected by the depth limitation of optical tweezers. The experiment process is described as follows: First, the program searches for cells around the initial position; then, the identified cells are driven to the destination by the proposed controller and reach a stable state; finally, the optical trap returns to the initial position for another experiment. Each transport test

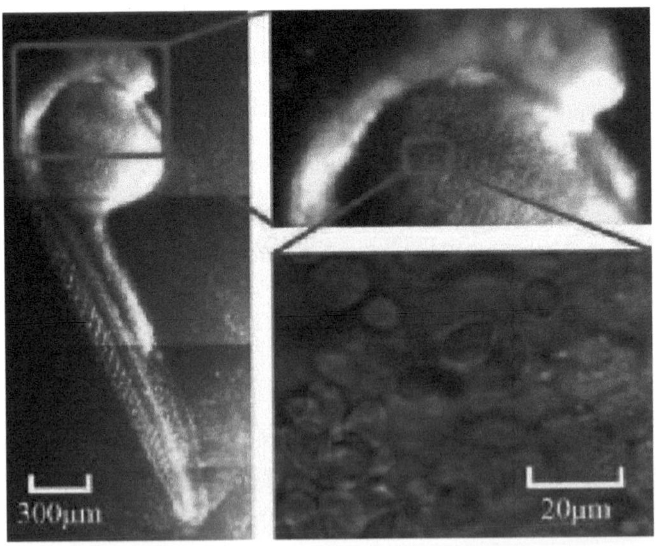

Figure 13.3 Venue of the cell movement experiment in the yolk of zebrafish (Li et al., 2017b).

is repeated more than 30 times. The laser output power in all experiments is set to 3 W (approximately 450 mW in the sample), which can provide 20 pN optical trapping power without causing significant thermal damage to the cells. In the experiment, two kinds of controllers, namely enhanced disturbance compensation controller and common position feedback (P-type) controller are implemented for comparison. The results of two sets of experiments are reported.

The environmental parameters in the first group of experimental results are: the flow velocity at the initial position is estimated to be $(-0.9254, -0.9623)\times 10^{-5}$ m/s, and the parameter $\overline{\beta}$ is estimated to be 0.125 s. The initial position of the trapped cell is $(0.7026, 0.4186) \times 10^{-4}$ m, the destination coordinate is $(0.2730, 0.3256) \times 10^{-4}$ m, and the measurement error is 1–2 μm. The parameters of the proposed controller are $b = 2$, $\alpha_0 = 0.5$, $\phi = 2$, and $\gamma = 3\times 10^{-7}$, and the parameter of the P-type controller is $k_p = 1$. The cell transport was repeated 10 times. Table 13.1 shows the average steady-state error and travel time for each trial. The average steady-state error is calculated by $\int_\Sigma \|e\| dt / \int_\Sigma 1 dt$, where t represents the time and $\Sigma = \{t \big| \|e\| < 1 \times 10^{-5}\}$. Using the proposed controller, nine cells successfully reached the destination, and one cell failed. Using the P-type controller, only six cells reached the destination, and four cells failed. This result confirms that the proposed controller can achieve a high success rate in transportation. Fig. 13.4 illustrates the position errors under the proposed controller and the P-type control of one trial for comparison. The travel time under the proposed controller is 3.31 s, which is less than the 4.78 s under the P-type controller. The average steady-state error under the proposed controller is 1.93 μm, which is less than the 2.90 μm under the P-type controller. Fig. 13.5 shows the cell transport trajectories with 10 experimental trials under the proposed disturbance compensation controller and the P-type controller, respectively. Obviously, the trajectory generated by the proposed controller is initially perpendicular to the flow direction and then turns to the destination. This phenomenon indicates that the proposed controller can keep the cells away from the cell flow at the beginning, and then successfully drive the cells to the destination.

The environmental parameters in the second group of experiments are: flow velocity at the initial position is $(-0.1389, -0.0851) \times 10^{-4}$ m/s, the estimated value of the parameter $\overline{\beta}$ is 0.125 s, the initial position coordinate of the trapped cell is $(0.6450, 0.2105) \times 10^{-4}$ m, and the destination coordinate is $(0.1334, 0.3905) \times 10^{-4}$ m. The parameters used for the proposal controller are $\phi = 2$ and $\gamma = 3 \times 10^{-7}$. Fig. 13.6 shows the experimental process of cell transportation with collision. The parameters of the proposed controller are $b = 2.5$ and $\alpha_0 = 0.2$. The control can manipulate the cell back to its original trajectory after colliding with other cells. Fig. 13.7 illustrates the cell transportation process under the proposed controller with three sets of parameters, namely $b = 1.5$ and $\alpha_0 = 0.2$, $b = 1.5$ and $\alpha_0 = 1$, $b = 0.5$ and $\alpha_0 = 0.2$, and a P-type controller ($k_p = 1$). As shown from

Table 13.1 Average steady-state error and travel time (Li et al., 2017b).

Experiments		1	2	3	4	5	6	7	8	9	10	Mean
Disturbance compensation controller	Average steady-state error (μm)	2.53	Fail	1.91	3.45	2.47	3.38	2.41	2.27	1.64	1.93	2.44
	Travel time (s)	5.80	Fail	4.30	3.72	6.34	5.73	6.08	3.47	4.77	3.31	4.84
P-type controller	Average steady-state error (μm)	2.90	3.94	Fail	3.14	2.41	2.14	Fail	Fail	Fail	2.89	2.90
	Travel time (s)	4.78	4.14	Fail	4.60	4.46	7.88	Fail	Fail	Fail	6.56	5.40

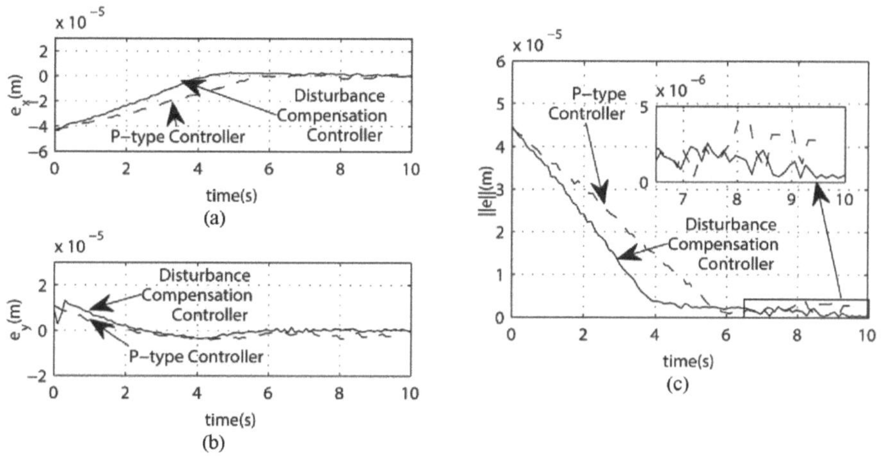

Figure 13.4 Position errors in cell transportation experiments (Li et al., 2017b). (A) Position error in x-axis. (B) Position error in y-axis. (C) The norm of the position error.

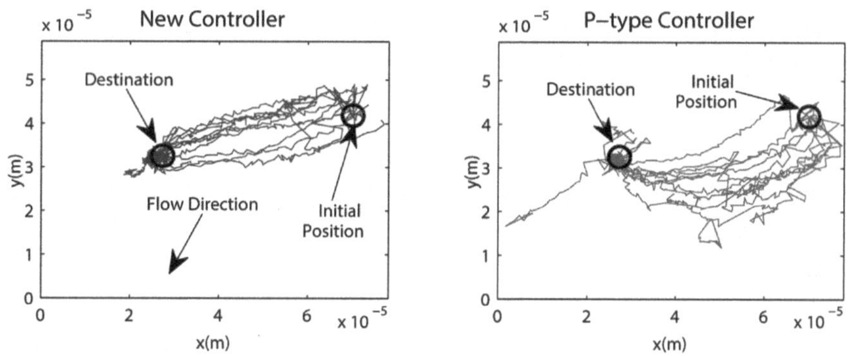

Figure 13.5 Cell transport trajectories (Li et al., 2017b).

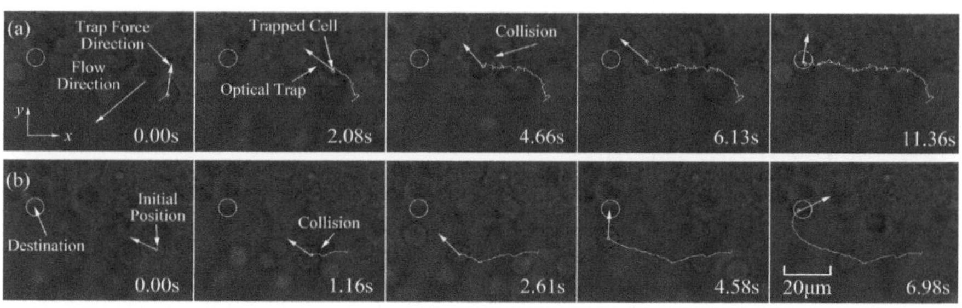

Figure 13.6 Cell transportation with collision (Li et al., 2017b). (A) Results under the disturbance compensation controller with $b = 2.5$ and $\alpha_0 = 0.2$. (B) Results under the P-type controller.

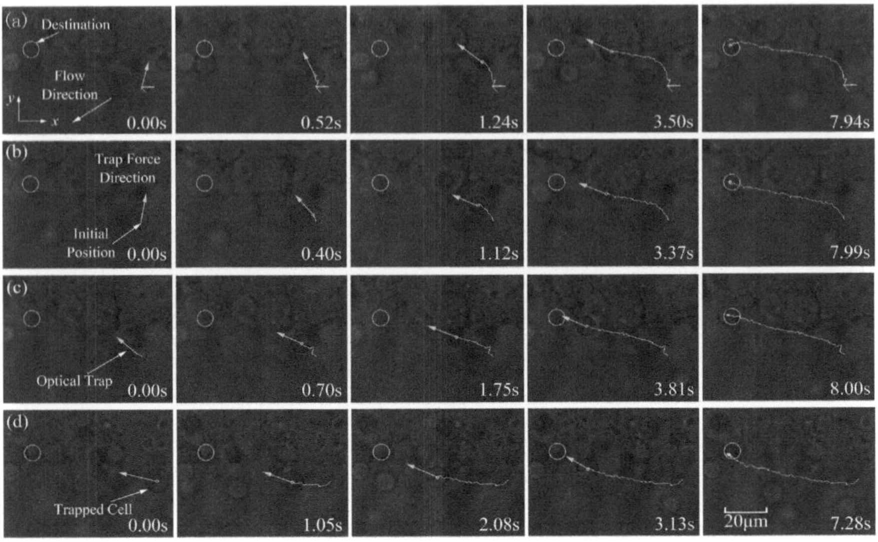

Figure 13.7 Cell transportation with different parameters (Li et al., 2017b). (A) Results under the disturbance compensation controller with $b = 1.5$ and $\alpha_0 = 0.2$. (B) Results under the disturbance compensation controller with $b = 1.5$ and $\alpha_0 = 1$. (C) Results under the disturbance compensation controller with $b = 0.5$ and $\alpha = 0.2$. (D) Results under the P-type controller.

the comparison of the initial trap force direction in Fig. 13.7C ($b = 0.5$) and that in Fig. 13.7A and B ($b = 1.5$), the increase of the b value makes the initial direction of cell movement deviate from the flow direction more significantly. Furthermore, the increased value of α minimizes the curvature of the trajectory. The steady-state error of the proposed controller with the three sets of parameters is similar, and they are all considerably lower than that under the P-type controller.

13.3 Magnetic microrobot for carrying and delivering cells in vivo

In this section, the design of magnetic microrobots that can carry and deliver cells in vivo is introduced.

13.3.1 Microrobot design

The designed microrobot employs a burr-like porous spherical structure to enhance magnetic drive and cell-carrying capacity. Fig. 13.8A shows the structural design of the microrobot before and after cell seeding. The distance between two burrs, expressed as the grid length (l_g), is determined based on the size of the cell carried. The length of each burr is denoted as the burr length (l_b), which is the same as the cell radius (r_c). The diameter (D) of the entire structure including burrs is determined

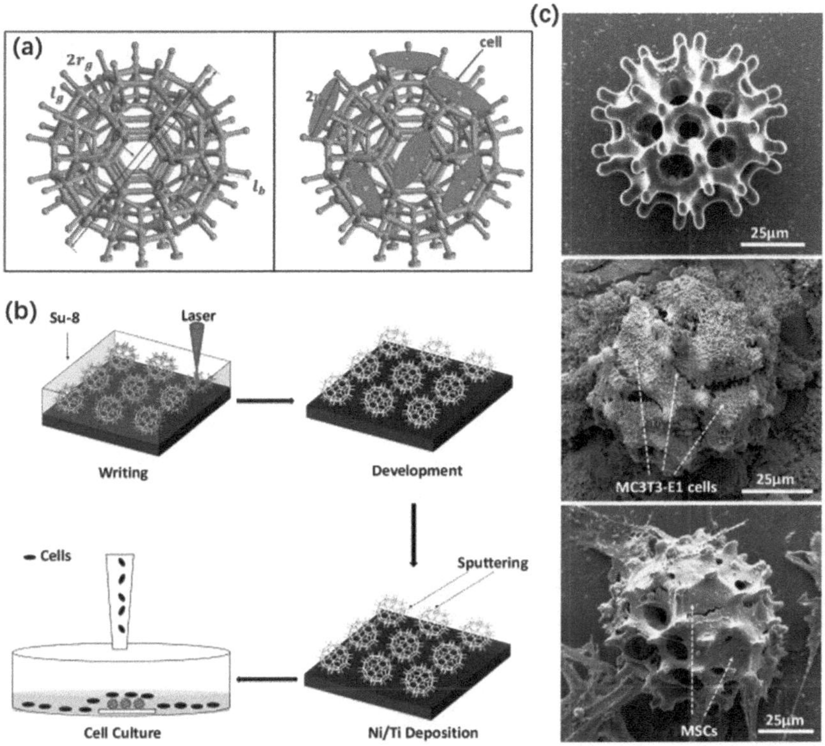

Figure 13.8 Design and fabrication of magnetic microrobots (Li et al., 2018). (A) Images of the designed burr-like porous spherical microrobot before and after cell seeding. (B) Fabrication procedures of the microrobots including writing, developing, Ni/Ti deposition, and cell culture process. (C) SEM images of a burr-like microrobot cultured with MC3T3-E1 cells and MSCs for 12 h. The laser power and scan speed of photoresist were set at 25 mW and 250 μm/s, respectively.

according to l_g, l_b, r_c, and the grid radius (r_g), which usually ranges between 70 and 100 μm for different cell types. Fig. 13.8B illustrates the fabrication process of the microrobot, including the steps of writing, developing, Ni/Ti deposition, and cell culture on the microrobot. Both l_g and l_b can be adjusted using 3D laser lithography to suit different cell types. Fig. 13.8C shows the scanning electron microscopy (SEM) image of the microrobot, in which MC3T3-E1 cells and mesenchymal stem cells (MSCs) are successfully cultured on the robot at a concentration of 1×10^6 cells/mL after 12 h. This robot design is justified as follows.

First, the spherical structure has the advantage of enhanced magnetic drive capability, in addition to that it can easily fuse the microrobot with the host tissue to promote the transfer of cells from the robot to the tissue (Danilevicius et al., 2015; Mironov et al., 2009; Agrawal et al., 2014). When the microrobot moves in blood vessels, the magnetic field gradient force is proportional to the thickness and cross-sectional area of the magnetically conductive material coated on the surface of the

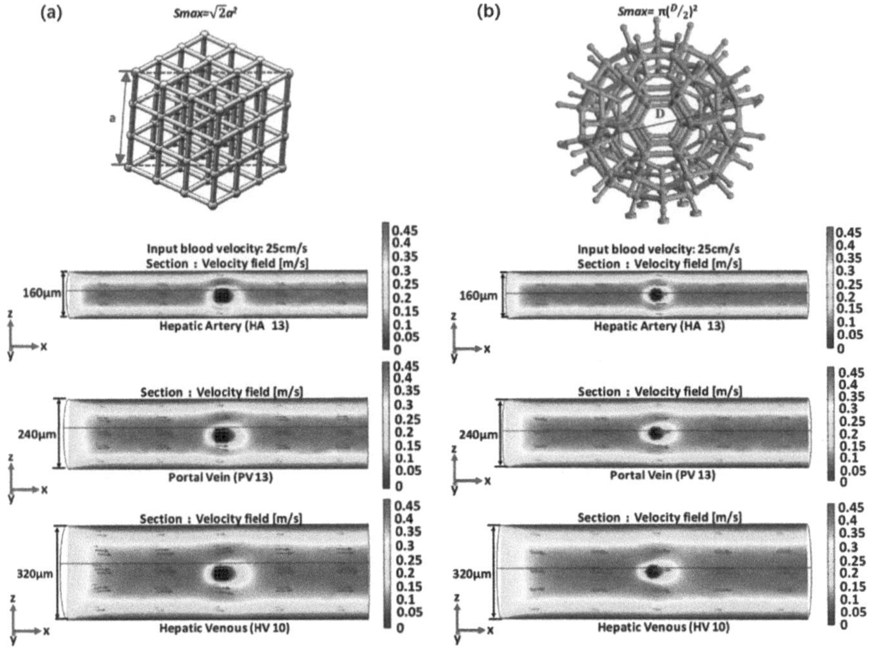

(c)

Ratios of surface area to viscous resistance of the structure(mm^2/N)	HA 13 Diameter: 160μm	PV 13 Diameter: 240μm	HV 10 Diameter: 320μm
Cubic structure Side length: 37μm Surface area: $0.010mm^2$	2801	3830	4315
Burr-like spherical structure Diameter: 50μm Surface area: $0.007mm^2$	3478	4320	4665

Figure 13.9 Simulation results of magnetic driving ability in hepatic artery, portal vein, and hepatic vein (Li et al., 2018). (A) Velocity fields of a cubic structure. (B) Velocity fields of a burr-like spherical structure. (C) Surface area-to-viscous resistance ratios of the two micro-robot structures.

robot, and it must be large enough to overcome the viscous resistance. Fig. 13.9A shows the numerical study results of the 3D cubic geometry and the spherical structure using the finite element method (Kim et al., 2013). The maximum cross-sectional area of the two robots with different structures is the same for easy comparison. Under the same coating thickness, the magnetic force increases with the increase in the surface area, and the increase in the ratio of the surface area to viscous resistance indicates an increase in the magnetic drive capability. Therefore, the surface area-to-resistance ratio can be used as a criterion for judging the magnetic drive capability. Similar to the study of Debbaut et al. (2014), hepatic artery, portal vein, and hepatic vein vessels with diameters of 160, 240, and 320 μm can be used, respectively. The flow velocity is uniformly set to 25 cm/s, which corresponds to normal hepatic artery and portal vein blood flow (Nakai et al., 2002). Fig. 13.9B illustrates the simulation results of the cross-sectional velocity fields of cubic and spherical structures in different environments. The calculation of the surface area-to-resistance ratio of the two structures is shown in Fig. 13.9C. The ratio of the proposed robot structure is higher than that of the cubic structure, which means that the designed robot with a spherical structure exhibits a stronger magnetic drive capability.

Second, the porous spherical structure can improve cell-carrying capacity. The porous scaffold structure mimics the extracellular matrix and can easily supply the nutrients needed for tissue vascularization, resulting in functional tissues and organs (Rouwkema et al., 2008; Ma, 2008) and cell growth (Hollister, 2005). The scaffold structure of fullerenes is characterized by the combination of pentagons and hexagons in the grid, which can facilitate cell attachment compared with triangular and square structures (Kawano et al., 2014). Using this porous scaffold, when the length of the grid is similar to the radius of the cells carried, the cell-loading capacity can be maximized. The size of the entire microrobot is mainly determined by the following two requirements in its application. The first requirement is effective cell loading, that is, the microrobots must have a large enough size that each robot can carry and deliver at least dozens of cells. The second requirement is efficient access. The microrobot should not be so large that the cell culture robot can enter various blood vessels. For example, the average diameter of the thinnest hepatic artery is 160 μm (Debbaut et al., 2014). To balance the above two requirements, choose the structure of the buckyball (C_{60}) for the proposed microrobot design, and the ratio of l_g to the structure diameter (D_o) is 1:4.8. Then determine the diameter of the entire microrobot as $D = D_o + 2l_b = 4.8(l_g + 2r_g) + 2r_g + 2l_b$. When the cell radius r_c is known, l_g is the key parameter to determine the cell-carrying capacity. Fig. 13.10A illustrates the

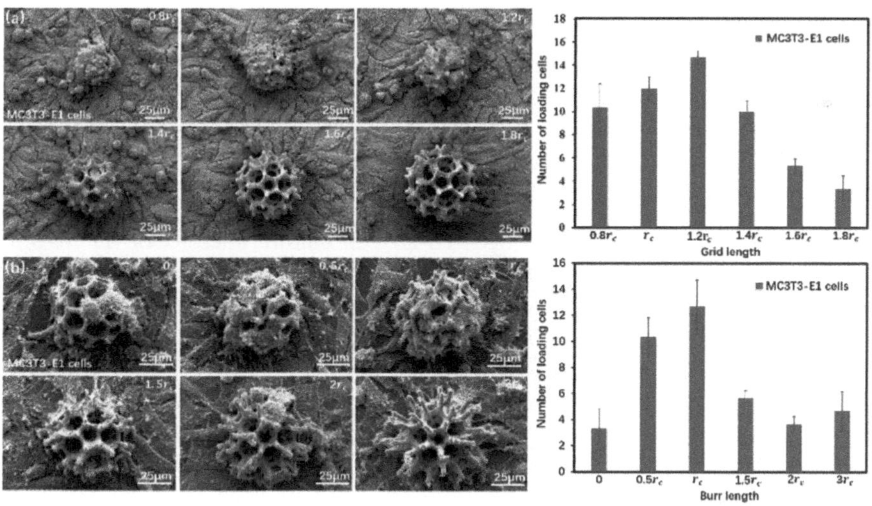

Figure 13.10 Microrobots with different cell-carrying capacities under different grid length (l_g) and burr length (l_b) (Li et al., 2018). (A) SEM images and statistical results of cell-cultured microrobots when $l_g = 0.8r_c, r_c, 1.2r_c, 1.4r_c, 1.6r_c, 1.8r_c$, where r_c is the mean radius of carried cells ($n = 3$). (B) SEM images and statistical results of cell-cultured microrobots when $l_b = 0, 0.5r_c, r_c, 1.5r_c, 2r_c, 3r_c$ ($n = 3$).

experimental results of loading and culturing MC3T3-E1 cells ($r_c = 7.5$ μm) when $l_g = 0.8r_c, r_c, 1.2r_c, 1.4r_c, 1.6r_c, 1.8r_c$, where $l_b = r_c$ and the scaffold grid radius $r_g = 1$ μm. When $l_g = 1.2r_c$, the microrobot shows the best cell-carrying capacity. Using these selected parameters, the microrobot has a diameter of approximately 70 μm and is used to carry MC3T3-E1 cells. In a similar way, the microrobot has a diameter of approximately 90 μm and is used to carry MSCs ($r_c = 10$ μm).

Third, adding a burr-like structure to the porous spherical microrobot can further improve the cell-carrying capacity. According to the cell culture performance of microrobots fabricated on the same glass substrate (within 200 μm), compare spherical porous microrobots with different burr sizes. Each microrobot carries the same number of cells for cultivation. Fig. 13.10B illustrates the results of the experiment performed on MC3T3-E1 cells when $l_b = 0, 0.5r_c, r_c, 1.5r_c, 2r_c, 3r_c$, where $l_g = 1.2r_c$, which is based on the previous selection. When $l_b = r_c$, the microrobot shows the best cell-loading ability.

Through the viability test of MC3TE-E1 cells and MSCs, the influence of coating materials Ni and Ti on cell culture was studied. MC3TE-E1 cells and MSCs were cultured on Ni- and Ti-coated flat square glass. Cells cultured on clean glass without Ni and Ti coatings were used as controls. Before cell seeding, the glass substrate was sterilized with ultraviolet light. The SEM images of MC3T3-E1 cells and MSCs cultured on a glass substrate on days 1, 3, and 5 are shown in Fig. 13.11A and B. After coating the glass surface with Ti, the cells showed a good morphology and proliferated. The survival rates of the two types of cells on days 1, 3, and 5 are shown in Fig. 13.11C. The negative and positive signs represent the PI regions of live cells and dead cells, respectively. Fig. 13.11D shows a histogram of the average survival rates of the two types of cells. These data indicate that the Ni and Ti materials coated on the surface of the microrobot are not cytotoxic to MC3T3-E1 cells and MSCs, which can be proved by their easy adhesion to the robot structure and subsequent proliferation.

13.3.2 Transport of cell-cultured microrobots

First, the in vitro transportation of MC3T3-E1 cell culture microrobot ($D = 70$ μm) was carried out to reach the desired position, which was controlled by a visual position feedback controller. A self-built electromagnetic coil system was used to drive the cell culture microrobot. Fig. 13.12A shows a microrobot carrying cultured MC3T3-E1 cells, moving along a rectangular path to four desired positions a, b, c, and d. The phase contrast image of the microrobot carrying MC3T3-E1 cells is also shown in Fig. 13.12A. Fig. 13.12B shows that the translational velocity of the microrobot increases with the increase of the applied magnetic field gradient. The relationship is almost linear in three different fluid environments, including phosphate-buffered saline (PBS), artificial cerebrospinal fluid [140.0 mM $NaCl$/3.0 mM KCl/1.0 mM $MgCl_2$/1.3 mM $CaCl_2$/2.0 mM Na_2HPO_4/2.0 mM NaH_2PO_4/10.0 mM glucose (pH 7.4)] and mouse serum (from 6-week-old Balb/C nude mice centrifuged at 300 g for 3 min). The increase in volume magnetization leads to an increase in the moving speed

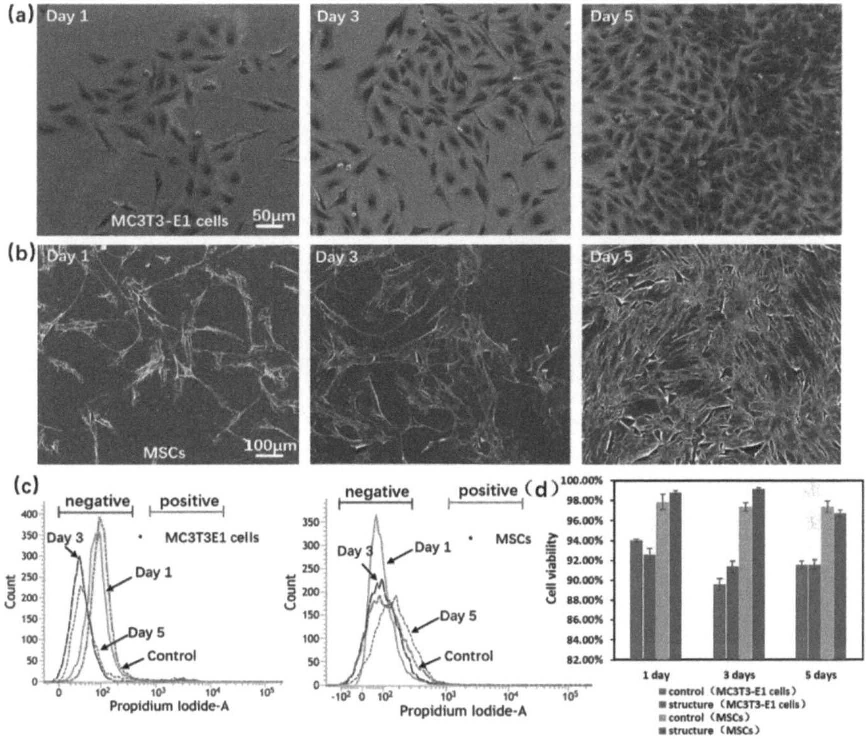

Figure 13.11 Cell viability tests (Li et al., 2018). SEM images of (A) MC3T3-E1 cells and (B) MSCs on days 1, 3, and 5 of culture. (C) Survival rates of MC3T3-E1 cells and MSCs in culture at 1, 3, and 5 days after PI staining. (D) Histogram representing the average viability of cells cultured for 1, 3, and 5 days ($n = 3$). Error bars indicate SD.

under the same magnetic gradient, which can be achieved by increasing the thickness of the coating material (Ni) (Kim et al., 2016). Fig. 13.12C illustrates that the position error of the cell culture microrobot when moving along the required rectangle converges to zero. In the experiment, the actual position of the robot was measured using image-processing technology, which includes three basic steps: threshold segmentation, connected region extraction, and position correlation (Li et al., 2017b). All data were obtained by repeating the experiment at least three times. The Reynolds number and related experimental parameters are shown in Table 13.2. The above results verify that the designed microrobot with cultured cells can be automatically and accurately transported to the desired location using the electromagnetic coil setup.

Then, the MSC-cultured microrobot ($D = 90$ μm) was transported in the yolk of the zebrafish embryo 30 h after fertilization. Zebrafish is widely used as an animal model due to its high genetic similarity to humans. The zebrafish's yolk is transparent, easy to monitor, and large enough for the movement of microrobots. The MSC-cultured microrobot was sucked by the air pressure of the needle tip and injected into the

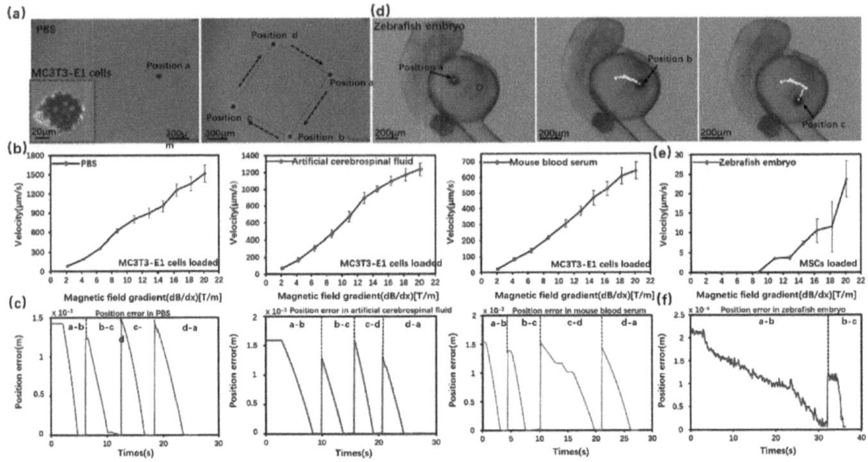

Figure 13.12 Control of a cell-cultured microrobot in vitro and in vivo (Li et al., 2018). (A) Movement of a microrobot cultured with MC3T3-E1 cells along a desired rectangular path in a clockwise direction in PBS. (B) Velocity of MC3T3-E1 cell-cultured microrobot against the magnetic field gradient in different fluid environments ($n = 4$). (C) Position errors of the MC3T3-E1 cell-cultured microrobot in different fluid environments (with a magnetic field gradient of 4–9 T/m). (D) Time-lapsed images of the MSC-cultured microrobot moving in the yolk of a zebrafish embryo. (E) Velocity of MSC-cultured microrobot against the magnetic field gradient in vivo ($n = 4$). (F) Positional errors of the MSC-cultured microrobot in vivo (with a magnetic field gradient of 20 T/m). Error bars indicate SD.

Table 13.2 The Reynolds numbers and related environmental parameters (Li et al., 2018).

		PBS	Artificial cerebrospinal fluid	Mouse blood serum
Density		0.998×10^3 kg/m^3	1.000×10^3 kg/m^3	1.050×10^3 kg/m^3
Robot maximum velocity		1.520×10^{-3} m/s	1.240×10^{-3} m/s	6.420×10^{-4} m/s
Dynamic viscosity μ		1.002×10^{-3} Pa s	1.230×10^{-3} Pa s	2.670×10^{-3} Pa s
Re	$D = 70$ μm	0.106	0.074	0.016
	$D = 90$ μm	0.136	0.095	0.021

yolk of the anesthetized zebrafish embryo. Fig. 13.12D shows the movement of the MSC-cultured microrobot in the yolk of zebrafish embryo from a to b and then from b to c. The heartbeat of the zebrafish can be clearly observed during the experiment, indicating that the zebrafish was still alive. Fig. 13.12E illustrates that the microrobot cannot move until the magnetic field gradient is large enough to overcome the threshold. Fig. 13.12F illustrates the position error of the microrobot. Due to the presence of biological macromolecules such as protein and nucleic acid in the zebrafish embryo's yolk, the velocity in the a–b interval was significantly slower than that in the b–c interval. Compared with other living environments, such as PBS, artificial cerebrospinal fluid, or mouse serum, the yolk of zebrafish embryos exhibits higher viscosity, greater viscous resistance, and uneven material distribution. Therefore, under the same gradient force, the navigation speed of the microrobot in the zebrafish embryo is much slower than in other media (Fig. 13.12B).

13.3.3 Delivery of cells from the microrobot to the site

After the cell-carrying microrobot reaches the destination, the transfer of the cells from the microrobot to the desired site determines the successful delivery of the cells of the designed microrobot. Cells, as living organisms, can be spontaneously released from microrobots to surrounding tissues. In order to verify this idea, first an in vitro experiment was performed to release cells from a microrobot onto a glass substrate. Fig. 13.13A shows a phase-contrast image of MC3T3-E1 cells carried by a microrobot in contact with a pure glass substrate. After the cells were cultured for 1 day, six 3T3 cells were released from the microrobot and firmly attached to the glass substrate. After the cells were cultured for 2 days, the released 3T3 cells differentiated, 11 of which

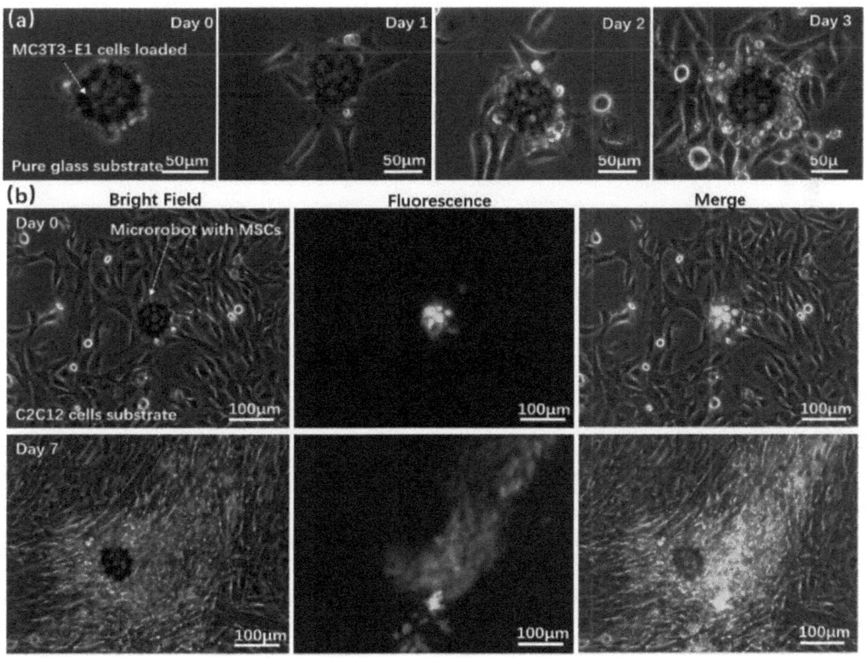

Figure 13.13 In vitro cell-release experiments on a glass substrate (Li et al., 2018). (A) MC3T3-E1 cells were released from the microrobot onto a pure glass substrate and proliferated at 3 days of cultivation. (B) MSCs transferred from the microrobot onto the glass substrate with precultured C2C12 cells at 7 days of cultivation.

were found on the glass substrate. After the cells were cultured for 3 days, 25 3T3 cells proliferated onto the substrate. These results confirm the successful delivery of microrobots and the growth of cells on the in vitro substrate. Then the microrobot carrying the cultured MSCs was placed on the glass substrate with precultured C2C12 cells to simulate the microtissue environment (Fig. 13.13B). The MSCs carried by the microrobot were labeled with the fluorescent reagent carboxyfluorescein diacetate succinimidyl ester (CFDA SE) before being released on the substrate. After 7 days of culture, the labeled MSCs proliferated on the substrate (Fig. 13.13B). These results once again verified that the cells carried by the developed microrobot can be successfully transferred to the desired site in vitro.

Second, an in vitro experiment was carried out, which involved the release of MC3T3-E1 cells from a microrobot in a microfluidic chip to simulate the transendothelial migration of released cells. The chip was composed of blood vessel-like microchannels that mimic the blood vessel network, an array of cell migration channels that mimic the endothelial layer, and tissue chambers that transport cells. Fig. 13.14A shows the schematic of the experiment, in which the cell culture microrobots were transferred along the microchannel to the docking area to release the cells, and the released cells reached the tissue chambers through the migration channels. Fig. 13.14B illustrates the experimental results of MC3T3-E1 cell migration across endothelium within 3 days. Some released cells were found in the tissue area, indicating that the released cells can successfully pass through the vascular endothelial layer to reach the target area.

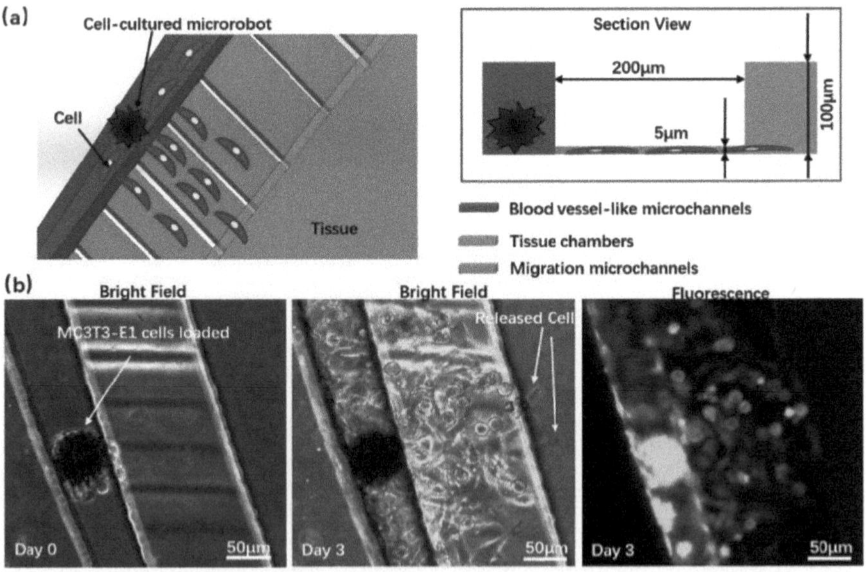

Figure 13.14 In vitro cell-release experiments in a microfluidic chip (Li et al., 2018). (A) Schematic of the cell-releasing process. (B) Results of the transendothelial migration of cells.

Finally, an in vivo experiment was performed to spontaneously release cells from the microrobots to the nude mouse. Since tumorigenic and tumor cells can be easily detected within a few weeks, HeLa cells were selected as sample cells to illustrate the in vivo release capability of the microrobot. A group of microrobots carrying HeLa GFP+ cells were injected subcutaneously into the left dorsum of nude mice. These cells were dispersed in 100 μL PBS and 100 μL Matrigel (1000 microrobots in 200 μL). The same number of microrobots without HeLa cells were also injected into the right dorsum of the same mouse as a control. After culturing for 4 weeks, the area of increased fluorescence intensity was clearly observed on the left dorsum of the mouse (Fig. 13.15A), indicating that the tumor was caused by the injection of HeLa cells. After injecting the microrobot without HeLa cells, no tumor was found on the right dorsum of the mouse. In order to verify that the tumor was caused by the HeLa cells released from the microrobot to the surrounding tissues, and not caused by the cells left on the microrobot, the mouse was sacrificed 4 weeks after the injection to obtain the in vivo histological results (Fig. 13.15B). The optical micrographs in these sections clearly show that the microrobots are located on the edge of the tumor tissue, which indicates that the tumor is formed by the HeLa cells released by the injected microrobot onto the tissue.

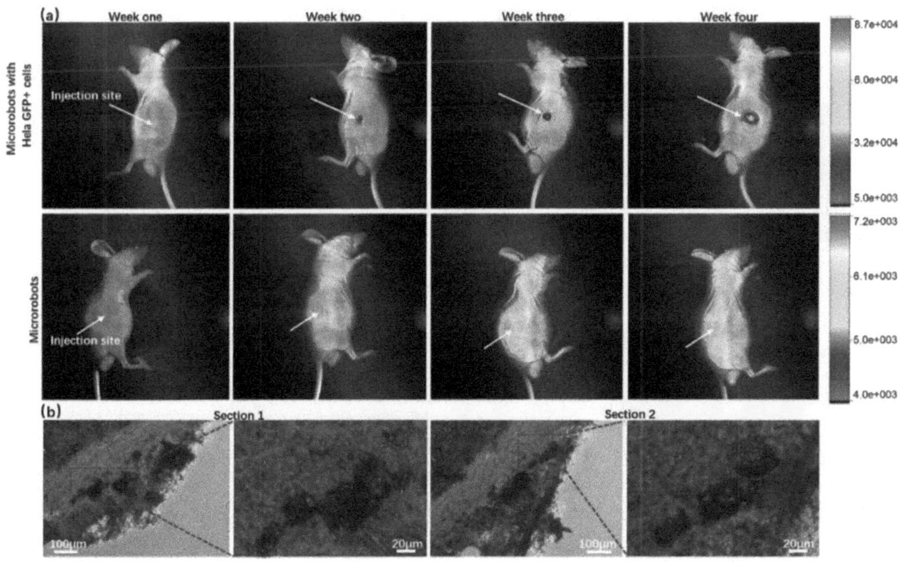

Figure 13.15 In vivo cell-release experiments on nude mice (Li et al., 2018). (A) In vivo fluorescence imaging of a swarm of microrobots. The microrobots with HeLa GFP+ cells were injected into the left dorsum of the nude mice. The microrobots not carrying any cells were injected into the right dorsum of the nude mice. The arrows represent the position of the injection. (B) Two different hematoxylin & eosin-stained sections of HeLa tumor with the injected microrobots. The positions of the microrobots are marked by the dashed lines.

13.4 Precise delivery of stem cells for cancer therapy using magnet-driven and image-guided degradable microrobots

13.4.1 Degradable microrobot design

Using the burr-like porous spherical structure shown in Fig. 13.16A, the microrobot can be made of degradable materials to potentially reduce immune activation and thrombosis. Polyethylene glycol (PEG) exhibits high mechanical strength and high resolution during the manufacturing process (Chin et al., 2017; Lee and Lee, 2017).

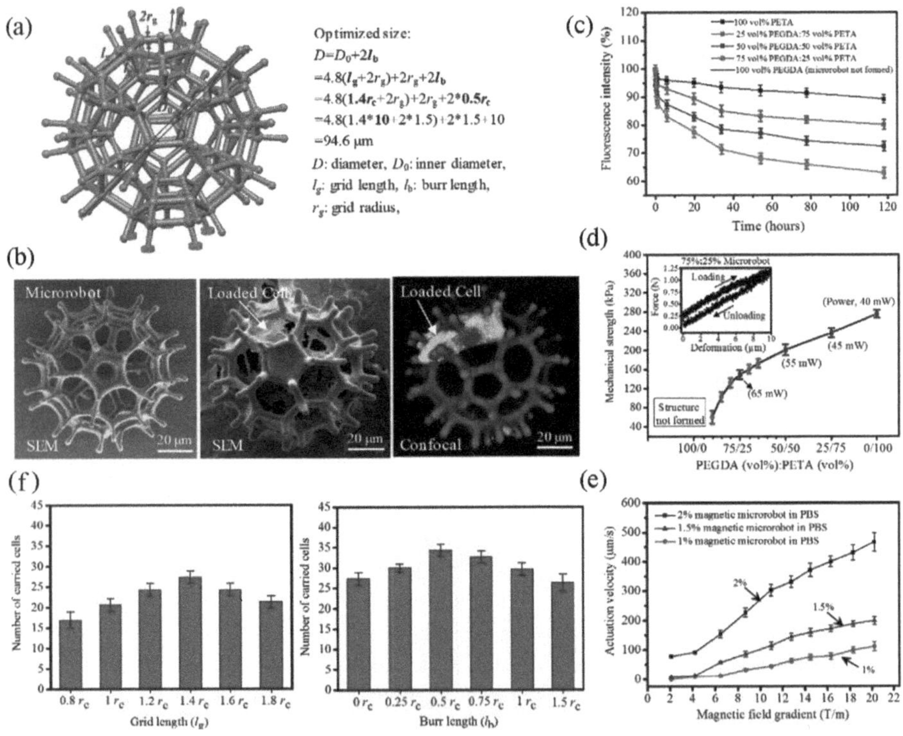

Figure 13.16 Degradable microrobot design and size determination (Wei et al., 2020). (A) Calculation of the model of the burr-like porous microrobot with optimized size. (B) SEM images of microrobot structure (left), cell-loaded microrobot (center), and confocal scan of GFP-MSCs cultured on the microrobot (right). In the confocal image, cell nuclei were stained with Hoechst 33,342. (C) Fluorescence intensity of microrobots with different compositions of PEGDA and PETA in PBS with time. (D) Mechanical strength of microrobots with different compositions of PEGDA and PETA. The inset shows the mechanical test of the microrobot in 75 vol%:25 vol% of PEGDA to PETA by deforming the microrobot by using measurable force. (E) Magnetic actuation test of microrobots with different compositions of super-paramagnetic particles with 75 vol% PEGDA and 25 vol% PETA. (F) Statistical results of MSC-loaded microrobots with different grid lengths (l_g) and burr lengths (l_b).

PEG is easily oxidized and can be oxidatively degraded by the ether framework under relevant biological conditions (Ulbricht et al., 2014). PEG diacrylate (PEGDA) is a derivative of PEG and has been used as a degradable material for various drug delivery and tissue engineering-based applications. The combination of PEGDA and pentaerythritol triacrylate (PETA) can be used to make microrobots while ensuring its degradability and mechanical strength. The composite can be hydrolyzed into small molecules, and the degradation products can be excreted from the body.

3D lithography can be used to manufacture microrobots made of synthetic composite materials. Fig. 13.16B shows an SEM image of the microrobot structure (left), the microrobot loaded with MSCs (center), and the confocal scan of the visible GFP-labeled MSCs cultured on the microrobot (right). The cells carried are MSCs derived from human induced pluripotent stem cells, which can deliver glutathione peroxidase 3 (hiPSC-MSC-GPx3). These engineered MSCs can inhibit the growth of cancer cells in cancer treatment (Qi et al., 2016).

Microrobots made of different material compositions can be studied in terms of degradability, mechanical strength, and magnetic actuation ability. First, based on the degradability assessment, a microrobot constructed with different PEGDA ratios was used. Fig. 13.16C shows that the microrobots with high PEGDA ratios show signs of rapid degradation. This result is consistent with the report (Peters et al., 2016). Second, the mechanical strength of microrobots with different PETA ratios was examined. Fig. 13.16D shows that the mechanical strength of the microrobot increases as the PETA ratio increases, and high PETA compositions require low laser power for manufacturing. These results indicate that high PETA composition is beneficial to the structural integrity of the microrobot. To determine the lowest PETA composition for microrobot manufacturing, materials with different PETA ratios were tested based on structural integrity. A minimum composition of 10 vol% PETA is required to integrally form the microrobot. In a test using the microrobot to carry hiPSC-MSC-GPx3, it was also found that a microrobot containing at least 25 vol% PETA can remain stable and intact after loading cells. Therefore, ingredients of 75 vol% PEGDA and 25 vol% PETA are recommended here. Third, the Fe_3O_4 nanoparticles in the material were determined based on the magnetic drive. Fig. 13.6E shows that when the proportion of Fe_3O_4 increases, the microrobot can achieve a higher driving speed. The proportion of magnetic components should be limited to less than 2 vol%, because a higher proportion of components will hinder the penetration of the laser, resulting in defects in the microrobot (Wei et al., 2020). Finally, a composition of 74 vol% PEGDA, 24 vol% PETA, and 2 vol% Fe_3O_4 nanoparticle solution was selected for the proposed microrobot prototype.

The size of the microrobot is determined based on the load capacity of the cell. Under the condition that the diameter of the microrobot is less than 100 μm so that the microrobot can access most blood vessels, the key parameters of the microrobot, namely the grid length (l_g) and the burr length (l_b) (Fig. 13.16A), can be optimized based on the maximum loading of cells. In the study of Wei et al. (2020), the grid length of 1.4 r_c and burr length of 0.5 r_c were chosen, the size of the microrobot was finally calculated to be 94.6 μm, and the radius of the scaffold grid r_g was 1.5 μm. With these parameters, each microrobot can load about 35 cells (Fig. 13.6F).

The degradability and biocompatibility of the designed microrobot were also evaluated. Fig. 13.17A illustrates the fluorescence signal of the microrobots made of degradable 75 vol% PEGDA:25 vol% PETA hydrogel and hard-to-degrade 100 vol% PETA hydrogel in NaOH solution and PBS environment, respectively. The results show that the degradable 75 vol% PEGDA:25 vol% PETA microrobot has a 92% reduction in fluorescence intensity within 24 h in NaOH solution, while the fluorescence intensity of 100 vol% PETA microrobot is only reduced by 13% (Fig. 13.17A, top). In the PBS environment, the fluorescence intensity of the degradable microrobot dropped by 40% after 2 weeks of incubation, while the fluorescence intensity of the hard-to-degrade microrobot remained almost unchanged (Fig. 13.17A, bottom). These results indicate that the designed microrobots are degradable and the degradation rate in an alkaline environment is faster than in PBS. The complete degradation of the microrobot in NaOH solution can predict the degradation of the microrobot in PBS. In vivo experiments were carried out on the degradability of microrobots in the subcutaneous (SC) tissues of nude mice, which provided an

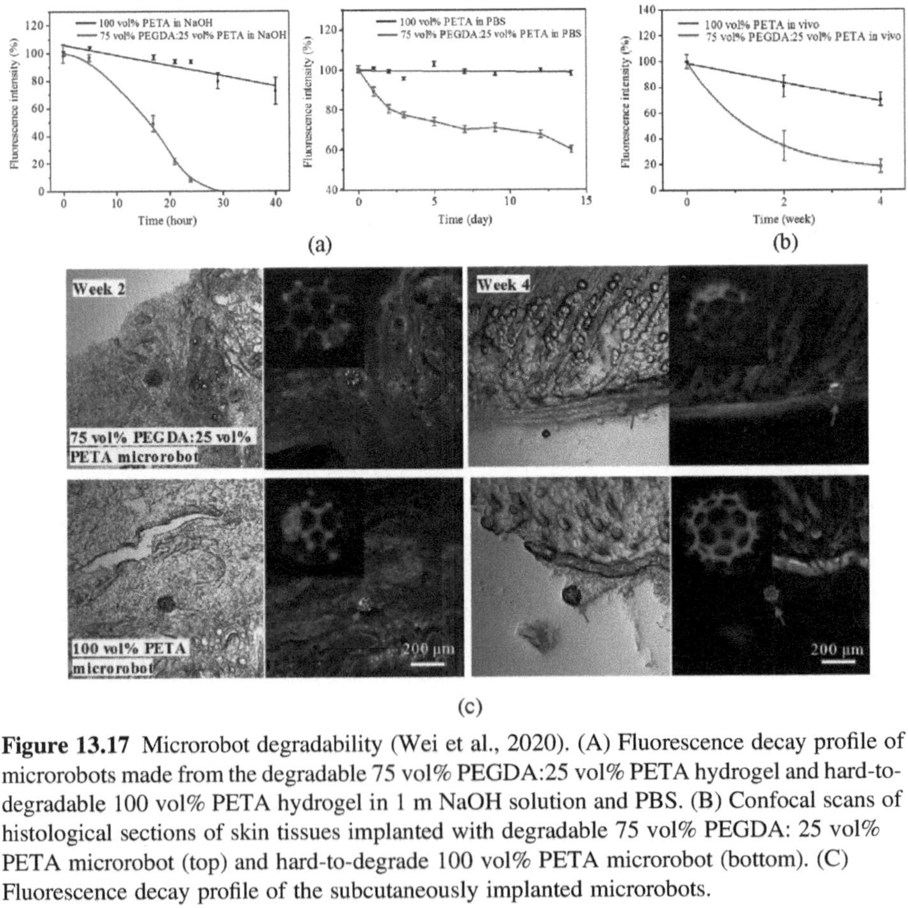

Figure 13.17 Microrobot degradability (Wei et al., 2020). (A) Fluorescence decay profile of microrobots made from the degradable 75 vol% PEGDA:25 vol% PETA hydrogel and hard-to-degradable 100 vol% PETA hydrogel in 1 m NaOH solution and PBS. (B) Confocal scans of histological sections of skin tissues implanted with degradable 75 vol% PEGDA: 25 vol% PETA microrobot (top) and hard-to-degrade 100 vol% PETA microrobot (bottom). (C) Fluorescence decay profile of the subcutaneously implanted microrobots.

environment close to reality for studying the degradation of microrobots. Degradable 75 vol% PEGDA:25 vol% PETA microrobots and hard-to-degrade 100 vol% PETA microrobots were implanted subcutaneously on the left and right flanks of each mouse. Fig. 13.17B shows a histological section of tissue implanted with the microrobot. The confocal scan image showed that the microrobot was not washed away. The fluorescence signal of rhodamine B only existed in or near the microrobot. No rhodamine B leaked in a large area. The fluorescence signal of rhodamine B on the microrobot was also characterized. Fig. 13.17C shows that the fluorescence intensity of the degradable 75 vol% PEGDA:25 vol% PETA microrobot is reduced by approximately 65% at 2 weeks after implantation, and by 82% at 4 weeks. The hard-to-degrade 100 vol% PETA microrobot has been reduced by 19% and 30%, respectively.

13.4.2 In vivo imaging of microrobots

To facilitate in vivo experiments, real-time imaging of microrobots at a depth of several millimeters to several centimeters is required. Wei et al. (2020) combined the microrobots and customized photoacoustic (PA) tomography to achieve in vivo microrobot imaging. Microrobots can be designed with light-absorbing materials to ensure high optical absorption coefficient and high contrast with hemoglobin molecules in the visible spectrum. By adjusting the optical excitation wavelength, the contrast of the microrobot in the blood is optimized, and the blood and the microrobot are quantified. To visualize the tissue environment, registered PA and ultrasound (US) images can be acquired simultaneously.

The absorption of blood in the near-infrared spectrum is weaker than that in the visible spectrum. In order to enhance the PA signal of the microrobot and improve the contrast between the microrobot and blood, 1064 nm was selected for in vivo imaging (Wei et al., 2020). The microrobot is coated with a 10 nm thick layer of gold to further enhance absorption while ensuring good biocompatibility. To provide more therapeutic cells to the diseased site, a group (from a few to hundreds) of microrobots is always used in one treatment. A large number of microrobots increases the PA signal. Fig. 13.18A shows that under the 1064 nm laser wavelength, the PA amplitude is positively correlated with the number of microrobots. Compared with uncoated microrobots under the same excitation, gold-coated microrobots can generate five times stronger signals. To demonstrate microrobot imaging in deep tissues, two sets of microrobots were imaged in chicken tissue (Fig. 13.18B). One group was composed of 10 gold-coated microrobots, and the other group was composed of 10 non-gold-coated microrobots. Compared with uncoated microrobots, coated microrobots show stronger PA signals at various tissue thicknesses. The gold-coated microrobot group can be clearly imaged at a depth of 2 cm, while the uncoated microrobot group is almost undetectable at this depth. This experiment shows that the microrobot has good contrast in deep PA imaging.

Microrobot imaging was further detected in mouse liver (Wei et al., 2020). Two hundred microrobots were injected into the left lateral lobe (LLL) through the portal vein, then harvested and fixed in paraformaldehyde (PFA), and imaged with US and PAT. Fig. 13.18C shows the imaging result. The US image shows the morphology

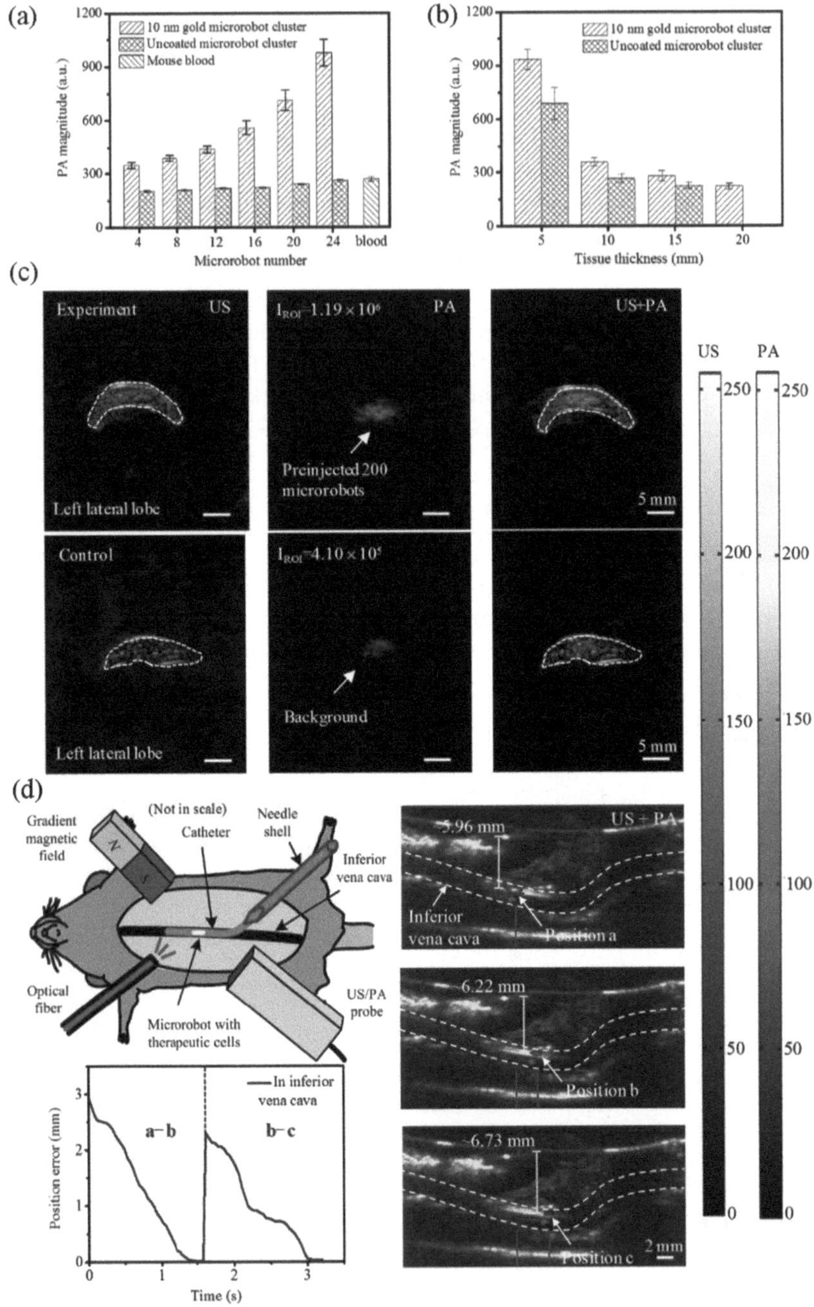

Figure 13.18 PA imaging of the microrobots (Wei et al., 2020). (A) PA magnitude of the microrobot cluster with different numbers of microrobots. (B) PA magnitude of the microrobot clusters against tissue thickness. (C) US and PA images of microrobots in LLL. Experimental LLL was injected with 200 gold-coated microrobots, and control LLL was not injected with any microrobots. The US mode detected the LLL morphology, whereas the PA mode captured the microrobot signal. The merged images show the distribution of microrobots in LLL. The depth of microrobot imaging was 6 mm. (D) Image-guided navigation of cell-loaded microrobots in the inferior vena cava of the mouse and its position error.

of LLL, and the PA image shows the absorption contrast of the liver tissue by the microrobot. The merged US and PA images show the location of the microrobots in the LLL. The signal amplitude of the LLL with 200 injection microrobots is 2.8 times that of the control. The experiment was repeated three times.

Finally, PA imaging guided in vivo navigation of the cell-loaded microrobots was conducted at a depth of 6 mm of the inferior vena cava in nude mice (male, 6–8 weeks) (Fig. 13.18D). The microrobot group consists of five gold-coated microrobots. Using a sharp needle catheter, a group of microrobots carrying cells were delivered to the inferior vena cava. Under the guidance of real-time PA and US imaging (20 frames/s per imaging mode), the microrobots in the catheter were activated by a gradient magnetic field in the vein. A PID controller was used in motion control to obtain position feedback through visual processing of the PA image. During navigation of the microrobots, two target positions were set and marked as b and c (Fig. 13.18D). The group of microrobots with cells moved from starting position a to target position b, and then from b to target position c. The total displacement was 5.1 mm. The position error of the microrobot (Fig. 13.18D) shows that the microrobot with cells can accurately navigate in the vascular environment to transport therapeutic cells.

13.4.3 Preclinical tests of microrobots carrying MSCs for liver tumor treatment

To verify the therapeutic effect of the developed microrobot for cell delivery, an experiment of delivering hiPSC-MSC-GPx3 via the microrobots was performed on nude mice implanted with orthotopic liver tumors at the LLL (Wei et al., 2020). The hiPSCMSC-GPx3 carried was plasmid engineered to produce GPx3 protein, which inhibits epithelial–mesenchymal transition through the extracellular signal-regulated kinase-nuclear factor κB-Smad interaction protein 1 signaling pathway, thereby inhibiting tumor growth and invasiveness. Cells that do not overexpress GPx3 (such as hiPSC-MSC-pCDH) cannot show inhibitory effects on cancer cells (Qi et al., 2016, 2018). Nude mice were divided into three groups, namely, a treatment group that delivered MSCs by microrobots, a nontreatment group that delivered only microrobots without MSCs, and a control group. In the treatment group, each mouse implanted with a tumor was injected with 200 MSC-carrying microrobots. In the nontreatment group, each mouse was injected with the same number of microrobots without MSCs. In the control group, each mouse was injected with PBS only. All injections were performed in the mouse portal vein and delivered to the tumor site through the vascular circulation. To guide the treatment of LLL, the right and middle branches of the portal vein that separates the right and middle liver lobes were clamped during the operation.

In the animal model of the treatment group, the ability of the microrobot to release MSCs in vivo was evaluated. As shown in Fig. 13.19A, by using the confocal image on day 5, a large number of GFP-labeled MSCs were found to penetrate into the sinusoidal space of the LLL tissue. These findings indicate that MSCs were released from the microrobots and migrated into the diseased tissue. The therapeutic effect of the

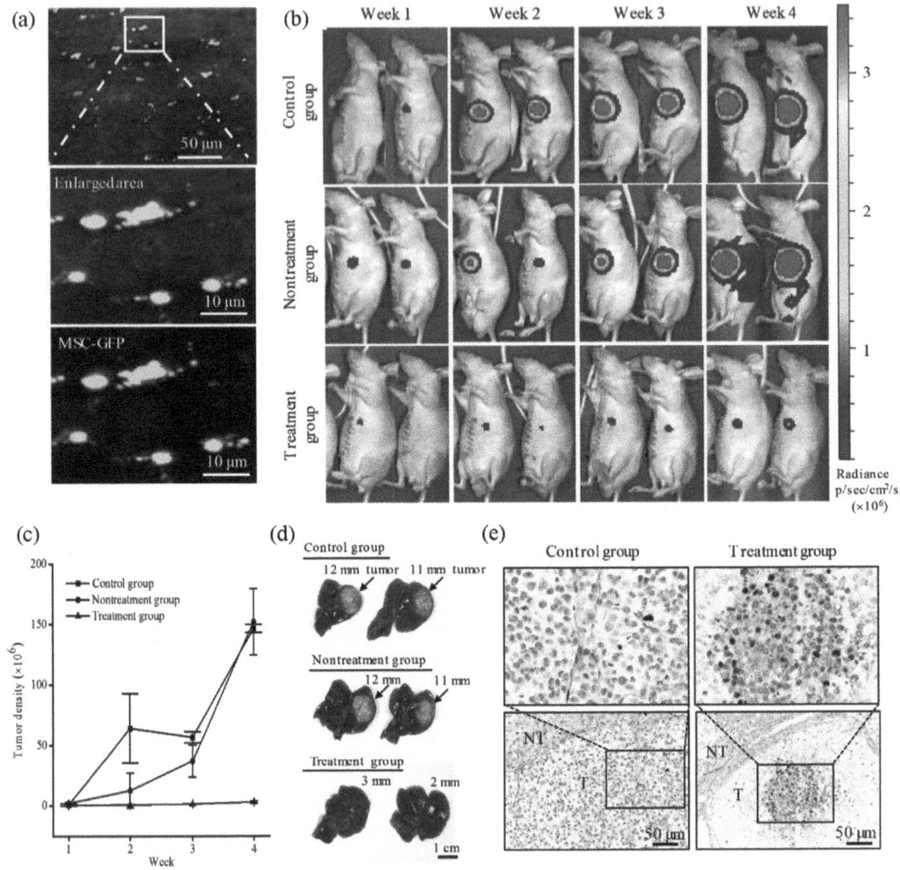

Figure 13.19 In vivo experiment of delivering hiPSC-MSC-GPx3 via the microrobots for liver tumor treatment (Wei et al., 2020). (A) Intravital images of GFP-labeled MSCs in liver parenchyma at day 5. The liver cells and nuclei were stained with MitoTracker Red and Hoechst, respectively. (B) Luminescence dynamics of tumor growth on nude mice in the three groups. (C) Tumor density of the three groups. The treatment group received an injection of 200 microrobots carrying MSCs with 100 μL PBS. The nontreatment group received an injection of 200 microrobots without MSCs with 100 μL PBS. The control group received an injection of 100 μL PBS only. (D) Comparison of ex vivo tumor size in the three groups. (E) Histological examination of the tumor and adjacent nontumor tissue by using TUNEL staining. *NT*, nontumor tissue; *T*, tumor.

released cells on tumor growth was then evaluated based on the bioluminescence intensity. Fig. 13.19B shows the tumor dynamics of the three groups within 4 weeks. The tumor size in the control group and the nontreatment group expanded rapidly. In contrast, the tumor size in the treatment group expanded slightly within 4 weeks. The quantitative results of the three groups of tumor density are shown in Fig. 13.19C. After 4 weeks, three groups of mice were scratched to obtain tumor samples. Fig. 13.19D shows that after the slice histological examination, the tumors of the control group and the nontreatment group protruded on the surface of the liver, with an average size of 11.5 mm, while the average size of the tumors in the treatment group was only 2.5 mm. The harvested tumors were further sectioned and stained with terminal deoxynucleotidyl transferase dUTP nick end labeling (TUNEL) to detect tumor cell apoptosis. As can be seen from Fig. 13.19E, the treatment group showed more severe tumor cell apoptosis than the control group. All these results indicate that the developed microrobot can effectively transport cells to the tumor site for cancer treatment. Notably, there is a minimal difference in tumor size between the control group and the nontreatment group, which indicates that the microrobot has little effect on the tumor.

Cell therapy is effective on the host with few side effects; however, traditional cell therapy relies heavily on the transfer of large numbers of cells in situ. Using the high positioning ability of the magnetic field, magnetic microrobots have become a viable solution that can transport and deliver cells to the target site, thereby greatly reducing the use of a large number of cells that overproduce cytokines and cause excessive immune responses. Using the microrobot approach, cells can be stably attached to the microrobot. Since the magnitude of shear stress and cell exposure time in the static environment in vitro are usually negligible, the side effects of the microrobot on the differentiation of the stem cells carried may be small. Biological modification of microrobots with extracellular matrix can further reduce stem cell differentiation.

13.5 Conclusions

This chapter introduced cell navigation and delivery from the following three perspectives.

First, an automated in vivo cell transport driven by an optical tweezers manipulator is introduced. A disturbance compensation controller is developed to overcome the influence of fluid (for example, blood flow) on cells. The controller can adjust the trajectory of the cells online to improve the success rate of transportation, and minimize the steady-state error by compensating for disturbances caused by blood flow. Simulation and experimental results show that the proposed controller can effectively and automatically transfer a single trapped cell to the desired position. This research can be useful for many precision medical applications, such as precise transportation of target cancer cells to selected destinations to simulate metastasis, drug delivery, in vivo cell sorting and extraction, and in vivo manipulation of microrobots and microsensors.

Second, a magnetic burr-like spherical porous microrobot is designed to carry and transport the target cells to the desired site in vivo under the magnetic gradient field-driven mechanism. 3D laser lithography is used to fabricate microrobots with sufficiently flexible robot structure design. Different cell types, including MC3T3-E1 cells and MSCs, are selected for testing. MC3T3-E1 cells can potentially differentiate into osteocytes. MSCs can potentially differentiate into various cell types of host tissues, such as adipocytes, chondrocytes, and myocytes. By transferring cells to a glass substrate, simulating the transendothelial migration of released cells, and releasing cells in nude mice, it has been demonstrated that the cells can be released from the designed microrobot successfully. The automatic navigation of cell culture microrobots is demonstrated in zebrafish embryos. The above results support the feasibility of using magnetically driven microrobots to accurately deliver targeted cells in vivo.

Third, an image-guided magnetically driven degradable microrobot is further designed to deliver engineered stem cells to the desired site in vivo for precise targeted therapy. Microrobots must meet the requirements of degradability, mechanical strength, and magnetic actuation simultaneously. Carrying cells can be spontaneously released from the microrobot in a living environment. By using unique photoacoustic imaging technology, the microrobot can be visualized at a penetration depth of several centimeters. Preclinical tests have been performed on nude mice to prove that the microrobot releases loaded cells, delivers these cells to the target site, and the cells significantly inhibit tumor growth. All the results reveal the feasibility of using the designed microrobot to transport and deliver the therapeutic cells to the desired site, and prove that its therapeutic effect on tumor treatment is successful.

References

Agrawal, H., Shang, H., Sattah, A.P., Yang, N., Peirce, S.M., Katz, A.J., 2014. Human adipose-derived stromal/stem cells demonstrate short-lived persistence after implantation in both an immunocompetent and an immunocompromised murine model. Stem Cell Res. Ther. 5.

Aijaz, A., Li, M., Smith, D., Khong, D., LeBlon, C., Fenton, O.S., Olabisi, R.M., Libutti, S., Tischfield, J., Maus, M.V., Deans, R., Barcia, R.N., Anderson, D.G., Ritz, J., Preti, R., Parekkadan, B., 2018. Biomanufacturing for clinically advanced cell therapies. Nat. Biomed. Eng. 2, 362.

Ahmed, D., Baasch, T., Blondel, N., Läubli, N., Dual, J., Nelson, B.J., 2017. Neutrophil-inspired propulsion in a combined acoustic and magnetic field. Nat. Commun. 8, 770.

Arcese, L., Fruchard, M., Ferreira, A., 2013. Adaptive controller and observer for a magnetic microrobot. IEEE Trans. Robot. 29 (4), 1060–1067.

Ceylan, H., Yasa, I.C., Sitti, M., 2017. 3D chemical patterning of micromaterials for encoded functionality. Adv. Mater. 29, 1605072.

Ceylan, H., Yasa, I.C., Yasa, O., Tabak, A.F., Giltinan, J., Sitti, M., 2019. 3D-printed biodegradable microswimmer for theranostic cargo delivery and release. ACS Nano 13, 3353.

Chin, S.Y., Poh, Y.C., Kohler, A.C., Compton, J.T., Hsu, L.L., Lau, K.M., Kim, S., Lee, B.W., Lee, F.Y., Sia, S.K., 2017. Additive manufacturing of hydrogel-based materials for next-generation implantable medical devices. Sci. Robot. 2, eaah6451.

Danilevicius, P., Rezende, R.A., Pereira, F.D., Selimis, A., Kasyanov, V., Noritomi, P.Y., da Silva, J.V., Chatzinikolaidou, M., Farsari, M., Mironov, V., 2015. Burr-like, laser-made 3D microscaffolds for tissue spheroid encagement. Biointerphases 10, 021011.

Debbaut, C., Segers, P., Cornillie, P., Casteleyn, C., Dierick, M., Laleman, W., Monbaliu, D., 2014. Analyzing the human liver vascular architecture by combining vascular corrosion casting and micro-CT scanning: a feasibility study. J. Anat. 224, 509–517.

Evensen, L., Johansen, P.L., Koster, G., Zhu, K., Herfindal, L., Speth, M., Fenaroli, F., Hildahl, J., Bagherifam, S., Tulotta, C., Prasmickaite, L., Maelandsmo, G.M., Snaar-Jagalska, E., Griffiths, G., 2016. Zebrafish as a model system for characterization of nanoparticles against cancer. Nanoscale 8, 862–877.

Felfoul, O., Mohammadi, M., Taherkhani, S., de Lanauze, D., Xu, Y.Z., Loghin, D., Essa, S., Jancik, S., Houle, D., Lafleur, M., Gaboury, L., Tabrizian, M., Kaou, N., Atkin, M., Vuong, T., Batist, G., Beauchemin, N., Radzioch, D., Martel, S., 2016. Magneto-aerotactic bacteria deliver drug-containing nanoliposomes to tumour hypoxic regions. Nat. Nanotechnol. 11, 941.

Fukuda, T., Nakajima, M., Liu, P., ElShimy, H., 2009. Nanofabrication, nanoinstrumentation and nanoassembly by nanorobotic manipulation. Int. J. Robot. Res. 28, 537–547.

Hollister, S.J., 2005. Porous scaffold design for tissue engineering. Nat. Mater. 4, 518.

Hong, G., Antaris, A.L., Dai, H., 2017. Near-infrared fluorophores for biomedical imaging. Nat. Biomed. Eng. 1, 10.

Hu, S., Sun, D., 2011. Automatic transportation of biological cells with a robot-tweezer manipulation system. Int. J. Robot Res. 30 (14), 1681–1694.

Iacovacci, V., Blanc, A., Huang, H., Ricotti, L., Schibli, R., Menciassi, A., Behe, M., Pané, S., Nelson, B.J., 2019. High-resolution SPECT imaging of stimuli-responsive soft microrobots. Small 15, 1900709.

Jeon, S., Kim, S., Ha, S., Lee, S., Kim, E., Kim, S.Y., Park, S.H., Jeon, J.H., Kim, S.W., Moon, C., Nelson, B.J., Kim, J., Yu, S.W., Choi, H., 2019. Magnetically actuated microrobots as a platform for stem cell transplantation. Sci. Robot. 4, eaav4317.

Johansen, P.L., Fenaroli, F., Evensen, L., Griffiths, G., Koster, G., 2016. Optical micromanipulation of nanoparticles and cells inside living zebrafish. Nat. Commun. 7, 10974.

Jun, Y., Tripathy, S.K., Narayanareddy, B.R., Mattson-Hoss, M.K., Gross, S.P., 2014. Calibration of optical tweezers for in vivo force measurements: how do different approaches compare? Biophys. J. 107, 1474–1484.

Kawano, T., Sato, M., Yabu, H., Shimomura, M., 2014. Honeycomb-shaped surface topography induces differentiation of human mesenchymal stem cells (hMSCs): uniform porous polymer scaffolds prepared by the breath figure technique. Biomater. Sci. 2, 52–56.

Kim, H., Ali, J., Cheang, U.K., Jeong, J., Kim, J.S., Kim, M.J., 2016. Micro manipulation using magnetic microrobots. J. Bionic Eng. 13, 515–524.

Kim, S., Qiu, F., Kim, S., Ghanbari, A., Moon, C., Zhang, L., Nelson, B.J., Choi, H., 2013. Fabrication and characterization of magnetic microrobots for three-dimensional cell culture and targeted transportation. Adv. Mater. 25, 5863–5868.

Labanieh, L., Majzner, R.G., Mackall, C.L., 2018. Programming car-T cells to kill cancer. Nat. Biomed. Eng. 2, 377.

Lee, K.C., Lee, S., 2017. Drug delivery: brushing off antigenicity. Nat. Biomed. Eng. 1, 0019.

Li, J., de Ávilladde, B.E.F., Gao, W., Zhang, L., Wang, J., 2017a. Micro/nanorobots for biomedicine: delivery, surgery, sensing, and detoxification. Sci. Robot. 2, eaam6431.

Li, J., Li, X., Luo, T., Wang, R., Liu, C., Chen, S., Li, D., Yue, J., Cheng, S., Sun, D., 2018. Development of a magnetic microrobot for carrying and delivering targeted cells. Sci. Robot. 3, eaat8829.

Li, X., Liu, C., Chen, S., Wang, Y., Cheng, S.H., Sun, D., 2017b. In vivo manipulation of single biological cells with an optical tweezers-based manipulator and a disturbance compensation controller. IEEE Trans. Robot. 33 (5), 1200–1212.

Liba, O., de la Zerda, A., 2017. Photoacoustic tomography: breathtaking whole-body imaging. Nat. Biomed. Eng. 1, 0075.

Lu, Y., Xu, Y.J., Zhang, G., Ling, D., Wang, M., Zhou, Y., Wu, Y.D., Wu, T., Hackett, M.J., Kim, B.H., Chang, H., Kim, J., Hu, X.T., Dong, L., Lee, N., Li, F., He, J.C., Zhang, L., Wen, H.Q., Yang, B., Choi, S.H., Hyeon, T., Zou, D.H., 2017. Iron oxide nanoclusters for T_1 magnetic resonance imaging of non-human primates. Nat. Biomed. Eng. 1, 637.

Ma, P.X., 2008. Biomimetic materials for tissue engineering. Adv. Drug Deliv. Rev. 60, 184−198.

Medina-Sánchez, M., Schmidt, O.G., 2017. Medical microrobots need better imaging and control. Nat. News 545, 406.

Mironov, V., Visconti, R.P., Kasyanov, V., Forgacs, G., Drake, C.J., Markwald, R.R., 2009. Organ printing: tissue spheroids as building blocks. Biomaterials 30, 2164−2174.

Nakai, A., Sekiya, I., Oya, A., Koshino, T., Araki, T., 2002. Assessment of the hepatic arterial and portal venous blood flows during pregnancy with Doppler ultrasonography. Arch. Gynecol. Obstet. 266, 25−29.

Nelson, B.J., Kaliakatsos, I.K., Abbott, J.J., 2010. Microrobots for minimally invasive medicine. Annu. Rev. Biomed. Eng. 12, 55−85.

Oskarsson, T., Batlle, E., Massagué, J., 2014. Metastatic stem cells: sources, niches, and vital pathways. Cell Stem Cell 14, 306−321.

Palagi, S., Mark, A.G., Reigh, S.Y., Melde, K., Qiu, T., Zeng, H., Parmeggiani, C., Martella, D., Sanchez-Castillo, A., Kapernaum, N., Giesselmann, F., Wiersma, D.S., Lauga, E., Fischer, P., 2016. Structured light enables biomimetic swimming and versatile locomotion of photoresponsive soft microrobots. Nat. Mater. 15, 647.

Pan, H., Sun, W., Gao, H., Jing, X., 2016. Disturbance observer-based adaptive tracking control with actuator saturation and its application. IEEE Trans. Autom. Sci. Eng. 13 (2), 868−875.

Park, S.J., Gazzola, M., Park, K.S., Park, S., Santo, V.D., Blevins, E.L., Lind, J.U., Campbell, P.H., Dauth, S., Capulli, A.K., Pasqualini, F.S., Ahn, S., Cho, A., Yuan, H., Maoz, B.M., Vijaykumar, R., Choi, J.W., Deisseroth, K., Lauder, G.V., Mahadevan, L., Parker, K.K., 2016. Phototactic guidance of a tissue-engineered soft-robotic ray. Science 353, 158.

Peters, C., Hoop, M., Pané, S., Nelson, B.J., Hierold, C., 2016. Degradable magnetic composites for minimally invasive interventions: device fabrication, targeted drug delivery, and cytotoxicity tests. Adv. Mater. 28, 533.

Qi, X., Ng, K.T., Shao, Y., Li, C.X., Geng, W., Ling, C.C., Ma, Y.Y., Liu, X.B., Liu, H., Liu, J., Yeung, W.H., Lo, C.M., Man, K., 2016. The clinical significance and potential therapeutic role of GPx3 in tumor recurrence after liver transplantation. Theranostics 6 (11), 1934.

Qi, X., Ng, K.T., Lian, Q., Li, C.X., Geng, W., Ling, C.C., Yeung, W.H., Ma, Y.Y., Liu, X.B., Liu, H., Liu, J., Yang, X.X., Lo, C.M., Man, K., 2018. Glutathione peroxidase 3 delivered by hiPSC -MSCs ameliorated hepatic IR injury via inhibition of hepatic senescence. Theranostics 8, 212−222.

Rouwkema, J., Rivron, N.C., van Blitterswijk, C.A., 2008. Vascularization in tissue engineering. Trends Biotechnol. 26, 434−441.

Segers, V.F.M., Lee, R.T., 2008. Stem-cell therapy for cardiac disease. Nature 451, 937.

Sitti, M., 2018. Miniature soft robots − road to the clinic. Nat. Rev. Mater. 3, 74.

Steager, E.B., Selman Sakar, M., Magee, C., Kennedy, M., Cowley, A., Kumar, V., 2013. Automated biomanipulation of single cells using magnetic microrobots. Int. J. Robot. Res. 32, 346.

Stephan, S.B., Taber, A.M., Jileaeva, I., Pegues, E.P., Sentman, C.L., Stephan, M.T., 2015. Biopolymer implants enhance the efficacy of adoptive T cell therapy. Nat. Biotechnol. 33, 97.

Tang, J., Su, T., Huang, K., Dinh, P.U., Wang, Z., Vandergriff, A., Hensley, M.T., Cores, J., Allen, T., Li, T., Sproul, E., Mihalko, E., Lobo, L.J., Ruterbories, L., Lynch, A., Brown, A., Caranasos, T.G., Shen, D., Stouffer, G.A., Gu, Z., Zhang, J., Cheng, K., 2018. Targeted repair of heart injury by stem cells fused with platelet nanovesicles. Nat. Biomed. Eng. 2, 17.

Tottori, S., Zhang, L., Qiu, F., Krawczyk, K.K., Franco-Obregón, A., Nelson, B.J., 2012. Magnetic helical micromachines: fabrication, controlled swimming, and cargo transport. Adv. Mater. 24, 811.

Ulbricht, J., Jordan, R., Luxenhofer, R., 2014. On the biodegradability of polyethylene glycol polypeptoids and poly(2-oxazoline)s. Biomaterials 35 (17), 4848–4861.

Wang, X., Qin, X.H., Hu, C., Terzopoulou, A., Chen, X.Z., Huang, T.Y., Maniura-Weber, K., Pané, S., Nelson, B.J., 2018. 3D printed enzymatically biodegradable soft helical microswimmers. Adv. Funct. Mater. 28, 1804107.

Williams, B.J., Anand, S.V., Rajagopalan, J., Saif, M.T.A., 2014. A self-propelled biohybrid swimmer at low Reynolds number. Nat. Commun. 5, 3081.

Wang, X., Chen, S., Kong, M., Wang, Z., Costa, K.D., Li, R.A., Sun, D., 2011. Enhanced cell sorting and manipulation with combined optical tweezer and microfluidic chip technologies. Lab Chip 11, 3656–3662.

Wei, T., Liu, J., Li, D., Chen, S., Zhang, Y., Li, J., Fan, L., Guan, Z., Lo, C.M., Wang, L., Man, K., Sun, D., 2020. Development of magnet-driven and image-guided biodegradable microrobots for the precise delivery of engineered stem cells for cancer therapy. Small 16 (41), 1906908.

Wen, J., Wu, D., Qin, M., Liu, C., Wang, L., Xu, D., Vinters, H.V., Liu, Y., Kranz, E., Guan, X., Sun, G., Sun, X., Lee, Y., Martinez-Maza, O., Widney, D., Lu, Y., Chen, I.S.Y., Kamata, M., 2019. Sustained delivery and molecular targeting of a therapeutic monoclonal antibody to metastases in the central nervous system of mice. Nat. Biomed. Eng. 3, 706.

Wu, Z., Li, L., Yang, Y., Hu, P., Li, Y., Yang, S.Y., Wang, L.V., Gao, W., 2019. A microrobotic system guided by photoacoustic computed tomography for targeted navigation in intestines in vivo. Sci. Robot. 4, eaax0613.

Xie, H., Haliyo, D.S., Régnier, S., 2009. A versatile atomic force microscope for three-dimensional nanomanipulation and nanoassembly. Nanotechnology 20, 215301.

Xie, M., Wang, Y., Feng, G., Sun, D., 2014. Automated pairing manipulation of biological cells with a robot-tweezers manipulation system. IEEE/ASME Trans. Mechatron. 20 (5), 2242–2251.

Yan, X., Sun, D., 2015. Multilevel-based topology design and cell patterning with robotically controlled optical tweezers. IEEE Trans. Control Syst. Technol. 23 (1), 176–185.

Yan, X., Zhou, Q., Vincent, M., Deng, Y., Yu, J., Xu, J., Xu, T., Tang, T., Bian, L., Wang, Y.X.J., Kostarelos, K., Zhang, L., 2017. Recent progress on micro- and nano-robots: towards in vivo tracking and localization. Sci. Robot. 2, eaaq1155.

Yasa, I.C., Tabak, A.F., Yasa, O., Ceylan, H., Sitti, M., 2019. 3D-printed microrobotic transporters with recapitulated stem cell niche for programmable and active cell delivery. Adv. Funct. Mater. 29, 1808992.

Zhong, M.C., Wei, X.B., Zhou, J.H., Wang, Z.Q., Li, Y.M., 2013. Trapping red blood cells in living animals using optical tweezers. Nat. Commun. 4, 1768.

Organelle biopsy and gene editing of single cells

14

14.1 Introduction

The study of bulk tissues only provides statistical averages of several behaviors that occur in different cells. Single-cell studies may reveal that genetic changes caused by tumorigenesis-related signaling pathways cause healthy cells to transform into cancer cells (Liu et al., 2015). In order to study diseases and their causes, single-cell surgery at the subcellular level, such as manipulating or removing subcellular components or organelles from single cells (Pertoft and Laurent, 1977), is increasingly needed (Schubert, 2011). Techniques related to single-cell surgery include preimplantation and diagnosis (Braude et al., 2002), characterization of organelle and subcellular activities (Liu et al., 2015), and cloning (Campbell et al., 1996), to name a few.

Over the past few decades, several micro/nanomanipulation tools for intracellular surgery have been developed. A scanning ion conductance microscope-based nanobiopsy system used electrowetting to draw cytoplasmic samples into glass nanopipettes in a minimally invasive manner, and then used high-throughput sequencing technology to analyze the extracted cell material (Actis et al., 2014). Atomic force microscopy (AFM) tip was used to extract specific mRNA from living cells (Osada et al., 2003), and a nanorobot was created for puncturing cells (Hayakawa et al., 2014). Similarly, carbon nanotubes placed at the tip of a glass pipette were used at the single-cell level to transfer fluids, interrogate cells, and perform optical and electrochemical diagnoses (Singhal et al., 2011).

These subcellular-level cellular surgery tasks are currently performed by skilled operators. Depending on the skill of the operator, various cell surgery tasks, such as positioning the tip of the micropipette relative to the cell position, inserting the tip into a specific position in the cell after the membrane is perforated, and extracting the micropipette from the cell, are very tedious and time consuming. To manipulate biological cells, numerous robotic micromanipulation systems have been reported in the literature. Several studies have tested the automation of embryo biopsy, such as force measurement during micropipette insertion (Kim et al., 2004), contact detection (Huang et al., 2009), automatic position selection for zona pellucida dissection (Wang et al., 2007), and automatic micropipette control and embryo rotation tracking (Wang and Ang, 2016). Some studies have attempted to automate this mechanical enucleation process using different micromanipulation tools, such as micropipettes (Wong and Mills, 2016), magnetically driven microtools (Ichikawa et al., 2010), and microfluidic chips (Hagiwara et al., 2013). Note that all of the above methods are applicable to large cells of ~ 80 μm. Single-cell biopsies of small cells, such as many human cells (~ 20 μm), are more challenging because of their small size, irregular shape, and flexible membrane, all of which require high-precision manipulation.

Robotic Cell Manipulation. https://doi.org/10.1016/B978-0-323-85259-3.00013-1

Cell biopsy is related to cell injection, but they are different. Cell injection is the process of inserting foreign materials into cells. Several cell injection systems that allow semi- (Sun and Nelson, 2002; Xie et al., 2010; Kallio et al., 2007) and fully automatic (Huang et al., 2009; Liu et al., 2009; Chow et al., 2016) injection processes have been proposed. Cell biopsy differs from cell injection in several ways. First, cell injection is done anywhere within the cell, usually in the center (Chow et al., 2016). In cell biopsy, the tip of the micropipette must be inserted precisely into the desired organelle position within the cell. Accurately accessing the spatial location of organelles within a cell, especially for small suspension cells, such as most human cells with a size of about 20 μm, is challenging. Therefore, cell biopsy requires highly precise positioning control. Secondly, cell biopsy requires some additional operations, such as aspiration control of the organelles in the micropipette and maintenance control of the cells during the extraction process. Therefore, organelle biopsy is more complicated than cell injection.

Shakoor et al. (2019) proposed a robotic single-cell organelle biopsy system for small cells of less than 20 μm in size. The system can perform complete automated single-cell biopsy tasks, including cell positioning, organelle detection, aspiration, and organelle release. To meet the high requirements for the positioning accuracy of organelles, a microfluidic single-cell patterning device was designed, which can compress and pattern cells in a rectangular channel in a one-dimensional (1D) array, thereby simplifying the automation process. Under the vision-based robust control algorithm, the system can be applied to biopsy a wide range of cells with high manipulation accuracy, while solving the uncertainty of the model and external interference. To demonstrate that the proposed system can be applied for organelle biopsy of different types of cells (such as cancer and human cell lines), suspension cells (NB4 cancer cells), and adherent cells [human dermal fibroblasts (HDFs)] were used in their experiments. Cell biopsy research is of great benefit to precision medicine. For example, biopsy of mitochondria can be used to restore the metabolite profile in mammalian cells after mitochondrial transfer (Wu et al., 2016) and to study cell degenerative mutations. Cells that survived mitochondrial biopsy can be used to interrogate live cells (Actis et al., 2014). Biopsy nuclei can be used for genome sequencing (Lin et al., 2014), RNA sequencing (Habib et al., 2016), cloning (Campbell et al., 1996; Li et al., 2016), and gene expression detection (Wada et al., 2004). The single nucleus obtained using the organelle biopsy system can be used for mitochondrial replacement therapy (Greenfield et al., 2017) and can also help to improve gene sequencing at the single-nucleus level.

The development of automated systems and enabling technologies to enhance organelle biopsy can greatly benefit its clinical application. For example, embryo biopsy during early embryonic development provides an alternative to pregnancy termination for parents who may transmit a genetic disease to their offspring (Vermeesch et al., 2016). Organelle biopsy can help improve therapeutic cloning or reproductive cloning (Li et al., 2016; Greggains et al., 2015). This technique can help identify the compartmentalization of mRNA. This is important after injury, because changes in the spatial distribution of mRNA can lead to neurodegenerative diseases and mental retardation. Organelle biopsy can also provide a basis for the development of drugs to reduce neurodegeneration, and can be used as a platform for clinical management and cancer research (Clark et al., 2006).

Robotic microinjection also shows significant advantages in single-cell gene editing. In view of their pluripotent differentiation potential and immunomodulatory properties, mesenchymal stem cells (MSCs) have been intensively studied and are a promising cell source for cell/gene-based therapy, regenerative medicine, and tissue engineering (Galipeau and Sensébé, 2018). However, MSCs gradually lose their biological functions after being separated from the original tissue, long-term cell culture, and massive expansion of cell populations in vitro. After MSCs are injected into patients, the phenotype of MSCs is comprehensively regulated by various physical, chemical, and biological factors (Galipeau and Sensébé, 2018; Robey et al., 2008). Due to the harsh environment in tissue lesions, their survival rate is low, and the cell apoptosis rate is high. Therefore, manipulating the cell fate transition of MSCs is a key challenge for the success of regenerative medicine and tissue engineering. By introducing foreign genes into MSCs as the main strategy to control the fate of MSCs, the obstacles that limit the performance of MSCs in treatment are solved (Oggu et al., 2017). Many genes have been studied for this purpose, including prosurvival genes and lineage-specific genes for cell differentiation (Frith et al., 2018). However, the key to the success of gene transfer depends on the gene delivery strategy, which aims to increase DNA uptake and subsequent protein expression as much as possible (Kay, 2011). Therefore, research has been devoted to methods that can effectively transfer genes to MSCs. The gene-delivery methods of engineered MSCs include viral vectors, chemical vectors, and physical delivery methods. Viral vectors are widely used due to their high transduction efficiency and stable gene expression (Yin et al., 2017). However, their limited packaging capabilities and safety issues, such as virus-induced insertion mutations and immunogenicity, hinder their clinical application. The addition of polybrene also severely inhibits the differentiation potential and proliferation of MSCs. Chemical carriers are attractive alternatives to transfection and have considerable advantages in terms of serum stability, cargo compatibility, and targeting ability. However, due to cytotoxicity and sensitivity to serum and antibiotics, their application in tissue engineering faces great challenges (Yin et al., 2014). As a typical example of physical delivery, microinjection uses microneedles to inject cargo such as proteins, DNA, and chemical molecules directly into the nucleus (Huang et al., 2009; Liu et al., 2014; Chow et al., 2016; Pan et al., 2020). Microinjection has a higher transfection efficiency than other cell transfection methods, but has the disadvantage of low throughput, especially when compared with scalable chemical delivery methods.

Guan et al. (2021) compared the ability of four gene-delivery vectors (calcium phosphate coprecipitation, PEI, Lipofectamine, and robotic microinjection) to transfect adult MSCs, and therefore evaluated the effects of these delivery vectors on cell viability, morphology, and bias in the differentiation potential of MSCs. They used the above four delivery vehicles to further knock out the osteoblast differentiation negative regulator PPARγ gene, and measured the effects of the four methods on gene function and stem cell differentiation. Their results indicate that the prejudice against commitment to osteogenesis or adipogenesis depends to a large extent on exposure to different delivery vehicles. Moreover, the function of therapeutic genes is differently interfered by gene carriers. Their research results further show that robotic microinjection is a promising method for generating transgenic MSCs, which will not destroy the differentiation commitment and gene function of MSCs.

As an important case study of organelle biopsy and manipulation, mitochondrial transfer is considered a potential method to restore the metabolic function of mitochondrial mutations (Sartori-Rupp et al., 2019). Mitochondria are essential organelles known as the powerhouse of cells (Friedman and Nunnari, 2014). Mitochondrial mutations play a key role in aging and neurodegenerative diseases, and they are known to be important regulators of cell death and survival (Shadel and Horvath, 2015). The malfunction of mitochondrial DNA (mtDNA) leads to the net production of reactive oxygen species, which is associated with various aging diseases, such as Alzheimer disease or amyotrophic lateral sclerosis (Sahin and Depinho, 2010). In senescence-related diseases, on-site senescent cells cause functional degradation through the senescence-related secretory phenotype (SASP) (Rhinn et al., 2019). Some previous studies have shown that the secretome of human fMSCs can improve the aging phenotype of human aMSCs in in vitro and in vivo models (Wang et al., 2016). These findings indicate that fMSC may have a unique metabolite profile and antiaging ability in the secretory group. Given that mitochondria are well-known metabolic regulators (Spinelli and Haigis, 2018), whether aMSCs can be transformed into fMSC-like cells by mitochondrial transfer is a common question. To replace endogenous mitochondria, microneedles can be used to inject isolated exogenous mitochondria into individual cells (King and Attardi, 1988). However, the transfer of mitochondria by direct microinjection with glass microneedles usually exhibits an inefficiency of only 0.3% (King and Attardi, 1988). In addition, the microneedle-based cell injection method has several limitations, such as blockage of the glass microneedle tip, physical damage to the cell, and restrictions on repeated injections of the same cell. To solve these problems, the thermal nanoblade method was developed (Wu et al., 2016), which uses microneedles >3 μm in diameter to prevent clogging. This method uses a pulsed laser to induce bubble cavitation to open holes in the cell membrane, and then uses a synchronous fluid to pump the mitochondria. However, the microneedle is only placed on the surface of the cell membrane and is not tightly wrapped inside the cell membrane, so the injection efficiency of this method is only 2%–3%.

Endocytosis and microcytosis are natural cell membrane phagocytosis processes. Cells can absorb particles ranging in size from nanometers to a few microns (Patel et al., 2017). Mitochondrial transfer via endocytosis is widely used as a high-throughput mitochondrial transfer process (Islam et al., 2012). To improve the absorption efficiency of mitochondria, a method has been proposed to force mitochondria into cells through centrifugation (Caicedo et al., 2015) and pressure-driven methods (Sercel et al., 2021). To improve the transfer efficiency of mitochondria, a method of using mitochondria combined with magnetic beads and then using an external magnetic field to press them into the cell has been proposed (Macheiner et al., 2016). However, using this method, the magnetic beads will also be transferred with the mitochondria, which may damage the host cell. All these methods make it difficult to control the quality and quantity of isolated mitochondria before they are transferred to cells. These methods also ignore mitochondrial heterogeneity, including mitochondrial functions that represent another level of mitochondrial complexity (Kuznetsov and Margreiter, 2009). Impurities in the isolated mitochondria can cause fragments and dead mitochondria (due to the long duration of the isolation process) to be transferred to the cell, which may harm the host cell (Wieckowski et al., 2009).

Shakoor et al. (2021) proposed a new micromanipulation system that integrates optical tweezers (OT), microfluidic chips, and automation technology to realize the precise and automated transportation of isolated mitochondria to single cells, and then investigated whether the transfer of fMSC (young) to aMSC (old) can improve the senescence of aMSC (old). A microfluidic device is used to pattern cells and mitochondria, OT is used to transport a predetermined number of mitochondria into the cell, and the cell absorbs these mitochondria through endocytosis. Using the automatically controlled OT can automatically and accurately collect the exact number of mitochondria and deliver them to the cells efficiently. Mitochondria isolated from fMSCs can be transferred to aMSCs and 293T kidney cells, indicating that the proposed transfer method can be applied to different cell types. The results show that the transfer of isolated mitochondria from fMSCs to aMSCs can significantly increase the antiaging and metabolic gene expression levels of aMSCs, thereby transforming aMSC into an fMSC-like phenotype.

The remainder of this chapter introduces three main methods. The first method is to use a microneedle-based cellular surgery robotic system for automated organelle biopsy of small single cells (Shakoor et al., 2019). The second method is to study gene-delivery effects regarding the differentiation potential and gene function of MSCs, in which a robotic microinjection system is used to inject CRISPR/Cas9 encoding plasmids to knock out the PPARγ gene in MSCs (Guan et al., 2021). The third method is to use automated optical tweezers to transfer mitochondria from fetal MSCs to adult MSCs to improve antiaging gene expression (Shakoor et al., 2021).

14.2 Automated organelle biopsy of single cells using microneedles

14.2.1 Genetic single-cell biopsy system

Fig. 14.1 shows a single-cell biopsy system, which contains three modules for execution, control, and sensing. The execution module includes an X−Y−Z positioning stage with a resolution of 10 nm along the X−Y direction, and a z-axis that controls the height of the objective lens. A micropipette used for organelle extraction is mounted on the in-house assembled 3-degrees of freedom (DOF) micromanipulator, which is connected to a modified microinjector based on the original product of Eppendorf (Cell Tramvario). The execution module also includes a microfluidic cell patterning device and a self-made pressure regulator for generating a vacuum inside the cell patterning device. The control module includes two motion controllers for controlling the 3-DOF manipulator and the X−Y−Z positioning platform. The sensing

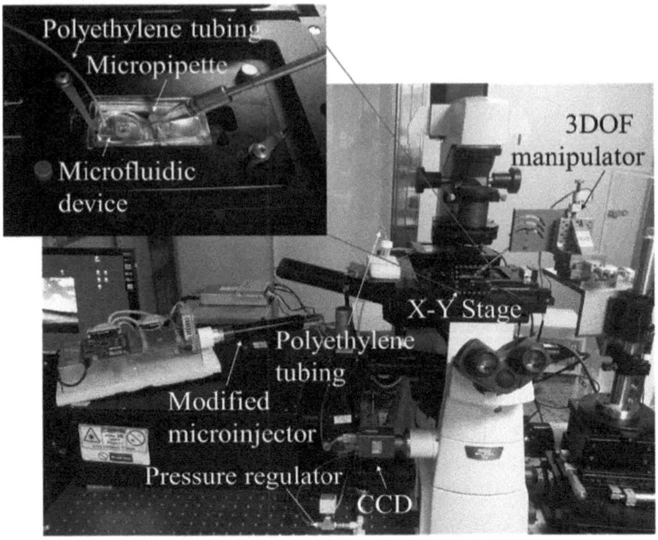

Figure 14.1 An automated single-cell biopsy system (Shakoor et al., 2019).

module includes a CCD camera and a microscope with a 60× objective lens. A graphical unit interface (GUI) is developed with Visual C++. All mechanical settings are supported by the antivibration table.

To simplify the cell manipulation process, cells are patterned in a 1D array. The PDMS-based microfluidic cell patterning device (MCPD) is designed by placing many rectangular channels in parallel. This design eliminates the need for a second manipulator (for cell retention) and simplifies the cell/organelle search and extraction process. Fig. 14.2 shows a schematic design of the microfluidic device. MCPD consists of an aspirating layer and a cell pattern layer. The arrangement of these two layers creates a rectangular hole to firmly pattern and fix each cell. As shown in Fig. 14.2, a small cylindrical gap called "storage" is added near the front of the channel to accommodate and store biopsy samples. "Storage" was created to save the extracted organelles in a defined location for repositioning for further analysis and to prevent them from being lost due to drift. In addition, the PDMS before "storage" helps to remove cell debris from the tip of the micropipette when it penetrates into the PDMS to eject the cell organelle into the "storage". Two adjacent channels are separated by a distance of 100 μm to ensure that only one channel and one "storage" can be seen in the field of view, which simplifies the image-processing perspective for detecting the location of the organelles of cells present in the field of view.

The microfluidic device was fabricated using soft lithography. First, a layer of 5 μm SU-8 photoresist (GM1050, Gersteltec Sarl) was spin-coated on the silicon wafer and prebaked on an electric furnace (AccuPlate, Labnet). The structure was exposed to ultraviolet (UV) light with the mask on top. The second layer with a thickness of 15 μm was fabricated following the same process. Then a mixture of PDMS and curing agent at a ratio of 10:1 was dropped onto the master mold, baked in an oven for 1.5 h, and

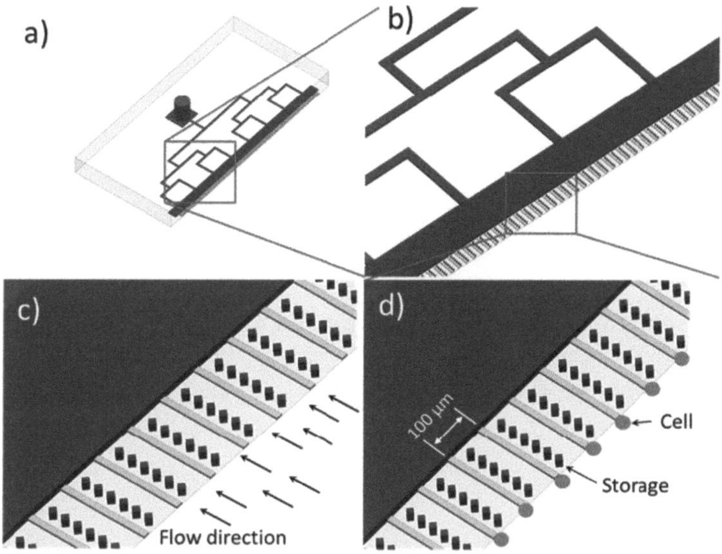

Figure 14.2 Schematic design of the cell patterning microfluidic device (Shakoor et al., 2019). (A) Full view of the microfluidic device. (B) Close-up view of the inset. (C) Flow direction. (D) Cell trapping.

finally peeled off the master mold. The bake time of PDMS should not exceed 1.5 h, because overbaking will harden the PDMS, which may prevent the microneedles from penetrating it. As shown in Fig. 14.3, a sharp microneedle beveled at 15 ~ 45 degrees can easily penetrate this soft PDMS without breaking.

After fabrication, the microfluidic cell patterning device was plasma-combined with a glass slide, washed with cell culture medium, and exposed to UV light for half an hour. Without this step, the liquid may not flow smoothly through the channel, and unwanted bubbles may be generated in front of the channel. The cell patterning device was connected to the slide rack, and the slide rack was fixed on the X–Y–Z positioning table. To generate fluid flow, the outlet of the cell holder was connected to the digital microinjector through polyethylene tubing. A pressure of −124.6 Pa was initially applied, and the cells were placed near the channel with a pipette. Within a few minutes, the cells were trapped in front of the channel, and the pressure was adjusted to squeeze the cells in the channel or maintain their position at the channel opening. When cells were present at the opening of the channel, a pressure of 24.9 Pa was considered to be sufficient to maintain the cell position. Increasing the pressure to 250 Pa for about 10 s would aspirate 90% of the cells into the channel, while reducing the pressure to 24.9 Pa would keep the cells in this state. To ensure that there is only one cell in the field of view, the nontrapped cells near the channel were removed by gently flushing the cell culture medium with a pipette.

Figs. 14.4 and 14.5 illustrate cell assembly that uses hydrodynamic drag force in the channel for organelle positioning. Depending on the size of the organelle to be biopsied, the cells can be trapped in the opening of the PDMS channel or compressed

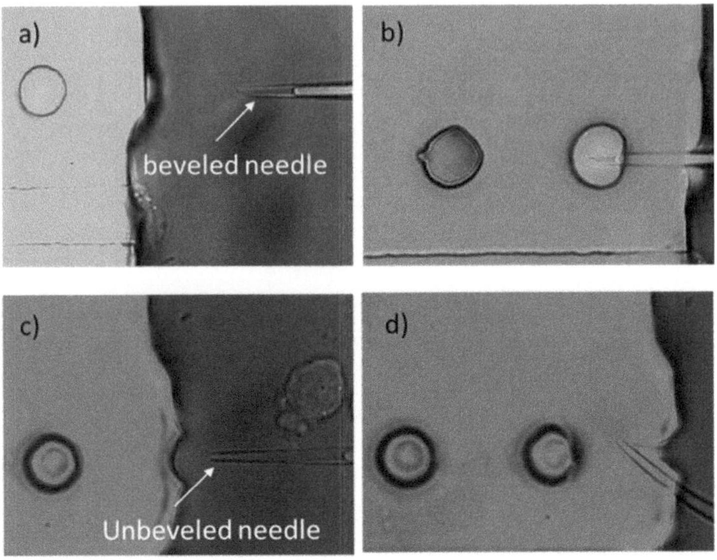

Figure 14.3 Microneedle penetration into PDMS (Shakoor et al., 2019). (A) Microneedle beveled at 20 degree. (B) Successful penetration of the beveled microneedle. (C) Unbeveled microneedle. (D) Microneedle unable to penetrate into the PDMS.

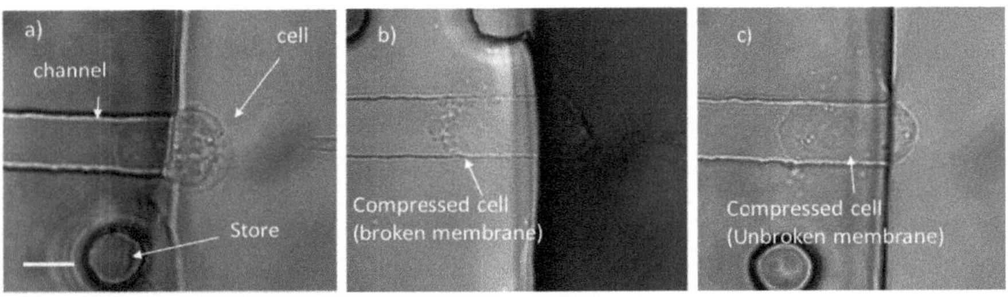

Figure 14.4 Cell (NB4) patterning by a microfluidic device (Shakoor et al., 2019). (A) The cell is trapped in front of the channel. (B) The cell is compressed in a channel of 2 μm height. The *arrow* is pointing at the bubble formation due to membrane opening. (C) Compressed cell, with unbroken membrane, in a channel with height of 5 μm. Scale bar is 15 μm.

in the PDMS channel. For a large organelle such as the nucleus (7−9 μm) of NB4 cells, its position within the ~20 μm cell can be easily accessed. Therefore, after holding the cells at the opening of the channel, automatic biopsy of large organelles can be realized. However, for small organelles, the cells must be compressed to limit the 3D position for the following reasons. First, unlike the nucleus, small organelles such as mitochondria (~2 μm) are distributed in the 3D space inside the cell. The 2D image obtained by a fluorescence microscope (see Fig. 14.5A) is a combination of stacked images obtained at different depths along the z-axis. To perform a mitochondrial biopsy in an automated manner, it is challenging to precisely position the tip of a

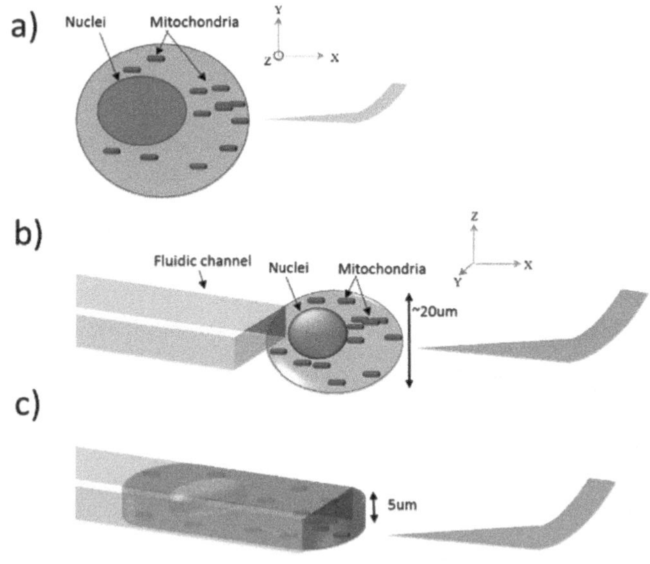

Figure 14.5 Confining the position of the mitochondria along the z-axis by compressing the cell (Shakoor et al., 2019). (A) 2D camera image view (top view). (B) 3D representation of the cell before compression. (C) 3D representation of the cell after compression inside the fluidic channel.

1–2 μm micropipette to coincide with the position of the mitochondria along the z-axis (see Fig. 14.5B), which requires the use of complex image-processing algorithms to obtain the exact position of the small organelle along the z-axis. Second, compressing the cells helps to accurately determine the negative pressure applied by the motor-controlled injector, which aspirates the mitochondria into the micropipette. If the tip of the micropipette is inserted into a cell where the mitochondria is relatively far from the tip of the micropipette along the z-axis (this is common for cells in suspension), then a large amount of cytoplasm must also be aspirated with the mitochondria, which can cause significant damage to the cell. Without limiting the position of the small organelle along the z-axis, the negative pressure applied by the computer-controlled injector to aspirate the organelle may vary from cell to cell, resulting in inconsistent biopsy results or requiring manual operations to control the amount of aspiration content.

Considering that adherent cells contain organelles at restricted locations along the cell height, careful compression of suspended cells can limit the location of small organelles without damaging the cells. Therefore, by compressing the cells, the distance along the z-axis between the tip of the micropipette and the small organelle is limited by the height of the channel, which is only 5 μm, as shown in Fig. 14.5C.

In addition, the beveled micropipette and the compression mode of the cells, which tighten the cell membrane, promote perforation of the cell membrane. For the above reasons, it is recommended to simplify the organelle biopsy process by aspirating approximately 95% of the cell into the channel of the microfluidic device (see Fig. 14.5C), rather than using complex image-processing algorithms to determine the 3D position of the mitochondria and the complex motion control of the biopsy injector along the z-axis. Experiments were performed to observe how different heights and widths of rectangular channels affect cell trapping and cell viability. It was found that a channel with a height of 5 μm and a width of 15 μm can accommodate and compress cells with a diameter of 20 μm without damaging their cell membranes (Fig. 14.4C).

14.2.2 Cell biopsy process

The procedure of performing automatic organelle extraction is outlined below. First, the micropipette tip and the cell in the microfluidic channel are brought into the same focal plane. After alignment, the position of the micropipette remains fixed along the z-axis throughout the organelle extraction process. After that, the X−Y stage to which the cell patterning device is attached is controlled by an algorithm developed to automatically perform organelle extraction tasks. Fig. 14.6 shows a schematic diagram of the automated extraction process of organelles (such as mitochondria).

The system uses image-processing algorithms to detect the location of fluorescently labeled organelles, such as the nucleus or mitochondria. Then, the stage automatically moves along the y-axis to align the organelle with the tip of the micropipette, as shown in Fig. 14.6A and B. After alignment, the stage approaches the tip of the micropipette along the x-axis to ensure that the expected organelle coincides with the tip of the micropipette (Fig. 14.6C). Then, the microinjector aspirates the organelle into the tip of the micropipette (Fig. 14.6D). The controller then moves the stage away from the micropipette to extract the micropipette from the cell (Fig. 14.6E). The aspirated organelles can be automatically placed in "storage" (see Fig. 14.6F−I) for further analysis. To release the organelles in the "storage," the stage is moved 15 μm along the y-axis, and the "storage" is placed in the microscope field of view (Fig. 14.6F). Image-processing technology is used to detect the center of the storage, and the stage moves the cell patterning device along the y-axis to align the micropipette with the center of the storage (Fig. 14.6G). The stage moves further along the x-axis, perforating the tip of the micropipette into the PDMS so that the center of the storage coincides with the tip of the micropipette (Fig. 14.6H). Finally, the microinjector automatically ejects the organelle into the storage area (Fig. 14.6I).

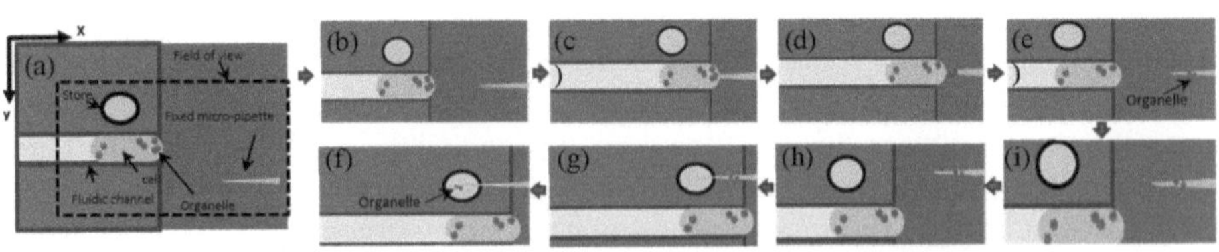

Figure 14.6 Schematic of organelle extraction (Shakoor et al., 2019). (A−E) Steps of the organelle extraction process and (F−I) steps of releasing the organelle into the storage.

In the process of manipulation, due to external disturbances (such as mechanical vibration) and model uncertainty, failures are prone to occur. Therefore, it is very important to design a robust controller that can compensate for external disturbances. In addition, the controller also needs to resolve the uncertainty of the dynamic model so that it can precisely control the microneedle toward the target organelle. To achieve these goals, Shakoor et al. (2019) proposed a robust sliding mode nonlinear controller.

14.2.3 Experiments

Biological tests were performed on the extracted organelles to characterize their biological functions. Mitochondrial membrane potential has been widely used as an indicator of mitochondrial health (Kluza et al., 2016). A significant decrease in mitochondrial membrane potential is an indicator of mitochondrial death. Using the organelle biopsy system described above, it can be verified that the membrane potential of the extracted mitochondria can remain the same as before the mitochondrial biopsy, thereby proving that the extracted mitochondria have survived. Actis et al. (2014) reported the invasiveness of the cell biopsy process through calcium imaging before and after mitochondrial biopsy. Shakoor et al. (2019) carried out a set of experiments to show that the membrane potential of the mitochondria extracted after mitochondrial biopsy and the calcium flux of the remaining cells can maintain almost unchanged. The following are the experimental details of Shakoorr et al. (2019).

14.2.3.1 Material preparation

NB4 and HDF cells were used in the organelle biopsy experiments. NB4 cells were kept in a Petri dish containing RPMI 1640 with 2 mM L-glutamine inside a humidified incubator with an atmosphere of 37°C and 5% CO_2. HDF cells were kept in Dulbecco's modified Eagle's medium (DMEM, Gibco), 100 U/mL penicillin supplemented with 10% fetal bovine serum (FBS, Gibco), and 100 U/mL streptomycin inside a humidified incubator with an atmosphere of 37°C and 5% CO_2. The cells were then stained with MitoTracker Red CMXRos (M7512, Thermo Fisher Scientific) and Hoechst (33342, Thermo Fisher Scientific) for fluorescence labeling of mitochondria and nucleus, respectively. The HDF cells were treated with trypsin (Sigma) for detachment from the Petri dish, while the NB4 cells were used directly in suspension.

A micropipette puller (P-2000, Sutter Instrument) was used to pull the glass micropipette (O.D. 1 mm and I.D. 0.78 mm) to obtain a gradual taper with a final tip size of 0.5 μm. To ensure perforation of the flexible cell membrane and to minimize the damage to the cells (for mitochondrial biopsy), a BV-10 microelectrode beveller (Sutter Instrument) was used to bevel the tip of the micropipette at 30 degrees. The final tip size was approximately 1–3 μm for mitochondrial biopsy, and 5–8 μm for nuclear biopsy. The micropipette was bent 4–5 mm from the tip to ensure that the tip could reach the cell-docking area of the microfluidic device.

Images (640 × 480) were captured using a CCD camera under 60× magnification. The physical size of each pixel was approximately 0.12 μm. To evaluate motion performance, the position tracking errors of the X–Y–Z stage were measured during the experiment.

14.2.3.2 Detection of mitochondria, nucleus, and storing space

As shown in Figs. 14.7A and 14.8A, by staining the organelles with the corresponding dyes, the organelles can be observed and distinguished from the cells and the background under the fluorescence microscope. Organelle biopsy or surgery requires complete 3D location information of the organelle. Therefore, instead of using complex image-processing algorithms to find the organelle and developing a controller for positioning the needle along the z-axis, it is better to restrict the organelle position to the z-axis in the microfluidic channel, as shown in Fig. 14.5. Using a cell-holding device to fix a single cell in a channel can greatly simplify the organelle search and biopsy process through the developed image-processing algorithm. In the image-processing

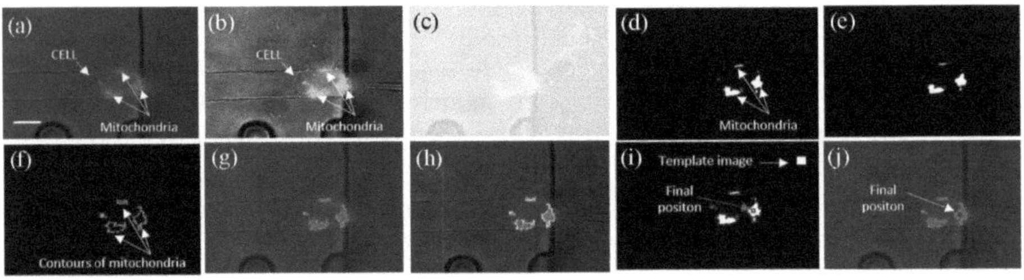

Figure 14.7 Automatic mitochondria detection (Shakoor et al., 2019). (A) Cell compressed inside the channel and stained with a MitoTracker as indicated by the *arrows*. (B) Grayscale image of (A) (for better visualization). (C) Image in the HSV plane. (D) Image after applying thresholding. (E) Image after applying Gaussian and Median filters. (F–H) Extracting the contours from the thresholding image and imposing contours on the original image. (H) Grayscale representation of (G). (I and J) Final selected position of mitochondria, as indicated by an *arrow*, after applying the template matching algorithm and using the template image shown in the inset of (I). Scale bar is 15 μm.

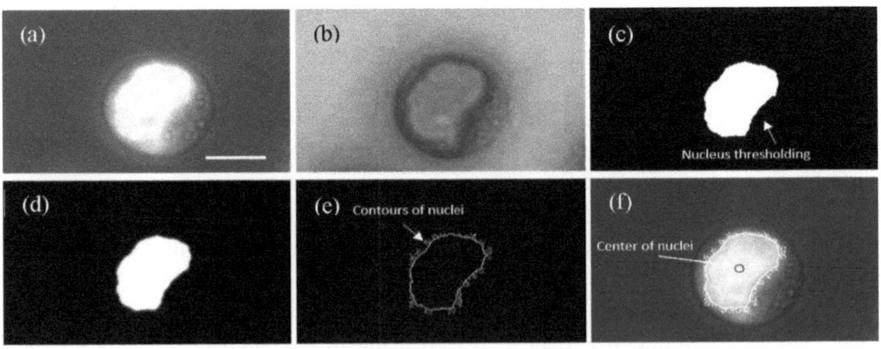

Figure 14.8 Automatic detection of the nucleus center (Shakoor et al., 2019). (A) Image of the cell stained with Hoechst 3342. (B) Threshold image. (C) Image after applying Gaussian low-pass filter. (D and E) Contours extracted from the threshold image. (F) Detection of the center of the nucleus as represented by a small *circle* (also pointed at by an *arrow*) and imposing the contour on the original image.

algorithm, fluorescence-labeled organelles can be detected by finding their HSV (hue, saturation, and value) range values in the 2D image, and they can be found through calibration experiments. Track bars were created in the GUI settings to observe the effect of HSV range changes. The change of HSV value will create the corresponding threshold image, as shown in Figs. 14.7D and 14.8C. To test whether the threshold image segmented the organelle area correctly, contours were extracted from the threshold image and imposed on the original image representing the position of the organelle. For certain types of stained organelles, the HSV value remains unchanged under a fixed brightness and exposure. Therefore, to obtain optimal results of organelle detection and subsequent organelle biopsy, experiments can be performed under a fluorescence microscope with zero brightness.

To detect the location of the mitochondrial region, an image was captured by a combination of fluorescence and brightfield microscopy, as shown in Fig. 14.7A, before converting to the HSV plane (Fig. 14.7C). Changing the HSV values created a corresponding threshold image, as shown in Fig. 14.7C, and these values remained unchanged for a fixed brightness and exposure time. The mitochondrial region, hue, saturation, and value of the image were represented by HSV values of 0–10, 160–179, 0–255, and 0–179, respectively. By applying these HSV values on the HSV plane image, a threshold image was obtained to distinguish the mitochondria marked with red fluorescence from other parts of the image, as shown in Fig. 14.7D. For verification purposes, contours were extracted and imposed on the original image to confirm the accurate threshold of the mitochondrial region (Fig. 14.7F–H). To reduce the high frequency and pepper noise in the image, Gaussian and median filters were applied (Fig. 14.7E). As shown in the right corner of Fig. 14.7I, a small image with a few white pixels was used as the template image. The normalized cross-correlation template matching method (CCORR_NORMED) was applied to detect one of the mitochondrial regions present in the threshold image (represented by the *arrow* in Fig. 14.7D). This method slides the template image over the threshold image to find the position that best matches the template image. The algorithm then draws a rectangle on the best matching area in the image, and finally selects the center of this rectangle (see Fig. 14.7I and J) as the position of the mitochondria. Compared with other mitochondrial regions, the size of the template image can help identify cell regions that contain more mitochondria. It was found that a template image with a size of 4×4 μm can find areas with high mitochondrial abundance in the image. The final position obtained by CCORR_NORMED is represented by the small black squares and *arrows* in Fig. 14.7I and J.

To detect the nucleus, cell images were captured by a combination of fluorescence and bright-field microscopy (Fig. 14.8A), and then converted to HSV plans (Fig. 14.8B). With HSV values ranging from 0 to 100 hue, 0–255 saturation and 0–179 values, a threshold image was obtained to distinguish the nucleus marked with blue fluorescence from the rest of the image (Fig. 14.8C). The image was then passed through a Gaussian and median filter to reduce noise (Fig. 14.8D). To find the center of the nucleus, the contour of the nucleus was detected (see Fig. 14.8E), and then the center of the nucleus was located by finding the central moment of the bounded area (Fig. 14.8F).

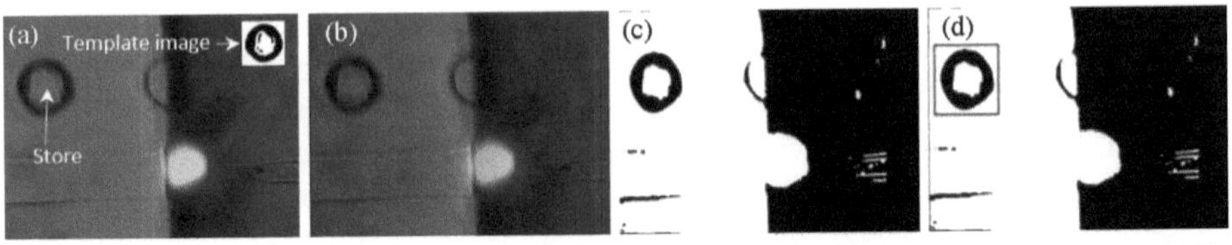

Figure 14.9 Automatic detection of the organelle storage place (Shakoor et al., 2019). (A) The original image containing the store as indicated by an *arrow*. The inset template image is used to find the positions of the storages in the images. (B) The image is converted to grayscale and filtered with a low-pass Gaussian filter to reduce noise. (C) Threshold image of the grayscale image. (D) Detection of the position of the organelle storage by using a template matching algorithm as indicated by the rectangle around the storage.

A template matching algorithm was utilized to automatically detect organelle storage space, as shown in Fig. 14.9. The image containing the cell storage space (Fig. 14.9A) was converted to a grayscale image (Fig. 14.9B). Then the image was passed through a low-pass Gaussian filter, and a threshold was applied to convert the image into a binary image (Fig. 14.9C). A template image, as shown in the inset in Fig. 14.9A, was used to match the region in the binary image. CCORR_NORMED was applied to locate the area with the highest matching probability. The rectangle in Fig. 14.9D represents the result of CCORR_NORMED. The vertex length of the rectangle was used to determine the center of the rectangle or the center of the cell storage space.

The image-processing technology used here is a simple and versatile method that can be used to detect many other organelles, such as lysosomes and Golgi apparatus. The organelles can be observed by simply changing the HSV value of the image to suit the respective dye color under a fluorescent microscope. In addition, the presented image-processing algorithm can distinguish between functional and nonfunctional organelles before biopsy. For example, because red (functional) mitochondria have different HSV values from green (nonfunctional) mitochondria, the image-processing algorithm can distinguish them based on their membrane potential. Therefore, the proposed system can also perform biopsy of organelles according to their real-time functional status.

14.2.3.3 Organelle extraction

The biopsy of the mitochondria and nucleus of individual cells depends on the successful extraction of these organelles from the cell. Fig. 14.10 shows images of the automatic extraction of mitochondria from HDF cells. These images were converted to grayscale for better visualization. To perform mitochondrial extraction in a minimally invasive manner, a beveled and almost cylindrical micropipette with a tip size of approximately 2–3 μm was used (Fig. 14.10A). The position of the mitochondria (Fig. 14.10B) was automatically identified using the proposed image-processing algorithm and aligned with the tip of the micropipette along the x-axis, as shown in Fig. 14.10C. Then, the cell patterning device was moved toward the tip of the

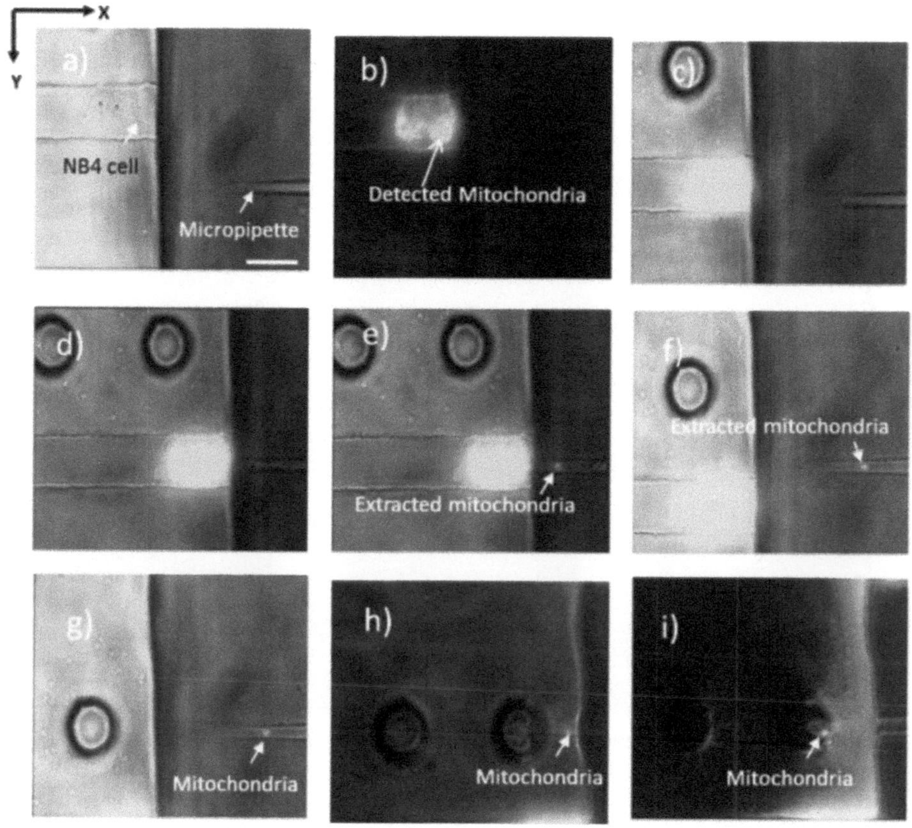

Figure 14.10 Automatic extraction of the mitochondria (Shakoor et al., 2019). The image is presented in grayscale for better visualization. (A) Micropipette and cell before biopsy. Scale bar is 10 μm. (B) Mitochondria detection. The small *square* pointed at with an *arrow* shows the detected position of the mitochondria. (C) Moving the stage to the aligned micropipette with the detected mitochondria. (D) Moving the stage toward the micropipette. (E) Aspirated mitochondria. (F) Moving the stage back to extract the micropipette out of the cell and moving the stage 15 μm along the y-axis to bring the "storage" within the field of view. (G) Moving the stage along the y-axis to align the micropipette with the center of the "storage." (H) The micropipette reaching the center of the storage. (I) Releasing the mitochondria.

micropipette until the tip of the micropipette coincided with the position of the mitochondria detected after perforating the cell membrane (Fig. 14.10D). The injector aspirated mitochondria into the micropipette (Fig. 14.10E), and the cell patterning device was moved to its original position (along the x-axis) to extract the micropipette from the cells. To ensure that the "storage" completely appeared in the field of view, the stage was moved 15 μm along the y axis (Fig. 14.10I) and positioned along the y axis to align the center of the storage with a micropipette tip. The stage moved along the x-axis so that the center of the storage coincided with the tip of the micropipette. The injector ejected the aspirated mitochondria by applying positive pressure on the back of the micropipette (Fig. 14.10I).

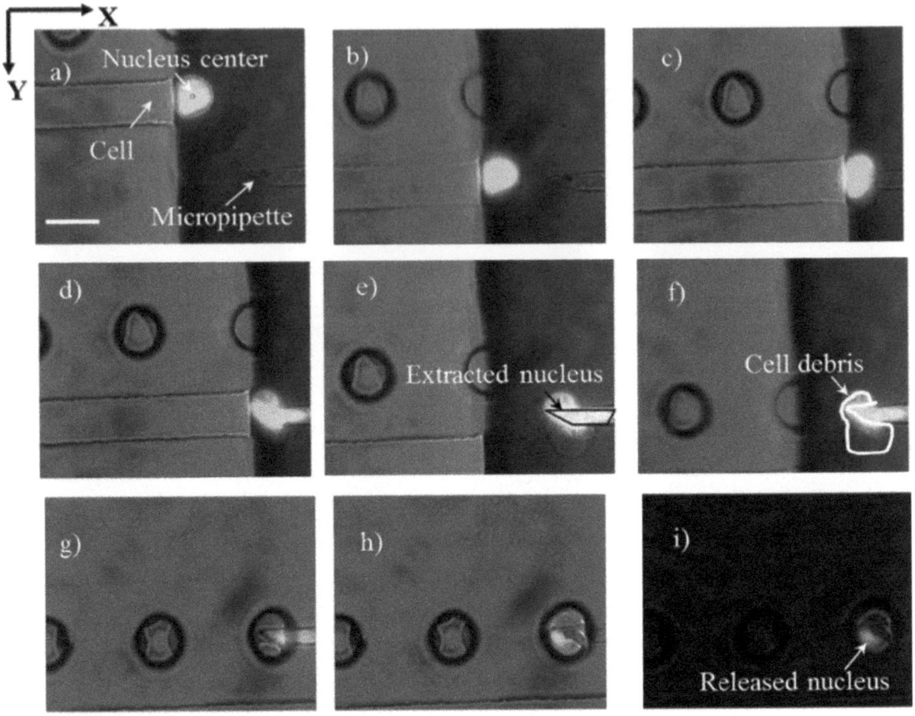

Figure 14.11 Automated extraction of nucleus from NB4 cell (Shakoor et al., 2019). (A) Automatic detection of the nucleus center via image processing. Scale bar is 15 μm. (B) The nucleus aligned with the tip of the micropipette by moving the stage along the y-axis. (C) Moving the stage toward the micropipette (along the x-axis). (D) Aspirating part of the nucleus. (E) Moving the stage toward its original position (along the x-axis) and 15 μm along the y-axis to bring the storage within the field of view. (F) Moving the stage along the y-axis to align the micropipette with the center of the storage. (F) Penetrating the micropipette tip by moving the stage along the x-axis. (H and I) Releasing the nucleus.

Fig. 14.11 shows the automatic extraction of nuclei from NB4 cells. In view of the large ratio of organelles to cell size, nuclear biopsy does not need to compress the cells, and the cells can be trapped at the entrance of the channel. The image-processing algorithm was used to automatically identify the center of the cell nucleus and align it with the tip of the micropipette along the x-axis, as shown in Fig. 14.11B. The cell patterning device was moved to the tip of the micropipette to perform perforation until the tip of the micropipette coincided with the center of the cell nucleus after perforating the cell membrane (Fig. 14.11C). The injector aspirated part of the cell nuclei into the micropipette (Fig. 14.11D). After that, the cell patterning device moved along the x-axis to its original position, while the stage moved 15 μm along the y-axis (Fig. 14.11E) to place the "storage" in the field of view. With the support of image-processing algorithms, the location of the organelle storage space was detected, and the cell patterning device was controlled to move along the y axis to align the storage center with the tip of the micropipette (Fig. 14.11F). Then the stage moved along the x-axis until the storage center meets the tip of the micropipette (Fig. 14.11G). During the micropipette tip perforation into the PDMS of the MCPD, cell debris was removed from the micropipette tip, and only the cell nucleus remained in the micropipette tip (Fig. 14.11G). The injector ejected the nucleus from the tip into the organelle storage space by applying positive pressure (Fig. 14.11H and I).

The micropipette can be easily pulled out of the cell if the extracted organelle is small (such as mitochondria), but this task is challenging if the extracted organelle is large (such as a nucleus). For aspirating large organelles, a greater negative pressure is applied to the micropipette during aspiration of the organelle, which may limit the separation of the micropipette and the cells. For example, when the cell nucleus occupies more than 60% of the cell volume, relatively high negative pressure is required to suck it into a micropipette tip ranging in size from 5 to 8 μm. If the same amount of negative pressure is applied to the back of the fluid channel, the cell will rupture during the extraction process of the micropipette, while some parts (cell debris) are still attached to the micropipette. Given the large size of the micropipette used for nuclear biopsy, the biopsy of the nucleus is very invasive, and the remaining part of the cell is considered to be cell debris. Therefore, instead of controlling the pressure on the back of the channel or extracting the micropipette from the cells, the cell debris is removed by penetrating the micropipette into the PDMS. This flushing process can be done automatically during the process of moving the micropipette to the storage (see Fig. 14.11F and G). The negative pressure required on the back of the micropipette during aspiration of the organelle depends on the amount of cell content to biopsy and the tip size of the micropipette. These control parameters are determined through calibration experiments.

14.2.3.4 Biological tests on extracted organelles and the remaining cells

After the organelles were extracted, a number of biological tests were performed on the extracted organelles and the remaining cells. The function of the extracted mitochondria was tested by observing the mitochondrial membrane potential before and after mitochondrial biopsy. Before the biopsy experiment, the cells were stained with JC-1 dye, a mitochondrial membrane potential probe (T3168, Thermo Fisher Scientific). According to the report (Yang et al., 2014; McCafferty et al., 2014), depolarized mitochondria show a change in fluorescence emission from yellow-orange or red-orange (depending on filter type) to green. After extraction from NB4 cells, the mitochondrial membrane potential remained unchanged, as shown in Fig. 14.12. Biopsy of mitochondria stained with JC-1 was performed from more than 25 NB4 cells. In all these cases, the mitochondrial membrane potential was observed, which indicated that the mitochondrial survival rate was 100%.

The survival rate of the remaining cell after mitochondrial extraction was also examined. Cells were stained with Fluo-4 calcium imaging (F10489, Thermo Fisher Scientific), and calcium flux was measured before and after mitochondrial extraction (Actis et al., 2014). Table 14.1 shows the extraction rate of mitochondria and nuclei

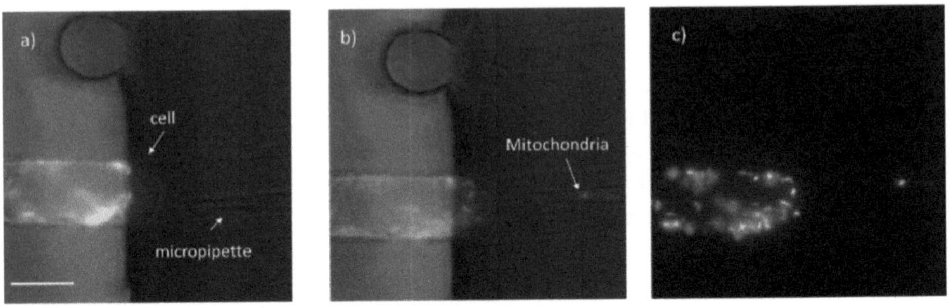

Figure 14.12 Functionality test of mitochondria after mitochondria biopsy (Shakoor et al., 2019). (A) Fluorescence image before biopsy (GFP filter). (B) Fluorescence image after biopsy. (C) Fluorescence image after biopsy (RFP filter).

Table 14.1 Organelle extraction rate (Shakoor et al., 2019).

Cell	Organelle	No. of cells used for organelle extraction	No. of cells with successful organelle extraction	Organelle extraction rate (%)
NB4	Mitochondria	125	78	62.4
NB4	Nuclei	125	86	68
HDF	Mitochondria	50	29	58
HDF	Nuclei	50	36	72

of NB4 and HDF cells using the automated organelle biopsy system. The organelle extraction rate was calculated from the ratio of the number of cells successfully biopsied to the total number of cells used in the experiment. Mitochondria and nuclear biopsy of NB4 cells can achieve extraction rates of 62.4% and 68%, respectively. Similarly, the organelle extraction rate of HDF cells was 58% of mitochondria and 72% of nuclei. The efficiency of mitochondrial biopsy is relatively low, because in some cases the detected mitochondria may be located near the back of the cell, and the micropipette may not be able to penetrate the nuclear membrane. Due to the relatively large size of the micropipette tip, the extraction rate of cell nuclei was affected by the sliding of the micropipette tip on the soft cell membrane. Fig. 14.13 summarizes the results of the mitochondrial extraction rate and cell survival rate of micropipette tips of different sizes. The cell survival rate was calculated from the ratio of the number of cells with successful biopsy to the number of cells surviving after mitochondrial biopsy. The negative pressure on the back of the micropipette was calibrated while monitoring the successful aspiration of the mitochondria into the micropipette. A larger negative pressure corresponded to a larger volume change in the micropipette, thereby aspirating more cell contents during the biopsy process, and increasing the mitochondrial extraction rate. According to the experimental calibration, two different aspiration pressures, P1 and P2, determined by the volume change per revolution, were used in all experiments to examine the mitochondrial biopsy and cell viability. The results are

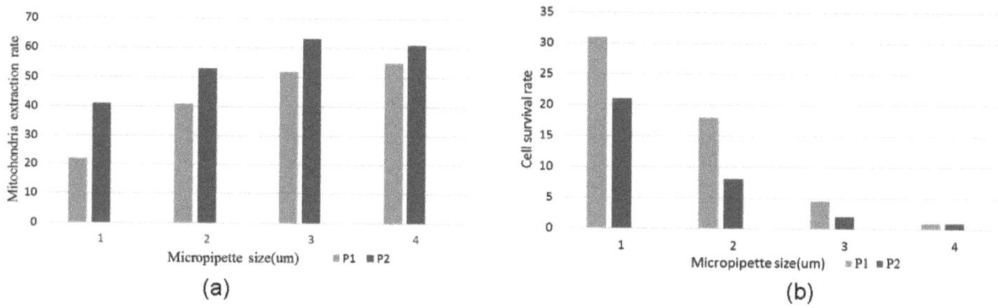

Figure 14.13 Comparison results with different sizes of the micropipette tip (Shakoor et al., 2019). (A) Mitochondria extraction rate. (B) NB4 cell survival rate.

summarized in Fig. 14.13. P1 and P2 represent the volume change when the injector was rotated 20 and 45 degrees, respectively. If the purpose of the biopsy is to analyze the biopsy cells, the same cell should not be extracted more than once, because a detectable difference in calcium flux can be observed in subsequent extractions. However, if the goal of the biopsy is to obtain mitochondria without regard to cell viability, the extraction process can be repeated multiple times on the same cell.

14.3 Gene-delivery approaches for MSC function improvement

This section compares the capability of the robotic microinjection method with that of three other gene-delivery vehicles, namely calcium phosphate coprecipitation, PEI, and Lipofectamine, in a case study of transfecting adult MSCs. The effects of these delivery vehicles on cell viability, morphology, and MSC multilineage differentiation potential are evaluated. Using the above four vectors, the osteoblast differentiation negative regulator PPARγ gene will be knocked out, and its effect on gene function and stem cell differentiation determined. The results indicate that the prejudice against osteogenesis or adipogenesis commitments largely depends on the exposure of different delivery vehicles. In addition, the function of therapeutic genes is differently interfered with by gene carriers. The results further show that robotic microinjection is a promising method for generating transgenic MSCs, which will not destroy the differentiation promise and gene function of MSCs.

14.3.1 Materials and methods

Four gene vectors were used to transfect human MSCs. After transfection of MSCs, their morphology and differentiation potential were tested to evaluate the effects of the four gene-delivery methods (Fig. 14.14). First, robotic microinjection-based transfection was performed with the optimal parameters as previously described (Chow et al., 2016; Pan et al., 2020). The optimal balance pressure was 0.8 lbf/in^2, and the insertion duration was 100 ms. Second, the calcium phosphate−DNA complex was

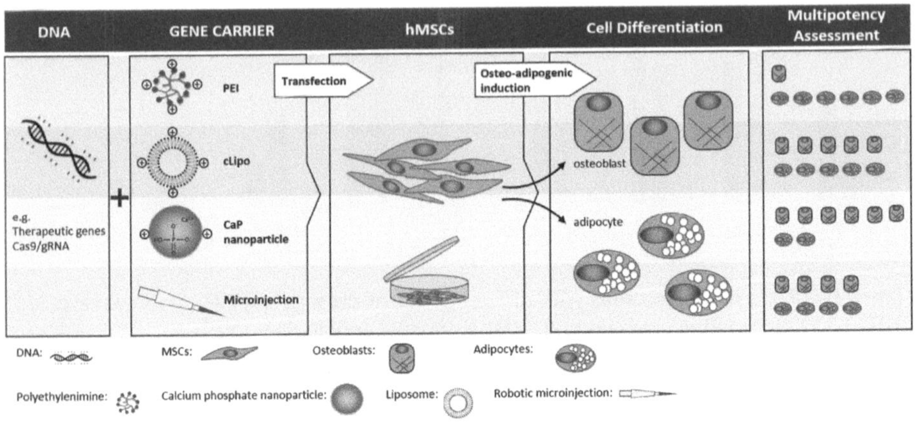

Figure 14.14 Schematic of transfection in MSCs using four delivery vehicles and differentiation potential assessment (Guan et al., 2021).

prepared by slowly dropping 0.5 μg DNA into 0.25 M $CaCl_2$, and then mixed with an equal volume of 2 × HEPES buffer (50 mM HEPES, 280 mM Na_3PO_4, 1.5 mM Na_2HPO_4) as described earlier (Jordan et al., 1996). The volume-to-weight ratios of $CaCl_2$-HEPES/DNA (μL/μg) were 10/1, 30/1, 50/1, 70/1, and 90/1. The mixture solution was incubated at room temperature for 20 min before transfection, and the cells were incubated with the complex for 6 h. Third, according to the manufacturer's protocol, Lipofectamine 3000 was transfected and optimized in MSCs. In short, Lipofectamine 3000 and 0.5 μg DNA were diluted in 50 μL blank medium, where the liposome/DNA volume ratios (μL/μg) were 0.25/1, 0.5/1, 1/1, 2/1, and 4/1. The cells were incubated with the complex for 4 h. Finally, the PEI−DNA complex was synthesized by mixing 0.5 μg DNA with PEI solution (1 mg/mL, Sigma−Aldrich), where the ratios of PEI/DNA were 0.5/1, 1/1, 2/1, 4/1, and 8/1. The cells were incubated with the complex for 4 h. Before CaP, cLipo PEI, and microinjection transfection, MSCs were seeded at a density of $1-2 \times 10^4$ cells/cm^2 and cultured to ~80% confluence. In all the above methods, the transfection efficiency was calculated by counting the positive cells in each view.

A dual-module microinjection system (Pan et al., 2020), which mainly consists of an inverted fluorescence microscope (Nikon), a CMOS camera (Tucsen Photonics), a motorized XY stage (Prior Scientific), two motorized XYZ micromanipulators (Sensapex), and a pressure provider (MicroData Instrument), was used to conduct cell injection (Fig. 14.15). High throughput can be achieved through automatic cell position detection, fast injection path optimization, adaptive penetration depth adjustment, and constant outflow injection. The optimization of the microinjector path was expressed as a symmetric traveling salesman problem, which can be solved by the Concord program. Two deep neural convolutional networks were used to detect cells. Cells for injection were cultured in a self-made chamber. The penetration interval was set to 1.7 s, so approximately 3000 cells could be injected in 1 h.

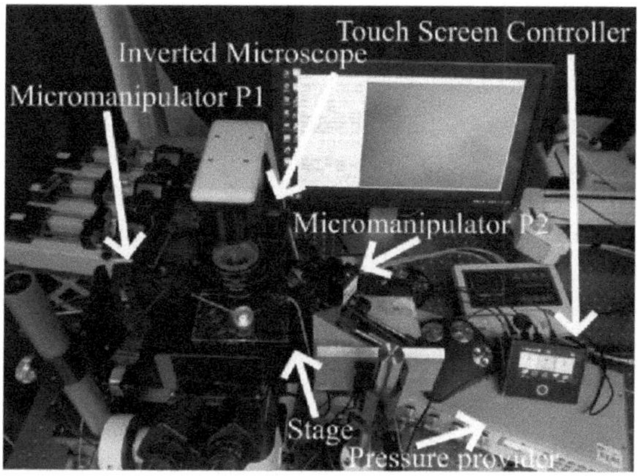

Figure 14.15 A dual-module microinjection system with two micromanipulators (Guan et al., 2021).

Human adult MSCs were cultured and expanded in αMEM medium (Gbico) supplemented with 10% FBS (Sigma–Aldrich) and 1% antibiotics (penicillin-streptomycin, Invitrogen). During the expansion process, cells were passaged at approximately 80% confluence using 0.25% trypsin and EDTA (Life Technologies). MSCs between the third and eighth generations were used. Four gene-delivery vectors were used to transfect MSCs, and adipogenic or osteogenic induction medium was added 24 h later. Osteogenic medium was StemPro osteocyte/chondrocyte differentiation basal medium supplemented with StemPro Osteogenic Supplement (Gbico). In the adipogenesis experiment, MSCs were fed StemPro adipocyte differentiation basal medium containing StemPro adipogenesis supplement. After transfection, MSCs were induced with differentiation medium for up to 14 days. During this period, the medium was changed every 3 days, and MSCs were harvested at each time point for evaluation of osteo-adipogenic potential by Alizarin red staining, Nile red staining, and/or RT-PCR.

Cell viability was tested using the MTT assay (Sigma–Aldrich). In short, cells were cultured in 100 μg/mL MTT PBS solution at 37°C and 5% CO_2 for 4 h. After that, the cells were washed twice with PBS and dissolved in DMSO. The absorbance at 560 nm was measured. The adult MSCs were transfected with reporter gene eGFP by CaP, cLipo, PEI, and microinjection, respectively. The transfected cells were cultured for 48 h and imaged using an inverted fluorescence microscope. Cell morphology was evaluated through the cell spreading area, circularity, and cell aspect ratio using the plug-in in ImageJ.

Immunofluorescence staining of actin and vinculin showed the actin cytoskeleton and focal adhesion complex in the transfected MSCs. The MSCs were spread on a cover glass, which was coated with 5 μg/mL fibronectin solution (R&G system). After transfection, MSCs were incubated for 48 h, and then fixed with 4% paraformaldehyde solution (Sigma–Aldrich) for 10 min at room temperature. Cell slides were blocked with 5% BSA solution at room temperature for at least 1 h, and then incubated with vinculin primary antibody (Abcam, ab129002) at 4°C overnight. After incubation, the samples were washed three times with PBS. Before incubating with the secondary antibody (Santa Cruz, sc-516250), the samples were permeabilized with 0.5% Triton X-100. Finally, the samples were stained with Alexa Fluor 488 Phalloidin (Invitrogen) for 1.5 h and DAPI for 15 min. A confocal microscope (Leica TCS SP8 confocal microscope system) was used to capture immunofluorescence images. The anisotropy of the actin fiber network was calculated using the FibrilTool plug-in in ImageJ to indicate cytoskeleton intensity (Boudaoud et al., 2014).

The DESKGEN website (http://deskgen.com) was used to design highly specific sgRNA targeting human PPARγ gene (NC_000003.12). sgRNA-U and sgRNA-E were made to target exon 5 of PPARγ. Lentiviral vectors expressing both Cas9 and sgRNA were constructed. The vectors were verified by Sanger sequencing. The other plasmid used encodes eGFP.

The PCR amplicon from specific primers (Table 14.2) was analyzed by 1.5% agarose gel electrophoresis. Sanger sequencing was performed by the BGI Group. For gene expression analysis, after 14 days of culture, total RNA was extracted from transfected and control MSCs using TRIzol (Invitrogen), and converted to cDNA using iScript Reverse Transcription Supermix (Bio-Rad). The CFX96 real-time PCR detection system (Applied Biosystems) and SYBR mix (Bio-Rad) were used to perform quantitative PCR to evaluate the expression level of marker genes (Table 14.2). WT and treated MSC cells were lysed by adding RIPA lysis buffer to test the PPARγ protein level. WB was performed on the lysate using PPARγ antibody (sc-7273, Santa Cruz).

Data were analyzed using one-way ANOVA with Tukey's post hoc test for comparison between groups. Data are shown as mean ± standard deviation (SD). Statistical significance was accepted when the *P*-value was less than 0.05.

Table 14.2 Nucleic acid sequence (Guan et al., 2021).

sgRNA-U	5′-AGTGTGCCCCATCATTGTTG tgg-3′
sgRNA-E	5′-TATGAGACATCCCCACTGCA agg-3′
PPARγ-F primer	5′-GCAGAATATTCAGTTGGCCTCAA-3′
PPARγ-R primer	5′-AGCAGAACGACACTACTGATACAC-3′
RUNX2-F primer	5′-TGGTTACTGTCATGGCGGGTA-3′
RUNX2-R primer	5′-TCTCAGATCGTTGAACCTTGCTA-3′
ALPL-F primer	5′-ACCACCACGAGAGTGAACCA-3′
ALPL-R primer	5′-CGTTGTCTGAGTACCAGTCCC-3′
LPL-F primer	5′-CTGCTGGCGTTGCAGGAAGT-3′
LPL-R primer	5′-GCTGGAAAGTACCTCCATTC-3′
FABP4-F primer	5′- AGCACCATAACCTTAGATGGGG -3′
FABP4-R primer	5′- CGTGGAAGTGACGCCTTTCA -3′

14.3.2 Results

14.3.2.1 Transfection efficiency and morphological disruptions in MSCs

The transfection conditions of different delivery methods with a series of *v/w* ratios (reagent/DNA, μL/μg) need to be optimized to deliver the eGFP plasmid to the MSC. When optimizing transfection conditions, the DNA dose is kept consistent through the delivery method. As shown in Fig. 14.16A, reducing the amount of transfection reagent (lower *v/w* ratio) can increase cell viability, while a large amount of reagent (higher *v/w* ratio) leads to a decrease in cell viability. On the other hand, transfection efficiency is significantly affected by the amount of transfection reagent. For example, while the PEI/DNA ratio is less than 2/1, the efficiency is extremely low and increases as the ratio increases. Unfortunately, a high PEI/DNA ratio (more than 2/1) will cause a sharp drop in transfection efficiency and cell viability (Fig. 14.16A). After considering transfection efficiency and cell viability, the best transfection conditions were determined as those of *v/w* ratio (μL/μg) of cLipo was 2/1, PEI was 2/1, and CaP was 50/1 (Fig. 14.16A). In the following experiments, only the optimal transfection conditions were used and compared. Fig. 14.16B shows that robotic microinjection can achieve the highest efficiency (50%–70%) of plasmid delivery to MSCs 48 h after transfection, while the efficiencies of PEI, cLipo, and CaP are lower, at about 10%–25%.

The cytotoxic effects of the four strategies were measured by MTT assay and crystal violet staining. Compared with the control group, the cell viability of MSCs in the microinjection group and the cLipo group showed similar performance 2 days after treatment, which did not significantly decrease (Fig. 14.16C). Interestingly, PEI caused a significant decrease in cell viability, while CaP treatment slightly increased cell viability. The cytopathic effects in control and treated MSCs were further studied using crystal violet staining. Morphological changes and cell numbers were assessed. Microinjection, cLipo, and CaP methods did not cause significant cytopathic effects, while PEI caused extreme fragmentation in cell culture and led to a decrease in cell number (Fig. 14.16D). Cell shrinkage occurred in PEI-treated MSCs, and shrinkage was also observed in CaP and cLipo groups, but to a lesser extent. A similar change was observed through a fluorescence microscope (Fig. 14.16E). The cell spreading area, cell circularity, and cell aspect ratio of GFP-positive MSCs were measured to quantify the morphological changes after transfection (Fig. 14.16F–H). Microinjection did not cause significant changes in MSCs, while MSCs transfected with cLipo and CaP became slightly more slender and showed a higher aspect ratio. However, PEI-treated MSCs showed a markedly round morphology with the highest circularity.

Immunofluorescence imaging was then used to evaluate the F-actin arrangement and focal adhesion distribution, based on which the cell morphology can be determined. Fig. 14.17A and B show that MSCs treated with microinjection and cLipo can maintain strong and dense actin stress fibers (phalloidin staining, green) and numerous adhesion complexes (represented by staining vinculin, red), which is similar to the control group. CaP-treated MSCs failed to form mature focal adhesion, and no

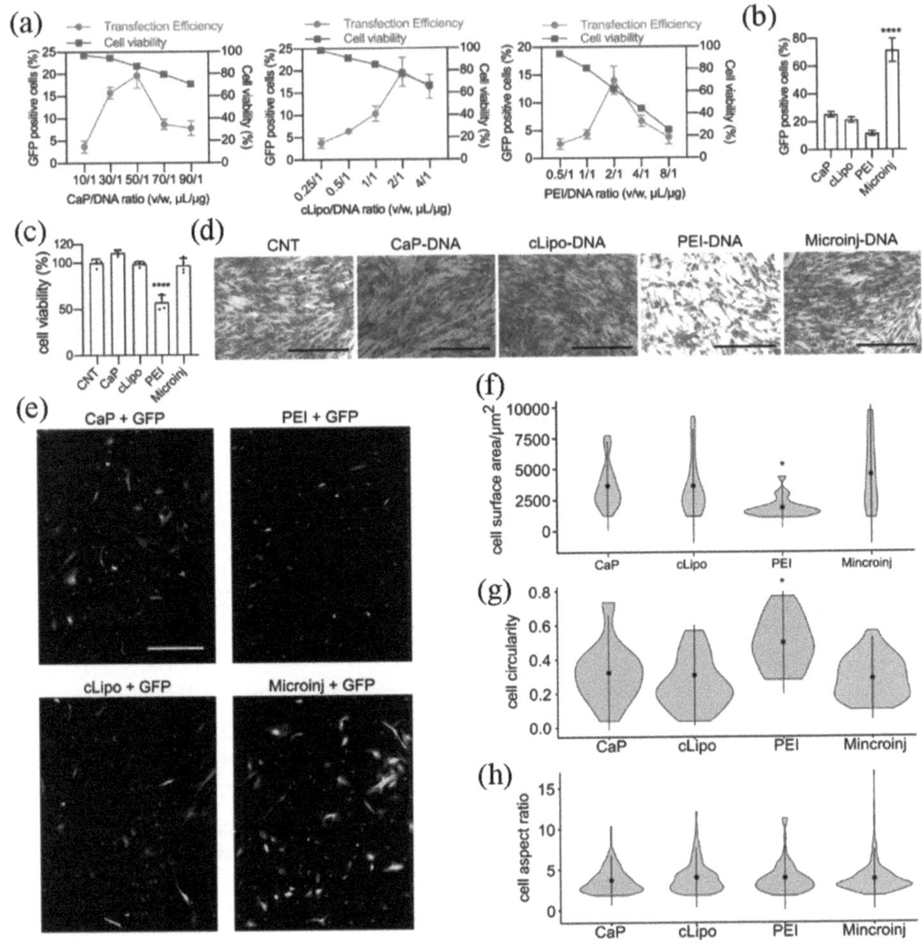

Figure 14.16 Transfection efficiency and morphology analysis in MSCs transfected via four delivery vehicles (Guan et al., 2021). (A) Optimization of cLipo, PEI, and CaP transfection in MSCs considering transfection efficiency and cell viability. Transfection efficiency was evaluated by the percentage of GFP-positive cells, and cell viability was measured by MTT assay at 48 h post transfection. Comparison of transfection efficiency (B) and cell viability (C) in MSCs via four delivery methods under optimal transfection conditions. (D) The cytopathic effect was estimated using crystal violet staining. Scale bar is 500 μm. (E) Fluorescent inverted microscopy images of positive cells (green) at 48 h after transfection. Scale bar is 500 μm. (F) Cell spread area, (G) cell circularity, and (H) cell aspect ratio of positive MSCs at 48 h post transfection. **** indicates the significance compared with all groups (n = 5 in B; n = 4 in C, $P < .0001$). * in F and G indicates the significance compared with all groups ($P < .05$).

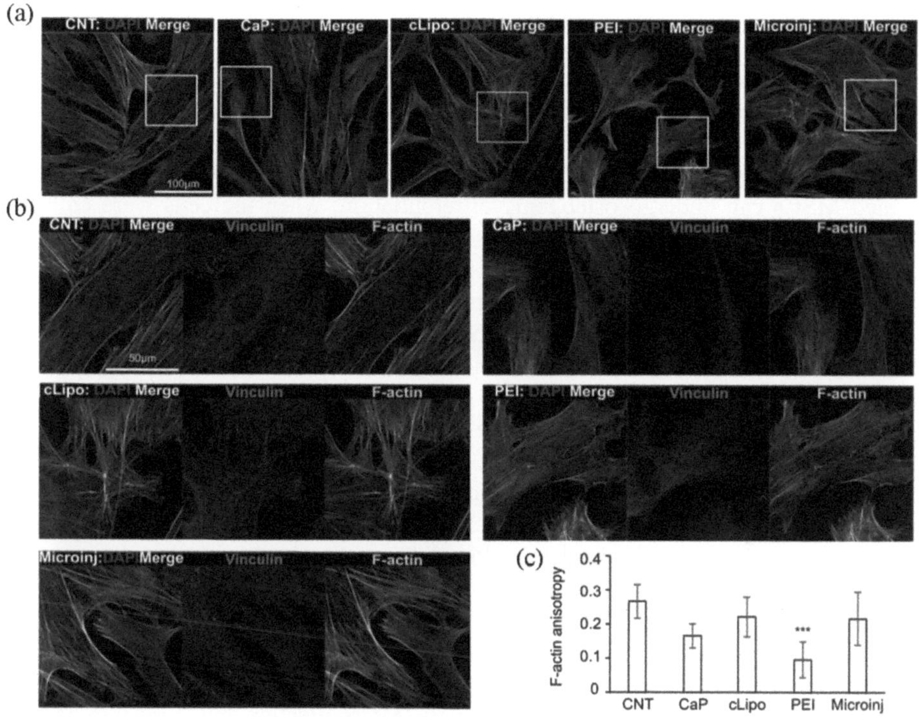

Figure 14.17 F-actin arrangement and focal adhesion distribution in MSCs exposed to different delivery vehicles (Guan et al., 2021). (A) Immunofluorescent images of MSCs stained for F-actin, vinculin, and nuclei at 48 h post transfection via microinjection, cLipo, CaP, and PEI. (B) Insets (white box in A) with high magnification shown details of F-actin arrangement and focal adhesion distribution. (C) Comparison of the mean anisotropy values of F-actin from MSCs. Control and transfected MSCs were stained with phalloidin. *** indicates a significance compared with the control group ($n = 4$, $P < .001$).

vinculin spots were observed at the ends of actin fibers. CaP-treated MSCs also showed a slight decrease in the tension of stress fibers. It is worth noting that PEI caused an extreme decrease in F-actin anisotropy, and no focal adhesion was observed in the PEI group, as shown in Fig. 14.17C.

14.3.2.2 Various forms of manipulation in osteo-adipogenic differentiation of MSCs

As the cytoskeleton organization, focal adhesion, and cell morphology have been shown to have a decisive influence on the differentiation of MSCs toward adipogenesis or osteoblasts, the influence of microinjection on the differentiation commitment of MSCs, in comparison with the other three delivery vehicles, was studied. A reliable feature of osteoblast formation is calcium accumulation in the extracellular matrix, also known as mineralization (Ducy et al., 1997). This can be evaluated by Alizarin

Red staining, which shows mineralized nodules in red. Transfected and untreated MSCs were cultured in osteogenic medium, and the osteogenic potential was detected by Alizarin Red staining after 14 days to determine the effect of the delivery method on the osteogenic ability. After induction, compared with the untreated control, CaP treatment resulted in a significant increase in calcium accumulation (calcium-ARS), as shown in Fig. 14.18A and C. Interestingly, even without induction medium, CaP-treated MSCs can undergo osteogenic differentiation; when the cells were cultured in basal medium, no mineralized nodules were observed in cLipo, microinjection, or the control group. The calcium levels in microinjected and cLipo-treated MSCs were similar to those in the control group after osteoinduction, while no mineralized nodules were observed in PEI-treated MSCs (Fig. 14.18A and C).

The potential of transfected MSCs to differentiate into adipocytes was evaluated using Nile Red staining after 14 days of culture in adipogenesis induction medium (Wang et al., 2009). Compared with the control, the adipogenesis ability of MSCs was inhibited after CaP treatment (Fig. 14.18B and D). In contrast, PEI-treated MSCs tended to differentiate into adipocytes. Among them, 11.6% of MSCs were Nile Red-positive and rich in lipid particles, while the control group had 6.9% Nile Red-positive cells. Robotic microinjection did not disrupt the adipogenic potential of MSCs, while cLipo had a slight effect on adipogenesis (Fig. 14.18B and D).

The above observations indicate that MSCs transfected with microinjection and other delivery vehicles exhibited a unique bias toward osteo-adipogenic differentiation potential. Exposure to CaP or PEI compelled multipotential MSCs to easily differentiate into osteoblasts or adipocytes, respectively. Microinjection and cLipo retained the pluripotency of MSCs, and no significant deviation was observed.

14.3.2.3 Similar capacity for gene editing in MSCs

As a nuclear receptor that regulates differentiation, PPARγ is a potential candidate as a drug target because the lack of PPARγ promotes osteogenic differentiation and inhibits adipogenesis (Sun et al., 2013). To genetically modify MSCs, the CRISPR/Cas9 system was used to knock out the PPARγ gene in adult MSCs. Two sgRNAs were designed to target exon 5 of PPARγ in human MSCs, as shown in Fig. 14.19A. Plasmid DNA expressing Cas9 and sgRNA was delivered to MSCs through four delivery vehicles: CaP, cLipo, PEI, and robotic microinjection. The efficiency of gene editing was evaluated by semiquantitative analysis of PCR products, and the protein level of PPARγ was detected by western blot analysis. It was found that all four delivery vehicles realized gene editing in MSCs. In the genotyping experiment, all treatments after gel electrophoresis showed short bands of PCR products (Fig. 14.19B). Microinjection, CaP, and cLipo groups resulted in a significant decrease in protein expression 4 days after CRISPR/Cas9 delivery (Fig. 14.19C). Although the PEI-based CRISPR/Cas9 component delivery achieved a similar level of gene mutation, it failed to reduce protein expression to the same level as the other three groups. In general, the four delivery vehicles did not cause significant differences in gene editing efficiency. Sanger sequencing and ICE analysis of PCR amplicons were performed to characterize indels. When sgRNA-E was introduced into MSCs, it was found that

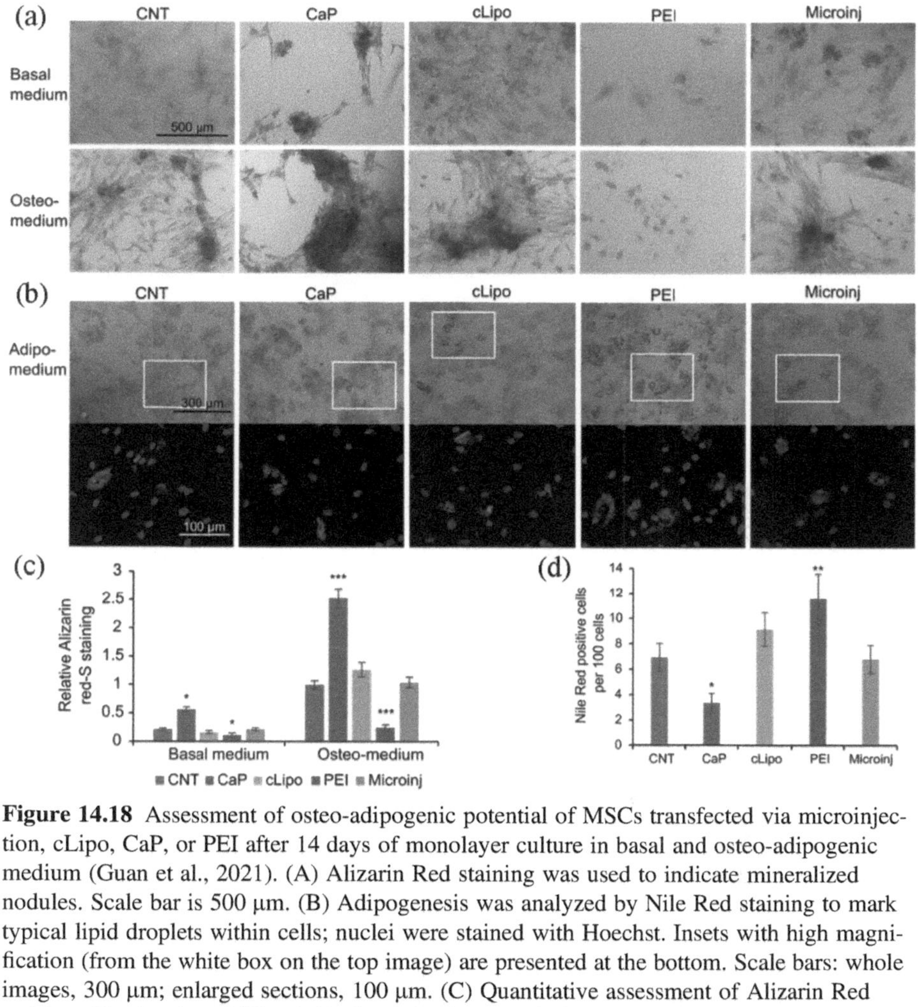

Figure 14.18 Assessment of osteo-adipogenic potential of MSCs transfected via microinjection, cLipo, CaP, or PEI after 14 days of monolayer culture in basal and osteo-adipogenic medium (Guan et al., 2021). (A) Alizarin Red staining was used to indicate mineralized nodules. Scale bar is 500 μm. (B) Adipogenesis was analyzed by Nile Red staining to mark typical lipid droplets within cells; nuclei were stained with Hoechst. Insets with high magnification (from the white box on the top image) are presented at the bottom. Scale bars: whole images, 300 μm; enlarged sections, 100 μm. (C) Quantitative assessment of Alizarin Red staining. The density of Alizarin Red staining in control MSCs after differentiation was set as 1. * indicates the significance compared with control group after culture in the basal medium (n = 3, $P < .05$). *** indicates the significance compared with the control group after osteo-induction (n = 3, $P < .001$). (D) Nile Red-positive cells were counted in each view for evaluating the effect of different treatments on the adipogenic potential of MSCs. Nile Red-positive cells were not detected under basal medium, and images are not shown. *, ** indicate the significance of CaP and PEI compared with control group, respectively (n = 4, $*P < .05$, $**P < .01$).

the gene editing efficiency was very high, at between 60% and 82% (robot microinjection, 71%; cLipo, 82%; CaP, 64%; and PEI, 60%). No special indel pattern was observed, indicating that the four delivery vehicles did not cause deviation of the gene KO mutation (Fig. 14.19D). The 10 off-target sites of sgRNA-U and sgRNA-E were also sequenced, and no indel events were detected.

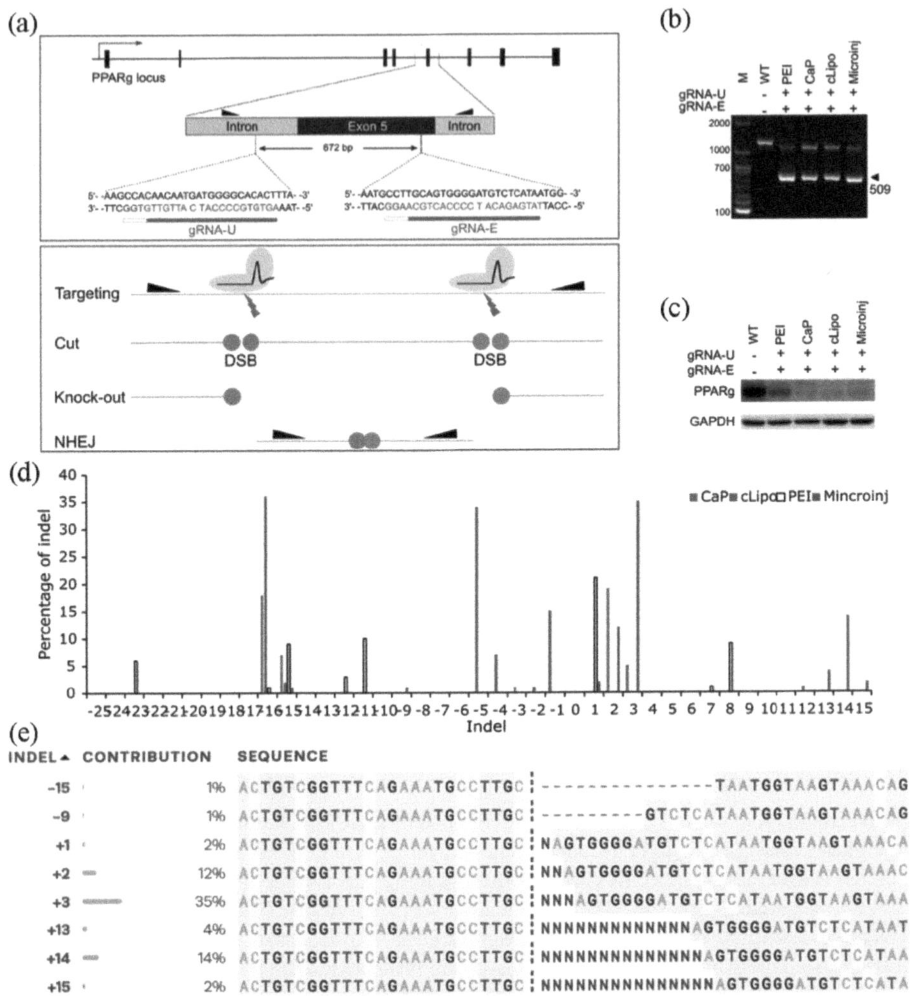

Figure 14.19 Knock-out of PPARγ gene in human MSCs using four methods for delivering CRISPR/Cas9 component (Guan et al., 2021). (A) Upper diagram of PPARγ gene locus and sgRNA target sites. Lower schematic for CRISPR/Cas9 KO and detecting KO event with PCR. Exons are shown as dark blocks. *Gray rectangles* and *lines* between blocks indicate introns. Two gRNA targeting sites were selected for the PPARγ locus to cut out 672 bp, and the sequence for each sgRNA (sgRNA-U and sgRNA-E) is shown in teal with the PAM sequence. *Triangles* indicate genotyping PCR primers used to confirm on-target deletion of PPARγ gene. PCR amplicon is 1181 bp from WT cell and 509 bp (1181 − 672 = 509 bp) from the knockout cell. DSB is the abbreviation for double strand break of DNA, and NHEJ for nonhomologous end joining. (B) Gel electrophoresis of PCR products to confirm gene knockout. After transfection, genomic DNA was extracted for amplification of the region spanning the deletion site. The short bands (arrowhead) indicate the occurrence of KO events. (C) Protein level was assessed by western blot analysis. GAPDH was the endogenous control. (D) Sequence analysis with ICE to calculate gene editing efficiency. The X axis indicates indel type, where the negative means deletion and the positive means insertion. (E) Representative sequence alignment. Data are from PCR amplicon after microinjection of sgRNA-E. N indicates any inserted nucleotide and the dashed line indicates deletion of a nucleotide.

14.3.2.4 Compromise of therapeutic gene function in MSCs

In view of the devastating impact of delivery methods on the differentiation promise of MSCs, further studies have been conducted on whether the choice of gene-delivery methods will affect the function of therapeutic genes. This is important for stem cell-based therapies, because therapeutic genes must be introduced into MSCs before infusion to patients to improve performance. Using a robotic microinjection system and three chemical, special sgRNAs and Cas9 were delivered to MSCs to knock out the PPARγ gene in MSCs to promote osteogenic differentiation. Four PPARγ$^{-/-}$ MSC cell cultures, namely PPARγ$^{-/-}$ CaP-MSCs, PPARγ$^{-/-}$ cLipo-MSC, PPARγ$^{-/-}$ PEI-MSC, and PPARγ$^{-/-}$ Microinj-MSC, were obtained.

To determine the ability of osteogenic differentiation, each of these cell cultures was individually cultured in osteogenic induction medium for 14 days. After osteogenic induction, PPARγ$^{-/-}$CaP-MSCs easily differentiated into osteoblasts and showed stronger Alizarin Red staining than PPARγ WT MSCs (Fig. 14.20A and D). PPARγ$^{-/-}$ cLipo-MSCs and PPARγ$^{-/-}$ Microinj-MSCs followed the same trend as PPARγ$^{-/-}$ CaP-MSCs, and the deposited calcium increased by two to three times compared with WT MSCs. In contrast, calcium accumulation in the PPARγ$^{-/-}$ PEI-MSCs group was not obvious. Alkaline phosphatase (ALP) activity is a distinctive feature of the osteoblast phenotype and is a well-known marker of new bone formation and differentiation into osteoblasts. The ALP activity was evaluated by alkaline phosphatase staining. Compared with WT MSCs after osteogenic differentiation, the ALP activity in PPARγ$^{-/-}$ CaP-MSC, PPARγ$^{-/-}$ cLipo-MSC, and PPARγ$^{-/-}$ Microinj-MSC also increased significantly (Fig. 14.20B). However, PPARγ$^{-/-}$ MSC from PEI showed lower ALP activity than other groups and WT MSCs.

To characterize the effects of different gene-delivery methods on the adipogenic potential of PPARγ$^{-/-}$ MSCs, knockout MSCs and WT MSCs were subjected to adipogenic differentiation medium for 14 days. After Nile Red staining, the ability of PPARγ knockout MSCs from CaP, cLipo, and microinjection to differentiate into adipocytes was impaired. Compared with about 8% in WT MSCs, less than 4% of cells were positive for Nile Red (Fig. 14.20C and E). In contrast, PPARγ knockout MSCs derived from PEI still exhibited high adipogenic capacity, with approximately 8% of cells rich in lipid droplets. This showed that even without the PPARγ gene, gene carriers like PEI can initiate adipogenic differentiation by themselves.

Since PPARγ is a key nuclear receptor for the transcriptional regulation of various genes in the osteo-adipogenesis of MSCs, the gene expression levels of differentiation markers were further examined using qRT-PCR. After osteogenic induction on the 14th day, the expression levels of osteoblast differentiation markers RUNX2 and ALPL in the CaP, cLipo, and microinjection KO groups were higher than for the PPARγ WT control (Fig. 14.20F). This finding is consistent with previous studies, which indicated that PPARγ acts as a negative regulator of osteogenesis (Wan et al., 2010). However, PEI suppressed the expression levels of RUNX2 and ALPL, indicating that PEI can mask the advantage of PPARγ in inhibiting osteogenic commitment. During the induction of adipogenesis, PPARγ knockout significantly downregulated the gene expression of adipogenic differentiation markers, such as

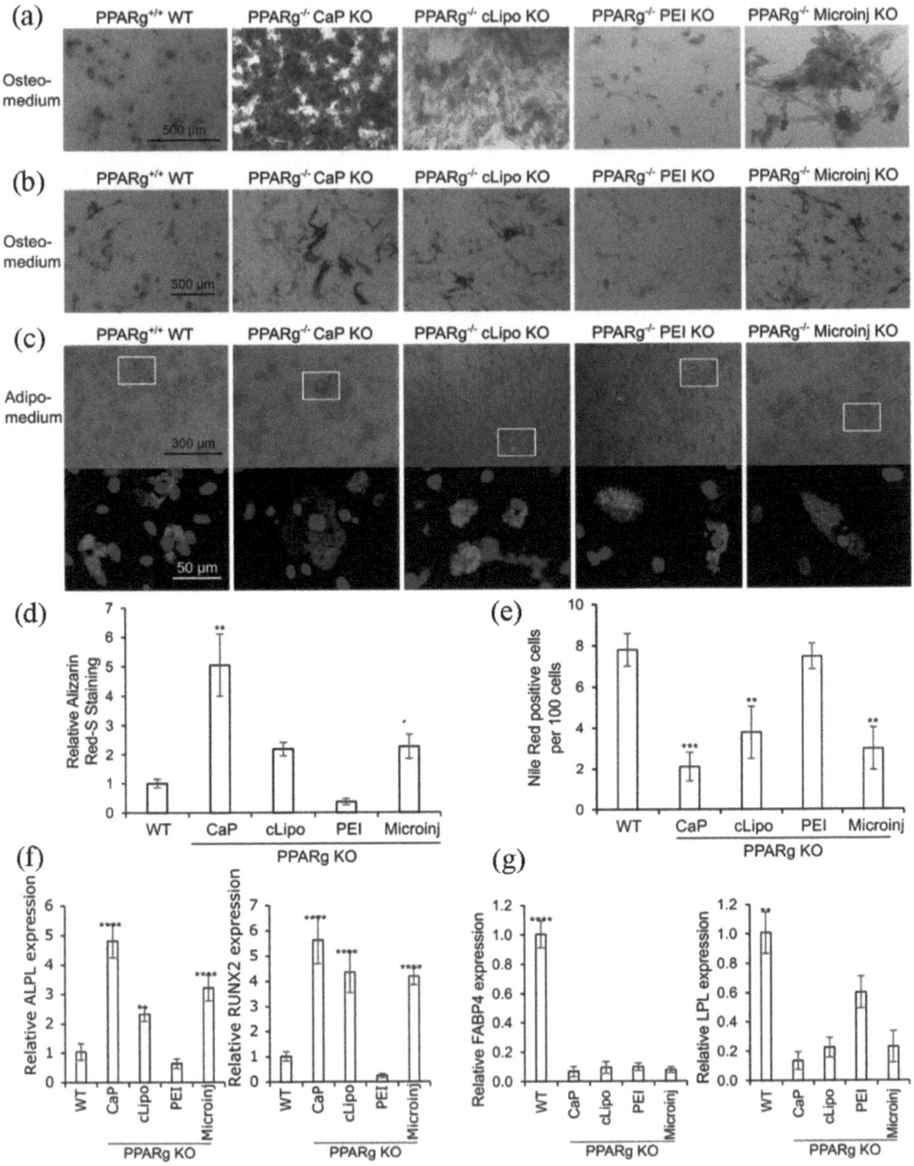

Figure 14.20 Assessment of the effects of the four delivery vehicles on PPARγ gene function in the differentiation commitment of MSCs (Guan et al., 2021). (A) Alizarin Red staining was used to characterized mineralized nodules in genetically modified MSC cultures after osteogenic induction. Scale bar is 500 μm. (B) ALP activity was evaluated by alkaline phosphatase staining. (C) Genetically modified MSCs underwent adipogenic differentiation. Lipid drop was stained by Nile Red staining and Nile Red-positive cells were counted. Insets with high magnification (from white box on the top image) are presented at the bottom. (D) Quantitative assessment of Alizarin Red staining. The density of Alizarin Red staining in

LPL and FABP4, in all PPARγ knockout groups (Fig. 14.20G). Although PEI induced higher adipogenesis, FABP4 expression was almost undetectable, and compared with WT MSCs, the expression level of LPL in PPARγ knockout MSCs derived from PEI was also extremely low.

These findings indicate that the function of therapeutic genes is impaired by gene-delivery methods. Transgenic MSCs using different delivery vectors exhibit different differentiation potentials, and the bias toward osteogenic or adipogenic differentiation depends to a large extent on the gene-delivery vector used.

14.3.2.5 Discussion

The use of genetically modified MSCs in cell therapy has shown attractive prospects for applications in many diseases, including osteoarthritis, diabetes, wounds, neurological diseases, and cancer (Galipeau and Sensébé, 2018; Ren et al., 2008; Sage et al., 2016). Unfortunately, MSCs fail to achieve their full therapeutic properties, partly because of gene-delivery vectors, which are used during the generation of transgenic MSCs. In fact, some studies have shown that the reagents used during viral transduction regulate the fate of MSC cells (Nidetz et al., 2020; Griukova et al., 2018; Lin et al., 2012). PEI is one of the chemical gene carriers, which manipulates the differentiation promise of transgenic MSCs, preferably toward the adipogenic lineage (Gonzalez-Fernandez et al., 2017). It is necessary to further study the effect of commonly used chemical gene carriers on the differentiation potential of MSCs. In addition, microinjection, as a typical physical delivery method, uses microneedles to inject cargo directly into the nucleus. No harmful chemicals are required during the transfection process.

Microinjection combined with robotics technology can achieve high-throughput capability and has broad application prospects in the genetic modification of MSCs. Table 14.3 summarizes the influence of robotic microinjection methods on MSCs compared with other delivery vehicles. By simultaneously using two microinjection modules and deep learning technology on the same cell processing platform to improve the efficiency of automatic cell detection and segmentation, high throughput can be achieved. Robotic microinjection can achieve about 60% transfection efficiency in MSCs, which is significantly higher than CaP, cLipo, and PEI. However, compared with the methods of CaP, cLipo, and PEI, the throughput of microinjection remains a

PPARγ WT MSCs after differentiation was set as 1. (E) Quantification of Nile Red-positive cells. The positive cells were counted in each view. (F) mRNA levels of osteogenic marker RUNX2 and ALPL were calculated after osteogenic differentiation medium in WT MSCs and PPARγ$^{-/-}$ MSCs. (G) mRNA levels of adipogenic marker genes LPL and FABP4 were calculated after adipogenic differentiation medium in WT MSCs and PPARγ$^{-/-}$ MSCs. mRNA levels of marker genes were measured by quantitative RT-PCR. The relative fold change was calculated against the transcript levels of the WT MSCs. GAPDH was used as the internal control. Gene expression level of respective gene was set as 1 in PPARγ WT MSCs. ** in (D and G) indicates the significance compared with all groups ($P < .01$). Asterisks in (E, F, and G) indicate significance compared with the WT group (**$P < .01$, ****$P < .0001$).

Table 14.3 Summary of the influence of the four delivery vehicles on MSCs (Guan et al., 2021).

Gene carriers	Transfection efficiency	Cytotoxicity		Bias of differentiation commitment	Effect on therapeutic gene function (e.g. PPARγ)	Throughput	Application
		Viability (%)	Morphology change				
Microinjection	High ~60%	96.98	Slight	Without bias	Not significant	Low: Capacity of 3000 cells per hour	In vitro cell culture, zygotes, ex vivo cell (Davis et al., 2000; Chaverra-Rodriguez et al., 2018)
Calcium phosphate nanoparticles	Low < 25%	110.82	Slight: Immature focal adhesion	Exaggerated osteogenesis Suppressed adipogenesis	Stir	High	In vitro cell culture (Litvinova et al., 2020)
Liposome	Low < 25%	98.74	Slight	Without bias	Not significant	High	In vitro, ex vivo cell culture (de Carvalho et al., 2018)
Polyethylenimine	Low < 25%	57.21	Severe: Rounded and loss of focal adhesion	Suppressed osteogenesis Exaggerated adipogenesis	Stir	High	In vitro cell culture (Pandey and Sawant, 2016)
MSCs without treatment	–	100	None	Full potential	–	–	–

major disadvantage. The transfection efficiency of chemical gene vectors is generally low, especially in primary cells, MSCs, and difficult-to-transfect cells. This phenomenon is due to their inability to control the transportation of cargo in the cell, where the transferred DNA passively travels from the outside to the cytoplasm, and then finally enters the nucleus. In contrast, microinjection uses microneedles to inject cargo directly into the nucleus of target cells. So far, transfection using chemical gene vectors is an empirical process, and its efficiency largely depends on many factors, including the gene/chemical reagent ratio, the uptake of the gene–chemical reagent complex by the target cell, the stability of the intracellular plasmid, and the plasmid entry into the nucleus.

Although microinjection is still difficult to produce a large number of transfected cells for in vivo applications, its high efficiency and low cost make it widely used in zygotes, in vitro cell culture, and even ex vivo cells. PEI and calcium phosphate nanoparticles are used extensively in in vitro research, but cytotoxicity hinders its further expansion into in vivo applications. Liposome-based transfection is commercially used for in vitro and ex vivo cells, but it still encounters the cytotoxicity problem.

14.4 Automated optical tweezers manipulation for mitochondrial transfer

14.4.1 Mitochondrial transfer through robot-assisted optical tweezers manipulation

Mitochondria are essential organelles of cells and known as the powerhouse of cells (Friedman and Nunnari, 2014). Mutations in mitochondria play a key role in aging and neurodegenerative diseases. The malfunction of mitochondrial DNA (mtDNA) and the net production of reactive oxygen species are associated with many aging diseases, such as Alzheimer disease and amyotrophic lateral sclerosis (Sahin and Depinho, 2010; Vafai and Mootha, 2012). Some previous studies have shown that human fetal MSCs (fMSCs) can improve the aging phenotype of adult MSCs (aMSCs) in both in vitro and in vivo models (Wang et al., 2016). These findings indicate that fMSC may have a unique metabolite profile in the secretory group and may have anti-aging capabilities. Given that mitochondria are a well-known metabolic regulator, whether aMSCs can be transformed into fMSC-like cells by mitochondrial transfer is an open question.

Mitochondrial transfer is considered a potential method to restore the cellular function of mitochondrial mutant cells (Clark and Shay, 1982). However, the transfer of isolated mitochondria through many traditional mitochondrial transfer methods, such as microinjection, endocytosis, and micropinocytosis, may cause potential damage to recipient cells (Frezza et al., 2007). Optical tweezers (OT) is a unique tool that uses a highly focused beam to provide force on the order of a pico-Newton trap (Ashkin et al., 1987). OT is used for many biological tasks, such as mitochondrial capture (Jeffries et al., 2007) and cell transport (Hu and Sun, 2011), because it can manipulate particles noninvasively, flexibly, and precisely. Several robotic strategies have been proposed in the past to automatically control cell transportation and manipulation through OT. The microfluidic chip was invented as a platform to simplify biological operations, such as single-cell manipulation and analysis (Shakoor et al., 2019).

Using a robotic optical tweezers system, Shakoor et al. (2021) developed a robot-assisted OT manipulation method for high-throughput single-cell mitochondrial transfer. Fig. 14.21A shows a schematic diagram of the process of mitochondrial transfer based on robot-assisted OT manipulation. A microfluidic device is designed to place mitochondria in nearby cells, which can greatly simplify the automated process of mitochondrial transport. The mitochondrial receptor cells will form a pattern in a 1D array of single-cell trapping channels, and the isolated mitochondria will be placed near the cells, as shown in Fig. 14.21B. After that, OT will trap and transport a predetermined number of healthy isolated mitochondria on the surface of each single cell, and then be taken up by the cell through endocytosis, as shown in Fig. 14.21C. Using holographic OTs, different numbers of mitochondria can be trapped at the same time. Following the same procedure, as described above, multiple mitochondria will be transported and transferred to aMSCs. Mitochondrial transfer in cells will be tested using 3D image reconstruction and confocal microscopy. By staining the cells with CFDA SE dye for 5 min before mitochondrial transfer, a 3D cell reconstruction under a fluorescence microscope will be obtained. After mitochondria are transferred, 2D stacked images of the transferred cells will be collected, and then 3D images will be reconstructed.

Fig. 14.21D and E illustrate the robot-assisted OT system setup and its schematic diagram, which contains three modules, namely execution, control, and sensing. The execution unit includes a holographic OT device that can create multiple traps simultaneously, a microfluidic device for patterning cells and mitochondria, an X−Y electric positioning platform (Prior Scientific, ProScan) for horizontally moving the microfluidic device, and a Z-axis stage to control the height of the objective lens. Two syringe pumps (LSP01-2A, longer pumps) used to control the internal pressure of the microfluidic device are also included in the execution module. The control module includes a motion controller for controlling the 3-DOF X−Y−Z positioning platform and a controller for OT. The sensor module contains a microscope (Nikon TE2000), a 60× objective lens, and a CCD camera (FO124SC, Foculus). Visual C++ will be used to build a GUI interface. All mechanical settings are supported by the antivibration table.

The microfluidic chip is composed of two inlets, three outlets, and a middle channel. Inlets 1 and 2 are used to introduce recipient cells and isolated mitochondria into the microfluidic device, respectively. Outlets 1 and 2 are designed as two tree structures. Outlet 1 is used for cell trapping, while outlet 2 is used to generate uniform fluid flow to ensure uniform cell trapping. Outlet 3 is used to collect cells from the microfluidic device for further analysis of the mitochondrion-transferred cells. The recipient cells will be loaded into a 1 mL syringe, and then introduced into the microfluidic device through a polyethylene tubing from inlet 1 to trap the cells in the U-shaped channel. Within a few minutes, single cells can be captured in 128 U-shaped trapping channels at outlet 1, as shown in Fig. 14.21F. After the cells are patterned into microfluidic channels, the isolated mitochondria of the donor cells are placed near the cell trapping channel to simplify the quality and quantity control of the mitochondrial transfer process. This process of mitochondrial transport will be repeated until the required number of mitochondria are placed on the cell surface. After processing,

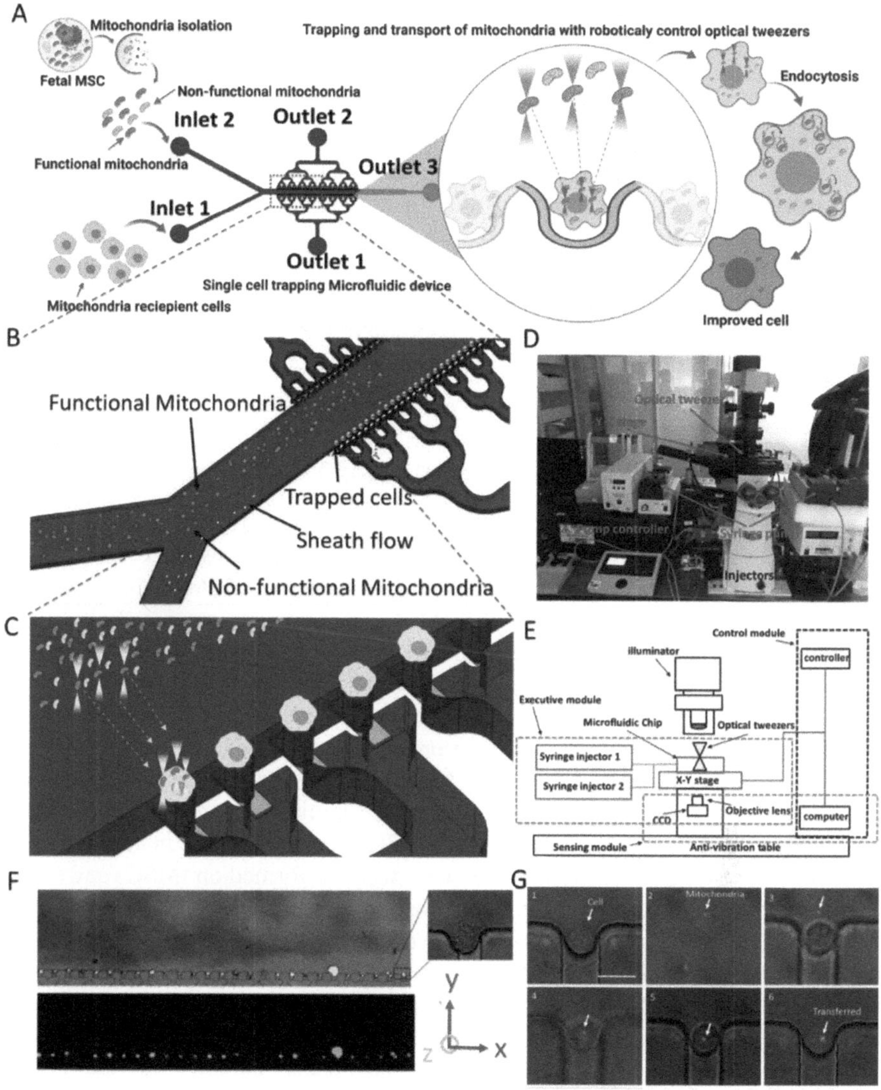

Figure 14.21 System setup and preliminary results of OT-based mitochondrial transfer method (Shakoor et al., 2021). (A) Schematic of isolated mitochondrial transfer in cells via OT-based mitochondrial transfer technique. (B) Schematic of cell patterning and mitochondrial placement in the microfluidic device. (C) Mechanism and procedure of mitochondrial transportation using OT. (D) Entire system setup. (E) Schematic of the robot-assisted OT system that includes execution, control and sensing, and executive modules. (F) Experimental results of single-cell patterning of GFP-stained cells patterned in the microfluidic device. (G) Experimental sequence of single fMSC isolated mitochondrial trapping, transportation, and transfer into aMSCs.

the transferred cells can be collected from the microfluidic chip. The same process can be repeated in order to obtain a therapeutic amount of mitochondria-transferred cells for clinical use.

Unlike the previous mitochondrial transfer methods that ignored the functional status of isolated mitochondria before the transfer process (Wu et al., 2016; Caicedo et al., 2015), this OT-based mitochondrial transfer can control the quantity and quality of mitochondria before transfer. To check the function of mitochondria before and after transfer, the donor cells will be stained with membrane potential staining dye (JC-1, Thermo Fisher). Subsequently, mitochondria with high membrane potential (functional) will show red or orange fluorescence, while mitochondria with low membrane potential will show green fluorescence (nonfunctional) emission. Image-processing methods (such as Shakoor et al., 2019) can be used to automatically detect isolated mitochondria and target cells.

14.4.2 Mitochondria transfer from fetal MSCs to adult MSCs to improve antiaging gene expression

Mitochondria mainly control energy metabolism in cells. Previous work has found that the secretome of fMSCs can improve the aging phenotype of aMSC in in vitro and in vivo models; therefore, it indicates that fMSCs may have unique metabolic characteristics in the secretome and antiaging ability (Wang et al., 2016). To fully understand the difference between fMSCs and aMSCs, Shakoor et al. (2021) used the high-throughput isobaric tags for relative and absolute quantification (iTRAQ) proteomics method to characterize the unique protein profile of cell lines, and then perform bioinformatics analysis based on the results. These processes can help to identify specific metabolic genes that are highly expressed in fMSCs compared to aMSCs, and to determine whether the mitochondrial function in fMSCs is highly active. In addition, quantitative polymerase chain reaction (qPCR) tests were performed on fMSCs and aMSCs to further verify the identified metabolic genes.

Fig. 14.22A shows the expression profile of secreted proteins of fMSCs and non-transferred aMSCs (control) by heat map. Based on the Pearson correlation, the fetal and adult secretomes were divided into two groups. A total of 1465 peptides were identified and aligned with unique proteins using MaxQuant. Fig. 14.22B illustrates two enriched items in the gene network. Enrichment means searching for the name of the protein in the database (pathway or spelling term) of gene signal transduction. Generally, every protein can be found in pathways that contain a large number of genes. The enrichment pathways are summarized in Fig. 14.22C and D. Due to mitochondria deficiency, senescent cells usually exhibit increased glycolytic activity (Kaplon et al., 2013). Therefore, the high activity of gluconeogenesis indicates that the mitochondria of fMSCs may exert a unique metabolic regulation effect, thereby reducing the aging phenotype. Metabolism-related genes *GOT2*, *PGAM1*, *PGK1*, *MDH2*, *ENO1*, *LDHB*, and *DLST* were selected as biofunctional markers from the iTRAQ comparison. Among them, *GOT2*, *PGAM1*, *PGK1*, *MDH2*, and *ENO1* are related to gluconeogenesis, *LDHB* and *DLST* are related to the TCA cycle, and *BCAT1* is involved in amino acid metabolism. These metabolic genes are highly expressed in fMSCs, indicating that fMSCs have high gluconeogenetic activity. Fig. 14.22E shows the qPCR test results of these highly expressed fMSC metabolic

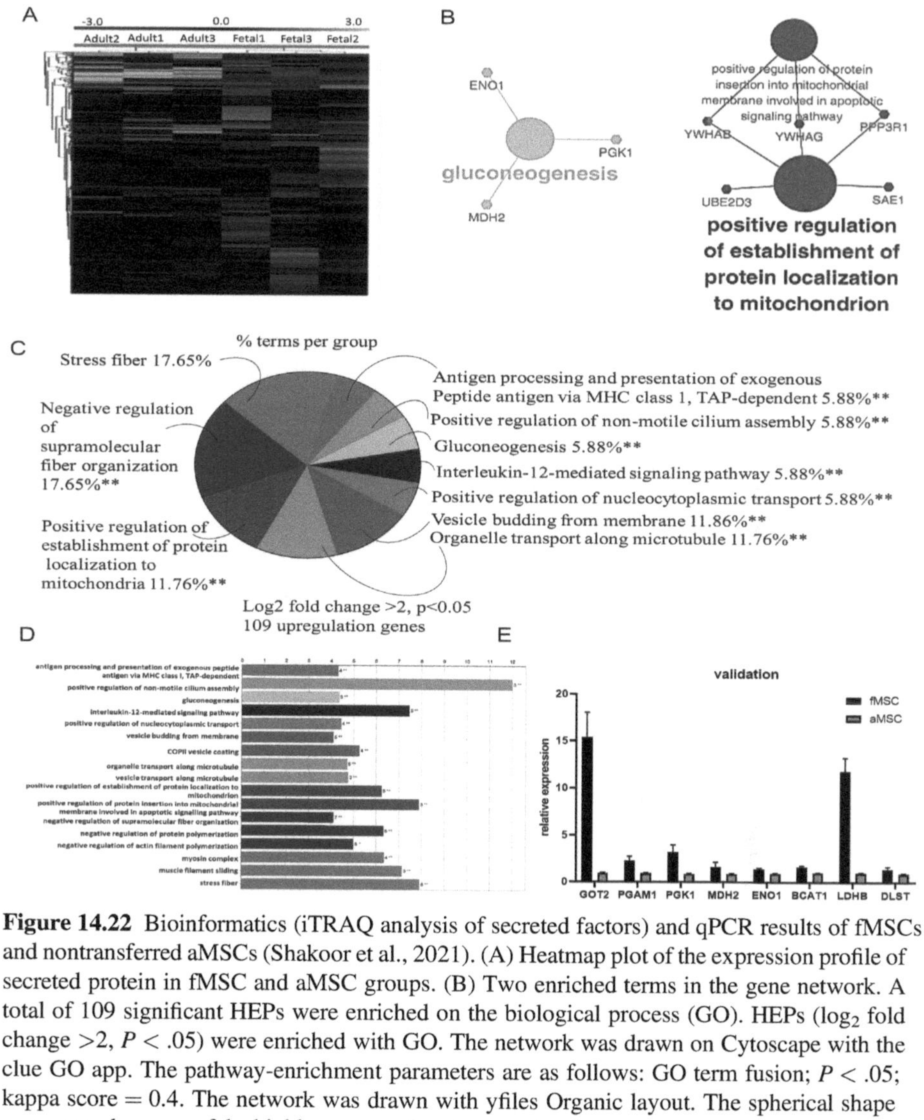

Figure 14.22 Bioinformatics (iTRAQ analysis of secreted factors) and qPCR results of fMSCs and nontransferred aMSCs (Shakoor et al., 2021). (A) Heatmap plot of the expression profile of secreted protein in fMSC and aMSC groups. (B) Two enriched terms in the gene network. A total of 109 significant HEPs were enriched on the biological process (GO). HEPs ($\log_2$ fold change >2, $P < .05$) were enriched with GO. The network was drawn on Cytoscape with the clue GO app. The pathway-enrichment parameters are as follows: GO term fusion; $P < .05$; kappa score = 0.4. The network was drawn with yfiles Organic layout. The spherical shape represents the name of the highly expressed pathway, whereas the hexagon represents the name of enriched HEP. (C) Comparison of protein-expression levels between fMSCs and aMSCs and GO enrichment. The ratio of the most significantly enriched GO term is shown in the pie chart (**$P < .05$). %Gene/Term is the quantitative index, also known as the arrival factor. The rich factor is the number of differentially expressed genes divided by the number of complete genes in the pathway. (D) Selected GO enrichment result of ClueGo. ClueGo is the name of the plugin in Cytoscape. The function of ClueGo is to visualize the relationship between genes and GO terms. (E) Validation of gene expressions of metabolic genes of fMSCs and aMSCs through qPCR. The tested genes were selected based on iTRAQ and bioinformatic analysis. High expression of these genes indicates high gluconeogenetic activity in fMSC. The calculated reference level is the CT value of GAPDH for each cell (fMSC and aMSC).

genes compared with aMSCs. Through the transfer of mitochondria from fMSCs to aMSCs, metabolic genes in aMSCs also became highly expressed, indicating that the phenotype of aMSCs can become fMSC-like.

Fig. 14.23 illustrates the qPCR results of the antiaging and metabolic gene expression levels of transferred and untransferred (control) aMSCs at different times (2, 24, and 72 h), in which six fMSC isolated mitochondria were transferred to aMSC in each

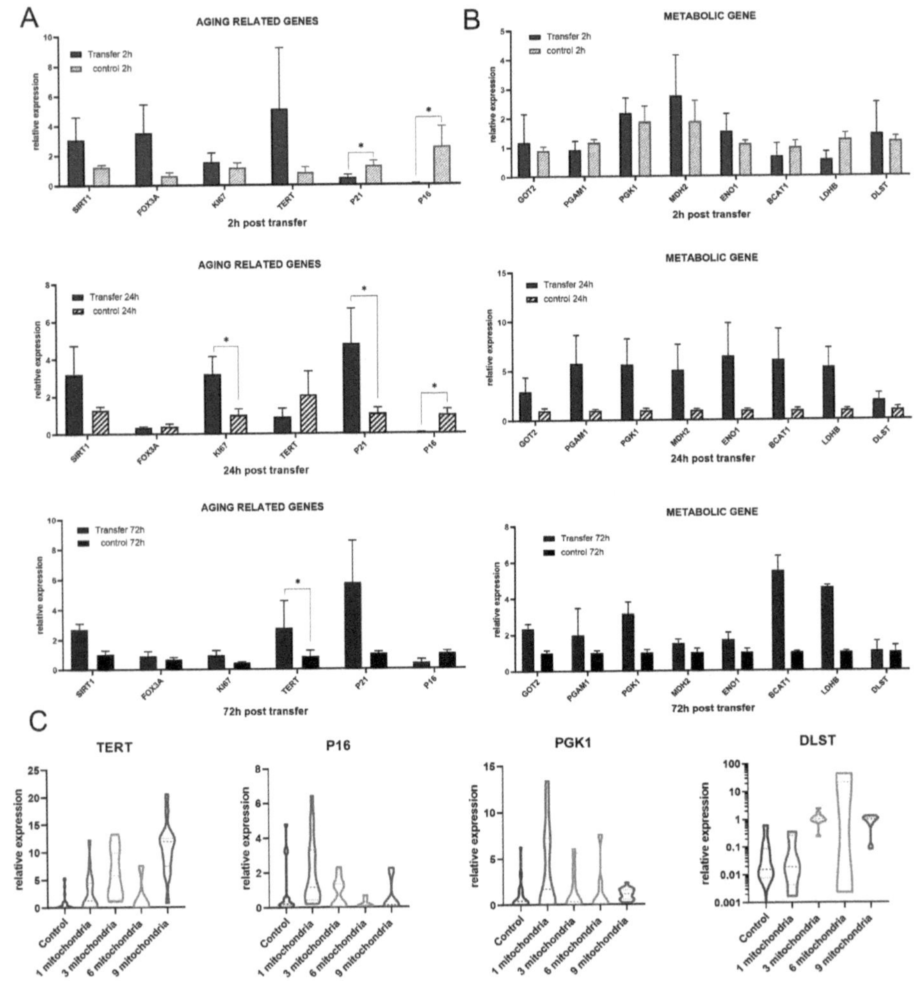

Figure 14.23 Gene-expression levels of aMSCs after 2, 24, and 72 h of fMSC mitochondrial transfer (Shakoor et al., 2021). (A) Expression levels of antiaging-related genes and cell-cycle inhibitors. Mean ± SEM, $*P < .05$. *SITR1*, *FOXO3A*, and *TERT* are antiaging-related genes. *Ki67*, *P21*, and *P16* are cell-cycle-related genes. (B) Expression levels of metabolic genes. Mean ± SEM (n = 4), $*P < .05$ and ~360 cells in each test. The reference level used for calculation was the CT value of GAPDH for each cell (fMSC and aMSC), where GAPDH served as an internal control. After normalizing gene expression with respect to GAPDH, the relative expression of genes in fMSCs was normalized to the expression of the same genes in aMSCs.

transfer group. Fig. 14.23A shows the expression levels of senescence genes and cell cycle inhibitors, and Fig. 14.23B shows the expression levels of metabolic genes. Compared with the control group, the antiaging and metabolic gene expression of transplanted aMSCs was significantly increased.

The above describes an automated OT manipulation method for mitochondrial transfer in single cells. The microfluidic cell positioning device is used to pattern cells and mitochondria, while the OT manipulation system is used to collect a predetermined number of healthy isolated mitochondria and automatically transport them to the top of the cell. The cells then absorb these mitochondria through endocytosis. Compared with the passive transfer method of coculture, the transfer method based on OT can effectively control the quantity and quality of mitochondria before transfer. The results of using qPCR analysis to check cell antiaging and metabolic gene expression show that the mitochondria of fMSCs have the potential to reverse the aging phenomenon of aMSCs. This OT-based automated mitochondrial transfer method can greatly promote precision medicine and cell therapy of mtDNA-related diseases.

14.5 Conclusions

This chapter introduced organelle biopsy and gene editing from the following three perspectives. First, a surgical system based on robotic microneedles is introduced to realize automated single-cell biopsy of small cells (diameter $< 20\ \mu m$). The cells are patterned with a microfluidic device, and image-processing algorithms based on template matching are used to automatically measure the positions of the desired organelles in the cells. The microfluidic device can be automatically controlled to a micropipette for organelle extraction. Mitochondrial and nuclear biopsy experiments on small suspension cells (NB4 $\sim$ 18 μm) and adherent cells (HDF $\sim$ 20 μm) can prove the proposed method. Second, the gene-delivery method using high-throughput robotic microinjection on MSCs is reported and compared with some existing chemical delivery methods in terms of pluripotency and therapeutic gene function. Studies have shown that robotic microinjection has high transfection efficiency, low cell damage, and the ability to retain MSC pluripotency and therapeutic gene functions. The PEI method may cause severe morphological changes, and the liposome method has a low transfection efficiency. Third, an automated optical tweezers-based manipulation method is introduced for mitochondrial transfer in single cells. This method uses a microfluidic cell positioning device to pattern cells and mitochondria, and then uses optical tweezers to collect a predetermined number of healthy isolated mitochondria and automatically transport them to the top of the cell. These mitochondria are taken up by the host cell through endocytosis. Compared with the passive transfer method of coculture, this method can effectively control the quantity and quality of mitochondria before transfer. A case study of transferring mitochondria from fetal MSCs to adult MSCs to improve antiaging and metabolic gene expression is reported. This method can greatly promote precision medicine and cell therapy for mtDNA-related diseases.

References

Actis, P., Maalouf, M.M., Kim, H.J., Lohith, A., Vilozny, B., Seger, R.A., Pourmand, N., 2014. Compartmental genomics in living cells revealed by single-cell nanobiopsy. ACS Nano 8 (1), 546–553.

Ashkin, A., Dziedzic, J.M., Yamane, T., 1987. Optical trapping and manipulation of single cells using infrared laser beams. Nature 330, 769–771.

Boudaoud, A., Burian, A., Borowska-Wykret, D., Uyttewaal, M., Wrzalik, R., Kwiatkowska, D., Hamant, O., 2014. FibrilTool, an ImageJ plug-in to quantify fibrillar structures in raw microscopy images. Nat. Protoc. 9 (2), 457–463.

Braude, P., Pickering, S., Flinter, F., Ogilvie, C.M., 2002. Preimplantation genetic diagnosis. Nat. Rev. Genet. 3 (12), 941–955.

Caicedo, A., Fritz, V., Brondello, J.M., Ayala, M., Dennemont, I., Abdellaoui, N., de Fraipont, F., Moisan, A., Prouteau, C.A., Boukhaddaoui, H., Jorgensen, C., Vignais, M.L., 2015. MitoCeption as a new tool to assess the effects of mesenchymal stem/stromal cell mitochondria on cancer cell metabolism and function. Sci. Rep. 5, 1.

Campbell, K.H., McWhir, J., Ritchie, W.A., Wilmut, I., 1996. Sheep cloned by nuclear transfer from a cultured cell line. Nature 380 (6569), 64–66.

Chaverra-Rodriguez, D., Macias, V.M., Hughes, G.L., Pujhari, S., Suzuki, Y., Peterson, D.R., Kim, D., McKeand, S., Rasgon, J.L., 2018. Targeted delivery of CRISPR-Cas9 ribonucleoprotein into arthropod ovaries for heritable germline gene editing. Nat. Commun. 9 (1), 3008.

Chow, Y.T., Chen, S., Liu, C., Liu, C., Li, L., Kong, C.W.M., Cheng, S.H., Li, R.A., Sun, D., 2016. A high-throughput automated microinjection system for human cells with small size. IEEE ASME Trans. Mechatron. 21 (2), 838–850.

Clark, M.A., Shay, J.W., 1982. Mitochondrial transformation of mammalian cells. Nature 295, 605.

Clark, I.E., Dodson, M.W., Jiang, C., Cao, J.H., Huh, J.R., Seol, J.H., Yoo, S.J., Hay, B.A., Guo, M., 2006. Drosophila pink1 is required for mitochondrial function and interacts genetically with parkin. Nature 441 (7097), 1162–1166.

Davis, B.R., Yannariello-Brown, J., Prokopishyn, N.L., Luo, Z., Smith, M.R., Wang, J., Carsrud, N.D., Brown, D.B., 2000. Glass needle–mediated microinjection of macromolecules and transgenes into primary human blood stem/progenitor cells. Blood 95 (2), 437–444.

de Carvalho, T.G., Pellenz, F.M., Laureano, A., Mariano da Rocha Silla, L., Giugliani, R., Baldo, G., Matte, U., 2018. A simple protocol for transfecting human mesenchymal stem cells. Biotechnol. Lett. 40 (3), 617–622.

Ducy, P., Zhang, R., Geoffroy, V., Ridall, A.L., Karsenty, G., 1997. Osf2/Cbfa1: a transcriptional activator of osteoblast differentiation. Cell 89 (5), 747–754.

Frezza, C., Cipolat, S., Scorrano, L., 2007. Organelle isolation: functional mitochondria from mouse liver, muscle and cultured fibroblasts. Nat. Protoc. 2, 287–295.

Friedman, J.R., Nunnari, J., 2014. Mitochondrial form and function. Nature 505, 335.

Frith, J.E., Kusuma, G.D., Carthew, J., Li, F., Cloonan, N., Gomez, G.A., Cooper-White, J.J., 2018. Mechanically-sensitive miRNAs bias human mesenchymal stem cell fate via mTOR signalling. Nat. Commun. 9 (1), 257.

Galipeau, J., Sensébé, L., 2018. Mesenchymal stromal cells: clinical challenges and therapeutic opportunities. Cell Stem Cell 22 (6), 824–833.

Gonzalez-Fernandez, T., Sathy, B.N., Hobbs, C., Cunniffe, G.M., McCarthy, H.O., Dunne, N.J., Nicolosi, V., O'Brien, F.J., Kelly, D.J., 2017. Mesenchymal stem cell fate following non-viral gene transfection strongly depends on the choice of delivery vector. Acta Biomater. 55, 226–238.

Greenfield, A., Braude, P., Flinter, F., Lovell-Badge, R., Ogilvie, C., Perry, A.C.F., 2017. Assisted reproductive technologies to prevent human mitochondrial disease transmission. Nat. Biotechnol. 35 (11), 1059–1068.

Greggains, G.D., Lister, L.M., Tuppen, H.A.L., Zhang, Q., Needham, L.H., Prathalingam, N., Hyslop, L.A., Craven, L., Polanski, Z., Murdoch, A.P., Turnbull, D., Herbert, M., 2015. Therapeutic potential of somatic cell nuclear transfer for degenerative disease caused by mitochondrial DNA mutations. Sci. Rep. 4 (1), 3844.

Griukova, A., Deryabin, P., Sirotkina, M., Shatrova, A., Nikolsky, N., Borodkina, A., 2018. P38 MAPK inhibition prevents polybrene-induced senescence of human mesenchymal stem cells during viral transduction. PLoS One 13 (12), e0209606.

Guan, Z., Chen, S., Pan, F., Fan, L., Sun, D., 2021. Effects of gene delivery approaches on differentiation potential and gene function of mesenchymal stem cells. IEEE Trans. Biomed. Eng. 68.

Habib, N., Li, Y., Heidenreich, M., Swiech, L., Avraham-Davidi, I., Trombetta, J.J., Hession, C., Zhang, F., Regev, A., 2016. Div-Seq: single-nucleus RNA-Seq reveals dynamics of rare adult newborn neurons. Science 353 (6302), 925–928.

Hagiwara, M., Kawahara, T., Iijima, T., Arai, F., 2013. High-speed magnetic microrobot actuation in a microfluidic chip by a fine V-Groove surface. IEEE Trans. Robot. 29 (2), 363–372.

Hayakawa, T., Fukada, S., Arai, F., 2014. Fabrication of an on-chip nanorobot integrating functional nanomaterials for single-cell punctures. IEEE Trans. Robot. 30 (1), 59–67.

Hu, S., Sun, D., 2011. Automatic transportation of biological cells with a robot-tweezer manipulation system. Int. J. Robot Res. 30 (14), 1681–1694.

Huang, H.B., Sun, D., Mills, J.K., Cheng, S.H., 2009. Robotic cell Injection system with position and force control: toward automatic batch biomanipulation. IEEE Trans. Robot. 25 (3), 727–737.

Ichikawa, A., Tamio, T., Kazutsugu, M., Seiya, T., Kohtaro, O., 2010. Automated cell-cutting for cell cloning. SICE J. Control Meas. Syst. Integr. 3 (2), 75–80.

Islam, M.N., Das, S.R., Emin, M.T., Wei, M., Sun, L., Westphalen, K., Rowlands, D.J., Quadri, S.K., Bhattacharya, S., Bhattacharya, J., 2012. Mitochondrial transfer from bone-marrow-derived stromal cells to pulmonary alveoli protects against acute lung injury. Nat. Med. 18, 759.

Jeffries, G.D.M., Edgar, J.S., Zhao, Y., Shelby, J.P., Fong, C., Chiu, D.T., 2007. Using polarization-shaped optical vortex traps for single-cell nanosurgery. Nano Lett. 7, 415–420.

Jordan, M., Schallhorn, A., Wurm, F.M., 1996. Transfecting mammalian cells: optimization of critical parameters affecting calcium-phosphate precipitate formation. Nucleic Acids Res. 24 (4), 596–601.

Kallio, P., Ritala, T., Lukkari, M., Kuikka, S., 2007. Injection guidance system for cellular microinjections. Int. J. Rot. Res. 26 (11/12), 1303–1313.

Kaplon, J., Zheng, L., Meissl, K., Chaneton, B., Selivanov, V.A., MacKay, G., Van Der Burg, S.H.E., Verdegaal, M.E., Cascante, M., Shlomi, T., Gottlieb, E., Peeper, D.S., 2013. A key role for mitochondrial gatekeeper pyruvate dehydrogenase in oncogene-induced senescence. Nature 498, 109.

Kay, M.A., 2011. State-of-the-art gene-based therapies: the road ahead. Nat. Rev. Genet. 12 (5), 316–328.

Kim, D.H., Sun, Y., Kim, B., 2004. Mechanical force response of single living cells using a microrobotic system. Proc. IEEE Int. Conf. Robot. Autom. 5013–5018.

King, M.P., Attardi, G., 1988. Injection of mitochondria into human cells leads to a rapid replacement of the endogenous mitochondrial DNA. Cell 52, 811.

Kluza, J., Gallego, M.A., Loyens, A., Beauvillain, J.C., Sousa-Faro, J.M.F., Cuevas, C., Marchetti, P., Bailly, C., 2016. Cancer cell mitochondria are direct proapoptotic targets for the marine antitumor drug lamellarin D. Cancer Res. 66 (6), 3177–3187.

Kuznetsov, A.V., Margreiter, R., 2009. Heterogeneity of mitochondria and mitochondrial function within cells as another level of mitochondrial complexity. Int. J. Mol. Sci. 10, 1911.

Li, H., Wang, G., Hao, Z., Zhang, G., Qing, Y., Liu, S., Qing, L., Pan, W., Chen, L., Liu, G., Zhao, R., Jia, B., Zeng, L., Guo, J., Zhao, L., Zhao, H., Lv, C., Xu, K., Cheng, W., Li, H., Zhao, H.Y., Wang, W., Wei, H.J., 2016. Generation of biallelic knock-out sheep via gene-editing and somatic cell nuclear transfer. Sci. Rep. 6 (33675).

Lin, P., Lin, Y., Lennon, D.P., Correa, D., Schluchter, M., Caplan, A.I., 2012. Efficient lentiviral transduction of human mesenchymal stem cells that preserves proliferation and differentiation capabilities. Stem Cells Transl. Med. 1 (12), 886–897.

Lin, K., Limpens, E., Zhang, Z., Ivanov, S., Saunders, D.G.O., Mu, D., Pang, E., Cao, H., Cha, H., Lin, T., Zhou, Q., Shang, Y., Li, Y., Sharma, T., van Velzen, R., de Ruijter, N., Aanen, D.K., Win, J., Kamoun, S., Bisseling, T., Geurts, R., Huang, S., 2014. Single nucleus genome sequencing reveals high similarity among nuclei of an endomycorrhizal fungus. PLoS Genet. 10 (1), e1004078.

Litvinova, L., Yurova, K., Shupletsova, V., Khaziakhmatova, O., Malashchenko, V., Shunkin, E., Melashchenko, E., Todosenko, N., Khlusovam, M., Sharkeev, Y., Komarova, E., Sedelnikova, M., Khlusov, I., 2020. Gene expression regulation and secretory activity of mesenchymal stem cells upon in vitro contact with microarc calcium phosphate coating. Int. J. Mol. Sci. 21 (20), 7682.

Liu, X., Kim, K., Zhang, Y., Sun, Y., 2009. Nanonewton force sensing and control in microrobotic cell manipulation. Int. J. Robot Res. 28 (8), 1065–1076.

Liu, J., Siragam, V., Gong, Z., Chen, J., Leung, C., Lu, Z., Ru, C., Xie, S., Luo, J., Hamilton, R.M., Sun, Y., 2014. Robotic adherent cell injection for characterizing cell-cell communication. IEEE Trans. Biomed. Eng. 62 (1), 119–125.

Liu, J., Wen, J., Zhang, J., Sun, Y., 2015. Voyage inside the cell: microsystems and nanoengineering for intracellular measurement and manipulation. Microsyst. Nanoeng. 1, 1–15.

Macheiner, T., Fengler, V.H.I., Agreiter, M., Eisenberg, T., Madeo, F., Kolb, D., Huppertz, B., Ackbar, R., Sargsyan, K., 2016. Magnetomitotransfer: an efficient way for direct mitochondria transfer into cultured human cells. Sci. Rep. 6, 1.

McCafferty, M.M., Burke, G.A., Meenan, B.J., 2014. Mesenchymal stem cell response to conformal sputter deposited calcium phosphate thin films on nanostructured titanium surfaces. J. Biomed. Mater. Res. 102 (10), 3585–3597.

Nidetz, N.F., McGee, M.C., Tse, L.V., Li, C., Cong, L., Li, Y., Huang, W., 2020. Adeno-associated viral vector-mediated immune responses: understanding barriers to gene delivery. Pharmacol. Ther. 207, 107453.

Oggu, G.S., Sasikumar, S., Reddy, N., Ella, K.K.R., Rao, C.M., Bokara, K.K., 2017. Gene delivery approaches for mesenchymal stem cell therapy: strategies to increase efficiency and specificity. Stem Cell Rev. Rep. 13 (6), 725–740.

Osada, T., Uehara, H., Kim, H., Ikai, A., 2003. mRNAanalysis of single living cells. J. Nanobiotechnol. 1 (2).

Pan, F., Chen, S., Jiao, Y., Guan, Z., Shakoor, A., Sun, D., 2020. Automated high-productivity microinjection system for adherent cells. IEEE Robot. Auto. Lett. 5 (2), 1167–1174.

Pandey, A.P., Sawant, K.K., 2016. Polyethylenimine: a versatile, multifunctional non-viral vector for nucleic acid delivery. Mater. Sci. Eng. C 68, 904–918.

Patel, D., Rorbach, J., Downes, K., Szukszto, M.J., Pekalski, M.L., Minczuk, M., 2017. Macropinocytic entry of isolated mitochondria in epidermal growth factor-activated human osteosarcoma cells. Sci. Rep. 7, 1.

Pertoft, H., Laurent, T., 1977. Isopycnic separation of cells and cell organelles by centrifugation inmodified colloidal silica gradients. Methods Cell Sep. 25–65 (New York, NY, USA: Springer).

Ren, G., Zhang, L., Zhao, X., Xu, G., Zhang, Y., Roberts, A.I., Zhao, R.C., Shi, Y., 2008. Mesenchymal stem cell-mediated immunosuppression occurs via concerted action of chemokines and nitric oxide. Cell Stem Cell 2 (2), 141–150.

Rhinn, M., Ritschka, B., Keyes, W.M., 2019. Cellular senescence in development, regeneration and disease. Development 146.

Robey, T.E., Saiget, M.K., Reinecke, H., Murry, C.E., 2008. Systems approaches to preventing transplanted cell death in cardiac repair. J. Mol. Cell. Cardiol. 45 (4), 567–581.

Sage, E.K., Thakrar, R.M., Janes, S.M., 2016. Genetically modified mesenchymal stromal cells in cancer therapy. Cytotherapy 18 (11), 1435–1445.

Sahin, E., Depinho, R.A., 2010. Linking functional decline of telomeres, mitochondria and stem cells during ageing. Nature 464, 520.

Sartori-Rupp, A., Cervantes, D.C., Pepe, A., Gousset, K., Delage, E., Corroyer-Dulmont, S., Schmitt, C., Krijnse-Locker, J., Zurzolo, C., 2019. Correlative cryo-electron microscopy reveals the structure of TNTs in neuronal cells. Nat. Commun. 10 (1).

Schubert, C., 2011. Single-cell analysis: the deepest differences. Nature 480 (7375), 133–137.

Sercel, A.J., Patananan, A.N., Man, T., Wu, T.H., Yu, A.K., Guyot, G.W., Rabizadeh, S., Niazi, K.R., Chiou, P.Y., Teitell, M.A., 2021. Stable transplantation of human mitochondrial DNA by high-throughput, pressurized isolated mitochondrial delivery. Elife 10, 1.

Shadel, G.S., Horvath, T.L., 2015. Mitochondrial ROS signaling in organismal homeostasis. Cell 163, 560.

Shakoor, A., Xie, M., Luo, T., Hou, J., Shen, Y., Mills, J.K., Sun, D., 2019. Achieving automated organelle biopsy on small single cells using a cell surgery robotic system. IEEE Trans. Biomed. Eng. 66 (8), 2210–2222.

Shakoor, A., Wang, B., Fan, L., Kong, L., Gao, W., Sun, J., Man, K., Li, G., Sun, D., 2021. Automated optical tweezers manipulation to transfer mitochondria from fetal to adult MSCs to improve anti-aging gene expressions. Small 17.

Singhal, R., Orynbayeva, Z., Sundaram, R.V.K., Niu, J.J., Bhattacharyya, S., Vitol, E.A., Schrlau, M.G., Papazoglou, E.S., Friedman, G., Gogotsi, Y., 2011. Multifunctional carbon-nanotube cellular endoscopes. Nat. Nanotechnol. 6 (1), 57–64.

Spinelli, J.B., Haigis, M.C., 2018. The multifaceted contributions of mitochondria to cellular metabolism. Nat. Cell Biol. 20, 745.

Sun, Y., Nelson, B.J., 2002. Biological cell injection using an autonomous microrobotics system. Int. J. Robot Res. 21, 861–868.

Sun, H., Kim, J.K., Mortensen, R., Mutyaba, L.P., Hankenson, K.D., Krebsbach, P.H., 2013. Osteoblast-targeted suppression of PPARγ increases osteogenesis through activation of mTOR signaling. Stem Cells 31 (10), 2183–2192.

Vafai, S.B., Mootha, V.K., 2012. Mitochondrial disorders as windows into an ancient organelle. Nature 491, 374.

Vermeesch, J.R., Voet, T., Devriendt, K., 2016. Prenatal and pre-implantation genetic diagnosis. Nat. Rev. Genet. 17 (10), 643–656.

Wada, M., Matsuda, Y., Fujita, K., Nanjo, A., 2004. RT-PCR amplification of mRNAs in nuclei or cytosol of single cells of tomato callus after micropipette extraction. Plant Cell Tissue Organ Cult. 79 (1), 109–114.

Wan, J., Xiong, S., Chao, S., Xiao, J., Ma, Y., Wang, J., Roy, S., 2010. PPARgamma gene C161T substitution alters lipid profile in Chinese patients with coronary artery disease and type 2 diabetes mellitus. Cardiovasc. Diabetol. 9, 13.

Wang, Z., Ang, W.T., 2016. Automatic dissection position selection for cleavage-stage embryo biopsy. IEEE Trans. Biomed. Eng. 63 (3), 563–570.

Wang, W.H., Liu, X.Y., Sun, Y., 2007. Contact detection in microrobotic manipulation. Int. J. Robot Res. 26 (8), 821–828.

Wang, W., Itaka, K., Ohba, S., Nishiyama, N., Chung, U., Yamasaki, Y., Kataoka, K., 2009. 3D spheroid culture system on micropatterned substrates for improved differentiation efficiency of multipotent mesenchymal stem cells. Biomaterials 30 (14), 2705–2715.

Wang, B., Lee, W.Y.W., Huang, B., Zhang, J.F., Wu, T.Y., Jiang, X., Wang, C.C., Li, G., 2016. Secretome of human fetal mesenchymal stem cell ameliorates replicative senescen. Stem Cells Dev. 25, 1755.

Wieckowski, M.R., Giorgi, C., Lebiedzinska, M., Duszynski, J., Pinton, P., 2009. Isolation of mitochondria-associated membranes and mitochondria from animal tissues and cells. Nat. Protoc. 4, 1582.

Wong, C.Y., Mills, J.K., 2016. Cleavage-stage embryo rotation tracking and automated micropipette control: towards automated single cell manipulation. Proc. IEEE Int. Conf. Intell. Robot. Syst. 2351–2356.

Wu, T.H., Sagullo, E., Case, D., Zheng, X., Li, Y., Hong, J.S., TeSlaa, T., Patananan, A.N., McCaffery, J.M., Niazi, K., Braas, D., Koehler, C., Graeber, T.G., Chiou, P.Y., Teitell, M.A., 2016. Mitochondrial transfer by photothermal nanoblade restores metabolite profile in mammalian cells. Cell Metabol. 23 (5), 921–929.

Xie, Y., Sun, D., Liu, C., Tse, H.Y., Cheng, S.H., 2010. A force control approach to a robot-assisted cell microinjection system. Int. J. Robot Res. 29 (9), 1222–1232.

Yang, H., Vonk, L.A., Licht, R., van Boxtel, A.M.G., Bekkers, J.E.J., Kragten, A.H.M., Hein, S., Varghese, O.P., Howard, K.A., Öner, F.C., Dhert, W.J.A., Creemers, L.B., 2014. Cell type and transfection reagent-dependent effects on viability, cell content, cell cycle and inflammation of RNAi in human primary mesenchymal cells. Eur. J. Pharmaceut. Sci. 53, 35–44.

Yin, H., Kanasty, R.L., Eltoukhy, A.A., Vegas, A.J., Dorkin, J.R., Anderson, D.G., 2014. Nonviral vectors for gene-based therapy. Nat. Rev. Genet. 15 (8), 541–555.

Yin, H., Kauffman, K.J., Anderson, D.G., 2017. Delivery technologies for genome editing. Nat. Rev. Drug Discov. 16 (6), 387–399.

Summary

15

15.1 Operation tools for cell manipulations

The operation tools and techniques used to manipulate cells are outlined in detail in Chapter 2; these include microneedles (or micropipettes), optical tweezers, electrokinetic manipulation tools, magnetic manipulators, atomic force microscopy (AFM), and a variety of imaging technologies for intracellular manipulation.

Microneedles (or micropipettes) are mostly used for microinjection of single cells, as detailed in Chapter 3. A microneedle perforates the cell membrane with its small and sharp tip and then injects materials into cells. By integrating robotics, the microneedle-based cell injection can be processed automatically and more accurately. Over the past few decades, many robot-assisted microneedle cell injection systems have been developed for suspension cells and adherent cells. With microneedles, hybrid position and force control for automated batch injection of cells can be realized. Microneedles can also be used to characterize the mechanical properties of cells, as discussed in Chapter 3. Piezo-driven pipettes represent another type of cell-piercing technique, where the injection pipette is driven by a series of piezoelectric pulses with adjustable frequency, amplitude, and duration. Microneedle-based cell injection has shown great potential in the application of highly efficient cell transfection for organelle biopsy and gene editing of single cells, as reported in Chapter 14.

Optical tweezers use highly focused low-power laser beams to manipulate dielectric spherical particles ranging from tens of nanometers to tens of micrometers. As the amount of force (in piconewtons) applied to the cell and its degree of deformation (in nanometers) can provide the information about its mechanical flexibility, optical tweezers have been widely used to stretch cells to characterize cell biomechanical properties, as reported in Chapter 4. In the stretching process, the beads are attached to the cell surface used as a handle, and the light traps of optical tweezers are used to move the beads and gradually increase the distance between them to stretch the cell. Optical tweezers are also used to translate and rotate single cells. Chapters 5 and 6 introduce the use of robotically controlled optical tweezers to automatically transport and rotate cells, respectively. Utilizing their high-precision transportation property, optical tweezers have also been used to isolate target cells from mixtures (Chapter 8) or control a group of cells to form the desired pattern (Chapter 10). Chapter 9 introduces the concept that optical tweezers can be used to trap chemoattractant-loaded microbeads, which release the stimulus and induce the target cells to migrate to the desired area. In Chapter 12, robotically controlled optical tweezers are used to achieve cell fusion that combines two or multiple cells to form a single entity. The other cell manipulation methods using optical tweezers include cell adhesion (Chapter 11) and organelle biopsy of single cells (Chapter 14). All the above examples indicate that optical tweezers are a unique and useful tool in cell manipulation.

Robotic Cell Manipulation. https://doi.org/10.1016/B978-0-323-85259-3.00016-7

Dielectrophoresis (DEP) is another useful tool to manipulate cells. The common applications of DEP include cell separation, cell trapping, and cell patterning. Considering that the DEP force acting on a cell is generally proportional to the size of the cell and the displacement of the cell deviating from the streamline depends on the cell size, cell separation can be achieved by integrating DEP with the microfluidic device. Chapter 8 introduces the use of a combined DEP manipulation and sheathless method to effectively separate cells based on the size or dielectric properties of cells. In cell trapping, the dielectric affinity column can be used to trap the targeted cells at the electrode tip through the DEP field. Chapter 4 introduces the use of DEP to stretch individual cells to characterize the biophysical properties of cells. Compared with the optical force, DEP can provide a larger stretching force on the cell. DEP force can also be used for cell patterning. Using an electric field to fix the position of the cells, the cells can be patterned through a fixation step using a cross-linking agent or cell adhesion protein. This method can be used in tissue engineering to create different cell patterns for culture and tissue development. Chapter 10 introduces the use of DEP to polarize cells to build 3D cell patterns on multilayer structures with high cell density. Studies have shown that DEP-based cell pattern technology can enhance cell seeding and develop high-quality artificial tissues.

A magnetic manipulator is a tool that uses magnetic gradient force or torque to manipulate or drive magnetic particles. In recent years, magnetic manipulators have been often used to drive magnetic microrobots or particles in in vivo applications because magnetic actuation has the advantages of noninvasiveness and good control ability, minimal tissue damage, and insensitivity to biological substances. Several methods using permanent magnets, Helmholtz and/or Maxwell coil pairs, and multiple electromagnets have been commonly used to design and construct magnetic steering systems. Electromagnetic coils have the advantage of providing a remotely controlled source for untethered agents with magnetic characteristics. The intensity and gradient of the magnetic field generated by the electromagnetic coils can be adjusted by changing the energized currents of the coils. Two common magnetic drive mechanisms are gradient field drive, which directly drags the microrobot by a magnetic-gradient force, and rotating torque drive, which actuates the microrobot by the locomotion force produced by oscillating the microrobot and squeezing ambient liquid. Chapter 13 introduces the use of a gradient field-based electromagnetic steering system to drive magnetic microrobots carrying cells to the desired position in vivo.

Atomic force microscopy (AFM) is a type of scanning probe microscopy, which uses a sharp tip mounted on the end of a flexible cantilever to scan. It has three major abilities: force measurement, topographic imaging, and manipulation. In force measurement, AFM can be used to measure the force between the probe and the sample as a function of their mutual separation. For imaging, the probe's response to the force applied to the sample can be used to form an image of the 3D shape (topography) of the sample surface with high resolution. In manipulation, the force between the needle tip and the sample can also be used to change the properties of the sample in a controlled manner.

Finally, the imaging technologies used for intracellular manipulation are introduced. The state-of-the-art microscopes on the market, including confocal fluorescence microscopy (CFM), two-photon fluorescence microscopy (TPFM), and light sheet fluorescence microscopy (LSFM), are first introduced. In CFM, the pinhole aperture placed in front of the microscope's photodetector focuses the illuminating light on the specimen, thereby eliminating most of the out-of-focus blur during the observation process. Many biological test results in this book were obtained using CFM. TPFM functions based on two-photon absorption and excitation, which can perform tomography to measure samples at different optical depths. In LSFM, the light sheet produced by the thin laser sampling beam is focused on only a part of the sample, and the fluorescence is collected perpendicularly from the illumination axis. Compared with CFM and TPFM, LSFM is more suitable for applications that require long-term measurement and careful exposure. The other imaging technologies such as photoacoustic microscopy (PAM), traditional wide-field fluorescence microscopy (WFFM), super-resolution microscopy (SIM), and stimulated emission depletion microscopy (STEDM) are also introduced. Chapter 14 introduces the use of the unique PAM technology to visualize the microrobots (diameter: about 80 μm) at a penetration depth of several centimeters in the tissue.

15.2 Cell manipulation types

Cell manipulation refers to the process of shaping and manipulating cells using the above-mentioned special technical tools to change cell functions, treat and resist diseases, and help cells rejuvenate. The ability to manipulate cells with high precision and high throughput is crucial and requires the combination of robotics and traditional cell physical manipulation. The types of robot-assisted cell manipulations introduced in this book are summarized below.

15.2.1 Cell microinjection

Chapter 3 introduces the robot-assisted microneedle-based microinjection of suspension cells and adherent cells. The size of the injected cells ranges from a large size of 500 μm^{-1} mm (such as zebrafish embryos) to a small size of less than 20 μm (such as most human cells). Traditional manual cell manipulation has many disadvantages such as artificial fatigue and poor reproducibility. By contrast, robotic cell injection can achieve higher efficiency and accuracy through automation. Chapter 3 introduces several topics of microinjection, including robotic cell microinjection settings, position and force control, and multiple methods to achieve high performance, high throughput, and high productivity in cell injection. Case studies of applying robotic microinjection methods to single-cell transfection and cell mechanical characterization are also discussed. In Chapter 14, the automatic organelle biopsy of small single cells is realized using microneedle injection, and the use of high-throughput robotic microinjection to deliver genes to MSCs is further introduced. Compared with traditional cell transfection methods such as polyethyleneimine (PEI), cationic liposomes (cLipo), and calcium phosphate nanoparticles (CaP), robotic microinjection has higher transfection efficiency, lower cell damage, and stronger ability to retain

MSC pluripotency and therapeutic gene function. Chapters 3 and 14 show that robotic microinjection technology can effectively deepen the understanding of cell function and promote cell therapy in precision medicine.

15.2.2 Cell stretching and compression

Cell deformation processes, such as cell stretching or compression, are an important cell manipulation method that can help characterize the biophysical characteristics of cells or achieve intracellular transmission. Chapter 4 introduces the integration of robotics and various micromanipulation tools, including optical tweezers, DEP, microfluidic channels, and magnetic devices, to stretch or compress individual cells to characterize cell characteristics or achieve in situ intracellular delivery. Optical tweezers and DEP can be used to stretch a single cell to characterize the mechanobiological properties of the cell. Optical tweezers can stretch cells accurately, while DEP can provide a high stretching force. Cell compression can be achieved by mechanical confinement. Compared with optical and DEP stretching methods, mechanical confinement can cause large cell deformations, thereby identifying cell biomechanical properties at different levels. In addition, intracellular delivery can be achieved by using magnetic force to deform cells. This unique method can help deliver different types of materials efficiently and rapidly to cells that are difficult to transfect.

15.2.3 Cell transportation and delivery

In many biomedical applications, cells require precise positioning. The huge demand for cell positioning accuracy and throughput highlights the need for automated cell transportation by combining robotics and microprocessing technology. Chapter 5 introduces the use of robot-controlled optical tweezers to automatically transport cells, including the basic theories and methods of the robotic optical tweezers system, the motion and path planning of cell transport, and the advanced controller that can simultaneously control cell positioning, cell trapping, and obstacle avoidance in cell transport. Chapter 13 introduces the use of robotic optical tweezers to control cell transport in vivo. An enhanced disturbance compensation controller is developed to minimize the influence of fluid on the cell. Simulations and experiments that track individual cells in live zebrafish embryos demonstrate the effectiveness of the proposed method in a dynamic in vivo environment. Chapter 13 further introduces the use of microrobots to carry and deliver target cells in vivo under the actuation of an electromagnetic drive system. When the microrobot reaches the target site, the carried cells can be spontaneously released from the microrobot to the surrounding tissues. The use of microrobots can enable the therapeutic dose of cells to access difficult-to-reach tissues or human cavities, making various medical treatments possible and minimally invasive.

15.2.4 Cell rotation

Cell rotation is a necessary process in many cell therapy applications, allowing operating tools to access target components within the cell with minimal damage to the cell.

Chapter 6 introduces the use of a robotic optical tweezers system to control cell rotation. The in-plane and out-of-plane rotations of the cell are introduced, including dynamics analysis, control development, and experimental evaluation. Cell rotation control represents an advancement in single-cell manipulation and has the potential to contribute to many cell-oriented therapeutic applications.

15.2.5 Intracellular surgery of cells

Intracellular surgery, such as intracellular component extraction and preimplantation genetic diagnosis, has aroused great interest in recent years. Chapter 7 introduces an accurate and automated intracellular delivery method that uses a robotic microscope system based on 3D image reconstruction. A series of optical sections along the vertical direction is obtained by microscope lens movement. A 3D reconstruction model of the specimen is established after several deconvolution, segmentation, and reconstruction processes. Intracellular delivery can be achieved based on the 3D information. An optimal delivery position can be acquired via geometric analysis based on the volume-based model. A robust controller that can compensate for external disturbances is utilized to manipulate micropipettes to deliver exogenous materials into single cells. Chapter 14 introduces organelle extraction using a robotic surgical system based on microneedles. Mitochondrial and nuclear biopsy experiments on small suspension cells and adherent cells (diameter: 20 μm) are performed successfully.

15.2.6 Cell sorting and separation

Many biomedical applications require effective separation of interesting cells from mixtures. Chapter 8 introduces two strategies for enhancing cell-sorting operations by combining robot-assisted cell manipulation with microfluidic chip technology. The first strategy is to combine optical tweezers and microwell array technology to achieve high-precision cell sorting and separation based on a small number of samples. The second strategy is to combine gravity-sedimentation-based sheathless prefocusing and DEP technology to separate cells with different sizes and dielectric properties without changing the design of the microfluidic chip. Experiments and case studies have been conducted to prove the effectiveness of these strategies.

15.2.7 Cell stimulation and migration control

Cell migration is a natural movement that occurs in response to stimuli in the living environment. Controlling cell migration by inducing appropriate stimuli is important for many biological applications. Chapter 9 introduces the cell migration model induced by chemical attractants and the control of the manipulation system based on robotic optical tweezers. The cell migration model is established based on the microbeads trapped by optical tweezers. The microbeads loaded with chemoattractant release the stimulus, thereby inducing target cells to follow the microbeads to migrate to the desired area. This model can quantitatively characterize the relationship among protrusion force, cell motility, and chemoattractant gradient. A potential field-based controller is developed to control the optical tweezers to manipulate the microbeads in stimulating cell migration. The cell behavior under electrical stimulation (ES) is also introduced in Chapter 9.

15.2.8 Cell patterning

Cell patterning refers to arranging cells in a desired shape at the desired position, which can be used in many biomedical applications, such as cell—cell interactions, drug screening, and tissue engineering. Chapter 10 introduces three cell patterning methods. The first method is to use robotically controlled optical tweezers to control cells to form a multilevel topology pattern. The second method is to use DEP to pattern cells onto a multilayer 3D engineering scaffold. The third method is to use a gravitational sedimentation-based method to pattern multiple cell types for cell coculture. Chapter 10 also introduces a case study of using cell patterning methods to automatically seed cells into multilayer honeycomb patterns for bone tissue engineering applications. In Chapter 14, mitochondrial receptor cells form a 1D array in microfluidic channels for automatic mitochondrial transfer.

15.2.9 Cell adhesion for cell—cell interaction

Cell adhesion is a process in which cells come into contact with one another or with their substratum through specialized protein complexes. Cell—cell interactions can be studied through the use of the synergy of adhesion molecules fixed on the cell membrane and the exchange of intercellular diffusion factors. Understanding the basic principles of this process is important for developing new therapeutic strategies. Chapter 11 introduces the use of optical tweezers to manipulate cell adhesion for the study of cell—cell interactions. A case study of the interaction between leukemia cancer cells and bone marrow stromal cells is reported, in which the adhesion characteristics of leukemia cells to stromal cells are characterized, and the fluorescence intensity used as a marker of the Wnt signaling pathway of leukemia cells is analyzed. The method of manipulating cell adhesion will provide a unique way to study inaccessible mechanisms of cell—cell interaction.

15.2.10 Cell fusion

Cell fusion is a cellular process of combining two or multiple cells to form a single entity. Artificially induced cell fusion in vitro has become a promising method of monoclonal antibody production, somatic cell reprogramming, cancer immunotherapy, and tissue regeneration. Chapter 12 introduces an engineering fusion approach through robotic manipulation with optical tweezers. The cells are manipulated with optical tweezers and then fused under 355 nm pulsed ultraviolet (UV) laser irradiation. The basic working principle of laser-induced fusion is demonstrated in fusing human embryonic stem cells (hESCs) at the single-cell level. By using a microfluidic chip with a microwell array, highly selective and controllable cell fusion can be achieved. The successful development of laser-induced single-cell fusion technology will benefit many fields of biomedical research such as cell differentiation, cell maturation, and cell reprogramming.

15.3 Potential medical applications

Cell manipulation has great potential in various medical applications. This book also introduces many case studies on microsurgery, gene editing, and cancer treatment, which are summarized below.

15.3.1 Cell transfection

Cell transfection is a process wherein foreign genetic substances (such as nucleic acids) are delivered into cells to produce genetically modified cells. Chapter 3 introduces the application of robotic microinjection technology to quantitatively control the delivered substance (such as modRNA encoding nuclear eGFP) to human foreskin fibroblast (HFF) cells to achieve single-cell transfection. The amount of mRNA can determine the expression level of protein in a cell, which indicates that the amount of protein synthesized in living cells can be controlled by quantitative microinjection of microRNA. The transfection efficiency of delivering different amounts of modRNA to HFF cells is further measured. Chapter 3 also reports that the mixture of plasmid encoding eGFP and plasmid encoding mCherry can be injected into HFF cells at different ratios, indicating that DNA can be successfully delivered into cells. This finding represents an important strategy in cell biology research. In Chapter 14, gene-delivery methods to transfect adult MSCs for functional improvement are investigated. The robotic microinjection method is compared with three other gene-delivery vehicles, namely, calcium phosphate coprecipitation, PEI, and lipofectamine, in terms of cell viability, morphology, and MSC multilineage differentiation potential. Using these vectors, the osteoblast differentiation negative regulator PPARγ gene is knocked out, and its effect on gene function and stem cell differentiation is determined. The results further show that robotic microinjection is a promising method for generating transgenic MSCs, which will not destroy the differentiation promise and gene function of MSCs. Chapter 4 also introduces the case study of using iron ball/rod-based magnetic force-driven intracellular delivery to deliver CXCR4 siRNAs into HepG2 cells to inhibit the proliferation and migration of cancer cells.

15.3.2 Probing mechanobiological properties of cells through cell stretching

Chapter 4 introduces two case studies to probe the mechanobiological properties of cells by using robotically controlled optical tweezers to stretch cells. The first case study stretches hematopoietic cells to verify the hypothesis that hematopoietic cells at different stages during normal and leukemia differentiation show distinctive biophysical properties. Hematopoiesis is a highly conserved key process, which is produced and maintained by rare hematopoietic stem cells (HSCs). Abnormal regulation of HSCs and their progenitor cells (HSPCs) can lead to diseases including acute myeloid leukemia (AML). Information on the biophysical properties of hematopoietic cells during their early differentiation under normal and leukemic conditions is crucial. This work shows that normal and leukemic hematopoietic cell populations with different primitives exhibit different forms of deformability, indicating that the biophysical properties may be related to stem cell or leukemia-initiating cell (LIC) capabilities. These findings also provide a solid foundation for studying normal and leukemia cell signals and their biophysical properties at the individual cell level. The second case study is stretches hESCs in cardiac differentiation. hESCs and hESC-derived cardiomyocytes (hESC-CMs) have broad prospects in the treatment of cardiovascular diseases. However, the mechanobiological properties of hESCs and hESC-CMs remain elusive. Any abnormal changes in biomechanics may lead to disorders of cell viability and pathological changes. The results of this case study indicate that the mechanical stiffness of hESC-CMs, which is characterized by dynamic and static responses, is significantly improved compared with that of undifferentiated hESCs. The findings lay the foundation for using hESC-CMs as a model to study mechanical and contractile defects in heart disease conditions such as Duchenne muscular dystrophy and heart failure.

15.3.3 Isolating targeted cells from mixtures

Stem cells offer unprecedented promise, especially in regenerative medicine. However, unpurified stem cells may form tumors after being transplanted into patients. Therefore, stem cell purification is important in the clinical application of stem cell therapy. Chapter 8 introduces a case study of isolation and deposition of hESCs from a mixture of different cells using automatically controlled optical tweezers on a microfluidic chip. Another case study reported in Chapter 8 involves isolating THP-1 cells from OCI-AML3 cells based on dielectric properties via a combined gravity sedimentation-based sheathless prefocusing and DEP method. THP-1 and OCI-AML3 cells are AML cells of similar size. They have different subtypes based on their maturity and the cell type that leukemia develops. These two types of cells can only be separated by their different dielectric properties. DEP force is related to cell diameter and dielectric properties, and it can be used to determine different dielectric properties based on intracellular heterogeneity.

15.3.4 Electrical stimulation of MSCs to improve osteogenic differentiation

MSCs are multipotent cells that can be differentiated into multiple cell types including osteoblasts. Electrical stimulation (ES) can promote bone healing and osteogenic differentiation of bone marrow MSCs. Direct current and alternating current (AC) are widely used to promote the osteogenic differentiation of MSCs in vivo and in vitro. Here, the information about effective differentiation is crucial. Chapter 9 introduces a case study of ES of MSCs with optimized ES parameters based on the calcium spike mode of MSC. Various ES parameters of AC, including voltage, signal shapes, frequency, and duty time, are tested and optimized through real-time monitoring of calcium spike patterns. Methods to optimize osteogenic differentiation are useful in clinical treatments, such as fractures.

15.3.5 Cell patterning for tissue engineering and coculture

Chapter 10 introduces the use of DEP to automatically seed cells into a multilayer honeycomb pattern for bone tissue engineering applications. The scaffold incorporates DEP for noncontact manipulation of cells, and the inherent honeycomb structure is integrated in each scaffold layer. When a voltage is applied to the stacked scaffold layers to generate a 3D electric field, the cells are manipulated to form a honeycomb cell pattern for subsequent culture. The honeycomb structure can effectively simulate the morphology of natural bone tissue and provide good mechanical stability to guide tissue formation. Chapter 10 also reports the second case study of the patterned coculture of multiple cell types in microfluidic channels via gravitational sedimentation. Hela-GFP cells are patterned with a mixture of human umbilical vein cell line and normal human dermal fibroblasts (HDFn) to study the interaction between cancer cells and normal stromal cells under well-organized coculture conditions. The established cell coculture models can be applied to various applications, such as drug screening and cell—cell interaction studies.

15.3.6 Cell adhesion characterization

Cell interaction occurs due to the secretion of diffusible factors and direct cell—cell contact. Information on how physical contact or adhesion molecules affect specific signaling pathways is crucial to understanding the interaction process. Chapter 11 introduces a case study of cell adhesion and migration mediated by the stroma-secreted chemokine SDF-1 and its cognate receptor CXCR4 at the single-cell level, based on optical tweezers manipulations. The study of the roles of SDF-1 and CXCR4 in the interaction of leukemia/bone marrow cells indicates that adhesion molecules can affect the adhesion of leukemia cells to stromal cells to a large extent and induce leukemia cells to migrate to the stromal cell layer. On the basis of the adhesion characteristics of Molm13 leukemia cells to the M210B4 stromal cell layer, three types of adhesion are defined: tight adhesion, loose adhesion, and free suspension. To verify whether SDF-1 secreted by M210B4 bone marrow stromal cells causes the directional migration of Molm13 cells expressing CXCR4, the relative movement between tightly adherent leukemia cells and stromal cells is examined. This method provides a new way to characterize and control cell adhesion and explore the mechanism of cell—cell interaction.

15.3.7 Generating artificial cancer stem cells through cell fusion manipulation

Cancer stem cells play an important role in cancer research and new drug development. Chapter 12 introduces a case study of laser-induced fusion of a single hepatocellular carcinoma cell (HepG2) and hESC to produce specific fusion cells to obtain stemness and carcinoid characteristics. Fusion cells exhibit increased tumorigenicity and resistance to drug treatments, and they are highly similar to tumor stem cells (TSCs) or tumor-initiating cells (TICs). TICs are important in tumorigenesis, aggravation, metastasis, and recurrence. In vivo tumorigenicity assays and drug resistance assays also prove that the fusion of cancer cells and stem cells results in cancer cells that are highly similar to cancer stem cells. The results of this research show that, on the one hand, some stem cell therapies may produce cancer stem cell-like cells and exacerbate cancer, rather than cure the disease; on the other hand, artificially generated tumor-initiating cells can be used to generate malignant cells for cancer stem cell drug screening and research into its mechanism of action.

15.3.8 Using magnetic microrobots to deliver stem cells for liver cancer treatment

A major challenge in clinical cell therapy is how to accurately and quantitatively deliver therapeutic cells to targets in vivo. Currently, systemic delivery through circulation can only enable a small percentage of cells to reach their target sites. Thus, a large number of cells are used to achieve the therapeutic effects, which may cause side effects of overproduction of inflammatory cytokines and excessive immune responses. The use of microrobots to facilitate precise cell delivery provides a new and promising solution to cell therapy applications. Chapter 13 introduces the use of image-guided magnetically driven degradable microrobots to deliver engineered stem cells to the site of liver tumor of mice to inhibit tumor growth. The carried cells can be spontaneously released from the microrobot in the living environment. By using unique photoacoustic imaging technology, the microrobot can be visualized at a penetration depth of several centimeters during transportation. All the results reveal the feasibility of using the designed microrobot to transport and deliver the therapeutic cells to the desired site in vivo, as well as prove that its therapeutic effect on tumor treatment is successful.

15.3.9 Mitochondrial transfer to improve antiaging gene expression

Mitochondrial mutations play a key role in aging and neurodegenerative diseases, and they are known to be important regulators of cell death and survival. The literature demonstrates that the secretome of human fetal MSCs (fMSCs) can ameliorate the senescent phenotype of human adult MSCs (aMSCs), suggesting that fMSCs may have a unique metabolite profile in the secretome and possess antisenescence ability. Chapter 14 introduces the use of an automated optical tweezers-based manipulation method to transfer mitochondria from mMSCs to aMSCs, thereby transforming aMSCs into fMSC-like cells. The results of the cell antiaging and metabolic gene expression based on qPCR analysis indicate that the mitochondria of fMSCs have the potential to reverse the aging phenomenon of aMSCs. This approach could considerably contribute to precision medicine for cell therapy of mtDNA-related diseases.

Index

Note: 'Page numbers followed by "f" indicate figures and "t" indicate tables.'

Q

R

S

T

U

V

Kolibri 360 GmbH
Ferdinand-Jühlke-Straße 7
99095 Erfurt, Deutschland
produktsicherheit@kolibri360.de